NORMAL TEMPERATURES IN CHILDREN

Age	F——Temperature——C	
3 months	99.4	37.5
6 months	99.5	37.5
1 year	99.7	37.7
3 years	99.0	37.2
5 years	98.6	37.0
7 years	98.3	36.8
9 years	98.1	36.7
11 years	98.0	36.7
13 years	97.8	36.6

Modified from Lowrey, G.H.: Growth and development of children, ed. 8. Copyright © 1986 by Year Book Medical Publishers, Inc., Chicago. (Modified and reproduced with permission.)

NORMAL BLOOD PRESSURE READINGS FOR CHILDREN

Girls

Age	Systolic Blood Pressure Percentile 5th	10th	50th	90th	95th	Age	Diastolic Blood Pressure* Percentile 5th	10th	50th	90th	95th
1 day	46	50	65	80	84	1 day	38	42	55	68	72
3 days	53	57	72	86	90	3 days	38	42	55	68	71
7 days	60	64	78	93	97	7 days	38	41	54	67	71
1 mo	65	69	84	98	102	1 mo	35	39	52	65	69
2 mo	68	72	87	101	106	2 mo	34	38	51	64	68
3 mo	70	74	80	104	108	3 mo	35	38	51	64	68
4 mo	71	75	90	105	109	4 mo	35	39	52	65	68
5 mo	72	76	91	106	110	5 mo	36	39	52	65	69
6 mo	72	76	91	106	110	6 mo	36	40	53	66	69
7 mo	72	76	91	106	110	7 mo	36	40	53	66	70
8 mo	72	76	91	106	110	8 mo	37	40	53	66	70
9 mo	72	76	91	106	110	9 mo	37	41	54	67	70
10 mo	72	76	91	106	110	10 mo	37	41	54	67	71
11 mo	72	76	91	105	110	11 mo	38	41	54	67	71
1 yr	72	76	91	105	110	1 yr	38	41	54	67	71
2 yr	71	76	90	105	109	2 yr	40	43	56	69	73
3 yr	72	76	91	106	110	3 yr	40	43	56	69	73
4 yr	73	78	92	107	111	4 yr	40	43	56	69	73
5 yr	75	79	94	109	113	5 yr	40	43	56	69	73
6 yr	77	81	96	111	115	6 yr	40	44	57	70	74
7 yr	78	83	97	112	116	7 yr	41	45	58	71	75
8 yr	80	84	99	114	118	8 yr	43	46	59	72	76
9 yr	81	86	100	115	119	9 yr	44	48	61	74	77
10 yr	83	87	102	117	121	10 yr	46	49	62	75	79
11 yr	86	90	105	119	123	11 yr	47	51	64	77	81
12 yr	88	92	107	122	126	12 yr	49	53	66	78	82
13 yr	90	94	109	124	128	13 yr	46	50	64	78	82
14 yr	92	96	110	125	129	14 yr	49	53	67	81	85
15 yr	93	97	111	126	130	15 yr	49	53	67	82	86
16 yr	93	97	112	127	131	16 yr	49	53	67	81	85
17 yr	93	98	112	127	131	17 yr	48	52	66	80	84
18 yr	94	98	112	127	131	18 yr	48	52	66	80	84

*K4 was used for ages less than 13; K5 was used for ages 13 and over.

Clinical Manual of Pediatric Nursing

Clinical Manual
of Pediatric Nursing

Donna L. Wong, RN, MN, PNP, CPN

Nurse Counselor in Private Practice;
Consultant, Children's Center,
Saint Francis Hospital,
Tulsa, Oklahoma

Lucille F. Whaley, RN, Ed D

Specialist, Parent-Child Nursing;
Professor Emeritus,
San Jose State University,
San Jose, California

With Home Care Instructions *by*

Christina Algiere Kasprisin, RN, MS

Quality Attainment Coordinator,
Saint Francis Hospital;
Assistant Clinical Professor,
University of Oklahoma College of Nursing,
Tulsa, Oklahoma

THIRD EDITION

with 235 illustrations

THE C. V. MOSBY COMPANY

St. Louis • Baltimore • Philadelphia • Toronto   1990

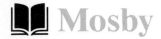

Editor William Grayson Brottmiller
Senior developmental editor Sally Adkisson
Production editor Richard Barber
Design Candace Conner

THIRD EDITION

Copyright © 1990 by The C. V. Mosby Company

Previous editions copyrighted 1981, 1986

Printed in the United States of America

The C. V. Mosby Company
11830 Westline Industrial Drive, St. Louis, Missouri 63146

ISBN: 0-8016-6144-7

GW/VH/VH   9 8 7 6 5 4 3 2 1

Preface

The third edition of Clinical Manual of Pediatric Nursing, like its previous editions, serves a unique function in the study and practice of pediatric nursing. It is a practical guide for nurses and students engaged in the care of children and their families, a compendious collection of clinical information, resources, and data packaged for convenient use and ease of access. For the practicing nurse, the book is a ready resource of material that is otherwise available only in a wide array of journal articles, texts, references, and brochures. For the student, it is an indispensable guide to the care of children and their families. It assumes the thorough preparation and basic theoretical knowledge only a textbook can provide, but it is not designed to accompany any particular textbook. Rather, it is an adjunct to clinical practice.

The Manual is authoritative and up to date. Its content reflects the latest research and current clinical practice. The number of care plans has been greatly expanded to improve the book's utility, and nursing diagnoses are fully integrated, reflecting current NANDA nomenclature. New content has been added, and the popular Home Care Instructions expanded and rewritten at a lower reading level than the previous edition. Users will appreciate access to the latest revision of the Denver Developmental Screening Test, the Denver II, and the latest in car seat safety design and regulations.

Perhaps the most visible change in this edition is the format, which has been re-thought and redesigned to ensure that specific information can be located quickly and easily, as it is needed. Color tabs printed on the back cover facilitate quick access to each of the book's six units, which have black tabs coordinated with those on the back cover. In addition to a new, highly detailed table of contents in the front of the book, unit table of contents with page references have been included on the front page of each unit. A guide to contents by topic is printed inside the back cover. Vital reference data appears inside the front covers, so it can be used at a moment's notice.

As in past editions, material designed for families of children is identified with the familiar teddy bear logo. Permission is given to photocopy this material and provide it to the family of the child to ensure that the family has access to accurate, current information; to improve the quality of home care; and to facilitate the nurse's teaching responsibilities.

Unit 1 focuses on the assessment of the child and family. It includes history taking, assessment of present and past physical health, and a summary of developmental achievement, both general and age-specific. New additions to this unit include guidelines for interviewing, a section on sleep assessment, and a greatly expanded family assessment section.

Unit 2 emphasizes health promotion in the areas of preventive care, nutrition, sleep, immunization, dental care, safety, parental guidance, and play. The material on immunization of well children is completely revised to reflect current recommendations, and a new section on sleep has been added. Some of the material on nutrition (including sample menus for specific age groups), sleep, dental care, injury prevention, and play may be photocopied and given to families.

Unit 3 outlines basic nursing procedures adapted for the pediatric client. This extensive collection of skills and procedures has been expanded to include positioning for extremity venipuncture, lumbar puncture, and bone marrow aspiration; collecting urine, stool, and nasal secretion specimens; administering medication via nasogastric, orogastric, or gastrotomy routes; discussion of long term venous access devices; invasive and noninvasive oxygen monitoring; and cardiopulmonary resuscitation.

Unit 4 is devoted to health problems, primarily those requiring hospitalization: 107 care plans are included. The format has been changed to better reflect the nursing process. Each nursing care plan consists of assessment guidelines specific to the condition, relevant nursing diagnoses, nursing goals, interventions, and expected patient and family outcomes. The nursing diagnoses conform to the nomenclature accepted by the North American Nursing Diagnosis Association (NANDA), and they are prioritized within the care plans. Nursing goals are addressed rather than patient goals because a large number of the health problems of children involve infants and very small children who are unable to actively participate in their own care. Nevertheless, in cases where patient and family goals are desired, they can be easily derived from the expected patient and family outcomes. These nursing care plans can be employed as standards of care for a nursing audit, and they can be readily individualized to meet the needs of specific patients and families.

The health problems were designed and selected to avoid repetition while including a large variety of disorders. Most commonly encountered disorders are included, and a variety of other health problems were chosen because they are frequently encountered in a variety of disorders. Cross references guide the user to generic care plans, such as the Child in Pain, or to commonly used nursing diagnoses, such as Noncompliance.

Unit 5 consists of a collection of instructions for those who provide care for a child in the home. These detailed Home Care Instructions are designed for duplication and distribution for the parent or other care provider. The instructions have been extensively rewritten in simple and clear language to accomodate users with a low reading level. They can be used for client teaching, facilitating discharge planning, or promoting continuity of care between home visits by health care professionals. New additions include caring for a child in a cast, preventing infection, instilling nose drops, suctioning the nose and mouth, performing cardiopulmonary resuscitation on an infant or child, or caring for a choking infant or child. All the instructions reflect research-based practice wherever possible. Where controversy exists or precise research data are lacking, the most convenient and practical suggestions are provided.

Unit 6 includes basic resource information for interpretation of laboratory data, including values in International Units. The extensive list of abbreviations and acronyms used in health care settings has been expanded and updated. A list of resources for families and health care professionals has been added. Every effort has been made to check the accuracy of the directory information as of January 1990.

Although the information in the manual is carefully researched, references are included only when citations are required to appropriately credit the work. The reader is directed to the current editions of NURSING CARE OF INFANTS AND CHILDREN and ESSENTIALS OF PEDIATRIC NURSING for more expanded references and discussion of material, especially for growth and development, interviewing, and health problems.

Every effort has been made to ensure that the information is accurate and up to date at the time of publication. However, as new research and experience broaden our practice, standards of care change accordingly. Therefore, the reader may find some differences in local and regional practices.

A number of people have contributed time and expertise to the preparation of the manuscript. We are especially grateful to Christina Algiere Kasprisin, R.N., M.S., for revising and expanding the Home Care Instructions in Unit 5. We appreciate the continuing contribution of Kristie Nix, R.N., Ed. D., for updating and rewriting the car seat safety material. The artistic illustrations of Marcia Williams are a special addition to the Home Care Instructions and car seat safety, and we appreciate her willingness to continue to work with us on this edition.

As always, we thank our families for their continued support and forbearance during the preparation of the manuscript. We are deeply indebted to our husbands, Ting and Bert, and to our children, Nina Wong and Kathleen and Maureen Whaley, whose presence enriches our lives immeasurably.

Donna L. Wong
Lucille F. Whaley

Reviewers

A number of colleagues provided reviews of specific content areas. Their constructive criticisms and suggestions have been invaluable in ensuring accurate and up-to-date material that reflects current clinical practice. To the following individuals we express our sincere gratitude:

Connie Morain Baker, M.S.
Consultant, Pediatric Program Development
Oklahoma City, OK

Jack A. Campbell
Certified Orthopedic Technician
Eastern Oklahoma Orthopedic Center
Tulsa, OK

Lynn Clutter, R.N., M.S.N.
Child Health and Parenting Consultant
Tulsa, OK

Judith P. Doll
Automotive Safety for Children
Indiana Highway Safety Leaders
Indianapolis, IN

Suzanne L. Feetham, Ph.D., R.N., F.A.A.N.
Director of Education and Research for Nursing and Operations
Children's Hospital National Medical Center
Washington, D.C.
Senior Fellow Distinguished Scholar
School of Nursing
University of Pennsylvania
Philadelphia, PA

Richard Ferber, M.D.
Director, Center for Pediatric Sleep Disorders
The Children's Hospital, Boston
Assistant Professor of Neurology
Harvard Medical School
Boston, MA

William K. Frankenburg, M.D., M.S.P.H.
Professor Pediatrics and Preventive Medicine
University of Colorado Health Sciences Center
Denver, CO

Barbara A. Hannah, R.M., M.S.
CPR Coordinator
Saint Francis Hospital
Affiliate Faculty Basic Life Support
Oklahoma Affiliate
American Heart Association
Tulsa Division
Tulsa, OK

Caryn Stoermer Hess, R.N., M.S.
Nursing Consultant
Englewood, CO

Marilyn Hockenberry-Eaton, RN, MSN, CPNP
Assistant Professor
Emory University
School of Nursing
Atlanta, GA

Debra P. Hymovich, Ph.D., R.N., F.A.A.N.
Post-Doctural Fellow
University of Pennsylvania
School of Nursing
Philadelphia, PA

Marguerite M. Jackson, R.N., M.S., C.I.C.
Director, Epidemiology Unit
University of San Diego Medical Center
San Diego, CA

Jacqueline C. Jones
Education Assistant
Automotive Safety for Children Program
James Whitcomb Riley Hospital
Indianapolis, IN

Edgar O. Ledbetter, M.D.
Director, Department of Maternal, Child, and Adolescent Health
American Academy of Pediatrics
Elk Grove Village, IL

Rosemary Liguori, M.S.N., R.N., CPNP/A
Formerly, Assistant Professor
University of Tulsa
School of Nursing
Nurse Consultant, Primary Health
Tulsa, OK

Margo McCaffery, M.S., R.N., F.A.A.N.
Consultant in the Nursing Care of People with Pain
Santa Monica, CA

Shirley W. Menard, R.N., M.S.N., C.P.N.P.
Assistant Professor
University of Texas Health Science Center
School of Nursing
San Antonio, TX

Myung, K. Park, M.D.
Department of Pediatrics
University of Texas Health Science Center
San Antonio, TX

Cecelia Shaw, R.N., B.S.N., O.C.N.
Clinical Supervisor/Research Coordinator
Cancer Care Associates
Tulsa, OK

Rosemarie E. Steffen, R.N., M.S.N.
Professor of Nursing
El Centro College
Dallas, TX

Karen Bruner Stroup, Ph.D.
Automotive Safety for Children Program
James Whitcomb Riley Hospital for Children
Indianapolis, IN

Contents

1

Assessment

HEALTH HISTORY

One of the most significant aspects of a health assessment is the health history. To take a thorough history, the nurse must be well versed in communication and interviewing principles. An overview of the process is presented in terms of general guidelines for communication and interviewing, with additional specific guidelines for children. Because of the frequent need for interpreters with non-English speaking families, guidelines for using interpreters are included.

The history furnishes information about the child's physical health since birth, details the events of the present problem, and comprises facts about social and family history that are essential for providing comprehensive care. The format summarized here resembles a medical history, but the objective of each assessment area is the identification of nursing diagnoses. The benefit of following the well-established medical approach is that it is systematic and familiar in sequence to members of the health team.

The summary is primarily intended for the recording of data, not the acquisition of information from the informant. Therefore, it is not meant to be used as a questionnaire. The right-hand column entitled "Comments" has been added to enhance and detail sections of the history, as well as emphasize areas of possible intervention. For a more comprehensive discussion of approaches to taking a history, see Chapter 6 in *Nursing Care of Infants and Children* or *Essentials of Pediatric Nursing.**

---

*Whaley L and Wong D: Nursing Care of Infants and Children, ed 3, St Louis, 1987, The CV Mosby Co; Whaley L and Wong D: Essentials of Pediatric Nursing, ed 3, St Louis, 1987, The CV Mosby Co.

General guidelines for communication and interviewing

Conduct the interview in a private, quiet area.
Begin the interview with appropriate introductions.
  Address each person by name.
Clarify the purpose of the interview.
Inform the interviewees of the confidential limits of the interview.
Demonstrate interest in the interview by sitting at eye level and close to interviewees (not across a desk), leaning slightly forward, and speaking in a calm, steady voice.
Begin with general conversation to put the interviewees at ease.
  Use comments, e.g., "How have things been since we talked last?" or (to the child) "What do you think is going to happen today?" to let the family express the main concern.
Include all parties in the interview.
  Direct age-appropriate questions to children, e.g., "What grade are you in school?" or "What do you like to eat?"
  Be sensitive to instances in which family members, such as adolescents, may wish to be interviewed separately.
Recognize and respect cultural patterns of communication, e.g., avoiding direct eye contact (American Indian) or nodding for courtesy—not actual agreement or understanding (many Asian cultures).
Use open-ended questions or statements that begin with "What," "How," "Tell me about," or "You were saying," and reflect back key words or phrases to encourage discussion.
  Encourage continued discussion with nodding, eye contact, saying "uh-huh," "I see," or "yes".
Use focused questions (questions that ask for a specific response, e.g., "What did you try next?") and closed questions (questions that ask for a single answer, e.g., "Did you call the doctor?") to direct the focus of the interview.
Ensure mutual understanding by frequently clarifying and summarizing information.
Use active listening to attend to the verbal and nonverbal aspects of the communication.
  Verbal cues to important issues include:
    Frequent reference to a topic
    Repetition of key words
    Special reference to an event or person

Nonverbal cues to important issues include:
  Changes in body position, e.g., looking away or leaning forward
  Changes in pitch, rate, intonation, and volume of speech, eg., speaking rapidly, frequent pauses, whispering, or shouting.
Use silence to allow persons:
  To sort out thoughts and feelings
  To search for responses to questions
  To share feelings expressed by another
Break silence constructively with statements, e.g., "Is there anything else you wish to say?", "I see you find it difficult to continue; how may I help?", or "I don't know what this silence means. Perhaps there is something you would like to put into words but find difficult to say."
Convey empathy by attending to the verbal and noverbal language of the interviewee and reflecting back the feeling of the communication, e.g., "I can see how upsetting that must have been for you."
Provide reassurance to acknowledge concerns and any positive efforts used to deal with problems.
Avoid blocks to communication
  Socializing
  Giving unrestricted and sometimes unasked-for advise
  Offering premature or inappropriate reassurance
  Giving overready encouragement
  Defending a situation or opinion
  Using stereotyped comments or cliches
  Limiting expression emotion by asking directed, close-ended questions
  Interrupting and finishing the person's sentence
  Talking more than the interviewee
  Forming prejudged conclusions
  Deliberately changing the focus
Close the interview with an opportunity for others to bring up overlooked or sensitive concerns with a statement such as, "Have we covered everything?"
Summarize the interview, especially if problems were identified or interventions were planned.
Discuss the need for follow-up and schedule a time.
Express appreciation for each person's participation.

Unit 1

Specific guidelines for communicating with children

Allow children time to feel comfortable with the nurse

Avoid sudden or rapid advances, broad smiles, extended eye contact, or other gestures that may be seen as threatening

Talk to the parent if child is initially shy

Communicate through transition objects such as dolls, puppets, or stuffed animals before questioning a young child directly

Give older children the opportunity to talk without the parents present

Assume a position that is at eye level with the child

Speak in a quiet, unhurried, and confident voice

Speak clearly, be specific, use simple words, and short sentences

State directions and suggestions *positively*

Offer choices only when one exists

Be honest with children

Allow them to express their concerns and fears

Use a variety of communication techniques

Guidelines for using an interpreter

Explain to interpreter reason for interview and type of questions that will be asked

Clarify whether a detailed or brief answer is required and whether the translated response can be general or literal

Introduce interpreter to family and allow some time before actual interview so that they can become acquainted

Communicate directly with family members when asking questions to reinforce interest in them and to observe nonverbal expressions

Refrain from interrupting family member and interpreter while they are conversing

Avoid commenting to interpreter about family members since they may understand some English

Respect cultural differences; it is often best to pose questions about sex, marriage, or pregnancy indirectly—ask about child's "father" rather than mother's "husband"

Allow time following interview for interpreter to share something that he or she felt could not be said earlier; ask about interpreter's impression of nonverbal clues to communication and family members' reliability or ease in revealing information

Arrange for family to speak with same interpreter on subsequent visits whenever possible

Outline of a health history

A. Identifying information
   1. Name
   2. Address
   3. Telephone number
   4. Age and birthdate
   5. Birthplace
   6. Race
   7. Sex
   8. Religion
   9. Nationality
   10. Date of interview
   11. Informant
B. Chief complaint
C. Present illness
   1. Onset
   2. Characteristics
   3. Course since onset
D. Past history
   1. Pregnancy (maternal)
   2. Labor and delivery
   3. Birth
   4. Previous illnesses, operations, or injuries
   5. Allergies
   6. Current medications
   7. Immunizations
   8. Growth and development
   9. Habits
E. Review of systems
   1. General
   2. Integument
   3. Head
   4. Eyes
   5. Nose

   6. Ears
   7. Throat
   8. Neck
   9. Chest
   10. Respiratory
   11. Cardiovascular
   12. Gastrointestinal
   13. Genitourinary
   14. Gynecologic
   15. Musculoskeletal
   16. Neurologic
   17. Endocrine
F. Nutrition history*
   1. Patterns of eating
   2. Dietary intake
G. Family medical history
   1. Family pedigree
   2. Familial diseases and congenital anomalies
   3. Geographic location
H. Family personal/social history*
   1. Family structure
   2. Family function
I. Sexual history
   1. Sexual concerns
   2. Sexual activity
J. Patient profile (summary)
   1. Health status
   2. Psychologic status
   3. Socioeconomic status

---

*Because of the importance of the nutrition history and family personal/social history, a separate section is devoted to assessment of these two topics on pp. 82 and 58, respectively.

Summary of a health history

Information	Comments
IDENTIFYING INFORMATION 1. Name 2. Address 3. Telephone number 4. Age and birthdate 5. Birthplace 6. Race 7. Sex 8. Religion 9. Nationality 10. Date of interview 11. Informant	Additional information appropriate to older adolescent may include occupation, marital status, and temporary and permanent address Under informant include subjective impression of reliability, general attitude, willingness to communicate, overall accuracy of data, and any special circumstances, such as use of an interpreter Informants should include parent and child, as well as others who may be primary caregivers, such as grandparent
CHIEF COMPLAINT (CC): to establish the major specific reason for the individual's seeking professional health attention	Record in patient's own words; include duration of symptoms If informant has difficulty isolating *one* problem, ask which problem or symptom led person to seek help *now* In case of routine physical examination, state CC as reason for visit

PRESENT ILLNESS (PI): to obtain all details related to the chief complaint
1. Onset
  a. Date of onset
  b. Manner of onset (gradual or sudden)
  c. Precipitating and predisposing factors related to onset (emotional disturbance, physical exertion, fatigue, bodily function, pregnancy, environment, injury, infection, toxins and allergens, or therapeutic agents)
2. Characteristics
  a. Character (quality, quantity, consistency, or other)
  b. Location and radiation (i.e., pain)
  c. Intensity or severity
  d. Timing (continuous or intermittent, duration of each, temporal relationship to other events)
  e. Aggravating and relieving factors
  f. Associated symptoms
3. Course since onset
  a. Incidence
    (1) Single acute attack
    (2) Recurrent acute attacks
    (3) Daily occurrences
    (4) Periodic occurrences
    (5) Continuous chronic episode
  b. Progress (better, worse, unchanged)
  c. Effect of therapy
	In its broadest sense, *illness* denotes any problem of a physical, emotional, or psychosocial nature
	Present information in chronologic order; may be referenced according to one point in time, such as *prior to admission* (PTA)
	Concentrate on reason for seeking help now, especially if problem has existed for some time

PAST HISTORY (PH): to elicit a profile of the individual's previous illnesses, injuries, or operations
1. Pregnancy (maternal)
  a. Number (gravida)
    (1) Dates of delivery
  b. Outcome (parity)
    (1) Gestation (full-term, premature, postmature)
    (2) Stillbirths, abortions
  c. Health during pregnancy
  d. Medications taken
2. Labor and delivery
  a. Duration of labor
  b. Type of delivery
  c. Place of delivery
  d. Medications
	Importance of perinatal history depends on child's age; the younger the child, the more important the perinatal history
	Explain relevance of obstetric history in revealing important factors relating to the child's health
	Assess parents' emotional attitudes toward the pregnancy and birth
	
	Assess parent's feelings regarding delivery; investigate factors affecting bonding, such as if awake and able to hold infant or if asleep and separated from infant

Summary of a health history—cont'd

Information	Comments

3. Birth
   a. Weight and length
   b. Time of regaining birth weight
   c. Condition of health
   d. Apgar score
   e. Presence of congenital anomalies
   f. Date of discharge from nursery
	If birth problems are reported, inquire about treatment, such as use of oxygen, phototherapy, surgery, and so on, and parents' emotional response to the event

4. Previous illnesses, operations, or injuries
   a. Onset, symptoms, course, termination
   b. Occurrence of complications
   c. Incidence of disease in other family members or in community
   d. Emotional response to previous hospitalization
   e. Circumstances and nature of injuries
	Make positive statements about diphtheria, scarlet fever, measles, chickenpox, mumps, tonsillitis, pertussis, and common illnesses such as colds, earaches, or sore throats
	Elicit a description of disease to verify the diagnosis
	Be alert to areas of injury prevention

5. Allergies
   a. Hay fever, asthma, or eczema
   b. Unusual reactions to foods, drugs, animals, plants, or household products
	Have parent describe the type of allergic reaction
	
	Note sensitivity to egg albumin and reactions to certain immunizations

6. Current medications a. Name, dose, schedule, duration, and reason for administration	Assess parents' knowledge of correct dosage of common drugs, such as acetaminophen; note underusage or overusage

7. Immunizations
   a. Name, number of doses, ages when given
   b. Occurrence of reaction
   c. Administration of horse or other foreign serum, gamma globulin, or blood transfusion
	May refer to immunizations as "baby shots"
	Whenever possible, confirm information by checking medical or school records

8. Growth and development
   a. Weight at birth, 6 months, 1 year, and present
   b. Dentition
      (1) Age of eruption/shedding
      (2) Number
      (3) Problems with teething
   c. Age of head control, sitting unsupported, walking, first words
   d. Present grade in school, scholastic achievement
   e. Interaction with peers and adults
   f. Participation in organized activities, such as scouts, sports, and so on
	Compare parents' responses with own observations of child's achievement and results from objective tests, such as DDST or DASE (see Figs. 1-57 and 1-58)
	
	School and social history can be more thoroughly explored under Family Assessment, p. 58

9. Habits
   a. Behavior patterns
      (1) Nail biting
      (2) Thumb sucking
      (3) Pica
      (4) Rituals, such as "security blanket"
      (5) Unusual movements (headbanging, rocking)
      (6) Temper tantrums
   b. Activities of daily living
      (1) Hour of sleep and arising
      (2) Duration of nocturnal sleep/naps
      (3) Age of toilet training
      (4) Pattern of stools and urination; occurrence of enuresis
      (5) Type of exercise
   c. Use/abuse of drugs, alcohol, coffee, or cigarettes
   d. Usual disposition; response to frustration
	Assess parents' attitudes toward habits and any remedies used to curtail them, such as punishment for bedwetting
	
	Record child's usual terms for defecation and urination
	
	With adolescents, estimate the quantity of drugs used

REVIEW OF SYSTEMS (ROS): to elicit information concerning any potential health problem 1. **_General_**—overall state of health, fatigue, recent and/or unexplained weight gain or loss, period of time for either, contributing factors (change of diet, illness, altered appetite), exercise tolerance, fevers (time of day), chills, night sweats (unrelated to climatic conditions), frequent infections, general ability to carry out activities of daily living	Explain relevance of questioning to parents (similar to pregnancy section) in comprising total health history of child Make positive statements about each system, for example, "Mother denies headaches, bumping into objects, squinting, or excessive rubbing of eyes" Use terms parents are likely to understand, such as "bruises" for ecchymoses

Information   **Comments**

2. **Integument**—pruritus, pigment or other color changes, acne, eruptions, rashes (location), tendency to bruising, petechiae, excessive dryness, general texture, disorders or deformities of nails, hair growth or loss, hair color change (for adolescent, use of hair dyes or other potentially toxic substances, such as hair straighteners)

3. **Head**—headaches, dizziness, injury (specific details)

4. **Eyes**—visual problems (ask about behaviors that indicate blurred vision, such as bumping into objects, clumsiness, sitting very close to television, holding a book close to the face, writing with head near desk, squinting, rubbing the eyes, bending the head in an awkward position), "cross-eye" (strabismus), eye infections, edema of lids, excessive tearing, use of glasses or contact lenses, date of last optic examination

5. **Nose**—nosebleeds (epistaxis), constant or frequent running or stuffy nose, nasal obstruction (difficulty in breathing), sense of smell

6. **Ears**—earaches, discharge, evidence of hearing loss (ask about behaviors such as need to repeat requests, loud speech, inattentive behavior), results of any previous auditory testing

7. **Mouth**—mouth breathing, gum bleeding, toothaches, toothbrushing, use of fluoride, difficulty with teething (symptoms), last visit to dentist (especially if temporary dentition is complete), response to dentist

8. **Throat**—sore throats, difficulty in swallowing, choking (especially when chewing food, which may be caused by poor chewing habits), hoarseness or other voice irregularities

9. **Neck**—pain, limitation of movement, stiffness, difficulty in holding head straight (torticollis), thyroid enlargement, enlarged nodes or other masses

10. **Chest**—breast enlargement, discharge, masses, enlarged axillary nodes (for adolescent female, ask about breast self-examination)

11. **Respiratory**—chronic cough, frequent colds (number per year), wheezing, shortness of breath at rest or on exertion, difficulty in breathing, sputum production, infections (pneumonia, tuberculosis), date of last chest x-ray examination; date of last tuberculin test and type of reaction, if any

12. **Cardiovascular**—cyanosis or fatigue on exertion, history of heart murmur or rheumatic fever, anemia, date of last blood count, blood type, recent transfusion

13. **Gastrointestinal**—(much of this in regard to appetite, food tolerance, and elimination habits has been asked elsewhere) concentrate on nausea, vomiting (if not associated with eating, it may indicate brain tumor or increased intracranial pressure), jaundice or yellowing skin or sclera, belching, flatulence, recent change in bowel habits (blood in stools, change of color, diarrhea, or constipation)

14. **Genitourinary**—pain on urination, frequency, hesitancy, urgency, hematuria, nocturia, polyuria, unpleasant odor of urine, direction and force of stream, discharge, change in size of scrotum, date of last urinalysis (for adolescent, sexually transmitted disease, type of treatment; for adolescent male, ask about testicular self-examination)

15. **Gynecologic**—menarche, date of last menstrual period, regularity or problems with menstruation, vaginal discharge, pruritus, date and result of last Pap test (include

Summary of a health history—cont'd

Information	Comments

obstetric history as discussed under birth history when applicable), if sexually active, type of contraception
16. *Musculoskeletal*—weakness, clumsiness, lack of coordination, unusual movements, back or joint stiffness, muscle pains or cramps, abnormal gait, deformity, fractures, serious sprains, activity level
17. *Neurologic*—seizures, tremors, dizziness, loss of memory, general affect, fears, nightmares, speech problems, any unusual habits
18. *Endocrine*—intolerance to weather changes, excessive thirst, excessive sweating, salty taste to skin, signs of early puberty

NUTRITION HISTORY: to elicit information about adequacy of child's dietary intake and eating patterns (see p. 82).

FAMILY MEDICAL HISTORY: to identify the presence of genetic traits or diseases that have familial tendencies; to assess family habits and exposure to a communicable disease that may affect family members
1. Family pedigree (Fig. 1-1) and guidelines for construction (boxed material)
2. Familial diseases and congenital anomalies, such as heart disease, hypertension, cancer, diabetes mellitus, obesity, congenital anomalies, allergy, asthma, tuberculosis, sickle cell disease, mental retardation, convulsions, insanity or other emotional problems, syphilis, or rheumatic fever; indicate symptoms, treatment, and sequelae
3. Family habits, such as smoking or chemical use
4. Geographic location, such as recent travel or contact with foreign visitors

Choose terms wisely when asking about child's parentage, for example, inquire about paternal history by referring to the child's "father" rather than mother's husband; use term "partner," rather than spouse
A pedigree is a pictorial representation or diagram of a family tree to visualize patterns of disease transmission

Important for identification of endemic diseases

FAMILY PERSONAL/SOCIAL HISTORY: to gain an understanding of the family's structure and function (see p. 58)

SEXUAL HISTORY: to elicit information concerning young person's concerns and/or activities and any pertinent data regarding adults' sexual activity that influences child
  a. Sexual concerns/activity of youngster
  b. Sexual concerns/activity of adults if warranted

Sexual history is an essential component of preadolescents' and adolescents' health assessment
Degree of investigation into parents' sexual history depends on its relevance to the child's health. It may be limited to family planning concerns or it may be more detailed if overt sexual activity or abuse is suspected
Investigate toward end of history when rapport is greatest
Respect sensitive and complex nature of questioning
  Give parents and youngster option of discussing sexual matters alone with nurse
  Assure confidentiality
  Clarify terms such as "sexually active" or "having sex?"
  Refer to sexual contacts as "partners" not "girlfriends" or "boyfriends" to avoid biasing discussion of homosexual activity
Discussion may flow easily after review of genitourinary tract, such as asking female about menstruation or male about urinary problems
Suggestions for beginning discussion include:
  "Tell me about your social life."
  "Who are your closest friends?"
  "Is there one very special friend?"
  "Some teenagers have decided to have sex. What do you think about that?"
Take detailed history of all contacts if sexually transmitted disease is suspected or diagnosed

Information	Comments
PATIENT PROFILE (P/P): to summarize the interviewer's overall impression of the child's and family physical, psychologic, and socioeconomic background 1. Health status 2. Psychologic status 3. Socioeconomic status	A comprehensive summary often identifies nursing diagnoses (see p. 242-243) based on subjective and objective findings

GUIDELINES FOR PEDIGREE CONSTRUCTION

1. Begin diagram in the middle of a large sheet of paper.
2. Represent males by a square placed to the left and females by a circle placed to the right.
3. Represent the proband (index case, original patient) with an arrow (if the counselee or patient is different, place a "C" under that person's symbol).
4. Use a horizontal line between a square and a circle for a mating or marriage.
5. Suspend offspring vertically from the mating line and place in order of birth with oldest to the left (regardless of sex).
6. Symbolize generations by Roman numerals with the earliest generation at the top.
7. Include three generations: grandparents, parents, offspring, siblings, aunts, uncles, and first cousins of proband.
8. Include name of each person (maiden names for married women), their date of birth, health problems, and date and cause of death.
9. Date the pedigree.

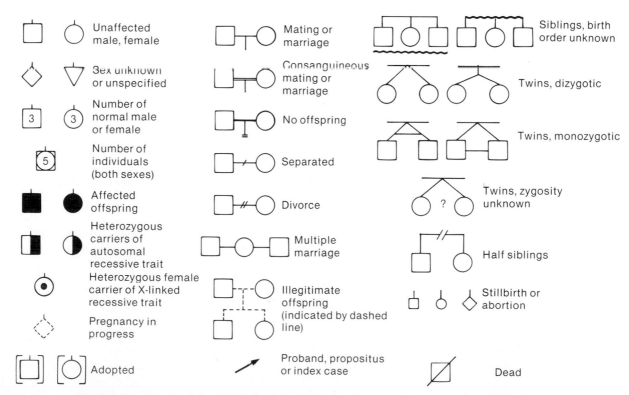

Fig. 1-1. Common pedigree symbols. If symbols other than these are used, add to the pedigree a key to explain their meaning.

PHYSICAL ASSESSMENT

Physical assessment is a continuous process that begins during the interview, primarily by using inspection or observation. During the more formal examination, the tools of percussion, palpation, and auscultation are added to enhance and refine the assessment of body systems. Like the health history, the summary of physical assessment resembles the systematic organization of the medical examination, but the objective is to formulate nursing diagnoses and evaluate the effectiveness of therapeutic interventions.

Because of important differences in physical assessment of the child and newborn, separate guidelines and summaries for conducting the physical examination of each age group are presented.

The summary of the physical assessment of the newborn is also presented in four sections: the area to be assessed, usual findings, common variations/minor abnormalities, and potential signs of distress/major abnormalities. Common variations/minor abnormalities should be recorded, but generally do not require further evaluation. Potential signs of distress/major ab-

normalities are recorded and need to be reported for further evaluation. The procedures for assessment are not presented here but in the summary of physical assessment of the child. In addition to the newborn summary, assessment of clinical gestational age is also described.

The summary of the physical assessment of the child is presented in four sections: the area to be assessed, the procedure for assessment, usual findings, and comments. The comments column includes findings that deviate from the normal and should be reported, special significance of certain findings, and areas for nursing intervention. This section includes detailed instructions for various assessment procedures.

For a more comprehensive discussion of performing a physical assessment, see Chapters 7 and 8 in *Nursing Care of Infants and Children* and *Essentials of Pediatric Nursing.**

---

*Whaley L and Wong D: Nursing Care of Infants and Children, ed 3, St Louis, 1987, The CV Mosby Co; Whaley L and Wong D: Essentials of Pediatric Nursing, ed 3, St Louis, 1989, The CV Mosby Co.

General guidelines for physical examination of the newborn

Provide a normothermic and nonstimulating examination area
  Undress only body area examined to prevent heat loss
Proceed in an orderly sequence (usually head to toe) with the following exceptions:
  Perform all procedures that require quiet first, such as auscultating the lungs, heart, and abdomen
  Perform disturbing procedures, such as testing reflexes, last
  Measure head, chest, and length at same time to compare results

Proceed quickly to avoid stressing the infant
  Check that equipment and supplies are working properly and are accessible
Comfort the infant during and after the examination if upset
  Talk softly
  Hold hands against chest
  Swaddle and hold
  Give pacifier

Summary of physical assessment of the newborn

Assessment	Usual findings	Common variations/ minor abnormalities	Potential signs of distress/ major abnormalities
GENERAL MEASUREMENTS	Head circumference 33-35 cm (13-14 inches) Chest circumference 30.5-33 cm (12-13 inches) Head circumference should be about 2-3 cm (1 inch) larger than chest circumference Crown-to-rump length 31-35 cm (12.5-14 inches) Crown-to-rump length approximately equal to head circumference Head-to-heel length 48-53 cm (19-21 inches) Birth weight 2700-4000 g (6-9 pounds)	Molding after birth may decrease head circumference Head and chest circumferences may be equal for first 1-2 days after birth Loss of 10% of birth weight in first week; regained in 10-14 days	Head circumference <10th or >90th percentile Birth weight <10th or >90th percentile

Summary of physical assessment of the newborn—cont'd

Assessment	Usual findings	Common variations/ minor abnormalities	Potential signs of distress/ major abnormalities
VITAL SIGNS			
Temperature	Axillary—36.5°-37° C (97.9°-98°F)	Crying may increase body temperature slightly Radiant warmer will increase axillary temperature	Hypothermia Hyperthermia
Heart rate	Apical—120-140 beats/minute	Crying will increase heart rate; sleep will decrease heart rate During first period of reactivity (6 to 8 hours), rate can reach 180 beats/minute	Bradycardia—Resting rate below 80-100 beats/minute Tachycardia—Rate above 160-180 beats/minute Irregular rhythm
Respirations	30-60 breaths/minute	Crying will increase respiratory rate; sleep will decrease respiratory rate During first period of reactivity (6 to 8 hours), rate can reach 80 breaths/minute	Tachypnea—Rate above 60 breaths/minute Apnea >15 seconds
Blood pressure	See inside front cover	Crying will increase blood pressure	Systolic pressure in calf <6-9 mm Hg than in upper extremity
GENERAL APPEARANCE	**Posture**—Flexion of head and extremities, which rest on chest and abdomen	**Frank breech**—Extended legs, abducted and fully rotated thighs, flattened occiput, extended neck	Limp posture, extension of extremities See also neuromuscular, p. 15
SKIN	At birth, bright red, puffy, smooth Second to third day, pink, flaky, dry Vernix caseosa Lanugo Edema around eyes, face, legs, dorsa of hands, feet, and scrotum or labia Normal color changes: **Acrocyanosis**—Cyanosis of hands and feet **Cutis marmorata**—Transient mottling when infant is exposed to decreased temperature	Neonatal jaundice after first 24 hours Ecchymoses or petechiae caused by birth trauma **Milia**—distended sebaceous glands that appear as tiny white papules on cheeks, chin, and nose **Miliaria** or **sudamina**—distended sweat (eccrine) glands that appear as minute vesicles, especially on face **Erythema toxicum**—Pink papular rash with vesicles superimposed on thorax, back, buttocks, and abdomen; may appear in 24 to 48 hours and resolve after several days **Harlequin color change**—Clearly outlined color change as infant lies on side; lower half of body becomes pink and upper half is pale	Progressive jaundice, especially in first 24 hours Cracked or peeling skin Generalized cyanosis Pallor Grayness Plethora Hemorrhage, ecchymoses, or petechiae that persist **Sclerema**—hard and stiff skin Poor skin turgor Rashes, pustules, or blisters **Café au lait spots**—light brown spots **Nevus flammeus**—port-wine stain

Unit 1

Summary of physical assessment of the newborn—cont'd

Assessment	Usual findings	Common variations/ minor abnormalities	Potential signs of distress/ major abnormalities
		Mongolian spots—Irregular areas of deep blue pigmentation, usually in the sacral and gluteal regions; seen predominantly in newborns of African, Asian, or Hispanic descent **Telangiectatic nevi ("stork bites")**—Flat, deep pink localized areas usually seen in back of neck	

HEAD

Fig. 1-2. Location of sutures and fontanels.

Assessment	Usual findings	Common variations/ minor abnormalities	Potential signs of distress/ major abnormalities
	Anterior fontanel—Diamond-shaped, 2.5-4.0 cm (1-1.75 inches) (Fig. 1-2) **Posterior fontanel**—Triangular-shaped 0.5-1 cm (0.2-0.4 inch) Fontanels should be flat, soft, and firm Widest part of fontanel measured from bone to bone, not suture to suture	Molding following vaginal delivery Third sagittal (parietal) fontanel Bulging fontanel because of crying or coughing **Caput succedaneum**—edema of soft scalp tissue **Cephalhematoma** (uncomplicated)—Hematoma between periosteum and skull bone	Fused sutures Bulging or depressed fontanels when quiet Widened sutures and fontanels **Craniotabes**—snapping sensation along lambdoid suture that resembles indentation of ping pong ball
EYES	Lids usually edematous Eyes usually closed Color—Slate gray, dark blue, brown Absence of tears Presence of red reflex Corneal reflex in response to touch Pupillary reflex in response to light Blink reflex in response to light or touch Rudimentary fixation on objects and ability to follow to midline	Epicanthal folds in Oriental infants Searching nystagmus or strabismus **Subconjunctival (scleral) hemorrhages**—Ruptured capillaries, usually at limbus	Pink color of iris Purulent discharge Mongoloid slant in non-Orientals Hypertelorism (3 cm or greater) Hypotelorism Congenital cataracts Constricted or dilated fixed pupil Absence of red reflex Absence of pupillary or corneal reflex Inability to follow object or bright light to midline Blue sclera Yellow sclera

Assessment	Usual findings	Common variations/ minor abnormalities	Potential signs of distress/ major abnormalities
EARS	Position—Top of pinna on horizontal line with outer canthus of eye Startle reflex elicited by a loud, sudden noise Pinna flexible, cartilage present	Inability to visualize tympanic membrane because of filled aural canals Pinna flat against head Irregular shape or size Pits or skin tags	Low placement of ears Absence of startle reflex in response to loud noise Minor abnormalities may be signs of various syndromes
NOSE	Nasal patency Nasal discharge—Thin white mucus Sneezing	Flattened and bruised	Nonpatent canals Thick, bloody nasal discharge Flaring of nares (alae nasi) Copious nasal secretions or stuffiness
MOUTH AND THROAT	Intact, high-arched palate Uvula in midline Frenulum of tongue Frenum of upper lip Sucking reflex—Strong and coordinated Rooting reflex Gag reflex Extrusion reflex Absent or minimal salivation Vigorous cry	Natal teeth (benign but may be aspirated) **Epstein pearls**—Small, white epithelial cysts along midline of hard palate	Cleft lip Cleft palate Large, protruding tongue or posterior displacement of tongue Profuse salivation or drooling **Candidiasis (thrush)**—White, adherent patches on tongue, palate, and buccal surfaces Inability to pass nasogastric tube Hoarse, high-pitched, weak, absent, or other abnormal cry
NECK	Short, thick, usually surrounded by skin folds Tonic neck reflex Neck-righting reflex Otolith-righting reflex	**Torticollis** (wry neck)— Head held to one side with chin pointing to opposite side	Excessive skinfolds Resistance to flexion Absence of tonic neck, neck-righting, or otolith-righting reflex Fractured clavicle
CHEST	Anteroposterior and lateral diameters equal Slight sternal retractions evident during inspiration Xiphoid process evident Breast enlargement	Funnel chest (pectus excavatum) Pigeon chest (pectus carinatum) Supernumerary nipples Secretion of milky substance from breasts ("witch's milk")	Depressed sternum Marked retractions of chin, chest, and intercostal spaces during respiration Asymmetric chest expansion or over-expansion Redness and firmness around nipples Wide-spaced nipples
LUNGS	Respirations chiefly abdominal Cough reflex absent at birth, present by 1-2 days Bilateral equal bronchial breath sounds	Rate and depth of respirations may be irregular, periodic breathing Crackles shortly after birth	Inspiratory stridor Expiratory grunt Retractions Persistent irregular breathing Periodic breathing with repeated apneic spells Deep sighing respirations Seesaw respirations Unequal breath sounds Persistent fine crackles Wheezing Diminished breath sounds Peristaltic sounds on one side, with diminished breath sounds on same side

Summary of physical assessment of the newborn—cont'd

Assessment	Usual findings	Common variations/ minor abnormalities	Potential signs of distress/ major abnormalities
HEART	Apex—Fourth to fifth intercostal space, lateral to left sternal border S_2 slightly sharper and higher in pitch than S_1	Sinus arrhythmia Transient cyanosis on crying or straining	Dextrocardia Displacement of apex Cardiomegaly Abdominal shunts Murmurs Thrills Persistent cyanosis
ABDOMEN	Cylindric in shape Liver—Palpable 2-3 cm below right costal margin Spleen—Tip palpable at end of first week of age Kidneys—Palpable 1-2 cm above umbilicus Umbilical cord—Bluish white at birth with two arteries and one vein Equal bilateral femoral pulses	Umbilical hernia **Diastasis recti**—Midline gap between recti muscles	Abdominal distention Localized bulging Distended veins Absent bowel sounds Enlarged liver and spleen Ascites Visible peristaltic waves Scaphoid or concave abdomen Green umbilical cord Presence of one artery in cord Urine or stool leaking from cord Palpable bladder distention following scanty voiding Absent femoral pulses
FEMALE GENITALIA	Labia and clitoris usually edematous Labia minora larger than labia majora Urethral meatus behind clitoris Vernix caseosa between labia Urinates within 24 hours	Blood-tinged or mucoid discharge (pseudomenstruation) Hymenal tag	Enlarged clitoris with urethral meatus at tip Fused labia Absence of vaginal opening Fecal discharge from vaginal opening No urination within 24 hours Masses in labia
MALE GENITALIA	Urethral opening at tip of glans penis Testes palpable in each scrotum Scrotum usually large, edematous, pendulous, and covered with rugae; usually deeply pigmented in dark-skinned ethnic groups Smegma Urinates within 24 hours	Urethral opening covered by prepuce Inability to retract foreskin Epithelial pearls Erection or priapism Testes palpable in inguinal canal Scrotum small	Hypospadias Epispadias Chordee Testes not palpable in scrotum or inguinal canal No urination within 24 hours Inguinal hernia Hypoplastic scrotum Hydrocele Masses in scrotum
BACK AND RECTUM	Spine intact, no openings, masses, or prominent curves Trunk incurvation reflex Anal reflex Patent anal opening Passage of meconium within 36 hours	Green liquid stools in infant under phototherapy	Anal fissures or fistulas Imperforate anus Absence of anal reflex No meconium within 36 hours Pilonidal cyst or sinus Tuft of hair along spine Spina bifida (any degree)

Assessment	Usual findings	Common variations/ minor abnormalities	Potential signs of distress/ major abnormalities
EXTREMITIES	Ten fingers and toes Full range of motion	Partial syndactyly between second and third toes	**Polydactyly**—Extra digits **Syndactyly**—Fused or webbed digits **Phocomelia**—Hands or feet attached close to trunk **Hemimelia**—Absence of distal part of extremity
	Negative scarf sign—Elbow does not reach midline Nail beds pink, with transient cyanosis immediately after birth Creases on anterior two thirds of sole	Second toe overlapping into third toe Wide gap between hallux and second toe Deep crease on plantar surface of foot between first and second toes	Hyperflexibility of joints Persistent cyanosis of nail beds Yellowing of nail beds Sole covered with creases Simian crease (see Fig. 1-7, *B*) Fractures

	Sole usually flat
	Symmetry of extremities
	Equal muscle tone bilaterally, especially resistance to opposing flexion
	Equal bilateral brachial pulses
		Asymmetric length of toes
		Dorsiflexion and shortness of hallux
			Dislocated or subluxated hip (Fig. 1-3)
			  Limitation in hip abduction
			  Unequal gluteal or leg folds
			  Unequal knee height (Allis or Galeazzi sign)
			  Audible click on abduction (Ortolani sign)
			Asymmetry of extremities
			Unequal muscle tone or range of motion

NEUROMUSCULAR SYSTEM	Extremities usually maintain some degree of flexion Extension of an extremity followed by previous position of flexion Head lag while sitting, but momentary ability to hold head erect Able to turn head from side to side when prone Able to hold head in horizontal line with back when held prone	Quivering or momentary tremors	**Hypotonia**—Floppy, poor head control, extremities limp **Hypertonia**—Jittery, arms and hands tightly flexed, legs stiffly extended, startles easily Asymmetric posturing (except tonic neck reflex) Opisthotonic posturing—arched back Signs of paralysis Tremors, twitches, and myoclonic jerks Marked head lag in all positions

Fig. 1-3. Signs of congenital dislocation of the hip. **A,** Asymmetry of gluteal and thigh folds. **B,** Limited hip abduction, as seen in flexion. **C,** Apparent shortening of the femur, as indicated by the level of the knees in flexion. **D,** Ortolani click (If infant is under 4 weeks of age.)

Unit 1

Assessment of reflexes

Reflex	Expected behavioral response	Deviation
LOCALIZED		
Eyes		
Blinking or corneal reflex	Infant blinks at sudden appearance of a bright light or at approach of an object toward the cornea; should persist throughout life	Absent or asymmetric blink suggests damage to cranial nerves II, IV, and V
Pupillary	Pupil constricts when a bright light shines toward it; should persist throughout life	Unequal constriction Fixed dilated pupil
Doll's eye	As the head is moved slowly to the right or left, eyes normally do not move; should disappear as fixation develops	Asymmetric in abducens paralysis
Nose		
Sneeze	Spontaneous response of nasal passages to irritation or obstruction; should persist throughout life	Absent or continuous sneezing
Glabellar	Tapping briskly on glabella (bridge of nose) causes eyes to close tightly	Absence
Mouth and throat		
Sucking	Infant should begin strong sucking movements of circumoral area in response to stimulation; should persist throughout infancy, even without stimulation, such as during sleep	Weak or absent suck
Gag	Stimulation of posterior pharynx by food, suction, or passage of a tube should cause infant to gag; should persist throughout life	Absence of gag suggests damage to glossopharyngeal nerve
Rooting	Touching or stroking the cheek along the side of the mouth will cause infant to turn the head toward that side and begin to suck; should disappear at about age 3-4 months, but may persist for up to 12 months	Absence, especially when infant is not satiated
Extrusion	When tongue is touched or depressed, infant responds by forcing it outward; should disappear by age 4 months	Constant protrusion of tongue may suggest Down syndrome
Yawn	Spontaneous response to decreased oxygen by increasing amount of inspired air; should persist throughout life	Absence
Cough	Irritation of mucous membranes of larynx or tracheobronchial tree causes coughing; should persist throughout life; usually present after first day of birth	Absence
Extremities		
Grasp	Touching palms of hands or soles of feet near base of digits causes flexion of hands and toes; palmar grasp should lessen after age 3 months, to be replaced by voluntary movement; plantar grasp lessens by 8 months of age	Asymmetric flexion may indicate paralysis
Babinski	Stroking outer sole of foot upward from heel and across ball of foot causes toes to hyperextend and hallux to dorsiflex; should disappear after age 1 year	Persistence indicates a pyramidal tract lesion
Ankle clonus	Briskly dorsiflexing foot while supporting knee in partially flexed position results in one to two oscillating movements ("beats"); eventually no beats should be felt	Several beats
MASS		
Moro	Sudden jarring or change in equilibrium causes sudden extension and abduction of extremities and fanning of fingers, with index finger and thumb forming a "C" shape, followed by flexion and abduction of extremities; legs may weakly flex; infant may cry; should disappear after age 3-4 months, usually strongest during first 2 months	Persistence of Moro reflex past age 6 months may indicate brain damage Asymmetric Moro reflex may suggest injury to brachial plexus, clavicle, or humerus

Reflex	Expected behavior response	Deviation
Startle	A sudden loud noise causes abduction of the arms with flexion of the elbows; the hands remain clenched; should disappear by age 4 months	Absence indicates hearing loss
Perez	While infant is prone on a firm surface, thumb is pressed along spine from sacrum to neck; infant responds by crying, flexing the extremities, and elevating the pelvis and head; lordosis of the spine, as well as defecation and urination, may occur; should disappear by age 4-6 months	Significance is similar to that of Moro reflex
Asymmetric tonic neck	When infant's head is quickly turned to one side, arm and leg extends on that side, and opposite arm and leg flex; should disappear by age 3-4 months, to be replaced by symmetric positioning of both sides of body	Absence or persistence may indicate central nervous system damage
Neck-righting	While infant is supine, head is turned to one side; shoulder and trunk turns toward that side, followed by pelvis; disappears at age 10 months	Absence; significance is similar to that of asymmetric tonic neck reflex
Otolith-righting	When body of an erect infant is tilted, head is returned to upright, erect position	Absence; significance is similar to that of asymmetric tonic neck reflex
Trunk incurvation (Galant)	Stroking infant's back alongside spine causes hips to move toward stimulated side; should disappear by age 4 weeks	Absence may indicate spinal cord lesion
Dance or step	If infant is held so that sole of foot touches a hard surface, there is a reciprocal flexion and extension of the leg, simulating walking; should disappear after age 3-4 weeks, to be replaced by deliberate movement	Asymmetry of stepping
Crawling	Infant, when placed on abdomen, makes crawling movements with the arms and legs; should disappear at about age 6 weeks	Asymmetry of movement
Placing	When infant is held upright under arms and dorsal side of foot is briskly placed against hard object, such as table, leg lifts as if foot is stepping on table; age of disappearance varies	Absence

Assessment of clinical gestational age

Assessment of gestational age is an important criterion because perinatal morbidity and mortality are related to gestational age and birth weight. One of the most frequently used methods of determining gestational age is based on physical and neurologic findings. The scale in Fig. 1-4, *A,* assesses six external physical and six neuromuscular signs. Each sign has a number score and the cumulative score correlates with a maturity rating from 26 to 44 weeks (see Maturity rating box on scale). The maturity rating is accurate within plus or minus 2 weeks of the infant's true age. Assessments can be performed anytime from birth to 42 hours of age but the greatest reliability is at 30 and 42 hours. Fig. 1-4, *B,* is a classification of newborns based on maturity and intrauterine growth. The newborn's length, weight, and head circumference are plotted according to the estimated gestational age. Values that fall within 10th to 90th percentile classify the newborn as appropriate for gestational age. Values that fall below the 10th percentile classify the newborn as small for gestational age. Values that fall above the 90th percentile classify the newborn as large for gestational age.

To facilitate the use of Fig. 1-4, *A,* the following tests and observations are described:

Test	Assessment/Description
Posture	With the infant quiet and in a supine position, observe the degree of flexion in the arms and legs. Muscle tone and degree of flexion increase with maturity. Full flexion of the arms and legs = 4.
Square window	With the thumb supporting the back of the arm below the wrist, apply gentle pressure with index and third fingers on dorsum of hand without rotating the infant's wrist. Measure the angle between the base of the thumb and forearm. Full flexion (hand lies flat on ventral surface of forearm) = 4.
Arm recoil	With the infant supine, fully flex both forearms on upper arms, hold for 5 seconds; pull down on hands to fully extend and rapidly release arms. Observe the rapidity and intensity of recoil to a state of flexion. A brisk return to full flexion = 4.
Popliteal angle	With the infant supine and the pelvis flat on a firm surface, flex lower leg on thigh and then flex thigh on abdomen. While holding knee with thumb and index finger, extend lower leg with index finger of other hand. Measure the degree of the angle behind the knee (popliteal angle). An angle less than 90° = 5.
Scarf sign	With the infant supine, support the head in the midline with one hand; use other hand to pull infant's arm across the shoulder so that infant's hand touches the shoulder. Determine location of elbow in relation to midline. Elbow does not reach midline = 4.
Heel to ear	With the infant supine and the pelvis flat on a firm surface, pull the foot as far as possible up toward the ear on the same side. Measure the distance of the foot from the ear and degree of knee flexion (same as popliteal angle). Knees flexed with a popliteal angle less than 10° = 4.

Unit 1

NEWBORN MATURITY RATING and CLASSIFICATION

ESTIMATION OF GESTATIONAL AGE BY MATURITY RATING
Symbols: X - 1st Exam   O - 2nd Exam

NEUROMUSCULAR MATURITY

	0	1	2	3	4	5
Posture						
Square Window (Wrist)	90°	60°	45°	30°	0°	
Arm Recoil	180°		100°-180°	90°-100°	< 90°	
Popliteal Angle	180°	160°	130°	110°	90°	< 90°
Scarf Sign						
Heel to Ear						

PHYSICAL MATURITY

	0	1	2	3	4	5
SKIN	gelatinous red, transparent	smooth pink, visible veins	superficial peeling &/or rash, few veins	cracking pale area, rare veins	parchment, deep cracking, no vessels	leathery, cracked, wrinkled
LANUGO	none	abundant	thinning	bald areas	mostly bald	
PLANTAR CREASES	no crease	faint red marks	anterior transverse crease only	creases ant. 2/3	creases cover entire sole	
BREAST	barely percept.	flat areola, no bud	stippled areola, 1–2 mm bud	raised areola, 3–4 mm bud	full areola, 5–10 mm bud	
EAR	pinna flat, stays folded	sl. curved pinna, soft with slow recoil	well-curv. pinna, soft but ready recoil	formed & firm with instant recoil	thick cartilage, ear stiff	
GENITALS Male	scrotum empty, no rugae		testes descending, few rugae	testes down, good rugae	testes pendulous, deep rugae	
GENITALS Female	prominent clitoris & labia minora		majora & minora equally prominent	majora large, minora small	clitoris & minora completely covered	

Gestation by Dates _____ wks

Birth Date _____ Hour _____ am / pm

APGAR _____ 1 min _____ 5 min

MATURITY RATING

Score	Wks
5	26
10	28
15	30
20	32
25	34
30	36
35	38
40	40
45	42
50	44

A

SCORING SECTION

	1st Exam=X	2nd Exam=O
Estimating Gest Age by Maturity Rating	_____Weeks	_____Weeks
Time of Exam	Date _____ am/pm Hour _____	Date _____ am/pm Hour _____
Age at Exam	_____ Hours	_____ Hours
Signature of Examiner	_____ M.D.	_____ M.D.

Fig. 1-4. A, Newborn maturity rating and classification.

Unit 1

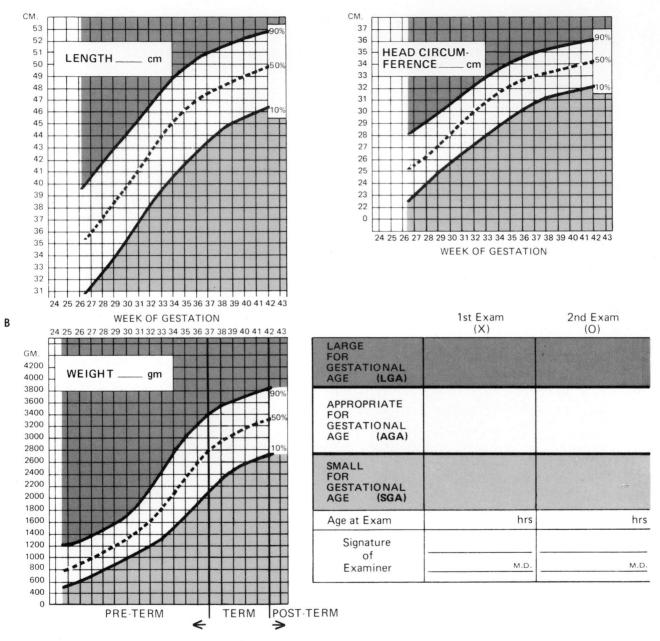

B

Fig. 1-4, cont'd. B, Classification of newborns based on maturity and intrauterine growth.
(Courtesy Mead Johnson & Company, Evansville, IN 47721. Scoring section modified from Ballard JL, et al: Pediatr Res 11:374, 1977. Figures modified from Sweet AY: Classification of the low-birth-weight infant. In Klaus MH and Fanaroff AA: Care of the high-risk infant, Philadelphia, WB Saunders Co., 1977.)

General guidelines for physical examination during childhood

Perform examination in appropriate, nonthreatening area.
  Have room well lit and decorated with neutral colors.
  Have room temperature comfortably warm.
  Place all strange and potentially frightening equipment out of sight.
  Have some toys, dolls, stuffed animals, and games available for the child.
  If possible, have rooms decorated and equipped for different age children.
  Provide privacy, especially for school-age children and adolescents.
  Check that equipment and supplies are working properly and are accessible to avoid disruption.
Provide time for play and becoming acquainted.
  Talking to the nurse.
  Making eye contact.
  Accepting the offered equipment.
  Allowing physical touching.
  Choosing to sit on examining table rather than parent's lap.
If signs of readiness are not observed, use the following techniques.
  Talk to the parent while essentially "ignoring" the child; gradually focus on the child or a favorite object, such as a doll.
  Make complimentary remarks about the child, such as his appearance, dress, or a favorite object.
  Tell a funny story or play a simple trick
  Have a nonthreatening "friend" available, such as a hand puppet to "talk" to the child for the nurse.
If the child refuses to cooperate, use the following techniques:
  Assess reason for uncooperative behavior; consider that a child who is unduly afraid of a male examiner may have had a previous traumatic experience, including sexual abuse.
  Try to involve child and parent in process or if appropriate, ask parent to leave.
  Avoid prolonged explanations about examining procedure.
  Use a firm, direct approach regarding expected behavior.
  Perform examination as quickly as possible.
  Have attendant gently restrain child.
  Minimize any disruptions or stimulation.
    Limit number of people in room.
    Use isolated room.
    Use quiet, calm, confident voice.

Begin the examination in a nonthreatening manner for young children or children who are fearful.
  Use those activities that can be presented as games, such as test for cranial nerves (p. 56) or parts of the Denver Developmental Screening Test (DDST) (p. 113).
  Use approaches such as "Simon says" to encourage child to make a face, squeeze a hand, stand on one foot, and so on.
  Use the "paper doll" technique.
    Lay the child supine on an examining table or floor that is covered with a large sheet of paper.
    Trace around the child's body outline.
    Use the body outline to demonstrate what will be examined, such as drawing a heart and listening with the stethoscope before performing the activity on the child.
If several children in the family will be examined, begin with the most cooperative child.
Involve child in the examination process:
  Provide choices, such as sitting on the table or in the parent's lap.
  Allow to handle or hold equipment.
  Encourage to use equipment on a doll, family member, or examiner.
  Explain each step of the procedure in simple language.
Examine child in a comfortable and secure position.
  Sitting in parent's lap.
  Sitting upright if in respiratory distress.
Proceed to examine the body in an organized sequence (usually head to toe) with following exceptions:
  Alter sequence to accommodate needs of different age children (see p. 22).
  Examine painful areas last.
  In emergency situation, examine vital functions (airway, breathing, and circulation) and injured area first.
Reassure child throughout examination, especially bodily concerns that arise during puberty.
Discuss the findings with the family at the end of the examination.
Praise child for cooperation during examination; give reward such as small toy or sticker.

Unit 1

Age-specific guidelines for physical examination during childhood

Age	Position	Sequence	Preparation
Infant	Before sits alone: supine or prone, preferably in parent's lap; before 4 to 6 months: can place on examining table After sits alone: use sitting in parent's lap whenever possible If on table, place with parent in full view	If quiet, auscultate heart, lungs, abdomen Record heart and respiratory rates Palpate and percuss same areas Proceed in usual head-toe direction Perform traumatic procedures last (eyes, ears, mouth [while crying], rectal temperature [if taken]) Elicit reflexes as body part examined Elicit Moro reflex last	Completely undress if room temperature permits Leave diaper on male Gain cooperation with distraction, bright objects, rattles, talking Smile at infant; use soft, gentle voice Pacify with bottle of sugar water or feeding Enlist parent's aid for restraining to examine ears, mouth Avoid abrupt, jerky movements
Toddler	Sitting or standing on/by parent Prone or supine in parent's lap	Inspect body area through play: "count fingers," "tickle toes" Use minimal physical contact intially Introduce equipment slowly Auscultate, percuss, palpate whenever quiet Perform traumatic procedures last (same as for infant)	Have parent remove outer clothing Remove underwear as body part examined Allow to inspect equipment; demonstrating use of equipment usually ineffective If uncooperative, perform procedures quickly Use restraint when appropriate; request parent's assistance Talk about examination if cooperative; use short phrases Praise for cooperative behavior
Preschool child	Prefer standing or sitting Usually cooperative prone/ supine Prefer parent's closeness	If cooperative, proceed in head-toe direction If uncooperative, proceed as with toddler	Request self-undressing Allow to wear underpants if shy Offer equipment for inspection: Briefly demonstrate use (may demonstrate on parent) Make up "story" about procedure: "I'm seeing how strong your muscles are" or "I am going to give your arm a hug with this special cloth" (blood pressure) Use paper-doll technique Give choices when possible Expect cooperation; use positive statements: "Open your mouth"
School-age child	Prefer sitting Cooperative in most positions Younger age prefer parent's presence Older age may prefer privacy	Proceed in head-toe direction May examine genitalia last in older child Respect need for privacy	Request self-undressing Allow to wear underpants Give gown to wear Explain purpose of equipment and significance of procedure, such as otoscope to see eardrum, which is necessary for hearing Teach about body functioning and care
Adolescent	Same as for school-age child Offer option of parent's presence	Same as older school-age child	Allow to undress in private Give gown Expose only area to be examined Respect need for privacy Explain findings during examination: "Your muscles are firm and strong" Matter-of-factly comment about sexual development: "Your breasts are developing as they should be" Emphasize normalcy of development Examine genitalia as any other body part; may leave to end May use mirror during examination of genitalia to allow youngster to view area examined and learn about personal anatomy

Outline of a physical assessment

A. Growth measurements
   1. Length/height
   2. Crown-to-rump length or sitting height
   3. Weight
   4. Head circumference
   5. Chest circumference
   6. Skinfold thickness and arm circumference
B. Physiologic measurements
   1. Temperature
   2. Pulse
   3. Respiration
   4. Blood pressure
C. General appearance
D. Skin
E. Accessory structures
F. Lymph nodes
G. Head
H. Neck
I. Eyes

J. Ears
K. Nose
L. Mouth and throat
M. Chest
N. Lungs
O. Heart
P. Abdomen
Q. Genitalia
   1. Male
   2. Female
R. Anus
S. Back and extremities
T. Neurologic assessment
   1. Mental status
   2. Motor functioning
   3. Sensory functioning
   4. Reflexes (deep tendons)
   5. Cranial nerves

Summary of physical assessment of the child

Assessment	Procedure
GROWTH MEASUREMENTS (Fig. 1-5)	Plot length, weight, and head circumference on standard percentile charts (pp. 102-110) Charts for 0 to 36 months and 2 to 18 years both include children ages 24 to 36 months; record only recumbent length on 0 to 36 month chart and only stature on 2 to 18 year chart Use weight-for-stature charts only for prepubescent children regardless of chronologic age

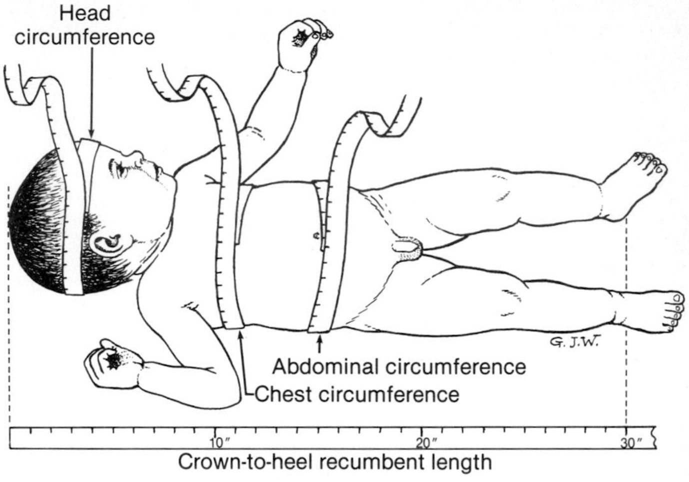

Fig. 1-5. Measurements.

MEASUREMENTS

Length/height	Recumbent length in children below 24 to 36 months:
	  Place supine with head in midline
	  Grasp knees and push gently toward table to *fully* extend legs
	  Measure from vertex (top) of head to heels of feet (toes pointing upward)
	Standing height (stature) in children over 24 to 36 months:
	  Remove socks and shoes
	  Have child stand as tall as possible, back straight, head in midline, and eyes looking straight ahead
	  Check for flexion of knees, slumping shoulders, raising of heels
	  Measure from top of head to standing surface
	  Measure to the nearest cm or ⅛ inch

Crown-to-rump length or sitting height	In infants, place on side with legs flexed at hips; measure from top of head to rump In children able to sit unsupported, sit against wall and measure from top of head to sitting surface
Weight	Weigh infants and young children nude on platform-type scale; protect infant by placing hand above body to prevent falling off scale Weigh older children in underwear (no shoes) on standing-type upright scale Check that scale is balanced before weighing Cover scale with clean sheet of paper for each child Measure to the nearest 10 g or ½ ounce for infants and 100 g or ¼ pound for children
Head circumference (HC)	Measure with paper or steel tape at greatest circumference, from slightly above the eyebrows and pinna of the ears to occipital prominence of skull
Chest circumference	Measure around chest at nipple line Ideally, take measurements during inhalation and expiration; record the average of the two values

Usual findings	Comments
Measurements of length, weight, and head circumference between the 25th and 75th percentiles are likely to represent normal growth Measurements between the 10th and 25th, and the 75th and 90th percentiles may or may not be normal, depending on previous and subsequent measurements and on genetic and environmental factors Growth curve remains generally within same percentile, except during rapid growth periods	Questionable results may include 1. Children whose height and weight are below the 5th or above the 95th percentile 2. Children whose height and weight percentiles are widely disparate, for example, height in the 10th percentile and weight in the 90th percentile, especially with above average skinfold thickness 3. Children who fail to show the expected gain in height and weight, especially during the rapid growth periods of infancy and adolescence 4. Children who show a sudden increase, except during puberty, or decrease in a previously steady growth pattern Compare findings with growth patterns of other family members; consider genetic influence on growth determination (see Chinese growth charts, p. 99)

Plot on growth chart (pp. 102-109)
Compare value with percentile for weight
Rule of thumb guide*:
    At 1 year = $1\frac{1}{2} \times$ birth length
    2 to 12 years = age (years) $\times 2\frac{1}{2} + 30$ = length (inches)
	If body length appears disproportionate, measure sitting height

Sitting height is 70% of total body length at birth, 60% at 2 years, and 52% at 10 years	Not a routine measurement Helpful in distinguishing dwarfism from small stature

Plot on growth chart (pp. 102-109)
Compare value with percentile for length
Rule of thumb guides*:
    At 1 year = $3 \times$ birth weight
    1 to 9 years: age (years) $\times 5 + 17$ = weight (pounds)
    9 to 12 years: age (years) $\times 9 - 20$ = weight (pounds)
	Compare weight with appearance, for example, excessive fat, well-developed musculature, flabby, loose skin, bony prominences (for skinfold measurement, see p. 111)
	Assess nutritional status; compare with weight

Plot on growth chart (pp. 103, 107, or 110)
Compare percentile with those of height and weight
Compare with chest circumference:
    At birth HC exceeds chest circumference by 2 to 3 cm (1 inch)
    At 1 to 2 years, HC equals chest circumference
    During childhood, chest circumference exceeds HC by about 5 to 7 cm (2 to 3 inches)
	Usually taken in children under 36 months of age
	Taken in any child whose head size appears abnormal

Compare with head circumference (see above)	May be measured during examination of chest

*Based on NCHS growth charts for boys, 50th percentile (p. 100).

Summary of physical assessment of the child—cont'd

Assessment	Procedure
Skinfold thickness and arm circumference	**MEASUREMENT OF TRICEPS SKINFOLD THICKNESS** With child's right arm flexed 90° at elbow, mark midpoint between acromion and olecranon on posterior aspect of arm With arm hanging freely, grasp a fold of skin between thumb and forefinger 1 cm above midpoint Gently pull fold away from underlying muscle and continue to hold until measurement is completed Place caliper jaws over skinfold at midpoint mark; if a plastic caliper (e.g., Ross Adipometer) is used, apply pressure with thumb to align lines on caliper; follow directions for using other calipers Estimate reading to nearest 1.0 mm, 2 to 3 seconds after applying pressure Take measurements until duplicates agree within 1 mm **MEASUREMENT OF MIDARM CIRCUMFERENCE** Follow same procedure as above, but instead of grasping a fold of skin and using calipers, wrap a paper or steel measuring tape around upper arm at midpoint Measure to nearest 1 cm
PHYSIOLOGIC MEASUREMENTS (Vital signs)	Ideally, record when child is quiet; otherwise, record value and note activity such as crying
Temperature*	Use axillary measurements in children under 4 to 6 years of age or in any child who is uncooperative, unconscious, seizure prone, or has had oral surgery; use rectal route when no other route is feasible because of risk of rectal perforation, especially in young infants For axillary temperature, place thermometer in axilla; press child's arm close to body; hold thermometer in place 3 minutes† For oral temperature, place the thermometer under the tongue in the right or left posterior sublingual pocket, not in the area in front of the tongue; have the child keep the mouth closed and refrain from biting on the glass thermometer; keep the thermometer in place for up to 7 minutes† For rectal temperature, position child supine, prone, or side-lying; insert well-lubricated tip of thermometer a maximum of 2.5 cm (1 inch) into rectum; hold in place for 4 minutes†
Pulse	Take apical pulse in children under 2 to 3 years Point of maximum intensity located lateral to nipple at fourth to fifth interspace at or near midclavicular line Take radial pulse in children over 2 to 3 years Count pulse for 1 full minute
Respiration	Observe rate of breathing for 1 full minute In infants and young children, observe abdominal movement In older children, observe thoracic movement

*For Home Care Instructions on taking temperature, see p. 533.

†There is no universal agreement on length of time for temperature taking; these values based on research findings may differ from those used in various practice settings.

Usual findings	Comments
Plot on percentile charts (pp. 111-112) For interpretation of measurements, see Comments	Skinfold thickness is an index of body fat Arm circumference is an indirect measure of muscle mass Measurements of skinfold thickness can be taken at triceps (most common site), subscapula, suprailiac, abdomen, or upper thigh with special calipers Percentiles for skinfold thickness and arm circumference may be used as reference data but should not be considered "standards" or "norms"; between 5th and 95th percentiles are not ranges of normal Because of lack of standard data, these measurements should probably not be used as a routine screening measurement in well child care, but rather in follow-up and monitoring of children who are identified as having potential or actual obesity or malnutrition
See inside front cover	Compare present value with past recordings Note obvious difference, such as sudden increase Assess possible physiologic/psychologic factors influencing the recordings
For average body temperatures in well children under basal conditions, see inside front cover	A fever is generally a rectal temperature above 38.0° C (100.4° F) and oral or axillary temperature above 37.8° C (100° F) Axillary readings differ by an average of 0.49° C (0.9° F) less than rectal readings Chart the route with the recorded temperature reading Temperature fluctuates markedly in young children Axillary measurements may be affected by poor peripheral circulation or use of radiant warmers Oral measurements may be affected by hot or cold beverages, smoking, and rapid breathing Rectal measurements may be affected by stool in the rectum Compare recordings with observations of child's dress, activity, and evidence of infection

For average pulse rates at rest, see inside front cover	Pulse rate may increase with inspiration and decrease with expiration
	See also Table 1-7
	May grade pulses
	  Grade 0 Not palpable
	  Grade +1 Difficult to palpate, thready, weak, easily obliterated with pressure
	  Grade +2 Difficult to palpate, may be obliterated with pressure
	  Grade +3 Easy to palpate, not easily obliterated with pressure (normal)
	  Grade +4 Strong, bounding, not obliterated with pressure

For average respiratory rates at rest, see inside front cover	See also pp. 41-43

Summary of physical assessment of the child—cont'd

| Assessment | Procedure |

Blood pressure

Table 1-1. COMMONLY AVAILABLE BLOOD PRESSURE CUFFS

Cuff name*	Bladder width (cm)	Bladder length (cm)
Newborn	2.5-4.0	5.0-9.0
Infant	4.0-6.0	11.5-18.0
Child	7.5-9.0	17.0-19.0
Adult	11.5-13.0	22.0-26.0
Large arm	14.0-15.0	30.5-33.0
Thigh	18.0-19.0	36.0-38.0

From Report of the Second Task Force on Blood Pressure Control in Children–1987, Pediatrics 79(1):1-25, 1987.

*Cuff name does not guarantee that the cuff will be appropriate size for a child within that age range.

Table 1-2. RECOMMENDED BLADDER DIMENSIONS FOR BLOOD PRESSURE CUFFS

Arm circumference at midpoint (cm)	Cuff name*	Bladder width (cm)	Bladder length (cm)
5-7.5	Newborn	3	5
7.5-13	Infant	5	8
13-20	Child	8	13
24-32	Adult	13	24
32-42	Wide adult	17	32
42-50	Thigh	20	42

From Frohlich ED and others: Recommendations for human blood pressure determination by sphygmomanometers: report of a special task force appointed by the Steering Committee, American Heath Association, Circulation 77:501A. 1988.

*Cuff name does not guarantee that the cuff will be appropriate size for a child within that age range.

Use an appropriately sized cuff (cuff size refers only to inner inflatable bladder, not cloth or plastic covering)

Report of the Second Task Force (1987) recommends (Table 1-1):
   Width sufficient to cover approximately 75% of upper arm between top of shoulder and olecranon (Fig. 1-6, *A*)
   Length sufficient to completely encircle circumference of limb with or without overlapping
   Enough room at antecubital fossa to place bell of stethoscope
   Enough room at upper edge of cuff to prevent obstruction of axilla

American Heart Association (Frohlich, 1988) recommends (Table 1-2):
   Width 40% to 50% limb circumference; measured at upper arm midway between top of shoulder and olecranon
   Length sufficient to completely or nearly completely encircle circumference of limb without overlapping
   For other measurement sites (see Fig. 1-6, *B, C,* and *D*) the above suggested guidelines can be used although the shape of the limb (i.e., conical shape of thigh) may prevent appropriate placement of the cuff

Use same position, e.g., lying down or preferably sitting, and right arm for measurement

Position limb at level of heart

Rapidly inflate cuff to about 20 mm Hg above point at which radial pulse disappears

Release cuff pressure at a rate of about 2 to 3 mm Hg per second during auscultation of artery

Read mercury-gravity manometer at eye level

Record systolic value as onset of a clear tapping sound (first Korotkoff sound)

Record diastolic pressure as both fourth Korotkoff sound (K4) (low-pitched, muffled sound) and fifth Korotkoff sound (K5) (disappearance of all sound) along with systolic pressure, limb, position, cuff size, and method, i.e., BP = 100/60/54 mm Hg, right arm, sitting, with child cuff by auscultation

If using electronic monitor, follow manufacturer's instructions and above guidelines for correct cuff size
   With oscillometric device (i.e., Dinamap), all four sites in Fig. 1-6 can be used, but reserve the thigh for last since it is most uncomfortable

Stabilize the limb during cuff deflation since movement interferes with the device's ability to measure blood pressure accurately

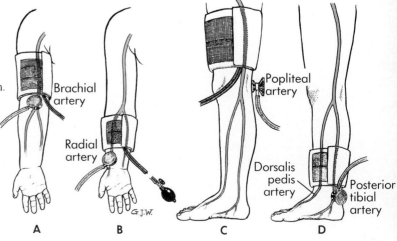

Fig. 1-6. Sites for measuring blood pressure. **A,** Upper arm. **B,** Lower arm or forearm. **C,** Thigh. **D,** Calf or ankle.

Usual findings

For blood pressure values at various ages using auscultation see inside front cover

These norms are based on:

K4 diastolic pressure for children up to 12 years

K5 diastolic pressure for adolescents 13 to 18 years

For blood pressure values at various ages using oscillometry see Table 1-3

Normal blood pressure: systolic and diastolic pressure less than 90th percentile for age and sex

Normal high blood pressure: systolic and diastolic pressure between the 90th and 95th percentile for age and sex

Table 1-3. NORMATIVE DINAMAP (OSCILLOMETRY) BP VALUES (SYSTOLIC/DIASTOLIC, MEAN IN PARENTHESES)

Age group	n	Mean	90th percentile	95th percentile
Newborn (1-3 days)	219	65/41(50)	75/49(59)	78/52(62)
1 month to 2 years	660	95/58(72)	106/68(83)	110/71(86)
2-5 years	631	101/57(74)	112/66(82)	115/68(85)

Normative oscillometric blood pressure values in the first five years in an office setting, Arch Dis Child. 143(7): 860-864, 1989

Table 1-4. CLASSIFICATION OF HYPERTENSION BY AGE-GROUP

Age group	Significant hypertension (mm Hg)	Severe hypertension (mm Hg)
Newborn (7 d)	Systolic BP ≥96	Systolic BP ≥106
(8-30 d)	Systolic BP ≥104	Systolic BP ≥110
Infant (<2 yr)	Systolic BP ≥112 Diastolic BP ≥74	Systolic BP ≥118 Diastolic BP ≥82
Children (3-5 yr)	Systolic BP ≥116 Diastolic BP ≥76	Systolic BP ≥124 Diastolic BP ≥84
Children (6-9 yr)	Systolic BP ≥122 Diastolic BP ≥78	Systolic BP ≥130 Diastolic BP ≥86
Children (10-12 yr)	Systolic BP ≥126 Diastolic BP ≥82	Systolic BP ≥134 Diastolic BP ≥90
Adolescents (13-15 yr)	Systolic BP ≥136 Diastolic BP ≥86	Systolic BP ≥144 Diastolic BP ≥92
Adolescents (16-18 yr)	Systolic BP >142 Diastolic BP ≥92	Systolic BP ≥150 Diastolic BP ≥98

From Report of The Second Task Force on Blood Pressure Control in Children—1987, Pediatrics 79(1): 1-25, 1987.

Comments

Blood pressure should be measured once a year in:

Children 3 years of age through adolescence

Children with symptoms of hypertension

Children in emergency rooms and intensive care units

High-risk infants

Low-risk neonates (not universal agreement)

Task Force guidelines using limb length for selecting cuff width may produce satisfactory blood pressure readings in children with average weight for height, but inaccurate readings in children with thick arms; using limb circumference for selecting cuff width more accurately reflects direct arterial blood pressure than using length

Using a small cuff causes a falsely elevated reading

Using a large cuff or compression of brachial artery by clothing pushed up on arm may result in lower reading; but, wide cuffs tend to affect blood pressure readings less than small cuffs

In choosing cuff sizes, use an oversized cuff rather than an undersized one when correct size is not available or use another site that more appropriately fits the cuff size:

Use larger size on thigh: place cuff above knee and auscultate popliteal artery (Fig. 1-6, *B*)

Use smaller size on forearm: place cuff above wrist and auscultate radial artery (Fig. 1-6, *C*)

Use larger size on calf: place cuff above malleoli or at midcalf and auscultate posterior tibial or dorsal pedal artery (Fig. 1-6, *D*)

Blood pressure differences between measurement sites vary depending on the type of measurement technique; generally, pressure in upper sites is less than the pressure in lower sites, i.e., systolic pressure in thigh is 10-20 mm Hg higher than in upper arm using noninvasive techniques

Compare blood pressure in upper and lower extremity at least once to detect abnormalities, e.g., coarctation of the aorta in which the lower extremity pressure is less than the upper extremity pressure

Repeat measurements above 90th percentile later during initial visit when child is least anxious; if a high reading persists, repeat measurements at least three times during subsequent visits to detect hypertension (Table 1-4):

Significant hypertension: blood pressure persistently between 95th and 99th percentile for age and sex

Severe hypertension: blood pressure persistently at or above 99th percentile for age and sex

Consider body size when blood pressure values are in normal high range because larger children have higher blood pressures than smaller children of same age; i.e., a tall child whose BP is at 90th percentile for age is considered normal

Refer children with consistently high blood pressure readings or significant differences in pressure between upper and lower extremities for further evaluation; i.e., in newborns a calf pressure less than 6 to 9 mm Hg compared to upper arm pressure (Park and Lee, 1989)

Blood pressure readings using oscillometry are generally higher than those using auscultation, but correlate better with direct radial artery blood pressure than auscultation readings (Park and Menard, 1987)

From Park M and Menard S: Normative arm and calf blood pressure values in the newborn, Pediatrics 83(2):240-243, 1989.

From Park M and Menard S: Accuracy of blood pressure measurement by the Dinamap monitor in infants and children, Pediatrics 79(6):907-914, 1987.

Summary of physical assessment of the child—cont'd

Assessment	Procedure
GENERAL APPEARANCE	Observe the following: Facies Posture Hygiene Nutrition Behavior Development State of awareness
SKIN	Observe skin in natural daylight or neutral artificial light *Color*—Most reliably assessed in sclera, conjunctiva, nail beds, tongue, buccal mucosa, palms, and soles *Texture*—Note moisture, smoothness, roughness, integrity of skin, and temperature *Temperature*—Compare each part of body for even temperature *Turgor*—Grasp skin on abdomen between thumb and index finger, pull taut, and release quickly Indent skin with finger
ACCESSORY STRUCTURES 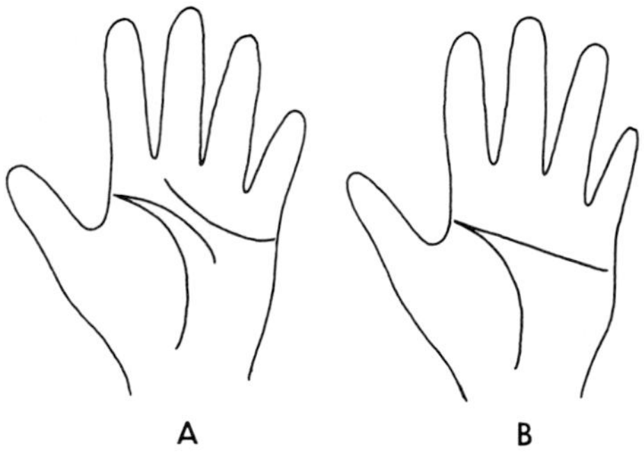 **Fig. 1-7. A,** Example of normal flexion crease on palm. **B,** Simian crease on palm.	*Hair*—Inspect color, texture, quality, distribution, elasticity, and hygiene *Nails*—Inspect color, texture, quality, distribution, elasticity, and hygiene *Dermatoglyphics*—Observe flexion creases of palm (Fig. 1-7)
LYMPH NODES (Fig. 1-8)	Palpate using distal portion of fingers Press gently but firmly in a circular motion Note size, mobility, temperature, tenderness, and any change in enlarged nodes *Cervical*—Tilt head slightly upward *Axillary*—Have arms relaxed at side but slightly abducted *Inguinal*—Place child supine

Usual findings	Comments
Evaluated in terms of a comprehensive assessment; often gives clues to underlying problems such as poor hygiene and nutrition from parental neglect or poverty	Record actual observations that lead to a conclusion such as signs of poor hygiene; give examples of present development milestones Follow up on clues that may indicate problems, for example, investigate feeding practices of family if child appears undernourished
	Reveals significant clues to problems such as poor hygiene, child abuse, inadequate nutrition, and serious physical disorders

Genetically determined
  Light-skinned—From milky white to rosy colored
  Dark-skinned—Various shades of brown, red, yellow, olive, and bluish tones
	Observe for abnormalities such as pallor, cyanosis, erythema, ecchymosis, petechiae, and jaundice (Table 1-5)
	Factors affecting color include natural skin tone, melanin production, edema, hygiene, hemoglobin levels of blood, amount of lighting, color of room, atmospheric temperature, and use of cosmetics

Smooth, slightly dry to touch, and even temperature	Note obvious changes such as clammy, oily skin, obvious lesions, excessive dryness
Usually same all over body, although parts exposed, such as hands, may be cooler	Note obvious differences such as warm upper extremities and cold lower extremities
Resumes shape immediately with no tenting, wrinkling, or prolonged depression	Turgor is an excellent indicator of adequate hydration and nutrition Note tenting suspension of the pulled skin, obvious pitting of skin upon indentation, or signs of swelling
Lustrous, silky, strong Genetic factors influence appearance; for example, black child's hair is usually coarser, duller, and curlier	Signs of poor nutrition include stringy, friable, dull, dry, depigmented hair Note areas of baldness, unusual hairiness, and any evidence of infestation During puberty, secondary hair growth indicates normal pubertal changes
Pink, convex in shape, smooth, and flexible, not brittle In dark-skinned child, color is darker	Note color changes such as blueness or yellow tint Observe for uncut or short ragged nails (nailbiting) Report any signs of clubbing (base of the nail becomes swollen and feels springy or floating when palpated)
Three flexion creases	If pattern differs, draw a sketch to describe it Observe for simian crease (one horizontal crease) (Fig. 1-7, *B*)
Generally not palpable, although small, nontender, movable nodes are normal	Note tender, enlarged, warm nodes, which are usually an indication of infection or inflammation *proximal* to their location

Summary of physical assessment of the child—cont'd

Table 1-5. DIFFERENCES IN COLOR CHANGES OF RACIAL GROUPS

Color change	Appearance in light skin	Appearance in dark skin
Cyanosis	Bluish tinge, especially in palpebral conjunctiva (lower eyelid), nail beds, earlobes, lips, oral membranes, soles, and palms	Ashen gray lips and tongue
Pallor	Loss of rosy glow in skin, especially face	Ashen gray appearance in black skin More yellowish-brown color in brown skin
Erythema	Redness easily seen anywhere on body	Much more difficult to assess; rely on palpation for warmth or edema
Ecchymosis	Purplish to yellow-green areas; may be seen anywhere on skin	Very difficult to see unless in mouth or conjunctiva
Petechiae	Purplish pinpoints most easily seen on buttocks, abdomen, and inner surfaces of the arms or legs	Usually invisible except in oral mucosa, conjunctiva of eyelids, and conjunctiva covering eyeball
Jaundice	Yellow staining seen in sclera of eyes, skin, fingernails, soles, palms, and oral mucosa	Most reliably assessed in sclera, hard palate, palms, and soles

Assessment	Procedure
HEAD	Note shape and symmetry Note head control (especially in infants) and head posture
	Evaluate range of motion (ROM)
	Palpate skull for fontanels, nodes, or obvious swellings
	Transilluminate skull in darkened room; firmly place rubber-collared flashlight against skull at various points
	Examine scalp for hygiene, lesions, infestation, signs of trauma, loss of hair, discoloration
	Percuss frontal sinuses in children over 7 years
NECK	Inspect size
	Trachea—Palpate for deviation; place thumb and index finger on each side and slide fingers back and forth
	Thyroid—Palpate noting size, shape, symmetry, tenderness, nodules; place pads of index and middle finger below cricoid cartilage; feel for isthmus rising during swallowing; feel each lobe laterally and posteriorly
	Carotid arteries—Palpate on both sides

Fig. 1-8. Location of superficial lymph nodes. Arrows indicate directional flow of lymph.

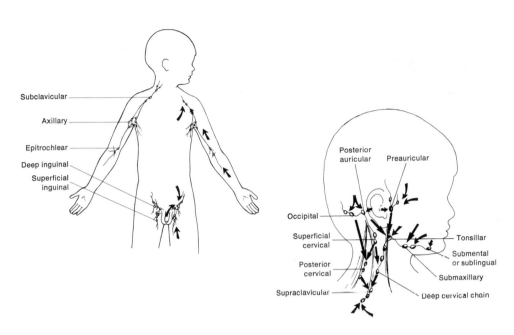

Usual findings	Comments

Even molding of head, occipital prominence
Symmetric facial features
Head control well-established by 6 months of age
Head in midline
 	
Moves head up, down, and from side to side
Smooth, fused except for fontanels (p. 12)
    Posterior fontanel closes by 2 months
    Anterior fontanel closes by 12 to 18 months
 	
Absence of halo around rubber collar
 	
Clean, pink (more deeply pigmented in dark-skinned children)
	Report any deviations from expected findings
	Clue to problems include the following:
	    Uneven molding—Premature closure of sutures
	    Asymmetry—Paralysis
	    Head lag—Retarded motor/mental development
	    Head tilt—Poor vision
	    Limited ROM—Torticollis (wryneck)
	    Resistance to movement and pain—Meningeal irritation
	    Halo of light through skull—Loss of cortex (hydrocephaly)
	    Ecchymotic areas on scalp—Trauma (possibly abuse)
	Loss of hair—Trauma (hair pulling), lack of stimulation (lying in same position)
	Painful sinuses—Infection

Resonant, nontender	
During infancy, normally short with skinfolds During early childhood, lengthens In midline; rises with swallowing In midline; rises with swallowing; lobes equal	Note any webbing Note any deviation, masses, or nodules when palpating neck structures Often thyroid is difficult to palpate Inquire if child ever received irradiation to neck or upper chest area
Equal bilaterally	Note unequal pulses and protruding neck veins

Summary of physical assessment of the child—cont'd

Assessment	Procedure

EYES

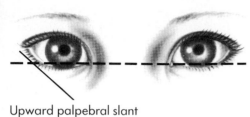

Upward palpebral slant

Fig. 1-9. Upward palpebral slant.

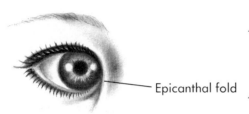

Epicanthal fold

Fig. 1-10. Epicanthal fold.

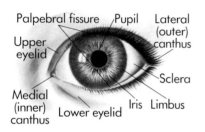

Fig. 1-11. Normal structure of the eye.

Inspect placement and alignment
If abnormality is suspected, measure inner canthal distance

Palpebral slant—Draw imaginary line through two points of medial (inner) canthi (Fig. 1-9)

Epicanthal fold—Observe for excess fold from roof of nose to inner termination of eyebrow (Fig. 1-10)

Lids—Observe placement, movement, and color (see Fig. 1-9)

Palpebral conjunctiva
Pull lower lid down while child looks up
Evert upper lid by holding lashes and pulling *down* and forward
Observe color

Bulbar conjunctiva—Observe color

Lacrimal punctum—Observe color

Eyelashes and ***eyebrows***—Observe distribution and direction of growth

Sclera—Observe color (Fig. 1-11)

Cornea—Check for opacities by shining light toward eye

Pupils (Fig. 1-11)
Compare size, shape, and movement
Test reaction to light; shine light source toward and away from eye
Test accommodation; have child focus on object from distance and bring object close to face

Iris—Observe shape, color, size, and clarity (Fig. 1-11)

Lens—Inspect

Fundus (Fig. 1-12)
Examine with ophthalmoscope set at 0; approach the child from a 15-degree angle; change to plus or minus diopters to produce clear focus
Measure structures in relationship to disc's diameter (DD)
To facilitate locating macula, have child momentarily look *directly* at light
Assess vision
(for visual acuity see pp. 124-129)

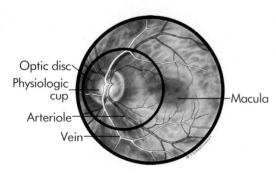

Fig. 1-12. Structures of the fundus. Interior circle represents approximate size of area seen with ophthalmoscope.

Usual findings	Comments
Placement is symmetric Inner canthal distance averages 3 cm (1.2 inches)	Note asymmetry, abnormal spacing (hypertelorism)
Usually palpebral fissures lie horizontally on imaginary line In Orientals, there may be an upward slant	Presence of upward slant and epicanthal folds in children who are not Oriental is significant finding in Down syndrome
Often present in Oriental children	May give false impression of strabismus

When eye is open, falls between upper iris and pupil
When eye is closed, sclera, cornea, and palpebral conjunctiva are completely covered
Symmetric blink
Color is same as surrounding skin
	Observe for deviations
	  Ptosis (upper lid covers part of pupil or lower iris)
	  Setting sun sign (upper lid above iris)
	  Inability to completely close eye
	  Malposition of lids; *ectropion* (turning out) or *entropion* (turning in)
	  Asymmetric, excessive, or infrequent blinking
	  Signs of inflammation along lid margin or on lid

Pink and glossy Vertical yellow striations along edge near hair follicle	Note any signs of inflammation Excessive pallor may indicate anemia
Transparent and white color of underlying sclera	A reddened conjunctiva may indicate eyestrain, fatigue, infection, or irritation such as from excessive rubbing or exposure to environmental irritants
Same color as lid	Excessive discharge, tearing, pain, redness, or swelling indicates dacryocystitis
Eyelashes curl away from eye Eyebrows are above eye, do not meet in midline	Note inward growth of lashes and unusual hairiness of brows
White Tiny black marks normal in deeply pigmented children Transparent	Note any yellow staining Note any opacities or ulcerations
Round, clear, and equal Pupils constrict when light approaches, dilate when light fades Pupils constrict as object is brought near face	PERRLA is common notation for "pupils equal, round, react to light and accommodation" Note any asymmetry in size and movement
Round, equal, clear Color varies from shades of brown, green, or blue	Note asymmetry in size, lack of clarity, cleft at edge (coloboma), absence of color (a pinkish glow is seen in albinism), or black and white speckling (Brushfield spots are commonly found in Down syndrome)
Should not be seen	Note any opacities

Red reflex—Brilliant, uniform reflection of red; appears darker color in deeply pigmented children, lighter in infants
Optic disc—Creamy pink but lighter than surrounding fundus, round or vertically oval
Physiologic cup—Small, pale depression in center of disc
Blood vessels—Emanate from disc; veins are darker and about one quarter larger than arteries; narrow band of light, the *arteriolar light reflex* is reflected from center of artery not vein; branches cross each other; may see obvious pulsations
Macula—One DD in size, darker in color than disc or surrounding fundus, located 2 DD temporal to the disc
Fovea centralis—Minute glistening spot of reflected light in center of macula
	Visualization of red reflex virtually rules out most serious defects of cornea, lens, and aqueous and vitreous chambers
	Observe for abnormalities
	  Partial red or white reflex
	  Blurring of disc margins
	  Bulging of disc
	  Loss of depression
	  Dilated blood vessels
	  Tortuous vessels
	  Hemorrhages
	  Absence of pulsations
	  Notching or indenting at crossing of vessels

Summary of physical assessment of the child—cont'd

Assessment	Procedure

EYES—cont'd

Use following tests for binocular vision:

Corneal light reflex test (also called red reflex gemini or Hirschberg test)— Shine a light directly into the eyes from a distance of about 40.5 cm (16 inches)

Cover test—Have child fixate on near (33 cm or 13 inches) or distant (50 cm or 20 inches) object; cover one eye and observe movement of the uncovered eye

Alternate cover test—Same as cover test except rapidly cover one eye then the other eye several times; observe movement of covered eye when it is uncovered

Peripheral vision—Have child look straight ahead; move an object, such as your finger, from beyond his field of vision into view; ask the child to signal as soon as he sees the object; estimate the angle from straight line of vision to first detection of peripheral vision

Color vision—Use Ishihara or Hardy-Rand-Rittler test

EARS

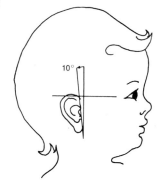

Fig. 1-13. Placement and alignment of pinna.

Pinna—Inspect placement and alignment (Fig. 1-13)
  1. Measure height of pinna by drawing an imaginary line from outer orbit of eye to occiput of skull
  2. Measure angle of pinna by drawing a perpendicular line from the imaginary horizontal line and aligning pinna next to this mark

Observe the usual landmarks of the pinna

Note presence of any abnormal openings, tags of skin, or sinuses

Inspect hygiene (odor, discharge, color)

Examine external canal and middle ear structures with otoscope
  Child below 3 years—Position prone with ear to be examined toward ceiling, lean over child, using upper portion of body to restrain arms and trunk, and examining hand to restrain the head
    Alternate position: seat child sideways in parent's lap; have parent hug child securely around trunk and arms and top of head
    Introduce speculum between 3 and 9 o'clock position in a *downward* and *forward* slant
    Pull pinna *downward* and *backward* to the 6 to 9 o'clock range (Fig. 1-14, *A*)
  Child over 3 years—Examine while seated with head tilted slightly away from examiner (if child needs restraining, use one of the previously mentioned positions)
    Pull pinna *upward* and *back* toward a 10 o'clock position (Fig. 1-14, *B*)
    Insert speculum ¼ to ½ inch; use widest speculum that easily accommodates diameter of canal

Usual findings	Comments
Binocularity is well established by 3 to 4 months of age	Refer any child with nonbinocular vision due to malalignment (strabismus) for further evaluation
Light falls symmetrically within each pupil	Light falls asymmetrically in each pupil
Uncovered eye does not move	Uncovered eye moves when other eye is covered
Neither eye moves when covered or uncovered In each quadrant, sees object at 50 degrees upward, 70 degrees downward, 60 degrees nasalward, and 90 degrees temporally	Covered eye moves as soon as occluder is removed Inability to see object until it is brought closer to straight line of vision indicates need for further evaluation
Able to see a letter or figure within the colored dots	Each test consists of cards on which a color field composed of spots of a certain "confusion" color is printed; against the field is a number (Ishihara) or symbol (Hardy-Rand-Rittler) similarly printed in dots but of a color likely to be confused with the field color and not seen by the person with a color vision deficit Counsel the affected child and parents about the practical inconveniences caused by the disorder, the mode of genetic transmission, and its irreversibility
Slightly crosses or meets this line	Low-set ears are commonly associated with renal anomalies or mental retardation
Lies within a 10-degree angle of the vertical line	
Extends slightly forward from the skull Prominences and depressions symmetric	Flattened ears may indicate infrequent change of positioning from a side-lying placement; masses or swelling may make the pinna protrude
Adherent lobule (normal variation)	Abnormal landmarks are often signs of possible middle ear anomalies If abnormal opening is present, note any discharge
Small amount of soft yellow cerumen	If ear needs cleaning, discuss hygiene with parent or child If ear is free of wax, ascertain the method of cleaning, especially advising against the use of cotton-tipped applicators or sharp or pointed objects in the canal
External canal—Pink (more deeply colored in dark-skinned child), outermost portion lined with minute hairs, some soft yellow cerumen	Note signs of irritation, infection, foreign bodies, and desiccated, packed wax (may interfere with hearing) If discharge is present, change speculum to examine other ear Note

Tympanic membrane (Fig. 1-15)
Translucent, light pearly pink or gray color
Slight redness seen normally in infants and children as a result of crying
Light reflex—Cone-shaped reflection, normally points away from face at 5 or 7 o'clock position
Bony landmarks present
	Red, tense, bulging drum
	  Dull transparent gray color
	  Black areas
	  Absence of light reflex or bony prominences
	  Retraction of drum with abnormal prominence of landmarks

Summary of physical assessment of the child—cont'd

Assessment	Procedure

Assess hearing (see also pp. 130 and 132)

Rinne test—Place vibrating stem and tuning fork against mastoid bone until child no longer hears sound; move prongs close to auditory meatus

Weber test—Hold tuning fork in midline of head or forehead

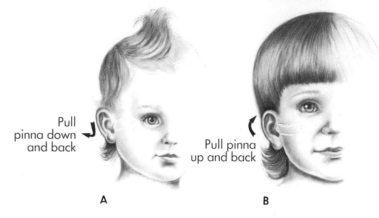

Fig. 1-14. Position of eardrum in **A,** Infant. **B,** Child over 3 years of age.

Pull pinna down and back

Pull pinna up and back

A   B

NOSE (Fig. 1-16)

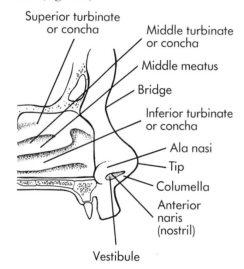

Superior turbinate or concha

Middle turbinate or concha

Middle meatus

Bridge

Inferior turbinate or concha

Ala nasi

Tip

Columella

Anterior naris (nostril)

Vestibule

Inspect size, placement, and alignment; draw imaginary vertical line from center point between eyes to notch of upper lip

Anterior vestibule—Tilt head backward, push tip of nose up, and illuminate cavity with flashlight; to detect perforated septum, shine light into one naris and observe for admittance of light through perforation

Fig. 1-16. External landmarks and internal structure of nose.

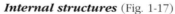

MOUTH AND THROAT

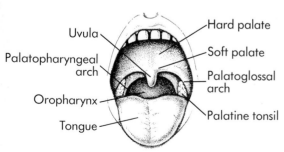

Uvula

Palatopharyngeal arch

Oropharynx

Tongue

Hard palate

Soft palate

Palatoglossal arch

Palatine tonsil

Lips—Note color, texture, any obvious lesions

Internal structures (Fig. 1-17)

Ask cooperative child to open mouth wide and say "Ahh"; usually not necessary to use tongue blade

Restrain young child by placing supine with both arms extended along side of head; have parent maintain arm position to immobilize head; may be necessary to use a tongue blade, but avoid eliciting gag reflex by depressing only toward the side of the tongue; use flashlight for good illumination

Fig. 1-17. Interior structure of mouth.

Usual findings	Comments
Hears sound when prongs are brought close to ear	Rinne and Weber tests distinguish between bone and air conduction; both tests require cooperation and are better suited to children of school age or older
Hears sound equally in both ears	Note abnormal results Rinne—Sound is not audible through ear Weber—Sound is heard better in *affected* ear

Fig. 1-15. Landmarks of tympanic membrane with "clock" superimposed.

Lies exactly vertical to imaginary line, with each side symmetric Both nostrils equal in size Bridge of nose flattened in black or Oriental children	Note any deviation to one side, unequalness in size of nostrils, or flaring of ala nasi (sign of respiratory distress) Usually do not use a nasal speculum to examine internal structures
Mucosal lining—Redder than oral membranes, moist, but no discharge	Note
Turbinate and meatus—Same color as mucosal lining	Abnormally pale, grayish pink, swollen, and boggy membranes Red, swollen membranes
Septum—In midline	Any discharge Foreign object in nose Deviated septum Perforated septum

More deeply pigmented than surrounding skin, smooth, moist	Note cyanosis, pallor, lesions, or cracks, especially at corners
Mucous membranes—Bright pink, glistening, smooth, uniform, and moist	Note lesions, bleeding, sensitivity, odor
Gingiva—Firm, coral pink, and stippled; margins are "knife-edged"	Note redness, puffiness (especially at margin), tendency to bleed
Teeth—Number appropriate for age, white, good occlusion of upper/lower jaw General rule for estimating number of teeth in children under 2 years: age (months) minus 6 months	Note loss of teeth, delayed eruption, malocclusion, obvious discoloration Compare dental findings with parental report of dental hygiene Assess need for further dental counseling Eating habits, such as bottle feeding at bedtime, excessive sugar Toothbrushing Sources of fluoride, need for supplementation Periodic, regular examinations by dentist
Tongue—Rough texture, freely movable, tip extends to lips, no lesions or masses under the tongue	Note smoothness, fissuring, coating on the tongue, excessive redness, swelling, or inability to move the tongue forward to lips; can interfere with speech

Summary of physical assessment of the child—cont'd

Assessment	Procedure

CHEST (Fig. 1-18)

Inspect size, shape, symmetry, movement, and breast development
Describe findings according to geographic and imaginary landmarks (Fig. 1-19)
Locate intercostal space (ICS), space directly below rib, by palpating chest inferiorly
   from 2nd rib
   Other landmarks:
      Nipples usually at 4th ICS
      Tip of 11th rib felt laterally
      Tip of 12th rib felt posteriorly
      Tip of scapula at 8th rib or ICS

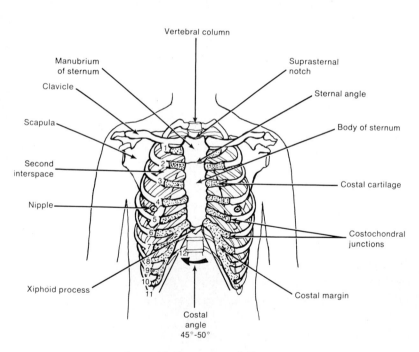

Fig. 1-18. Structures of rib cage.

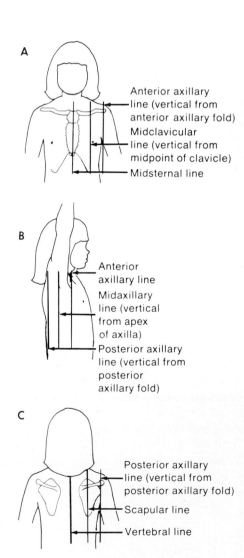

Fig. 1-19. Imaginary landmarks of chest.
A, Anterior. **B,** Right lateral. **C,** Posterior.

Usual findings	Comments
Palate—Intact, slightly arched	Note presence of any clefts
Uvula—Protrudes from back of soft palate, moves upward during gag reflex	Note if a bifid uvula is present
Palatine tonsils—Same color as surrounding mucosa, glandular rather than smooth, may be large in prepubertal children	Note exudate and enlargement that could become obstructive
Posterior pharynx—Same color as surrounding mucosa, smooth, moist	Assess for signs of infection
In infants, shape is almost circular; with growth, the lateral diameter increases in proportion to anteroposterior diameter	Measurement of chest and palpation of axillary nodes may be done here
Both sides of chest symmetric	Note deviations
Costal angle between 45 and 50 degrees	Barrel-shaped chest
Points of attachment between ribs and costal cartilage smooth	Asymmetry
Movement—During inspiration chest expands, costal angle increases, and diaphragm descends; during expiration, reverse occurs	Wide or narrow costal angle
	Bony prominences
	Pectus carinatum (pigeon breast)—sternum protrudes outward
Nipples—Darker pigmentation, located slightly lateral to midclavicular line between fourth and fifth ribs	Pectus excavatum (funnel chest)—lower portion of sternum is depressed
	Retractions (Fig. 1-20)
	Asymmetric or decreased movement
Breast development depends on age; no masses	Compare breast development with expected stage for age (see p. 96)
	Discuss importance of monthly breast self-examination with female adolescents

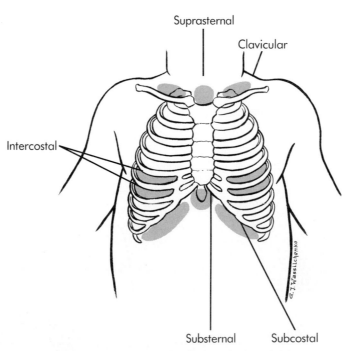

Fig. 1-20. Location of retractions.

Summary of physical assessment of the child—cont'd

Assessment	Procedure
LUNGS (Fig. 1-21)	Evaluate respiratory movements for rate, rhythm, depth, quality, and character
	With child sitting, place each hand flat against back or chest with thumbs in midline along lower costal margins
	Vocal fremitus—Palpate as above and have child say "99," "eee"
	Percuss each side of chest in sequence from apex to base (Fig. 1-22) For anterior lungs, child sitting or supine For posterior lungs, child sitting
	Auscultate breath and voice sounds for intensity, pitch, quality, relative duration of inspiration and expiration

Table 1-6. VARIOUS PATTERNS OF RESPIRATION

Tachypnea	Increased rate
Bradypnea	Decreased rate
Dyspnea	Distress during breathing
Apnea	Cessation of breathing
Hyperpnea	Increased depth
Hypoventilation	Decreased depth (shallow) and irregular rhythm
Hyperventilation	Increased rate and depth
Kussmaul breathing	Hyperventilation, gasping and labored respiration, usually seen in diabetic coma or other states of respiratory acidosis
Cheyne-Stokes respirations	Gradually increasing rate and depth with periods of apnea
Biot breathing	Periods of hyperpnea alternating with apnea (similar to Cheyne-Stokes except that the depth remains constant)
Seesaw (paradoxic) respirations	Chest falls on inspiration and rises on expiration

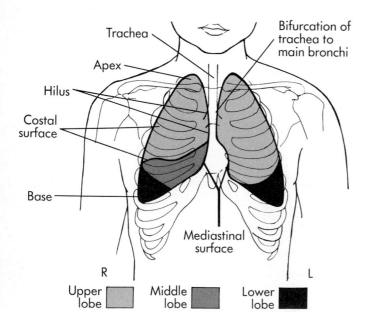

Fig. 1-21. Location of anterior lobes of lungs within thoracic cavity.

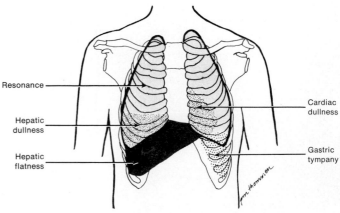

Fig. 1-22. Percussion sounds in thorax.

Usual findings	Comments
Rate expected for age (see inside front cover), regular, effortless, and quiet	Note abnormal rate, irregular rhythm, shallow depth, difficult breathing, or noisy, grunting respirations (Table 1-6)
Moves symmetrically with each breath; posterior base descends 5 to 6 cm (2 to 2.3 inches) during deep inspiration	
Vibrations are symmetric and most intense in thoracic area and least at base	Note asymmetric vibrations or sudden absence or decrease in intensity
	Note abnormal vibrations such as pleural friction rub or crepitation
Lobes are resonant except for (Fig. 1-22)	Note deviation from expected sounds
Dullness at fifth interspace right midclavicular line (liver)	
Dullness from second to fifth interspace over left sternal border to midclavicular line (heart)	
Tympany below left fifth interspace (stomach)	
Vesicular breath sounds	Note deviations from expected breath sounds, particularly if diminished; note absence of sounds
Heard over entire surface of lungs except upper intrascapular area and beneath manubrium	
Inspiration louder, longer, and higher pitched than expiration	Note adventitious sounds
Bronchovesicular breath sounds	
Heard in upper intrascapular area and manubrium	***Crackles***—Discrete noncontinuous crackling sound, heard primarily during inspiration from passage of air through fluid or moisture; if crackles clear with deep breathing, they are not pathologic
Inspiration and expiration almost equal in duration, pitch, and intensity	
Bronchial breath sounds	***Wheezes***—Continuous musical sounds; caused by air passing through narrowed passages, regardless of cause (exudate, inflammation, foreign body, spasm, tumor)
Heard only over trachea near suprasternal notch	
Expiration longer, louder, and of higher pitch than inspiration	***Sibilant wheeze***—Musical noise like a squeak; may be heard during inspiration or expiration; usually louder during expiration; occurs in smaller bronchi and bronchioles
	Sonorous wheeze—May be called rhonchi; loud, low, coarse sound like a snore heard at any point of inspiration or expiration; occurs in trachea or large bronchi; may clear with coughing
	Audible inspiratory wheeze (stridor)—Sonorous, musical wheeze heard without a stethoscope; indicates a high obstruction, e.g., epiglottitis
	Audible expiratory wheeze—Whistling, sighing wheeze heard without a stethoscope; indicates a low obstruction
	Pleural friction rub—Crackling, grating sound during inspiration and expiration; occurs from inflamed pleural surfaces; not affected by coughing
Voice sounds—heard but syllables are indistinct	Consolidation of lung tissue produces three types of abnormal voice sounds:
	Whispered pectoriloquy—The child whispers words and the nurse hears the syllables
	Bronchophony—The child speaks words that are not distinguishable but the vocal resonance is increased in intensity and clarity
	Egophony—The child says "ee," which is heard as the nasal sound "ay" through the stethoscope

Summary of physical assessment of the child—cont'd

Assessment	Procedure
HEART (Fig. 1-23)	General Instructions Begin with inspection, followed by palpation, then auscultation Percussion is not done because it is of limited value in defining the borders or the size of the heart Inspect size with child in semi-Fowler position; observe chest wall from an angle Palpate for point of maximum impulse (PMI) Palpate skin for capillary filling time 　Lightly press skin on central site, such as forehead, and peripheral site, such as top of hand or foot, to produce slight blanching 　Assess time it takes for blanched area to return to original color Auscultate for heart sounds 　Listen with child in sitting and reclining positions 　Use both diaphragm and bell chest pieces 　Evaluate sounds for quality, intensity, rate, and rhythm (Table 1-7) Follow sequence (Fig. 1-24) 　***Aortic area***—Second right intercostal space close to sternum 　***Pulmonic area***—Second left intercostal space close to sternum 　***Erb point***—Second and third left intercostal space close to sternum 　***Tricuspid area***—Fifth right and left intercostal space close to sternum 　***Mitral or apical area***—Fifth intercostal space, left midclavicular line (third to fourth intercostal space and lateral to left midclavicular line in infants)

Table 1-7. VARIOUS PATTERNS OF HEART RATE OR PULSE

Tachycardia	Increased rate
Bradycardia	Decreased rate
Pulsus alternans	Strong beat followed by weak beat
Pulsus bigeminus	Coupled rhythm in which beat is felt in pairs because of premature beat
Pulsus paradoxus	Intensity or force of pulse decreases with inspiration
Sinus arrhythmia	Rate increases with inspiration, decreases with expiration
Water-hammer or Corrigan pulse	Especially forceful beat caused by a very wide pulse pressure (systolic blood pressure minus diastolic blood pressure)
Dicrotic pulse	Double radial pulse for every apical beat
Thready pulse	Rapid, weak pulse that seems to appear and disappear

Fig. 1-23. Position of heart within thorax.

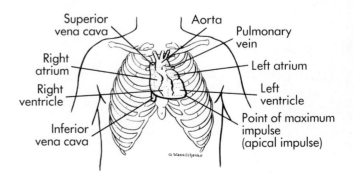

Superior vena cava
Aorta
Pulmonary vein
Right atrium
Left atrium
Right ventricle
Left ventricle
Inferior vena cava
Point of maximum impulse (apical impulse)

G. Wassilchenko

Usual findings	**Comments**

Symmetric chest wall

Apical impulse sometimes apparent (in thin children)

Infant—Fourth to fifth intercostal space and lateral to left sternal border

Child—Fifth intercostal space and left midclavicular line

Capillary refilling immediately or in 1 to 2 seconds

S_1S_2—Clear, distinct, rate equal to radial pulse; rhythm regular and even

Aortic area—S_2 heard louder than S_1

Pulmonic area—Splitting of S_2 heard best (normally widens on inspiration)

Erb point—Frequent site of innocent murmurs

Tricuspid area—S_1 louder sound preceding S_2

Mitral or apical area—S_1 heard loudest; splitting of S_1 may be audible

Quality—Clear and distinct

Intensity—Strong, but not pounding

Rate—Same as radial pulse

Rhythm—Regular and even

Usual findings of innocent murmurs

   Timing within S_1-S_2 cycle—Systolic, that is, they occur with or after S_1

   Quality—Usually of a low-pitched, musical, or groaning quality

   Loudness—Grade III or less in intensity and do not increase over time

   Area best heard—Usually loudest in the pulmonic area with no transmission to other areas of the heart

   Change with position—Audible in the supine position but absent in the sitting position

   Other physical signs—Not associated with any physical signs of cardiac disease

Comments:

Note obvious bulging

Infant's heart is larger in proportion to chest size and lies more centrally

PMI gives indication of size because it is usually located at apex; with cardiac enlargement, apex is displaced lower and more laterally

During palpation may feel abnormal vibrations called *thrills* that are similar to cat's purring; they are produced by blood flowing through narrowed or abnormal opening, such as stenotic valve or septal defect

Refilling taking longer than 3 seconds is abnormal and indicates impaired skin perfusion

To distinguish S_1 from S_2, palpate for carotid pulse, which is synchronous with S_1

A normal arrhythmia is *sinus arrhythmia,* in which heart rate increases with inspiration and decreases with expiration

Identify abnormal sounds; note presence of adventitious sounds such as pericardial friction rubs (similar to pleural friction rubs but not affected by change in respiration)

Record murmurs in relation to
   Area best heard
   Timing within S_1-S_2 cycle
   Change with position
   Loudness and quality

Grading of the intensity of heart murmurs
   I—Very faint, frequently not heard if child sits up
   II—Usually readily heard, slightly louder than grade I, audible in all positions
   III—Loud, but not accompanied by a thrill
   IV—Loud, accompanied by a thrill
   V—Loud enough to be heard with the stethoscope barely on the chest, accompanied by a thrill
   VI—Loud enough to be heard with the stethoscope not touching the chest, often heard with the human ear close to the chest, accompanied by a thrill

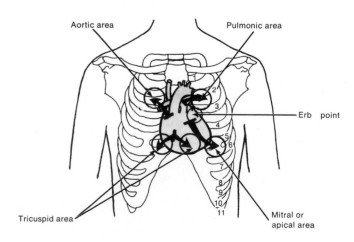

Fig. 1-24. Direction of heart sounds from anatomic valve sites.

Summary of physical assessment of the child—cont'd

Assessment	Procedure
ABDOMEN	**General instructions**
	Inspection, followed by auscultation, percussion, and palpation, which may distort the normal abdominal sounds
	Palpation may be uncomfortable for the child; deep palpation causes a feeling of pressure and superficial palpation causes a tickling sensation
	To minimize any discomfort and encourage cooperation, use the following:
	Position child supine with legs flexed at hips and knees
	Distract child with statements such as "I am going to guess what you ate by feeling your tummy"
	Have child "help" with palpation by placing own hand over examiner's palpating hand
	Have child place own hand on abdomen with fingers spread wide apart and palpate between the fingers
	Inspect contour, size, and tone
	Note condition of skin
	Note movement
	Inspect umbilicus for herniation, fistulas, hygiene, and discharge

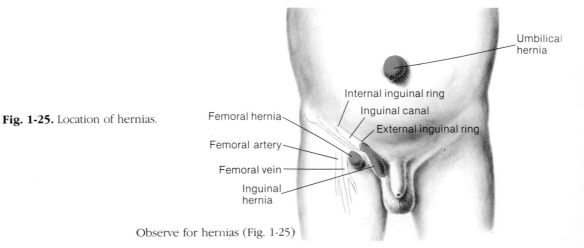

Fig. 1-25. Location of hernias.

Observe for hernias (Fig. 1-25)

    Inguinal—Slide little finger into external inguinal ring at base of scrotum; ask child to cough

    Femoral—Place finger over femoral canal (located by placing index finger over femoral pulse and middle finger against skin toward midline)

Auscultate for bowel sounds and aortic pulsations

Percuss the abdomen

Usual findings	Comments
Infants and young children—Cylindric and prominent in erect position, flat when supine	Contour, size, and tone are good indicators of nutritional status and muscular development
Adolescents—Characteristic adult curves, fairly flat when erect	Note deviations
Circumference decreases in relation to chest size with age	Prominent, flabby
Firm tone; muscular in adolescent males	Concave
	Tense, boardlike
	Loose, wrinkled
	Midline protrusion
	Silvery, whitish striae
	Distended veins
Smooth, uniformly taut	
In children under 7 or 8 years, rises with inspiration and synchronous with chest movement	Paradoxical respirations (chest rises while abdomen falls)
In older children, less respiratory movement	
Visible pulsations in epigastric region from descending aorta sometimes seen in thin children	Visible peristaltic waves
Flat to slight protrusion; no herniation or discharge	If herniation is present, palpate for abdominal contents
	Discuss with parents any "home" remedies used to reduce the herniation; discourage use of any
None	
Bowel sounds—Short metallic tinkling sounds like gurgles, clicks, or growls heard every 10 to 30 seconds	Bowel sounds may be stimulated by stroking abdominal wall with a fingertip
Aortic pulsations—Heard in epigastrium, slightly to left of midline	Note hyperperistalsis or absence of bowel sounds
Tympany over stomach on left side and most of abdomen, except for dullness or flatness just below right costal margin (liver)	Note percussion sounds other than those expected

Unit 1

Summary of physical assessment of the child—cont'd

Assessment	Procedure
ABDOMEN—cont'd	Palpate abdominal organs (Fig. 1-26)

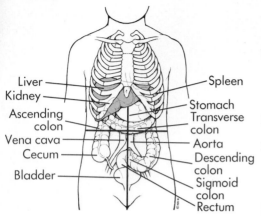

Liver
Kidney
Ascending colon
Vena cava
Cecum
Bladder

Spleen
Stomach
Transverse colon
Aorta
Descending colon
Sigmoid colon
Rectum

Palpate abdominal organs (Fig. 1-26)
  Place one hand flat against back and use palpating hand to "feel" organs between both hands
  Proceed from lower quadrants *upward*

Use imaginary lines at umbilicus to divide the abdomen into quadrants (Fig. 1-26)
  Right upper quadrant (RUQ)
  Right lower quadrant (RLQ)
  Left upper quadrant (LUQ)
  Left lower quadrant (LLQ)
Palpate femoral pulses—Place tips of two or three fingers about midway between iliac crest and pubic symphysis
Elicit abdominal reflex—Scratch skin from side to midline in each quadrant

Fig. 1-26. Location of structures in abdomen.

GENITALIA

Male (Fig. 1-27)

General instructions

Proceed in same manner as examination of other areas; explain procedure and its significance before doing it, such as palpating for testes
Respect privacy at all times
Use opportunity to discuss concerns about sexual development with older child and adolescent
Use opportunity to discuss sexual safety with young children, that this is their private area and if someone touches them in a way that is uncomfortable they should always tell their parent or some other trusted person
If sexually transmitted disease is suspected, wear gloves

Penis
  Inspect size

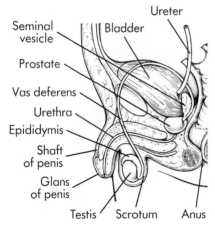

Ureter
Seminal vesicle
Prostate
Vas deferens
Urethra
Epididymis
Shaft of penis
Glans of penis
Bladder

Testis   Scrotum   Anus

Fig. 1-27. Major structures of genitalia in circumcised prepubertal male.

Glans and *shaft*—Inspect for signs of swelling, skin lesion, inflammation

Prepuce—Inspect in uncircumcised male

Urethral meatus—Inspect location and note any discharge

Scrotum—Inspect size, location, skin, and hair distribution

Testes—Palpate each scrotal sac using thumb and index finger

Usual findings	Comments
Liver—1 to 2 cm below right costal margin in infants and young children	Usually not palpable in older children Considered enlarged if 3 cm below costal margin Normally descends with inspiration; should not be considered a sign of enlargement
Spleen—Sometimes 1 to 2 cm below left costal margin in infants and young children	Usually not palpable in older children Considered enlarged if more than 2 cm below left costal margin; also descends with inspiration Other structures that sometimes are palpable include kidneys, bladder, cecum, and sigmoid colon; know their location to avoid mistaking them for abnormal masses
Equal and strong bilaterally	Most common palpable mass is feces
Umbilicus moves toward quadrant that was stroked	In sexually active females, consider a palpable mass in the lower abdomen a pregnant uterus Note absence of femoral pulse Normally may be absent in children under 1 year of age Note asymmetry or absence
	Examination may be anxiety producing for older children and adolescents; may be left to end of physical exam
Generally, size is insignificant in prepubescent male Compare growth to expected sexual development during puberty (see p. 95)	Note large penis, possible sign of precocious puberty In obese child, penis may be obscured by fat pad over pubic symphysis
None	
Easily retracted to expose glans and urethral meatus	In infants, prepuce is tight for several months and should not be retracted Discuss importance of hygiene
Centered at tip of glans No discharge	Note location on ventral or dorsal surface of penis, possible sign of ambiguous genitalia Whenever possible, note strength and direction of urinary stream
May appear large in infants Hangs freely from perineum behind penis One sac hangs lower than other Loose, wrinkled skin, usually redder and coarser in adolescents Compare hair distribution to that expected for pubertal stage; typical mature male pattern forms a diamond shape from umbilicus to anus (see p. 95)	Note scrota that are small, close to perineum, with any degree of midline separation Well-formed rugae indicate descent of testes

Small ovoid bodies about 1.5 to 2 cm long
Double in size during puberty
	Prevent cremasteric reflex by
	  Warming hands
	  Having child sit in tailor fashion
	  Block pathway of ascent by placing thumb and index finger over upper part of scrotal sac along inguinal canal
	Note failure to palpate testes after taking these precautions
	Discuss testicular self-examination with adolescent male

Summary of physical assessment of the child—cont'd

Assessment	Procedure
GENITALIA—cont'd	
Female (Fig. 1-28)	*External genitalia*—Inspect structures; place young child in semireclining position in parent's lap with knees bent and soles of feet in apposition

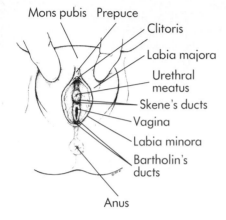

Mons pubis Prepuce
Clitoris
Labia majora
Urethral meatus
Skene's ducts
Vagina
Labia minora
Bartholin's ducts
Anus

Labia—Palpate for any masses

Urethral meatus—Inspect for location; identified as V-shaped slit by wiping downward from clitoris to perineum

Skene glands—Palpate or inspect

Vaginal orifice—Internal examination usually not performed; inspect for obvious opening

Bartholin glands—Palpate or inspect

Fig. 1-28. External structures of genitalia in prepubertal female. Labia are spread to reveal deep structures.

ANUS

Anal area—Inspect for general firmness, condition of skin

Anal reflex—Elicit by pricking or scratching perianal area gently

BACK AND EXTREMITIES

Inspect curvature and symmetry of spine

Test for scoliosis:
  Have child stand erect; observe from behind and note asymmetry of shoulders and hips
  Have child bend forward at the waist until back is parallel to floor; observe from side and note asymmetry or prominence of rib cage
Note mobility of spine

Inspect each extremity joint for symmetry, size, temperature, color, tenderness, mobility
Test for dislocated hip (p. 15)

Assess shape of bones:
  Measure distance between the knees when child stands with malleoli in apposition
  Measure distance between the malleoli when the child stands with knees together

Inspect position of feet; test if foot deformity at birth is result of fetal position or development by scratching outer, then inner, side of sole, if self-correctable, foot assumes right angle to leg
Inspect gait
  Have child walk in straight line
  Estimate angle of gait by drawing imaginary line through center of foot and line of progression (Fig. 1-29)

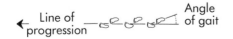

← Line of progression   Angle of gait

Fig. 1-29. Measurement of angle of gait.

Usual findings	Comments
Mons pubis—Fat pad over symphysis pubis; covered with hair in adolescence; usual hair distribution is inverted triangle (see p. 97)	
Clitoris—Located at anterior end of labia minora; covered by small flap of skin (prepuce)	Note evidence of enlargement (may be small phallus)
Labia majora—Two thick folds of skin from mons to posterior commissure; inner surface pink and moist	Note any palpable masses (may be testes), evidence of fusion, or enlargement
Labia minora—Two folds of skin interior to labia majora, usually invisible until puberty; prominent in newborn	
Located posterior to clitoris and anterior to vagina	Note opening from clitoris or inside vagina
Surround meatus; no lesions	Common sites of cysts and venereal warts (condylomata acuminata)
Located posterior to urethral meatus; may be covered by crescent-shaped or circular membrane (*hymen*); discharge usually clear or whitish	Note excessive, foul-smelling discharge
Surround vaginal opening, no lesions, secrete clear mucoid fluid	
Buttocks—Firm, gluteal folds symmetric	Note evidence of diaper rash; inquire about hygiene
	Note
Quick contraction of external anal sphincter; no protrusion of rectum	Fissures
	Polyps
	Rectal prolapse
	Warts
Rounded or C-shaped in the newborn	Note any abnormal curvatures and presence of masses or lesions
Cervical secondary curve forms about 3 months of age	Other signs of scoliosis include
Lumbar secondary curve forms about 12 to 18 months, resulting in typical double-S curve	Slight limp
	Crooked hem or waistline
Lordosis normal in young children but decreases with age	Complaint of backache
Shoulders, scapula, and iliac crests symmetric	
Flexible, full range of motion, no pain or stiffness	Note stiffness and pain upon movement of neck or back; requires immediate evaluation
Symmetric length	Note any deviations
Equal size	Note warmth, swelling, tenderness, and immobility of joints
Correct number of digits	
Nails pink (see assessment of skin, p. 30)	
Temperature equal, although feet may be cooler than hands	
Full range of motion	
Less than 5 cm (2 inches) in children over 2 years of age	Greater distance indicates *genu varum* (bowlegs) (Fig. 1-30)
Less than 7.5 cm (3 inches) in children over 7 years of age	Greater distance indicates *genu valgum* (knock-knees) (Fig. 1-31)
Held at right angle to leg; point straight ahead or turned slightly outward when standing	Note foot and ankle deformities (Table 1-8)
Fat pads on sole give appearance of flat feet; arch develops after child is walking	
"Toddling" or broad-base gait normal in young children; gradually assumes graceful gait with feet close together	Note abnormal gait
	Waddling
Feet turn outward less than 30° and inward less than 10°	Scissor
	Toeing-in
	Broad-based in older children

Summary of physical assessment of the child—cont'd

Assessment	Procedure

BACK AND EXTREMITIES—cont'd	***Plantar reflex***—Elicit reflex by stroking lateral sole from heel upward to little toe across to hallux
	Inspect development and tone of muscles
	
	Test strength:
	    Arms—Have child raise arms while applying counterpressure with your hands
	    Legs—Have child sit with legs dangling; proceed as with arms
	    Hands—Have child squeeze your fingers as tightly as he can
	    Feet—Have child plantar flex (push sole toward floor) while applying counterpressure to the soles

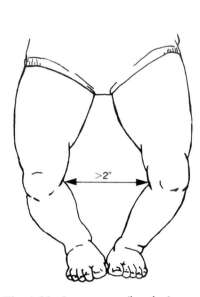

Fig. 1-30. Genu varum (bowleg).

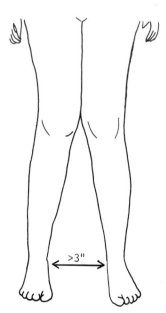

Fig. 1-31. Genu valgum (knock-knee).

Assessment	Procedure
NEUROLOGIC ASSESSMENT **Mental status**	Observe behavior, mood, affect, general orientation to surroundings, level of consciousness

Motor functioning	Test muscle strength, tone, and development (p. 113)
	Test cerebellar functioning:
	
	    Finger-to-nose test—With the child's arm extended, have touch nose with the index finger
	
	    Heel-to-shin test—With child standing, have run the heel of one foot down the shin of the other leg
	
	    Romberg test—Have child stand erect with feet together and eyes closed
	Have child touch tip of each finger with thumb in rapid succession
	Have child pat leg with first one side, then the other side of hand in rapid sequence
	Have child tap your hand with ball of foot as quickly as possible

Usual findings	Comments
Flexion of toes in children above 1 year	Babinski reflex seen in younger children (p. 16)
Symmetric Increase in tone during muscle contraction Equal bilaterally	Note atrophy, hypertrophy, spasticity, flaccidity, rigidity, or weakness

Table 1-8. TYPES OF FOOT AND ANKLE DEFORMITIES

Pes planus (flatfoot)—Normal finding in infancy; may be result of muscular weakness in older child

Pes valgus—Eversion of entire foot but sole rests on ground

Pes varus—Inversion of entire foot but sole rests on ground

Metatarsus valgus—Eversion of forefoot while heel remains straight. Also called toeing out or duck walk

Talipes valgus—Eversion (turning outward) of foot so that only inner side of foot rests on ground

Talipes varus—Inversion (turning inward) of foot so that only outer sole of food rests on ground

Talipes equinus—Extension or plantar flexion of foot so that only ball and toes rest on ground; commonly combined with talipes varus (most common of clubfoot deformities)

Talipes calcaneus—Dorsal flexion of foot so that only heel rests on ground

	Subjective impressions are based on observation throughout the examination Objective findings can be attained through developmental testing such as DDST
Performs each test successfully with eyes opened and closed	May be difficult to test in children younger than preschool age Note any awkwardness or lack of coordination in performance
Romberg test—Does not lean to side or fall	Falling or leaning to one side is abnormal and is called the _Romberg sign_

Unit 1

Summary of physical assessment of the child—cont'd

Assessment	Procedure
Sensory functioning	Test vision and hearing (pp. 124-132)
	Sensory intactness—Touch skin lightly with a pin and have child point to stimulated area while keeping eyes closed
	Sensory discrimination: Touch skin with pin and cotton; have child describe it as sharp or dull Touch skin with cold and warm object (such as metal and rubber heads of reflex hammer); have child differentiate between temperatures Using two pins, touch skin simultaneously with both or only one pin; have child discriminate when one or two pins are used
Reflexes (deep tendon)	*Biceps* Hold the child's arm by placing the partially flexed elbow in your hand with the thumb over the antecubital space; strike your thumbnail with the hammer
	Triceps Bend the arm at the elbow and rest the palm in your hand; strike the triceps tendon Alternate procedure—If the child is supine rest arm over chest and strike the triceps tendon
	Brachioradialis Rest the forearm on the lap or abdomen, with the arm flexed at the elbow and palm down; strike the radius about 1 inch (depending on child's size) above the wrist
	Knee jerk or patellar reflex Sit the child on the edge of the examining table or on parent's lap with the lower legs flexed at the knee and dangling freely; tap the patellar tendon just below the knee cap
	Achilles Use the same position as for the knee jerk; support the foot lightly in your hand and strike the Achilles tendon
	Ankle clonus—See p. 16
	Kernig sign Flex child's leg at hip and knee while supine; note pain or resistance
	Brudzinski sign With child supine, flex the head; note pain and involuntary flexion of hip and knees
Cranial nerves	See Assessment of cranial nerves, p. 56

Usual findings	Comments
Localizes pinprick	Use sterile pin or other sharp object (toothpick), being careful not to puncture skin
	Compare sensation in symmetric areas at both distal and proximal points
Able to distinguish types of sensation and temperature	Note difficulty in performing test, especially in older child
Minimal distance for discrimination on finger is about 2 to 3 mm	
Biceps—Partial flexion of forearm	Use reinforcement techniques to increase reflex activity:
	For upper extremity reflexes—ask child to clench teeth or to squeeze thigh with the hand on the side not tested
Triceps—Partial extension of forearm	For lower extremity reflexes—have child lock fingers and pull one hand against the other or grip hands together
	Usual grading of reflexes
	Grade 0 0 Absent
	Grade 1 + Diminished
	Grade 2 + + Normal
	Grade 3 + + + Brisker than normal
	Grade 4 + + + + Hyperactive (clonus)
	Note asymmetric, absent, diminished, or hyperactive reflexes
Brachioradialis—Flexion of the forearm and supination (turning upward) of the palm	
Patellar—Partial extension of lower leg	
Achilles—Plantar flexion of foot (foot pointing downward)	
Ankle clonus—Absence of beats	
Kernig—Absence of pain or resistance	These special reflexes are elicited when meningeal irritation is suspected
Brudzinski—Absence of pain or associated movements	Positive signs require immediate referral
	Testing of cranial nerves may be done as part of the neurologic examination or integrated into assessment of each system, such as cranial nerves II, III, IV, and VI with the eye
	Cranial nerves can usually be tested in children of preschool age and older
	Note inability to perform any of the items correctly

Assessment of cranial nerves

Cranial nerve	Distribution/Function	Test
I—Olfactory (S)*	Olfactory mucosa of nasal cavity	With eyes closed, have child identify odors such as coffee, alcohol from a swab, or other smells; test each nostril separately
II—Optic (S)	Rods and cones of retina, optic nerve	Check for perception of light, visual acuity, peripheral vision, color vision, and normal optic disc

III—Oculomotor (M)*	Extraocular muscles (EOM) of eye:
	    Superior rectus (SR)—Moves eyeball up and in
	    Inferior rectus (IR)—Moves eyeball down and in
	    Medial rectus (MR)—Moves eyeball nasally
	    Inferior oblique (IO)—Moves eyeball up and out
		Have child follow an object (toy) or light in the six cardinal positions of gaze (Fig. 1-32)

	Pupil constriction and accommodation	Perform PERRLA (see p. 35)
	Eyelid closing	Check for proper placement of lid (see p. 35)
IV—Trochlear (M)	Superior oblique muscle (SO)—Moves eye down and out	Have child look down and in (see Fig. 1-32)
V—Trigeminal (M, S)	Muscles of mastication	Have child bite down hard and open jaw; test symmetry and strength
	Sensory: face, scalp, nasal and buccal mucosa	With child's eyes closed, see if child can detect light touch in the mandibular and maxillary regions
		Test corneal and blink reflex by touching cornea lightly (approach child from the side so that child does not blink before cornea is touched)
VI—Abducens (M)	Lateral rectus (LR) muscle—Moves eye temporally	Have child look toward temporal side (see Fig. 1-32)
VII—Facial (M, S)	Muscles for facial expression	Have child smile, make funny face, or show teeth to see symmetry of expression
	Anterior two thirds of tongue (sensory)	Have child identify a sweet or salty solution; place each taste on anterior section and sides of protruding tongue; if child retracts tongue, solution will dissolve toward posterior part of tongue
	Nasal cavity and lacrimal gland, sublingual and submandibular salivary glands	Not tested
VIII—Auditory, acoustic, or vestibulocochlear (S)	Internal ear	Test hearing; note any loss of equilibrium or presence of vertigo

*S—sensory; M—motor.

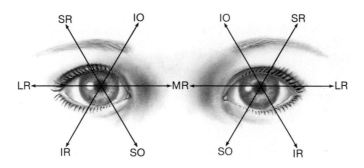

Fig. 1-32. Testing cardinal positions of gaze.

Cranial nerve	Distribution/Function	Test
IX—Glossopharyngeal (M, S)	Pharynx, tongue	Stimulate the posterior pharynx with a tongue blade; the child should gag
	Posterior one third of tongue (sensory)	Test sense of sour or bitter taste on posterior segment of tongue
X—Vagus (M, S)	Muscles of larynx, pharynx, some organs of gastrointestinal system, sensory fibers of root of tongue, heart, lung, and some organs of gastrointestinal system	Note hoarseness of the voice, gag reflex, and ability to swallow
		Check that uvula is in midline; when stimulated with a tongue blade, should deviate upward and to the stimulated side
XI—Accessory (M)	Sternocleidomastoid and trapezius muscles of shoulder	Have child shrug shoulders while applying mild pressure; with the hands placed on shoulders, have child turn head against opposing pressure on either side; note symmetry and strength
XII—Hypoglossal (M)	Muscles of tongue	Have child move tongue in all directions; have child protrude the tongue as far as possible; note any midline deviation
		Test strength by placing tongue blade on one side of tongue and having child move it away

FAMILY ASSESSMENT

Family assessment involves the collection of data about:

Family structure—The composition of the family—who lives in the home—and those social, cultural, religious, and economic characteristics that influence the child's and family's overall psychobiologic health; and

Family function—How the family behaves toward one another, the roles family members assume, and the quality of their relationships.

In its broadest sense the family refers to all those individuals who are significant to the nuclear unit, including relatives, friends, and other social groups, such as the school and church. The more common method of eliciting information on family structure and function is by interviewing family members. However, several family assessment tools can be used to collect and record graphically data about family composition, environment, and relationships. These tools include screening questionnaires and diagrams.

Theoretic framework

Family systems theory—The family is viewed as part of an open social system in that the family continually interacts with itself and the environment.

Key features include:

Ability of the family system to adapt

Change in any member causes a reciprocal change in other members ("ripple" effect)

No family member is identified as the "problem"; the problem lies in the type of interactions engaged in by the family

Change can occur at any point in the family system

Indications for comprehensive family assessment

Children receiving comprehensive well-child care

Children experiencing major stressful life events, such as chronic illness, disability, parental divorce, foster care, or death of a family member

Children requiring extensive home care

Children with developmental delays

Children with repeated accidental injuries and those with suspected child abuse

Children with behavioral or physical problems that suggest family dysfunction as the etiology

Family assessment interview

General guidelines for the family interview

Schedule the interview with the family at a time that is most convenient for all parties; include as many family members as possible; clearly state the purpose of the interview

Begin the interview by asking each person's name and their relationship to each other

Restate the purpose of the interview and the objective

Keep the initial conversation general to put members at ease and to learn the "big picture" of the family

Identify major concerns and reflect these back to the family

Restate the identified needs to be certain that all parties perceive the same message

Terminate the interview with a summary of what was discussed and a plan for additional sessions if needed

Assessment areas

Family composition

Immediate members of the household (names, ages, and relationships)

Significant extended family members

Previous marriages, separations, death of spouses, or divorces

Home and community environment

Type of dwelling

Number of rooms/occupants

Sleeping arrangements

Number of floors, accessibility of stairs, elevators

Adequacy of utilities

Safety features (fire escape, smoke detector, guardrails on windows, use of car restraint)

Environmental hazards (chipped paint, poor sanitation, pollution, heavy street traffic, and so on)

Availability and location of health facilities, schools, play areas

Relationship with neighbors

Recent crises or changes in home

Child's reaction/adjustment to recent stresses

Occupation and education of family members

Types of employment
Work schedules
Work satisfaction
Exposure to environmental/industrial hazards

Sources of income
Adequacy of income
Effect of illness on financial status
Highest degree or grade level attained

Cultural and religious traditions

Religious beliefs and practices
Cultural/ethnic beliefs and practices
Language spoken in home
Assessment questions include:
   Does the family identify with a particular religious/ethnic group?
   How is religion/ethnic background a part of the family's life?
   What religious/ethnic beliefs influence the family's perceptions of illness and its treatment?

What special religious/cultural traditions are practiced in the home (for example, food choices and preparation)?
Where were family members born and how long have they lived in this country?
Does the family rely on religious/cultural healers or remedies?
What language does the family speak most frequently?

Family interactions and roles

Refers to ways family members relate to each other
Chief concern is amount of intimacy and closeness among the members, especially spouses
Role refers to behaviors of people as they assume a different status or position
Involves general observations about
   Family members' responses to each other (cordial, hostile, cool, loving, patient, short-tempered)
   Obvious roles of leadership versus submission
   Support and attention shown to various members

Assessment questions include:
   What activities do the family perform together?
   Whom do family members talk to when something is bothering them?
   What are members' household chores?
   Who usually oversees what is happening with the children, such as at school or concerning their health?
   How easy or difficult is it for the family to change or accept new responsibilities for household tasks?

Power, decision making, and problem solving

Power refers to individual member's control over others in family; manifest through family decision making and problem solving
Chief concern is clarity of boundaries of power between parents and children
One method of assessment involves offering a hypothetical conflict or problem, such as a child with failing school grades, and asking family how they would handle this situation

Assessment questions include:
   Who usually makes the decisions in the family?
   If one parent makes a decision, can child appeal to other parent to change it?
   What input do children have in making decisions or discussing rules?
   Who makes and enforces the rules?
   What happens when a rule is broken?

Communication

Concerned with clarity and directness of communication patterns
Assessment involves observing:
   Who speaks to whom
   If one person speaks for another or interrupts
   If members appear disinterested when certain individuals speak
   If there is agreement between verbal and nonverbal messages

Further assessment includes periodically asking family members if they understood what was just said and to repeat the message
Assessment questions include:
   How often do family members wait until others are through talking before "having their say"?
   Do parents or older siblings tend to lecture and preach?
   Do parents tend to talk "down" to the children?

Expression of feelings and individuality

Concerned with personal space and freedom to grow with limits and structure needed for guidance
Observing patterns of communication offers clues to how freely feelings are expressed
Assessment questions include:
   Is it OK for family members to get angry or sad in the home?

Who gets angry most of the time? What do they do?
If someone is upset, how do other family members try to comfort him/her?
Who comforts specific family members?
When someone wants to do something new, such as try out for a new sport or get a job, what is family's response (offer assistance, discouragement, or no advice)?

Unit 1

Family assessment questionnaires
General guidelines for administration

Be familiar with the questionnaire, especially training requirement, complexity of questions, and expected length of time for completion

Explain to the family why the questionnaire is being administered and how the information will be used

Discuss the results with the family

Use the responses to help the family clarify and define what they perceive as a concern or need

Restate the needs to be certain that all parties perceive the same message

Family APGAR (Smilkstein, 1978)

Brief screening questionnaire designed to reflect a family member's satisfaction with the functional state of the family to record members of household (Fig. 1-33)

Acronym APGAR is for Adaptability, Partnership, Growth, Affection, and Resolve (commitment) (see box below)

Can be used with nuclear families, as well as families with alternative life-styles

Requires about 5 minutes to complete

Training to administer the Family APGAR is not required

Scoring: One of three choices are scored as follows: "Almost always"—2; "Some of the time"—1; "Hardly ever"—0. Scores for the five statements are totaled. Scores of 7 to 10 suggest a highly functional family; 4 to 6, a moderately dysfunctional family; 0 to 3 a severely dysfunctional family.

FAMILY APGAR

Definition	Functions measured by the Family APGAR	Relevant open-ended questions*
Adaptation is the use of intrafamilial and extrafamilial resources for problem solving when family equilibrium is stressed during a crisis.	How resources are shared, or the degree to which a member is satisfied with the assistance received when family resources are needed.	How have family members aided each other in time of need? In what way have family members received help or assistance from friends and community agencies?
Partnership is the sharing of decision making and nurturing responsibilities by family members.	How decisions are shared, or the member's satisfaction with mutuality in family communication and problem solving.	How do family members communicate with each other about such matters as vacations, finances, medical care, large purchases, and personal problems?
Growth is the physical and emotional maturation and self-fulfillment that is achieved by family members through mutual support and guidance.	How nurturing is shared, or the member's satisfaction with the freedom available within the family to change roles and attain physical and emotional growth or maturation.	How have family members changed during the past years? How has this change been accepted by family members? In what ways have family members aided each other in growing or developing independent life-styles? How have family members reacted to your desires for change?
Affection is the caring or loving relationship that exists among family members.	How emotional experiences are shared, or the member's satisfaction with the intimacy and emotional interaction that exists in the family.	How have members of your family responded to emotional expressions such as affection, love, sorrow, or anger?
Resolve is the commitment to devote time to other members of the family for physical and emotional nurturing. It also usually involves a decision to share wealth and space.	How time (and space and money) is shared, or the member's satisfaction with the time commitment that has been made to the family by its members.	How do members of your family share time, space, and money?

Modified from Smilkstein G: The Family APGAR: a proposal for a family function test and its use by physicians, J Fam Pract 6(6):1231-1239, 1978.

*Suggested questions to be used with Family APGAR form.

Feetham Family Functioning Survey* (Feetham and Humenick, 1982; Roberts and Feetham, 1982)

Provides information about family members' *perception* of relationships that contribute to or are affected by family functioning

Consists of questions relating to (1) relationships between the family and individuals, (2) relationships between the family and subsystems, such as housework and division of labor, and (3) relationships between the family and broader social units; 27 questions specifically address family functioning in terms of household tasks, child care, sexual and marital relationship, interaction with family, children, and friends, community involvement, and sources of emotional support

Developed as research instrument; for clinical use the items should not be scored to determine a family's functional state but to identify areas that may be of concern

Questions are answered on a 7-point scale that rates "what is," "what should be," and "how important it is" (box); discrepancy between the first two ratings, together with degree of importance, contributes to clinical assessment of the family members' perceptions of those family functions included in the survey

Requires less than 10 minutes to complete, but persons with less than high school education may have some difficulty with format

Training to administer the Survey is not required provided the user has general knowledge of administering measurement instruments; instructions for administration for research and clinical use purposes are included with the Survey forms

*The Survey is available for a fee from Suzanne Feetham, PhD., RN, FAAN, Director of Education and Research for Nursing and Operations, Children's Hospital National Medical Center, 111 Michigan Ave., NW, Washington, DC 20010 or call 202-939-4980.

SAMPLE QUESTIONS FROM THE FEETHAM FAMILY FUNCTIONING SURVEY

1. The amount of talk with your *friends* regarding your concerns and problems.

   (15) a. How much is there now?

   LITTLE   MUCH
   1   2   3   4   5   6   7

   (16) b. How much should there be?

   LITTLE   MUCH
   1   2   3   4   5   6   7

   (17) c. How important is this to me?

   LITTLE   MUCH
   1   2   3   4   5   6   7

2. The amount of talk with your *relatives* (do not include your spouse) regarding your concerns and problems.

   (18) a. How much is there now?

   LITTLE   MUCH
   1   2   3   4   5   6   7

   (19) b. How much should there be?

   LITTLE   MUCH
   1   2   3   4   5   6   7

   (20) c. How important is this to me?

   LITTLE   MUCH
   1   2   3   4   5   6   7

Reproduced with the permission of Suzanne L. Feetham, PhD, RN, FAAN, Children's Hospital National Medical Center, Washington, DC. Developed from research funded by Division of Nursing, HRA, HHS, NU00632, Wayne State University, Detroit, MI, 1977–1980.

Parent Perception Inventory (PPI)† (Hymovich, 1989)

Designed for use with families of children who have long-term disabilities or chronic illness; a modified form, Parent Perception Inventory-Modified (PPI-M) is available for use with families of healthy children

Consists of the following six instruments: concerns, beliefs and feelings, coping, general information, siblings, and spouse concerns and coping; the entire Inventory or selected scales can be administered

Length of time to complete the entire Inventory is approximately 30 to 45 minutes

Developed as a research instrument but can be used to identify areas that may be of concern to the family

Training to administer the Inventory is not required

†The Inventory is available for a fee from Debra P. Hymovich, PhD, RN, FAAN, 929 Longview Road, King of Prussia, PA 19406 or call 215-525-4289.

Unit 1

Family APGAR questionnaire

PART I

The following questions have been designed to help us better understand you and your family. You should feel free to ask questions about any item in the questionnaire.

The space for comments should be used when you wish to give additional information or if you wish to discuss the way the question is applied to your family. Please try to answer all questions.

Family is defined as the individual(s) with whom you usually live. If you live alone, your "family" consists of persons with whom you now have the strongest emotional ties.*

For each question, check only one box

	Almost always	Some of the time	Hardly ever
I am satisfied that I can turn to my family for help when something is troubling me. Comments: _____	☐	☐	☐
I am satisfied with the way my family talks over things with me and shares problems with me. Comments: _____	☐	☐	☐
I am satisfied that my family accepts and supports my wishes to take on new activities or directions. Comments: _____	☐	☐	☐
I am satisfied with the way my family expresses affection and responds to my emotions, such as anger, sorrow, and love. Comments: _____	☐	☐	☐
I am satisfied with the way my family and I share time together. Comments:	☐	☐	☐

*According to which member of the family is being interviewed the interviewer may substitute for the word 'family' either spouse, significant other, parents, or children.

Fig. 1-33. Family APGAR questionnaire. (Modified from Smilkstein G: The Family APGAR: A proposal for a family function test and its use by physicians, J Fam Pract 6(6):1231-1239, 1978. May be photocopied for clinical use.)

Family APGAR questionnaire

PART II

Who lives in your home?* List by relationship (eg, spouse, significant other,** child, or friend).

Please check below the column that best describes how you now get along with each member of the family listed.

Relationship	Age	Sex	Well	Fairly	Poorly
_____	__	__	☐	☐	☐
_____	__	__	☐	☐	☐
_____	__	__	☐	☐	☐
_____	__	__	☐	☐	☐
_____	__	__	☐	☐	☐
_____	__	__	☐	☐	☐

If you don't live with your own family, please list below the individuals to whom you turn for help most frequently. List by relationship, (eg, family member, friend, associate at work, or neighbor).

Please check below the column that best describes how you now get along with each person listed.

Relationship	Age	Sex	Well	Fairly	Poorly
_____	__	__	☐	☐	☐
_____	__	__	☐	☐	☐
_____	__	__	☐	☐	☐
_____	__	__	☐	☐	☐
_____	__	__	☐	☐	☐
_____	__	__	☐	☐	☐

*If you have established your own family, consider home to be the place where you live with your spouse, children, or significant other; otherwise, consider home as your place of origin, eg, the place where your parents or those who raise you live.
***"Significant other" is the partner you live with in a physically and emotionally nurturing relationship, but to whom you are not married.

Fig. 1-33, cont'd.

Unit 1

Home Observation and Measurement of the Environment (HOME)* (Caldwell and Bradley, 1984)

Used to assess child's home environment and interactions with family members

Includes three separate forms for children ages birth to 3 years, 3 to 6 years, and 6 to 10 (Fig. 1-34); forms are also available for children with moderate to severe disabilities in each of the three age groups and for each of the following conditions: visual, auditory, orthopedic, and cognitive impairments

Requires semi-structured interview and direct observation of child and parent in the home

Requires approximately 1 hour to administer

All items are scored in binary (yes-no) fashion; scoring is based on total number of yes answers and compared to percentile scores for ages birth to 6 years (percentile scores are not available for children ages 6 to 10 years or for children with disabilities)

Training to administer the HOME is not required; with careful study and knowledge of child development and family dynamics, the manual serves as an instructional guide, although establishing reliability with a person trained in the use of the HOME is recommended

*An Administration Manual is available for a fee from the Center for Research on Teaching and Learning, College of Education, University of Arkansas at Little Rock, 2801 S. University Avenue, Little Rock, AK 72204 or call (501)569-3422.

Home Screening Questionnaire (HSQ)† (Frankenburg and Coons, 1986)

Used to assess child's home environment

Includes two separate forms for children ages birth to 3 years and 3 to 6 years (Fig. 1-35, A and B)

Completed by parent in any setting

Requires about 15 to 20 minutes for completion

Scoring is based on credits for different answers; for each age group there is a minimal score for determining suspect or nonsuspect results

Training to administer the HSQ is suggested but not required

†The forms and manual are available for a fee from Denver Developmental Materials, Inc., P.O. Box 6919, Denver, CO 80206-0919 or call (303)355-4729.

Family resource questionnaires‡ (Dunst, Trivette, and Deal, 1988)

Several scales are available to measure the adequacy of different resources in households with children, parents' needs for different types of help and assistance, and the helpfulness of sources of support to families with young children

‡A packet of family resource scales and family functioning scales are reprinted in the text by Dunst, Trivette, and Deal or may be purchased for a fee from Brookline Books, Inc., P.O. Box 1046, Cambridge, MA 02238-1046 or call (617)868-0360.

Infant/Toddler HOME Inventory

Bettye M. Caldwell and Robert H. Bradley

Family Name _____ Visitor _____ Date _____

Address _____ Phone _____

Child's Name _____ Birthdate _____ Age _____ Sex _____

Parent Present _____ If other than parent, relationship to child _____

Family Composition _____
(persons living in household, including sex and age of children)

Family Ethnicity _____ Language Spoken _____ Maternal Education _____ Paternal Education _____

Is Mother Employed? _____ Type of work when employed _____ Is Father Employed? _____ Type of work when employed _____

Current child care arrangements _____

Summarize past year's arrangement _____

Other persons present during visit _____

Comments: _____

_____

A

SUMMARY

Subscale		Score Fourth	Lowest Half	Middle Fourth	Upper
I.	RESPONSIVITY		0 - 6	7 - 9	10 - 11
II.	ACCEPTANCE		0 - 4	5 - 6	7 - 8
III.	ORGANIZATION		0 - 3	4 - 5	6
IV.	LEARNING MATERIALS		0 - 4	5 - 7	8 - 9
V.	INVOLVEMENT		0 - 2	3 - 4	5 - 6
VI.	VARIETY		0 - 1	2 - 3	4 - 5
	TOTAL SCORE		0 - 25	26 - 36	37 - 45

Fig. 1-34. Home Inventory Questionnaires. **A,** For families of infants and toddlers. (From Caldwell B and Bradley R: Manual of Home Observation for Measurement of the Environment, revised edition. University of Arkansas at Little Rock, 1984.)

Infant/Toddler HOME

Place a plus (+) or minus (-) in the box alongside each item if the behavior is observed during the visit or if the parent reports that the conditions or events are characteristic of the home invironment. Enter the subtotal and the total on the front side of the Record Sheet.

I. RESPONSITIVITY	24. Child has a special place for toys and treasures.
1. Parent spontaneously vocalizes to child at least twice.	25. Child's play environment is safe.
2. Parent responds verbally to child's vocalizations or verbalizations.	**IV. LEARNING MATERIALS**
3. Parent tells child name of object or person during visit.	26. Muscle activity toys or equipment.
4. Parent's speech is distinct, clear and audible.	27. Push or pull toy.
5. Parent initiates verbal interchanges with Visitor.	28. Stroller or walker, kiddie car, scooter, or tricycle.
6. Parent converses freely and easily.	29. Parent provides toys for child to play with during visit.
7. Parent permits child to engage in "messy" play.	30. Cuddly toy or role-playing toys.
8. Parent spontaneously praises child at least twice.	31. Learning facilitators—mobile, table and chair, high chair, play pen.
9. Parent's voice conveys positive feelings toward child.	32. Simple eye-hand coordination toys.
10. Parent caresses or kisses child at least once.	33. Complex eye-hand coordination toys.
11. Parent responds positively to praise of child offered by Visitor.	34. Toys for literature and music.
II. ACCEPTANCE	**V. INVOLVEMENT**
12. Parent does not shout at child.	35. Parent keeps child in visual range, looks at often.
13. Parent does not express overt annoyance with or hostility to child.	36. Parent talks to child while doing household work.
14. Parent neither slaps nor spanks child during visit.	37. Parent conciously encourages developmental advance.
15. No more than 1 instance of physical punishment during past week.	38. Parent invests maturing toys with value via personal attention.
16. Parent does not scold or criticize child during visit.	39. Parent structures child's play periods.
17. Parent does not interfere with or restrict child 3 times during visit.	40. Parent provides toys that challenge child to develop new skills.
18. At least 10 books are present and visible.	**VI. VARIETY**
19. Family has a pet.	41. Father provides some care daily.
III. ORGANIZATION	42. Parent reads stories to child at least 3 times weekly.
20. Child care, if used, is provided by one of three regular substitutes.	43. Child eats at least one meal a day with mother and father.
21. Child is taken to grocery store at least once a week.	44. Family visits relatives or receives visits once month or so.
22. Child gets out of house at least 4 times a week.	45. Child has 3 or more books of his/her own.

23. Child is taken regularly to doctor's office or clinic.	**I**	**II**	**III**	**IV**	**V**	**VI**	**TOTAL**
TOTALS							

Fig. 1-34, cont'd. A, For families of infants and toddlers.

HOME Inventory for Families of Preschoolers (Three to Six)

Bettye M. Caldwell and Robert H. Bradley

Family Name _____ Date _____ Visitor _____

Child's Name _____ Birthdate _____ Age _____ Sex _____

Caregiver for visit _____ Relationship to child _____

Family Composition _____
(persons living in household, including sex and age of children)

Family Ethnicity _____ Language Spoken _____ Maternal Education _____ Paternal Education _____

Is Mother Employed? _____ Type of work when employed _____ Is Father Employed? _____ Type of work when employed _____

Address _____ Phone _____

Current child care arrangements _____

Summarize past year's arrangement _____

Caregiver for visit _____ Other persons present _____

B

SUMMARY

Subscale	Score	Percentile Range		
		Lowest Fourth	Middle Half	Upper Fourth
I. LEARNING STIMULATION		0 - 2	3 - 9	10 - 11
II. LANGUAGE STIMULATION		0 - 4	5 - 6	7
III. PHYSICAL ENVIRONMENT		0 - 3	4 - 6	7
IV. WARMTH AND AFFECTION		0 - 3	4 - 5	6 - 7
V. ACADEMIC STIMULATION		0 - 2	3 - 4	5
VI. MODELING		0 - 1	2 - 3	4 - 5
VII. VARIETY IN EXPERIENCE		0 - 4	5 - 7	8 - 9
VIII. ACCEPTANCE		0 - 2	3	4
TOTAL SCORE		0 - 29	30 - 45	46 - 55

For rapid profiling of a family, place an X in the box that corresponds to the raw score.

Fig. 1-34, cont'd. Home Inventory Questionnaire **B,** For families of preschoolers.

HOME Inventory (Preschool)

Place a plus (+) or minus (-) in the box alongside each item if the behavior is observed during the visit or if the parent reports that the conditions or events are characteristic of the home invironment. Enter the subtotals and the total on the front side of the Record Sheet.

I. LEARNING STIMULATION

1. Child has toys which teach color, size, shape.
2. Child has three or more puzzles.
3. Child has record player and at least five children's records.
4. Child has toys permitting free expression.
5. Child has toys or games requiring refined movements.
6. Child has toys or games which help teach numbers.
7. Child has at least 10 children's books.
8. At least 10 books are visible in the apartment.
9. Family buys and reads a daily newspaper.
10. Family subscribes to at least one magazine.
11. Child is encouraged to learn shapes.

Subtotal

II. LANGUAGE STIMULATION

12. Child has toys that help teach the names of animals.
13. Child is encouraged to learn the alphabet.
14. Parent teaches child simple verbal manners (please, thank you).
15. Mother uses correct grammar and pronunciation.
16. Parent encourages child to talk and takes time to listen.
17. Parent's voice conveys positive feeling to child.
18. Child is permitted choice in breakfast or lunch menu.

Subtotal

III. PHYSICAL ENVIRONMENT

19. Building appears safe.
20. Outside play environment appears safe.
21. Interior of apartment not dark or perceptually monotonous.
22. Neighborhood is esthetically pleasing.

23. House has 100 square feet of living space per person.
24. Rooms are not overcrowded with furniture.
25. House is reasonably clean and minimally cluttered.

Subtotal

IV. WARMTH AND ACCEPTANCE

26. Parent holds child close 10-15 minutes per day.
27. Parent converse with child at least twice during visit.
28. Parent answers child's questions or requests verbally.
29. Parent usually responds verbally to child's speech.
30. Parent praises child' qualities twice during visit.
31. Parent caresses, kisses, or cuddles child during visit.
32. Parent helps child demonstrate some achievement during visit.

Subtotal

V. ACADEMIC STIMULATION

33. Child is encouraged to learn colors.
34. Child is encouraged to learn patterned speech (songs, etc.).
35. Child is encouraged to learn spatial relationships.
36. Child is encouraged to learn numbers.
37. Child is encouraged to learn to read a few words.

Subtotal

VI. MODELING

38. Some delay of food gratification is expected.
39. TV is used judiciously.
40. Parent introduces visitor to child.
41. Child can express negative feelings without reprisal.
42. Child can hit parent without harsh reprisal.

Subtotal

Fig. 1-34, cont'd.

VII.	VARIETY IN EXPERIENCE	
43.	Child has real or toy musical instrument.	
44.	Child is taken on outing by family member at least every other week.	
45.	Child has been on trip more than fifty miles during last year.	
46.	Child has been taken to a museum during past year.	
47.	Parent encourages child to put away toys without help.	
48.	Parent uses complex sentence structure and vocabulary.	
49..	Child's art work is displayed some place in the house.	
50.	Child eats at least one meal per day with mother and father.	
51.	Parent lets child choose some foods or brands at grocery store	
	Subtotal	

VIII.	ACCEPTANCE	
52.	Parent does not scold or derogate child more than once.	
53.	Parent does not use physical restraint during visit.	
54.	Parent neither slaps nor spanks child during visit.	
55.	No more than one instance of physical punishment during past week.	
	Subtotal	

COMMENTS _____

_____

_____

_____

_____

Fig. 1-34, cont'd.

HOME Inventory for Families of Elementary Children

Bettye M. Caldwell and Robert H. Bradley

Family Name _____ Date of Visit _____

Observed Child's Name _____ Birthdate _____ Age _____ Sex _____

Caregiver for visit _____ Relationship to child _____

Family Composition _____
(persons living in household, including sex and age of children)

| Family Ethnicity _____ | Maternal Education _____ | Paternal Education _____ | Home Visitor _____ |

Is Mother Employed? _____ Type of work when employed _____   Is Father Employed? _____ Type of work when employed _____

Address _____ How long? _____ Phone _____

Current child care arrangements _____

Summarize past year's arrangement _____

Persons in home at time of visit _____

Observation of Summary

		Score
I.	Emotional & Verbal Responsivity	
II.	Encouragement of Maturity	
III.	Emotional Climate	
IV.	Growth Fostering Materials & Experiences	
V.	Provision for Active Stimulation	
VI.	Family Participation in Developmentally Stimulating Experiences	
VII.	Paternal Involvement	
VIII.	Aspects of the Physical Environment	

COMMENTS _____

_____

_____

_____

_____

Fig. 1-34, cont'd. Home Inventory Questionnaire **C,** For families of elementary children.

HOME Inventory (Elementary)

Place a plus (+) or minus (-) in the box alongside each item if the behavior is observed during the visit or if the parent reports that the conditions or events are characteristic of the home invironment. Enter the subtotals and the total on the front side of the Record Sheet.

I. EMOTIONAL & VERBAL RESPONSIBILITY

1. Family has fairly regular & predictable daily schedule for child (meals, daycare, bedtime, TV, homework, etc.).

2. Parent sometimes yields to child's fears or rituals (allows nightlight, accompanies child to new experiences, etc.).

3. Child has been praised at least twice during past week for doing something.

4. Child is encouraged to read on his own.

5. *Parent encourages child to contribute to the conversation during visit.

6. *Parent shows some positive emotional responses to praise of child by visitor.

7. *Parent responds to child's questions during interview.

8. *Parent uses complete sentence structure and some long words in conversing.

9. *When speaking of or to child, parent's voice conveys positive feelings.

10. *Parent initiates verbal interchanges with visitor, asks questions, makes spontaneous comments.

Subtotal

II. ENCOURAGEMENT OF MATURITY

11. Family requires child to carry out certain selfcare routines, e. g., makes bed, cleans room, cleans up after spills, bathes self. (A YES requires 3 out of 4).

12. Family requires child to keep living & play area reasonably clean & straight.

13. Child puts his outdoor clothing, dirty clothes, night clothes in special place.

14. Parents set limits for child & generally enforce them (curfew, homework before TV, or other regulations that fit family pattern).

15. Parent introduces interviewer to child.

16. *Parent is consistent in establishing or applying family rules.

17. *Parent does not violate rules of common courtesy.

Subtotal

III. EMOTIONAL CLIMATE

18. Parent has not lost temper with child more than once during previous week.

19. Mother reports no more than one instance of physical punishment occurred during past month.

20. Child can express negative feelings toward parents without harsh reprisals.

21. Parent has not cried or been visbly upset in child's presence more than once during past week.

22. Child has a special place in which to keep his possessions.

23. *Parent talks to child during visit (beyond correction and introduction).

24. *Parent uses some term of endearment or some dimunitive for child's name when talking about child at twice during visit.

25. *Parent does not express over annoyance with or hostility toward child—complains, describes child as "bad", says he won't mind, etc.

Subtotal

IV. GROWTH FOSTERING MATERIALS & EXPERIENCES

26. Child has free access to record player or radio.

27. Child has free access to musical instrument (piano, drum, ukelele, or guitar, etc.).

28. Child has free access to at least ten appropriate books.

29. Parents buys and reads a newspaper daily

30. Child has free access to desk or other suitable place for reading or studying.

31. Family has a dictionary and encourages child to use it.

32. Child has visited a friend by him/herself in the past week.

33. *House has at least two pictures or other type of artwork on the walls.

Subtotal

V. PROVISION FOR ACTIVE STIMULATION

34. Family has a television, and it is used judiciously, not left on continuously. (No TV requires an automatic NO – any scheduling scores YES).

35. Family encourages child to develop or sustain hobbies.

36. Child is regularly included in family's recreational hobby.

37. Family provides lessons to organizational membership to support child's talents (especially Y membership, gymnastic lessons, Art Center, etc.).

Subtotal

Fig. 1-34, cont'd.

V.	PROVISION FOR ACTIVE STIMULATION (Cont'd.)	
38.	Child has ready access to at least two pieces of playground equipment in the immediate vacinity.	
39.	Child has access to a library card, and family arranges for child to go to library once a month.	
40.	Family member has taken child, or arranged for child to go to a scientific, historical or art museum within the past year.	
41.	Family member has taken child, or arranged for child to take a trip on a plane, train, or bus within the last year.	
	Subtotal	

VI.	FAMILY PARTICIPATION IN DEVELOPMENTALLY STIMULATING EXPERIENCES	
42.	Family visits or recieves visits from relatives or friends at least once every other week.	
43.	Child has accompanied parent on a family business venture 3-4 times within the past year; e.g., to garage, clothing shop, appliance repair shop, etc.	
44.	Family member has taken child, or arranged for child to attend some type of live musical or theatre performance.	
45.	Family member has taken child, or arranged for child to go on a trip of more than 50 miles from his home (fifty mile radial distance, not total distance).	
46.	Parents discuss television programs with child.	
47.	Parent helps child to achieve motor skills—ride a two-wheel bicycle, roller skate, ice skate, play ball, etc.	
	Subtotal	

VII.	PATERNAL INVOLVEMENT	
48.	Father (or father substitute) regularly engages in outdoor recreation with child.	
49.	Child sees and spends some time with father or father figure, 4 days a week.	
50.	Child eats at least one meal per day, on most days, with mother and father (or mother and father figures).(One parent families rate an automatic NO).	
51.	Child has remained with this primary family group for ALL his life aside from 2-3 week vacations, illnesses of mother, visits of grand-mother, etc. (A YES requires no changes in mother's, father's, grandmother's or grandfather's presence since birth).	
	Subtotal	

VIII.	ASPECTS OF THE PHYSICAL ENVIRONMENT	
52..	Child's room has a picture or wall decoration appealing to children.	
53.	*The interior of the apartment is not dark or perceptually monotonous.	
54.	*In terms of available floor space, the rooms are not overcrowded with furniture.	
55.	*All visible rooms of the house are reasonably clean and minimally cluttered.	
56.	*There is at least 100 square feet of living space per person in the house.	
57.	*House is not overly noisy—television, shouts of children, radio, etc.	
58.	*Building has no potentially dangerous structural or health defects (e.g., plaster coming down from ceiling, stairway with boards missing, rodents, etc.)	
59.	* Child's outside play environment appears safe and free of hazards. (No outside play area requires an automatic NO).	
	Subtotal	

*To be scored on the basis of observation.

Fig. 1-34, cont'd.

SAMPLE

Child's Name _____ Bithdate _____ Age _____

Parent's Name _____ Phone No. _____

Address _____ Date _____

HOME SCREENING QUESTIONNAIRE
Ages 0-3 Years

Please answer **all** of the following questions about how your child's time is spent and some of the activities of your family. On some questions, you may want to check more than one blank.

FOR OFFICE USE ONLY	

_____ 1. How often do you and your child see relatives?
    _____ never
    _____ at least once a year
    _____ at least 6 times a year
    _____ at least once a month
    _____ at least once a week

_____ 2. Do you subscribe to any magazines?
    YES   NO If yes, what kind?
    _____ home and family magazines
    _____ news magazines
    _____ children's magazines
    _____ other

_____ 3. About how many hours each day does your child spend in a playpen, jumpchair, infant swing or infant seat?
    _____ none
    _____ up to 1 hour
    _____ 1 to 3 hours
    _____ more than 3 hours

_____ 4. Does your child have a toybox or other special place where he/she keeps his/her toys? YES NO

_____ 5. How many children's books does your child have of his/her *own?*
    _____ 0: too young
    _____ 1 or 2
    _____ 5-9
    _____ 10 or more

_____ 6. How many books do you own?
    _____ 0-9
    _____ 10-20
    _____ more than 20

    Where do you keep them?
    _____ in boxes
    _____ on a bookcase
    _____ other — explain _____
    _____

_____ 7. How often does someone take your child into a grocery store?
    _____ hardly ever; prefer to go alone
    _____ at least once a month
    _____ at least twice a month
    _____ at least once a week

_____ 8. How many different babysitters or day care centers have you used in the past three months? _____

_____ 9. Do you have any pets? YES NO
    (include dog, cat, fish, birds, etc.)

_____ 10. About how many times in the past week did you have to spank or slap your child to get him/her to mind? _____

_____ 11. Did you start talking to your child when he/she was
    _____ 0-3 months
    _____ 3-9 months
    _____ 9-15 months
    _____ when he/she was old enough to understand?

_____ 12. Most of the time do you feel that your child
    _____ is usually smiling and pleasant
    _____ prefers to be by himself/herself
    _____ responds readily to affection
    _____ gets angry when he/she doesn't get his/her way
    _____ is often cranky

_____ 13. Do you talk to your child as you are doing the housework?
    YES NO TOO YOUNG

Fig. 1-35. Sample Home Screening Questionnaires. **A,** Age 0-3 years. (Reprinted with permission of William K. Frankenburg, M.D. Copyright 1981, 1988, WK Frankenburg.)

SAMPLE

Child's Name _____ Bithdate _____ Age _____

Parent's Name _____ Phone No. _____

Address _____ Date _____

HOME SCREENING QUESTIONNAIRE
Ages 3-6 Years

Please answer **all** of the following questions about how your child's time is spent and some of the activities of your family. On some questions, you may want to check more than one blank.

FOR OFFICE USE ONLY

1. a) Do you get any magazines in the mail?
      YES   NO
    b) If yes, what kind?
      _____ home and family magazines
      _____ news magazines
      _____ children's magazines
      _____ other

2. Does your child have a toy box or other special place where he/she keeps his/her toys?   YES   NO

3. How many children's books does your family own?
      _____ 0 to 2
      _____ 3 to 9
      _____ 10 or more

4. How many books do you have besides children's books?
      _____ 0 to 9
      _____ 10 to 20
      _____ more than 20

5. How often does someone take your child into a grocery store?
      _____ hardly ever; I prefer to go alone
      _____ at least once a month
      _____ at least twice a month
      _____ at least once a week

6. About how many times in the past week did you have to spank your child? _____

7. Do you have a T.V.?   YES   NO
    About how many hours is the T.V. on each day? _____

FOR OFFICE USE ONLY

8. How often does someone get a chance to read stories to your child?
      _____ hardly ever
      _____ at least once a week
      _____ at least 3 times a week
      _____ at least 5 times a week

9. Do you ever sing to your child when he/she is nearby?   YES   NO

10. Does your child put away his/her toys by himself/herself *most of the time?*
      YES   NO

11. Is your child allowed to walk or ride his tricycle by himself/herself to the house of a friend or relative?   YES   NO

12. What do you do with your child's art work?
      _____ let him/her keep it
      _____ put it away
      _____ hang it somewhere in the house
      _____ throw it away shortly after looking at it

13. In the space below write you might say if you child said, "Look at that big truck".

14. What do you usually do when a friend is visiting you in your home and your child has nothing to do?
      _____ suggest something for him/her to do
      _____ offer him/her a toy
      _____ give him/her a cookie or something to eat
      _____ put him/her to bed for a nap
      _____ play with him/her

Fig. 1-35, cont'd.

Family assessment diagrams

General guidelines for administration

Be familiar with the diagram, especially directions for its use

Explain to the family why the diagram is being administered and how the information will be used

Discuss the diagram with the family

Use the diagram to help the family clarify and define what they perceive as a concern or need

Restate the needs to be certain that all parties perceive the same message

Genogram (family tree, family diagram)

Modified pedigree (see p. 9) that records composition of family members, usually from three generations

Uses symbols (Fig. 1-36) to represent attachment or intensity of relationship; if symbols other than these are used, add to the genogram a key to explain their meaning

Nuclear family or family members living in household may be designated by drawing a broken line around them

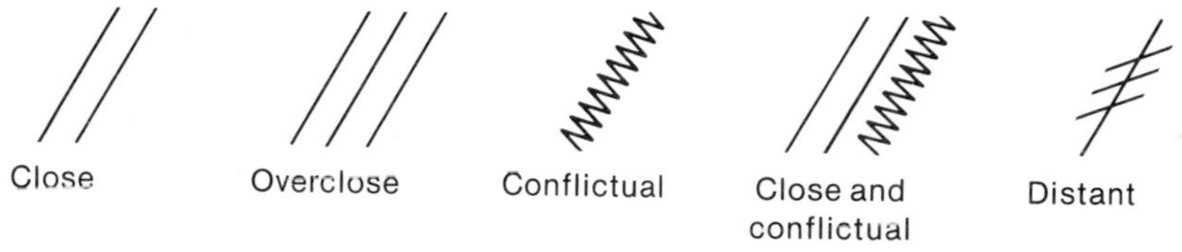

Close   Overclose   Conflictual   Close and conflictual   Distant

Fig. 1-36. Symbols of attachment or intensity of relationship. If symbols other than these are used, add to the genogram a key to explain their meaning.

Sociogram

Use of drawing to identify significant persons in individual's life

Instructions: "Draw a circle to represent you. Around the circle draw circles to represent the most significant persons in your life and label each. Draw the circles in proximity to your circle to represent closeness. For example, the most significant person is the circle closest to you."

Family circle (Thrower, Bruce, and Walton, 1982)

Purpose is same as sociogram but directions differ slightly: "Draw a circle to represent your family. Draw in smaller circles to represent you and the most significant persons in your life. People can be inside or outside the family circle. Draw the circles large or small depending on their significance or influence to you."

In either drawing, family members can label relationships as supportive with a plus sign or negative with a minus sign

Both drawings can be used with children as young as 5 years of age

Questions for discussion of either drawing include:

How would you change the circles to improve relationships?

How do you think you could accomplish these changes?

If one person in the circle were to change, how do you think that would affect others?

Ecomap (Hartman, 1979)

Visual presentation of family's support system outside the home

Begins with genogram of immediate family inside one circle and uses other smaller circles to represent each member's relationship with other significant people, agencies, or institutions (Fig. 1-37)

Size of circles is not important

Symbols of attachment (see Fig. 1-36) are used to signify the type of relationship

Arrows may be drawn along connecting lines to denote flow of energy or resources

Role rating scale

Parental rating of percentage of investment in three areas of their life: individual, parent, spouse

Instructions: "In the box, circle if you are the husband or wife. Imagine that your life as an individual, parent, and spouse

makes up 100 points. In the appropriate space, write in how many of the 100 points you devote to each part of your life. In the opposite space write in how many points you think your spouse devotes to each part of his/her life." (Fig. 1-38)

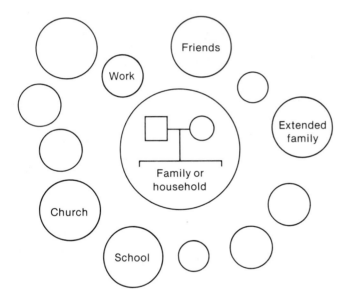

Fig. 1-37. Ecomap. Genogram is completed for immediate family members and circles are labeled as appropriate. (Modified from Hartman A: Finding families: an ecological approach to family assessment in adoption, Beverly Hills, CA, 1979, Sage Publications.)

SPOUSES' ROLE RATING SCALE		
	Husband	Wife
Individual		
Parent		
Spouse		

Fig. 1-38. Spouses' role rating scale.

REFERENCES

Caldwell B and Bradley R: Home Observation and Measurement of the Environment, revised edition, Little Rock, Ark., 1984, University of Arkansas.

Dunst C, Trivette C, and Deal A: Enabling and empowering families: principles and guidelines for practice, Cambridge, Mass., 1988, Brookline Books.

Feetham S and Humenick S: Feetham Family Functioning Survey. In Humenick S, (editor): Analysis of current assessment strategies in the health care of young children and childbearing families, Norwalk, Conn., 1982, Appleton-Century-Crofts.

Frankenburg W and Coons C: Home Screening Questionnaire: its validity in assessing home environment, J Pediatr 108(4):624-626, 1986.

Hartman A: Finding families: an ecological approach to family assessment in adoption, Beverly Hills, Calif., 1979, Sage Publications.

Hymovich D: Personal communication, 1989.

Roberts C and Feetham S: Assessing family functioning across three areas of relationship, Nurs Res 31(4):231-235, 1982.

Smilkstein G: The family APGAR: a proposal for a family function test and its use by physicians, J Fam Pract 6(6):1231-1239, 1978.

Thrower S, Bruce W, and Walton R: The Family Circle Method for integrating family systems concepts in family medicine, J Fam Pract 15(3):451-457, 1982.

ASSESSMENT OF TEMPERAMENT

Temperament is the *behavioral style* or the *how* rather than the what or why of behavior. Nine temperament variables have been identified:

1. **Activity level**—The activity level of the child.
   Scored in terms of motility during bathing, eating, playing, dressing, handling, reaching, crawling, walking, and sleep-wake cycles.
   High activity refers to high motor activity, such as preference for running or inability to sit still.
   Low activity refers to low motor activity, such as preference for reading or other quiet games and ability to sit still for prolonged periods.

2. **Rhythmicity**—The predictability and/or unpredictability of the child's functions.
   Scored in terms of sleep-wake cycles, hunger, feeding pattern, and elimination schedule.
   High rhythmicity refers to a child with regular bodily habits.
   Low rhythmicity refers to a child with irregular bodily habits.

3. **Approach-withdrawal**—The initial response of the child to a new stimulus.
   Scored in terms of response to new food, toy, person, or experience, such as first day at school.
   Approach refers to predominantly positive response, such as smiling, verbalizations, and reaching for the stimulus.
   Withdrawal refers to predominantly negative response, such as fussing, crying, and moving away from or refusing the stimulus.

4. **Adaptability**—The child's ability to adapt or adjust the routine to fit a new situation.
   Scored in terms of ease of adjusting to new situation (similar to approach-withdrawal), but is concerned with the nature of the initial response.
   High adaptability refers to the ability to settle in easily.
   Low adaptability refers to the inability to adjust easily.

5. **Intensity**—The energy level of response, irrespective of its quality or direction.
   Scored in terms of reactions to sensory stimuli, environmental objects, and social contacts.
   High intensity refers to behavioral reactions such as loud crying or laughing in response to a stimulus, such as receiving a new toy.
   Low intensity refers to behavioral reactions such as whimpering or failing to react to a stimulus, such as banging the head.

6. **Threshold**—How much stimulus is required before the child reacts to a given situation.
   Scored in terms of level of sensory stimuli needed before child responds.

Low threshold indicates high intensity to slight stimuli, such as waking up to soft sounds.
High threshold indicates low intensity to moderate to strong stimuli, such as lack of discomfort with a wet diaper.

7. **Mood**—The amount of happy, joyful behavior in contrast to unhappy, crying, whining behavior.
   Scored in terms of response to sensory stimuli, environmental objects, and social contacts.
   Positive mood refers to child who is generally pleasant and cooperative.
   Negative mood refers to child who is generally fussy and complaining.

8. **Attention-persistence**—The length of time that a given activity is pursued by the child and the continuation of an activity in spite of obstacles.
   Scored in terms of the child's ability to pursue an activity, such as read a book, or try to master a skill without giving up.
   Long attention–high persistence refers to a child who can pay attention for prolonged periods and continues working on a project or playing despite obstacles, such as parent telling him to stop or someone interrupting his activity.
   Short attention–low persistence refers to a child who has difficulty paying attention and gives up easily.

9. **Distractibility**—The effectiveness of outside stimuli in diverting the child's behavior or attention.
   Low distractibility refers to the child who is not easily distracted.
   High distractibility refers to the child who is easily distracted.

The three most common patterns of child temperament, which describe most but not all children, are described in Table 1-7.

Approximately 35% of children do not fall into the above categories, but are characterized by a variety of combinations of temperament variables.

Samples of questionnaires that can be used to assess children's temperament are presented on p. 78-81. The questionnaires focus on the nine temperament variables through questions that relate to activities appropriate to each age group, such as sleep, feeding, play, diapering, dressing, and response to new experiences. Low scores refer to low activity, high rhythmicity, approachability, adaptability, mild intensity, high threshold, positive mood, high attention-persistence, and low distractibility. High scores reflect the opposite temperament variables. The purpose of the questionnaires is to acquaint parents with their child's type of temperament and to guide them regarding appropriate child-rearing techniques.

Table 1-9. THREE COMMON PATTERNS OF CHILD TEMPERAMENT

Pattern (% of children)	Temperament variables				
	Rhythmicity	Approach/withdrawal	Adaptability	Intensity	Mood
Easy (40%)	High	Approach	High	Low	Positive
Difficult (10%)	Low	Withdrawal	Low	High	Negative
Slow to warm up (15%)	Moderate	Withdrawal	Low	Low	Negative

SAMPLE*

INFANT TEMPERAMENT QUESTIONNAIRE (ITQ)
(FOR 4 TO 8 MONTH OLD INFANTS)

Child's Name _____ **Sex** _____

Date of Birth _____ **Present Age** _____
              Month   Day   Year

Rater's Name _____ **Relationship to Child** _____

Date of Rating _____
                Month   Day   Year

The purpose of this questionnaire is to determine the general pattern of your infant's reactions to his/her environment.

The questionnaire consists of several pages of statements about your infant. Please circle the number indicating the frequency with which you think the statement is true for your infant. Although some of the statements seem to be similar, they are not the same and should be rated independently. If any item cannot be answered or does not apply to your infant, just draw a line through it. If your infant has changed with respect to any of the areas covered, use the response that best describes the recently established pattern. There are no good and bad or right and wrong answers, only descriptions of what your infant does. When you have completed the questionnaire, which will take about 25-30 minutes, you may make any additional comments at the end.

USING THE FOLLOWING SCALE, PLEASE CIRCLE THE NUMBER THAT INDICATES HOW OFTEN THE INFANT'S RECENT AND CURRENT BEHAVIOR HAS BEEN LIKE THAT DESCRIBED BY EACH ITEM.

	Almost never 1	Rarely 2	Variable usually does not 3	Variable usually does 4	Frequently 5	Almost always 6	
1. The infant eats about the same amount of solid food (within 1 oz.) from day to day.	almost never	1	2	3	4	5	6	almost always
2. The infant is fussy on waking up and going to sleep (frowns, cries).	almost never	1	2	3	4	5	6	almost always
3. The infant plays with a toy for under a minute and then looks for another toy or activity.	almost never	1	2	3	4	5	6	almost always
4. The infant sits still while watching TV or other nearby activity.	almost never	1	2	3	4	5	6	almost always
5. The infant accepts right away any change in place or position of feeding or person giving it.	almost never	1	2	3	4	5	6	almost always
6. The infant accepts nail cutting without protest.	almost never	1	2	3	4	5	6	almost always
7. The infant's hunger cry can be stopped for over a minute by picking up, pacifier, putting on bib, etc.	almost never	1	2	3	4	5	6	almost always
8. The infant plays continuously for more than 10 min. at a time with a favorite toy.	almost never	1	2	3	4	5	6	almost always
9. The infant accepts his/her bath any time of the day without resisting it.	almost never	1	2	3	4	5	6	almost always
10. The infant takes feedings quietly with mild expression of likes and dislikes.	almost never	1	2	3	4	5	6	almost always
11. The infant indicates discomfort (fusses or squirms) when diaper is soiled with bowel movement.	almost never	1	2	3	4	5	6	almost always
12. The infant lies quietly in the bath.	almost never	1	2	3	4	5	6	almost always
13. The infant wants and takes milk feedings at about the same times (within one hour) from day to day.	almost never	1	2	3	4	5	6	almost always
14. The infant is shy (turns away or clings to mother) on meeting another child for the first time.	almost never	1	2	3	4	5	6	almost always

*The first page of the scale is reprinted by permission of the authors.

A copy of the complete questionnaire can be obtained by sending a check for $10.00 to Dr. William B. Carey, Division of General Pediatrics, Children's Hospital of Philadelphia, PA, 19104, 34th St. and Civic Center Blvd., USA or call (215) 590-2319 or (215) 590-2168.

From Carey W and McDevitt S: Revision of the Infant Temperament Questionnaire, Pediatrics 61:735-739, 1978.

SAMPLE*

TODDLER TEMPERAMENT QUESTIONNAIRE (TTQ)
(FOR 1 TO 3 YEAR OLD CHILDREN)

DATA SHEET

Child's Name _____ Sex _____

Date of Birth _____ Present Age _____
　　　　　　　Month　　　　　　　　　　Day　　　　　　　　　Year

Rater's Name _____ Relationship to Child _____

Date of Rating _____
　　　　　　　Month　　　Day　　　Year

RATING INFORMATION

1. Please base your rating on the child's *recent* and *current* behavior (the last *four* to *six* weeks).
2. Consider only *your own* impressions and observations of the child.
3. Rate each question *independently*. Do not purposely attempt to present a consistent picture of the child.
4. Use *extreme ratings* where appropriate. Avoid rating only near the middle of the scale.
5. Rate each item *quickly*. If you cannot decide, skip the item and come back to it later.
6. *Rate every item*. Circle the number of any item that you are unable to answer due to lack of information or any item that does not apply to your child.

USING THE SCALE SHOWN BELOW, PLEASE MARK AN "X" IN THE SPACE THAT TELLS HOW OFTEN THE CHILD'S RECENT AND CURRENT BEHAVIOR HAS BEEN LIKE THE BEHAVIOR DESCRIBED BY EACH ITEM.

	Almost never 1	Rarely 2	Variable usually does not 3	Variable usually does 4	Frequently 5	Almost always 6	
1. The child gets sleepy at about the same time each evening (within ½ hour).	almost never	1	2	3	4	5	6	almost always
2. The child fidgets during quiet activities (story telling, looking at pictures).	almost never	1	2	3	4	5	6	almost always
3. The child takes feedings quietly with mild expression of likes and dislikes.	almost never	1	2	3	4	5	6	almost always
4. The child is pleasant (smiles, laughs) when first arriving in unfamiliar places.	almost never	1	2	3	4	5	6	almost always
5. A child's initial reaction to seeing the doctor is acceptance.	almost never	1	2	3	4	5	6	almost always
6. The child pays attention to game with parent for only a minute or so.	almost never	1	2	3	4	5	6	almost always
7. The child's bowel movements come at different times from day to day (over one hour difference).	almost never	1	2	3	4	5	6	almost always
8. The child is fussy on waking up (frowns, complains, cries).	almost never	1	2	3	4	5	6	almost always
9. The child's initial reaction to a new babysitter is rejection (crying, clinging to mother, etc.)	almost never	1	2	3	4	5	6	almost always
10. The child reacts to a disliked food even if it is mixed with a preferred one.	almost never	1	2	3	4	5	6	almost always
11. The child accepts delays (for several minutes) for desired objects or activities (snacks, treats, gifts).	almost never	1	2	3	4	5	6	almost always
12. The child moves little (stays still) when being dressed.	almost never	1	2	3	4	5	6	almost always
13. The child continues an activity in spite of noises in the same room.	almost never	1	2	3	4	5	6	almost always
14. The child shows strong reactions (cries, stamps feet) to failure.	almost never	1	2	3	4	5	6	almost always

*The first page of the scale is reprinted by permission of the authors.

A copy of the complete questionnaire can be obtained by sending a check for $10.00 to Dr. William Fullard, Department of Educational Psychology, Temple University, Philadelphia, PA 19122, USA or call (215) 787-6022.

From Fullard W, McDevitt S, and Carey W: Assessing temperament in one to three year old children, J Pediatr Psychol 9:205-217, 1984.

SAMPLE*

BEHAVIORAL STYLE QUESTIONNAIRE (BSQ)
(FOR 3 TO 7 YEAR OLD CHILDREN)

DATA SHEET

Child's Name _____ Sex _____

Date of Birth _____ Present Age _____
           Month   Day   Year

Rater's Name _____ Relationship to Child _____

Date of Rating _____
           Month   Day   Year

RATING INFORMATION

1. Please base your rating on the child's *recent* and *current* behavior (the last *four* to *six* weeks).
2. Consider only *your own* impressions and observations of the child.
3. Rate each question *independently*. Do not purposely attempt to present a consistent picture of the child.
4. Use *extreme ratings* where appropriate. Avoid rating only near the middle of the scale.
5. Rate each item *quickly*. If you cannot decide, skip the item and come back to it later.
6. *Rate every item*. Circle the number of any item that you are unable to answer due to lack of information or any item that does not apply to your child.

USING THE SCALE SHOWN BELOW, PLEASE MARK AN "X" IN THE SPACE THAT TELLS HOW OFTEN THE CHILD'S RECENT AND CURRENT BEHAVIOR HAS BEEN LIKE THE BEHAVIOR DESCRIBED BY EACH ITEM.

	Almost never 1	Rarely 2	Variable usually does not 3	Variable usually does 4	Frequently 5	Almost always 6
1. The child is moody for more than a few minutes when corrected or disciplined.	almost never	1 2	3	4	5 6	almost always
2. The child seems not to hear when involved in a favorite activity.	almost never	1 2	3	4	5 6	almost always
3. The child can be coaxed out of a forbidden activity.	almost never	1 2	3	4	5 6	almost always
4. The child runs ahead when walking with the parent.	almost never	1 2	3	4	5 6	almost always
5. The child laughs or smiles while playing.	almost never	1 2	3	4	5 6	almost always
6. The child moves slowly when working on a project or activity.	almost never	1 2	3	4	5 6	almost always
7. The child responds intensely to disapproval.	almost never	1 2	3	4	5 6	almost always
8. The child needs a period of adjustment to get used to changes in school or at home.	almost never	1 2	3	4	5 6	almost always
9. The child enjoys games that involve running or jumping.	almost never	1 2	3	4	5 6	almost always
10. The child is slow to adjust to changes in household rules.	almost never	1 2	3	4	5 6	almost always
11. The child has bowel movements at about the same time each day.	almost never	1 2	3	4	5 6	almost always
12. The child is willing to try new things.	almost never	1 2	3	4	5 6	almost always
13. The child sits calmly while watching TV or listening to music.	almost never	1 2	3	4	5 6	almost always
14. The child leaves or wants to leave the table during meals.	almost never	1 2	3	4	5 6	almost always

*The first partial page of the scale is reprinted by permission of the authors.

A copy of the complete questionnaire can be obtained by sending a check for $10.00 to Dr. Sean C. McDevitt, Westbridge Center for Children, Western Behavioral Associates, 4626 E. Shea Blvd., Phoenix, AZ 85028 USA or call (602) 494-0224.

From McDevitt S and Carey W: The measurement of temperament in 3-7 year old children, J Child Psychol Psychiatr 19:245-253, 1978.

Unit 1

SAMPLE*

MIDDLE CHILDHOOD TEMPERAMENT QUESTIONNAIRE
(FOR 8 TO 12 YEAR OLD CHILDREN)

DATA SHEET

Child's Name _____ Sex _____

Date of Birth _____ Present Age _____
          Month   Day   Year

Rater's Name _____ Relationship to Child _____

Date of Rating _____
          Month   Day   Year

INSTRUCTIONS TO PARENT

1. There are *no right or wrong* or good or bad answers, only descriptions of your child.
2. Please base your rating on the child's *recent* and *current* behavior (the last *four* to *six* weeks).
3. Rate each question *separately*. Do not purposely try to present a consistent picture of your child.
4. Use *extreme ratings* where appropriate. Try to avoid rating only near the middle of each scale.

5. Rate each item *quickly*. If you cannot decide, skip the item and come back to it later.
6. *Rate every item*. Please circle any item you are unable to answer due to lack of information or any item that does not apply to your child.
7. Consider only *your own* impressions and observations of the child.

USING THE SCALE SHOWN BELOW, PLEASE MARK AN "X" IN THE SPACE THAT TELLS HOW OFTEN THE CHILD'S RECENT AND CURRENT BEHAVIOR HAS BEEN LIKE THE BEHAVIOR DESCRIBED BY EACH ITEM.

	Almost never 1	Rarely 2	Variable usually does not 3	Variable usually does 4	Frequently 5	Almost always 6	
1. Runs to get where he/she wants to go.	almost never	1	2	3	4	5	6	almost always
2. Avoids (stays away from, doesn't talk to) a new sitter on first meeting.	almost never	1	2	3	4	5	6	almost always
3. Easily excited by praise (laughs, claps, yells, etc.).	almost never	1	2	3	4	5	6	almost always
4. Frowns or complains when asked by the parent to do a chore.	almost never	1	2	3	4	5	6	almost always
5. Notices (looks toward) minor changes in lighting (changes in shadows, turning on lights, etc.).	almost never	1	2	3	4	5	6	almost always
6. Loses interest in a new toy or game the same day she/he gets it.	almost never	1	2	3	4	5	6	almost always
7. Has difficulty (asks for advice, takes a long time, etc.) making decisions.	almost never	1	2	3	4	5	6	almost always
8. Uncomfortable with wet or dirty clothes, wants to change right away.	almost never	1	2	3	4	5	6	almost always
9. Shows strong reactions (yells, shouts, etc.) when pleasantly surprised.	almost never	1	2	3	4	5	6	almost always
10. Responses to parent's instructions are predictable.	almost never	1	2	3	4	5	6	almost always
11. Remains pleasant (smiles, etc.) even when tired.	almost never	1	2	3	4	5	6	almost always
12. Looks up right away from play when telephone or doorbell rings.	almost never	1	2	3	4	5	6	almost always
13. Moves right into a new place (store, theater, playground).	almost never	1	2	3	4	5	6	almost always
14. Adjusts within a day or two to changes in routine (different bed time, new chores, etc.).	almost never	1	2	3	4	5	6	almost always

---

*The first page of the scale is reprinted by permission of the authors.

A copy of the complete questionnaire can be obtained by sending a check for $10.00 to Robin L. Hegvik, 138 Montrose Avenue, #14, Rosemont, PA 19010 USA or call (215) 527-8108.

From Hegvik R, McDevitt S, and Carey W: The Middle Childhood Temperament Questionnaire, J Develop Behavior Pediatr 3:197-200, 1982.

Unit 1

NUTRITIONAL ASSESSMENT

A nutritional assessment is an essential part of a complete health appraisal. Its purpose is to evaluate the child's nutritional status—the state of balance between nutrient intake and nutrient expenditure or need. A thorough nutritional assessment includes information about dietary intake, clinical assessment of nutritional status, and biochemical status.

Information about dietary intake usually begins with a dietary history (see below) and may be coupled with a more detailed account of actual food intake. Two methods of recording food intake are a food diary and food frequency record. The food diary is a record of every food and liquid consumed for a certain number of days, usually 2 weekdays and 1 weekend day p. 83). A food frequency record provides information about the number of times in a day or week items from the four food groups are consumed (p. 84).

Clinical assessment of nutritional status provides information regarding signs of adequate nutrition and deficient or excess nutrition. The overview on p. 85 also identifies specific nutrients that may be responsible for abnormal clinical findings. In addition, measurement of height, weight, head circumference, skinfold thickness, and arm circumference are assessed. Techniques for measurement are on p. 24-27 and expected norms are on p. 100-112.

A number of biochemical tests are available for studying nutritional status. Common laboratory procedures for nutritional status include measurement of hemoglobin, serum transferrin, total-iron binding capacity, albumin, creatinine, and nitrogen (see Normal laboratory tests in Unit 6).

Dietary history

What are the family's usual mealtimes?
Do family members eat together or at separate times?
Who does the family grocery shopping and meal preparation?
How much money is spent to buy food each week?
How are most foods prepared—baked, broiled, fried, other?
How often does the family or your child eat out?
  What kinds of restaurants do you go to?
  What kinds of food does your child typically eat at restaurants?
Does your child eat breakfast regularly?
Where does he eat lunch?
What are your child's favorite foods, beverages, and snacks?
  What are the average amounts eaten per day?
  What foods are artificially sweetened?
  What are your child's snacking habits?
  When are sweet foods usually eaten?
  What are your child's toothbrushing habits?
What special cultural practices are followed?
  What ethnic foods are eaten?
What foods and beverages does your child dislike?
How would you describe his usual appetite (hearty eater, picky eater)?
What are his feeding habits (breast, bottle, cup, spoon, eats by self, needs assistance, any special devices)?
Does he take vitamins or other supplements; do they contain iron or fluoride?
Are there any known or suspected food allergies; is your child on a special diet?
Has your child lost or gained weight recently?
Are there any feeding problems (excessive fussiness, spitting up, colic, difficulty sucking or swallowing); any dental problems or appliances, such as braces, that affect eating?
What types of exercise does your child do regularly?
Is there a family history of cancer, diabetes, heart disease, high blood pressure, or obesity?

Additional questions for infants?
What was the infant's birth weight; when did it double, triple?
Was the infant premature?
Are you breast-feeding or have you breast-fed your infant? For how long?
If you use a formula, what is the brand?
  How long has the infant been taking it?
  How many ounces does he drink a day?
Are you giving the infant cow's milk (whole, low-fat, skimmed)?
  When did you start?
  How many ounces does he drink a day?
Do you give your infant extra fluids (water, juice)?
If he takes a bottle to bed at nap or nighttime, what is in the bottle?
At what age did you start cereal, vegetables, meat or other protein sources, fruit/juice, finger food, table food?
Do you make your own baby food or use commercial foods, such as infant cereal?
Does the infant take a vitamin/mineral supplement? If so, what type?
Has the infant shown an allergic reaction to any food(s)? If so, list the foods and describe the reaction.
Does the infant spit up frequently, have unusually loose stools, or have hard, dry stools? If so, how often?
How often do you feed your infant?
How would you describe your infant's appetite?

Food diary

TOTAL FOOD INTAKE						COMMENTS
Meals and Snacks		Description of Food Items				Any Related Factors?—Associated Activity, Place, Persons, Money, Feelings, Hunger, etc.
Time	Place	Food	Amount	Type or Preparation	With Whom Eaten?	

From Williams S: Handbook of maternal and infant nutrition, Berkeley, Calif,
1976, SRW Productions, Inc.

Unit 1

Unit 1

Food frequency record*

Food group	Number of servings per day or week	Approximate serving size (Indicate amount of liquids, fruits, and vegetables in cup portions; proteins in tablespoons or ounces)
MILK/CHEESE		
Milk		
Cheese		
Yogurt		
Pudding		
Ice cream		
Other		
PROTEIN FOODS		
Meat		
Fish		
Poultry		
Egg		
Peanut butter		
Legumes (dried beans, peas)		
Nuts		
Other		
BREADS/CEREALS		
Bread, tortilla		
Cooked pasta, rice, hot cereal		
Dry cereal (not presweetened)		
Crackers		
Muffins		
Other		
VEGETABLES		
Yellow or orange		
Green/leafy		
Other		
FRUIT		
Citrus (orange, grapefruit, tangerine)		
Juice		
Noncitrus		
Juice		
Other		
FATS		
(butter, oil, margarine, mayonnaise, salad dressing)		
SWEETS		
Soda, punch		
Cake/cookie, etc.		
Candy		
Presweetened cereal		

*For comparison of actual intake with recommended intake, see p. 169.

Clinical assessment of nutritional status

Evidence of adequate nutrition	Evidence of deficient or excess nutrition	Deficiency/excess*
GENERAL GROWTH		
Within 5th and 95th percentiles for height, weight, and head circumference	Below 5th or above 95th percentiles for growth	Protein, calories, fats, and other essential nutrients, especially A, pyridoxine, niacin, calcium, iodine, manganese, zinc
Steady gain with expected growth spurts during infancy and adolescence	Absence of or delayed growth spurts; poor weight gain	
Sexual development appropriate for age	Delayed sexual development	
		Excess vitamin A, D
SKIN		
Smooth, slightly dry to touch	Hardening and scaling	Vitamin A
Elastic and firm	Seborrheic dermatitis	Excess niacin
Absence of lesions	Dry, rough, petechiae	Riboflavin
Color appropriate to genetic background	Delayed wound healing	Vitamin C
	Scaly dermatitis on exposed surfaces	Riboflavin, vitamin C, zinc
	Wrinkled, flabby	Niacin
	Crusted lesions around orifices, especially nares	Protein and calories
		Zinc
	Pruritus	Excess vitamin A, riboflavin, niacin
	Poor turgor	Water, sodium
	Edema	Protein, thiamin
		Excess sodium
	Yellow tinge (jaundice)	Vitamin B_{12}
		Excess vitamin A, niacin
	Depigmentation	Protein, calories
	Pallor (anemia)	Pyridoxine, folic acid, vitamin B_{12}, C, E (in premature infants), iron
		Excess vitamin C, zinc
	Paresthesia	Excess riboflavin
HAIR		
Lustrous, silky, strong, elastic	Stringy, friable, dull, dry, thin	Protein, calories
	Alopecia	Protein, calories, zinc
	Depigmentation	Protein, calories, copper
	Raised areas around hair follicles	Vitamin C
HEAD		
Even molding, occipital prominence, symmetric facial features	Softening of cranial bones, prominence of frontal bones, skull flat and depressed toward middle	Vitamin D
Fused sutures after 18 months	Delayed fusion of sutures	Vitamin D
	Hard tender lumps in occiput	Excess vitamin A
	Headache	Excess thiamin
NECK		
Thyroid not visible, palpable in midline	Thyroid enlarged; may be grossly visible	Iodine
EYES		
Clear, bright	Hardening and scaling of cornea and conjunctiva	Vitamin A
Conjunctiva—Pink, glossy	Burning, itching, photophobia, cataracts, corneal vascularization	Riboflavin
Good night vision	Night blindness	
EARS		
Tympanic membrane—Pliable	Calcified (hearing loss)	Excess vitamin D
NOSE		
Smooth, intact nasal angle	Irritation and cracks at nasal angle	Riboflavin
		Excess vitamin A

*Nutrients listed are deficient unless specified as excess.

Unit 1

Clinical assessment of nutritional status—cont'd

Evidence of adequate nutrition	Evidence of deficient or excess nutrition	Deficiency/excess*
MOUTH		
Lips—Smooth, moist, darker color than skin	Fissures and inflammation at corners	Riboflavin Excess vitamin A
Gums—Firm, coral pink color, stippled	Spongy, friable, swollen, bluish-red or black color, bleed easily	Vitamin C
Mucous membranes—Bright pink, smooth, moist	Stomatitis	Niacin
Tongue—Rough texture, no lesions, taste sensation	Glossitis	Niacin, riboflavin, folic acid
	Diminished taste sensation	Zinc
Teeth—Uniform white color, smooth, intact	Brown mottling, pits, fissures	Excess fluoride
	Defective enamel	Vitamin A, C, D, calcium, phosphorus
	Caries	Excess carbohydrates
CHEST		
In infants, shape is almost circular	Depressed lower portion of rib cage	Vitamin D
In children, lateral diameter increases in proportion to anteroposterior diameter	Sharp protrusion of sternum	
Smooth costochondral junctions	Enlarged costochondral junctions	Vitamin C, D
Breast development—Normal for age	Delayed development	See General growth, above, especially zinc
CARDIOVASCULAR SYSTEM		
Pulse and blood pressure (BP) within normal limits	Palpitations	Thiamin
	Rapid pulse	Potassium Excess thiamin
	Arrhythmias	Magnesium, potassium Excess niacin, potassium
	Increased BP	Excess sodium
	Decreased BP	Thiamin Excess niacin
ABDOMEN		
In young children, cylindric and prominent	Distended, flabby, poor musculature	Protein, calories
Older children, flat	Prominent, large	Excess calories
Normal bowel habits	Potbelly, constipation	Vitamin D
	Diarrhea	Niacin Excess vitamin C
	Constipation	Excess calcium, potassium
MUSCULOSKELETAL SYSTEM		
Muscles—Firm, well-developed, equal strength bilaterally	Flabby, weak, generalized wasting	Protein, calories
	Weakness, pain, cramps	Thiamin, sodium, chloride, potassium, phosphorus, magnesium Excess thiamin
	Muscle twitching, tremors	Magnesium
	Muscular paralysis	Excess potassium
Spine—Cervical and lumbar curves (double S curve)	Kyphosis, lordosis, scoliosis	Vitamin D
Extremities—Symmetric; legs straight with minimum bowing	Bowing of extremities, knock-knees	Vitamin D, calcium, phosphorus
	Epiphyseal enlargement	Vitamin A, D
	Bleeding into joints and muscles, joint swelling, pain	Vitamin C
Joints—Flexible, full range of motion, no pain or stiffness	Thickening of cortex of long bones with pain and fragility, hard tender lumps in extremities	Excess vitamin A
	Osteoporosis of long bones	Calcium Excess vitamin D

Clinical assessment of nutritional status—cont'd

Evidence of adequate nutrition	Evidence of deficient or excess nutrition	Deficiency/excess*
NEUROLOGIC SYSTEM		
Behavior—Alert, responsive, emotionally stable	Listless, irritable, lethargic, apathetic (sometimes apprehensive, anxious, drowsy, mentally slow, confused)	Thiamin, niacin, pyridoxine, vitamin C, potassium, magnesium, iron, protein, calories
		Excess vitamin A, D, thiamin, folic acid, calcium
	Masklike facial expression, blurred speech, involuntary laughing	Excess manganese
Absence of tetany, convulsions	Convulsions	Thiamin, pyridoxine, vitamin D, calcium, magnesium
		Excess phosphorus (in relation to calcium)
Intact peripheral nervous system	Peripheral nervous system toxicity (unsteady gait, numb feet and hands, fine motor clumsiness)	Excess pyridoxine
Intact reflexes	Diminished or absent tendon reflexes	Thiamin, vitamin E

RECOMMENDED DIETARY ALLOWANCES[a] DESIGNED FOR THE MAINTENANCE OF GOOD NUTRITION OF PRACTICALLY ALL HEALTHY PEOPLE IN THE UNITED STATES)

Category	Age (years) or condition	Weight[b] (kg)	Weight[b] (lb)	Height[b] (cm)	Height[b] (in)	Protein (g)	Fat-soluble vitamins Vitamin A (μg RE)[c]	Vitamin D (μg)[d]	Vitamin E (mg α-TE)[e]	Vitamin K (μg)
Infants	0.0-0.5	6	13	60	24	13	375	7.5	3	5
	0.5-1.0	9	20	71	28	14	375	10	4	10
Children	1-3	13	29	90	35	16	400	10	6	15
	4-6	20	44	112	44	24	500	10	7	20
	7-10	28	62	132	52	28	700	10	7	30
Males	11-14	45	99	157	62	45	1,000	10	10	45
	15-18	66	145	176	69	59	1,000	10	10	65
	19-24	72	160	177	70	58	1,000	10	10	70
	25-50	79	174	176	70	63	1,000	5	10	80
	51+	77	170	173	68	63	1,000	5	10	80
Females	11-14	46	101	157	62	46	800	10	8	45
	15-18	55	120	163	64	44	800	10	8	55
	19-24	58	128	164	65	46	800	10	8	60
	25-50	63	138	163	64	50	800	5	8	65
	51+	65	143	160	63	50	800	5	8	65
Pregnant						60	800	10	10	65
Lactating	1st 6 months					65	1,300	10	12	65
	2nd 6 months					62	1,200	10	11	65

From Food and Nutrition Board, National Academy of Sciences–National Research Council, Washington, D.C., 1989.

[a]The allowances, expressed as average daily intakes over time, are intended to provide for individual variations among most normal persons as they live in the United States under usual environmental stresses. Diets should be based on a variety of common foods in order to provide other nutrients for which human requirements have been less well defined.

[b]Weights and heights of Reference Adults are actual medians for the U.S. population of the designated age, as reported by NHANES II. The median weights and heights of those under 19 years of age were taken from Hamill et al. (1979). The use of these figures does not imply that the height-to-weight ratios are ideal.

[c]Retinol equivalents. 1 Retinol equivalent = 1μg retinol or 6 μg β-carotene.

[d]As cholecaliferol. 10 μg cholecalciferol = 400 IU vitamin D

[e]α-Tocopherol equivalents. 1 mg d-α-tocopherol = 1 α-TE.

[f]1 NE (niacin equivalent) is equal to 1 mg of niacin or 60 mg of dietary tryptophan.

Water-soluble vitamins							Minerals						
Vita-min C (mg)	Thiamin (mg)	Ribo-flavin (mg)	Niacin (mg NE)[f]	Vita-min B$_6$ (mg)	Folate (µg)	Vita-min B$_{12}$ (µg)	Calcium (mg)	Phos-phorus (mg)	Mag-nesium (mg)	Iron (mg)	Zinc (mg)	Iodine (µg)	Sele-nium (µg)
30	0.3	0.4	5	0.3	25	0.3	400	300	40	6	5	40	10
35	0.4	0.5	6	0.6	35	0.5	600	500	60	10	5	50	15
40	0.7	0.8	9	1.0	50	0.7	800	800	80	10	10	70	20
45	0.9	1.1	12	1.1	75	1.0	800	800	120	10	10	90	20
45	1.0	1.2	13	1.4	100	1.4	800	800	170	10	10	120	30
50	1.3	1.5	17	1.7	150	2.0	1,200	1,200	270	12	15	150	40
60	1.5	1.8	20	2.0	200	2.0	1,200	1,200	400	12	15	150	50
60	1.5	1.7	19	2.0	200	2.0	1,200	1,200	350	10	15	150	70
60	1.5	1.7	19	2.0	200	2.0	800	800	350	10	15	150	70
60	1.2	1.4	15	2.0	200	2.0	800	800	350	10	15	150	70
50	1.1	1.3	15	1.4	150	2.0	1,200	1,200	280	15	12	150	45
60	1.1	1.3	15	1.5	180	2.0	1,200	1,200	300	15	12	150	50
60	1.1	1.3	15	1.6	180	2.0	1,200	1,200	280	15	12	150	55
60	1.1	1.3	15	1.6	180	2.0	800	800	280	15	12	150	55
60	1.0	1.2	13	1.6	180	2.0	800	800	280	10	12	150	55
70	1.5	1.6	17	2.2	400	2.2	1,200	1,200	320	30	15	175	65
95	1.6	1.8	20	2.1	280	2.6	1,200	1,200	355	15	19	200	75
90	1.6	1.7	20	2.1	260	2.6	1,200	1,200	340	15	16	200	75

From Food and Nutrition Board, National Academy of Sciences–National Research Council, Washington, D.C., 1989.

[a]The allowances, expressed as average daily intakes over time, are intended to provide for individual variations among most normal persons as they live in the United States under usual environmental stresses. Diets should be based on a variety of common foods in order to provide other nutrients for which human requirements have been less well defined.

[b]Weights and heights of Reference Adults are actual medians for the U.S. population of the designated age, as reported by NHANES II. The median weights and heights of those under 19 years of age were taken from Hamill et al. (1979). The use of these figures does not imply that the height-to-weight ratios are ideal.

[c]Retinol equivalents. 1 Retinol equivalent = 1µg retinol or 6 µg β-carotene.

[d]As cholecaliferol. 10 µg cholecalciferol = 400 IU vitamin D

[e]α-Tocopherol equivalents. 1 mg d-α-tocopherol = 1 α-TE.

[f]1 NE (niacin equivalent) is equal to 1 mg of niacin or 60 mg of dietary tryptophan.

Unit 1

ESTIMATED SAFE AND ADEQUATE DAILY DIETARY INTAKES OF SELECTED VITAMINS AND MINERALS[a]

Category	Age (years)	Vitamins	
		Biotin (µg)	Pantothenic acid (mg)
Infants	0-0.5	10	2
	0.5-1	15	3
Children and adolescents	1-3	20	3
	4-6	25	3-4
	7-10	30	4-5
	11 +	30-100	4-7
Adults		30-100	4-7

Category	Age (years)	Trace elements[b]				
		Copper (mg)	Manganese (mg)	Fluoride (mg)	Chromium (µg)	Molybdenum (µg)
Infants	0-0.5	0.4-0.6	0.3-0.6	0.1-0.5	10-40	15-30
	0.5-1	0.6-0.7	0.6-1.0	0.2-1.0	20-60	20-40
Children and adolescents	1-3	0.7-1.0	1.0-1.5	0.5-1.5	20-80	25-50
	4-6	1.0-1.5	1.5-2.0	1.0-2.5	30-120	30-75
	7-10	1.0-2.0	2.0-3.0	1.5-2.5	50-200	50-150
	11 +	1.5-2.5	2.0-5.0	1.5-2.5	50-200	75-250
Adults		1.5-3.0	2.0-5.0	1.5-4.0	50-200	75-250

From Food and Nutrition Board, National Academy of Sciences-National Research Council, Washington, D.C., 1989.

[a]Because there is less information on which to base allowances, these figures are not given in the main table of RDA and are provided here in the form of ranges of recommended intakes.

[b]Since the toxic levels for many trace elements may be only several times usual intakes, the upper levels for the trace elements given in this table should not be habitually exceeded.

ESTIMATED SODIUM, CHLORIDE, AND POTASSIUM MINIMUM REQUIREMENTS OF HEALTHY PERSONS[a]

Age	Weight (kg)[a]	Sodium (mg)[a,b]	Chloride (mg)[a,b]	Potassium (mg)[c]
Months				
0-5	4.5	120	180	500
6-11	8.9	200	300	700
Years				
1	11.0	225	350	1,000
2-5	16.0	300	500	1,400
6-9	25.0	400	600	1,600
10-18	50.0	500	750	2,000
>18[d]	70.0	500	750	2,000

From Food and Nutrition Board, National Academy of Sciences-National Research Council, Washington, D.C., 1989.

[a]No allowance has been included for large, prolonged losses from the skin through sweat.

[b]There is no evidence that higher intakes confer any health benefit.

[c]Desirable intakes of potassium may considerably exceed these values (~3,500 mg for adults).

[d]No allowance included for growth. Values for those below 18 years assume a growth rate at the 50th percentile reported by the National Center for Health Statistics and averaged for males and females.

Median height and weights and recommended energy intake

Category	Age (year) or condition	Weight (kg)	Weight (lb)	Height (cm)	Height (in)	REE[a] (kcal/day)	Multiples of REE	Average Energy Allowance (kcal)[b] Per kg	Average Energy Allowance (kcal)[b] Per day[c]
Infants	0.0-0.5	6	13	60	24	320		108	650
	0.5-1.0	9	20	71	28	500		98	850
Children	1-3	13	29	90	35	740		102	1,300
	4-6	20	44	112	44	950		90	1,800
	7-10	28	62	132	52	1,130		70	2,000
Males	11-14	45	99	157	62	1,440	1.70	55	2,500
	15-18	66	145	176	69	1,760	1.67	45	3,000
	19-24	72	160	177	70	1,780	1.67	40	2,900
	25-50	79	174	176	70	1,800	1.60	37	2,900
	51+	77	170	173	68	1,530	1.50	30	2,300
Females	11-14	46	101	157	62	1,310	1.67	47	2,200
	15-18	55	120	163	64	1,370	1.60	40	2,200
	19-24	58	128	164	65	1,350	1.60	38	2,200
	25-50	63	138	163	64	1,380	1.55	36	2,200
	51+	65	143	160	63	1,280	1.50	30	1,900
Pregnant	1st trimester								+0
	2nd trimester								+300
	3rd trimester								+300
Lactating	1st 6 months								+500
	2nd 6 months								+500

[a]Resting energy expenditure.

[b]In the range of light to moderate activity, the coefficient of variation is ±20%.

[c]Figure is rounded.

From Recommended Dietary Allowances, Food and Nutrition Board National Academy of Sciences–National Research Council, Washington, D.C., 1989.

The data is this table have been assembled from the observed median heights and weights of children together with desirable weights for adults for the mean heights of men (70 inches) and women (64 inches) between the ages of 18 and 34 years as surveyed in the United States population (HEW/NCHS data). The energy allowances for the young adults are for men and women doing light work. The allowances for the two older age groups represent mean energy needs over these age spans, allowing for a 2% decrease in basal (resting) metabolic rate per decade and a reduction in activity of 200 kcal/day for men and women between 51 and 75 years, 500 kcal for men over 75 years and 400 kcal for women over 75. The customary range of daily energy output is shown for adults in parentheses and is based on a variation in energy needs of ±400 kcal at any one age, emphasizing the wide range of energy intakes appropriate for any group of people.

Energy allowances for children through age 18 are based on medium energy intakes of children these ages followed in longitudinal growth studies. The values in parentheses are 10th and 90th percentiles of energy intake, to indicate the range of energy consumption among children of these ages.

Ranges of daily water requirements at different ages under normal conditions

Age	Average body weight (kg)	Total water requirements per 24 hours (ml)	Water requirements per kg per 24 hours (ml)
3 days	3.0	250-300	80-100
10 days	3.2	400-500	125-150
3 months	5.4	750-850	140-160
6 months	7.3	950-1100	130-155
9 months	8.6	1100-1250	125-145
1 year	9.5	1150-1300	120-135
2 years	11.8	1350-1500	115-125
4 years	16.2	1600-1800	100-110
6 years	20.0	1800-2000	90-100
10 years	28.7	2000-2500	70-85
14 years	45.0	2200-2700	50-60
18 years	54.0	2200-2700	40-50

From Behrman RE and Vaughan VC, editors: Nelson textbook of pediatrics, ed 3, Philadelphia, 1987, WB Saunders Co, p 115.

Unit 1

SLEEP ASSESSMENT

A sleep history is usually taken during the general health history. However, when sleep problems are identified, a more detailed history of sleep and awake patterns is needed for planning appropriate intervention (see pp. 172-175). The following information includes a summary of a comprehensive sleep history and a chart for parents to record the child's sleep/awake habits.

Assessment of sleep problems in children*

General history of chief complaint

Ask parents/child to describe sleep problems; record in their words

Inquire about onset, duration, character, frequency, and consistency of sleep problems

Circumstances surrounding onset (birth of sibling, start of toilet training, death of significant other, move from crib to bed)

Circumstances that aggravate problem, i.e., overtiredness, family conflict, or disrupted routine (visitors)

Remedies used to correct problem and results of interventions

24-hour sleep history

Time and regularity of meals†
  Family members present
  Activities afterward, especially evening meal
Time of night and day sleep periods
  Hours of sleep and waking
  Hours of being put to bed and taken out of bed
  How bedtime is decided (when child looks tired or at a time decided by parent; do both parents agree on bedtime?)
Pre-bedtime or nap rituals (bath, bottle or breast-feeding, snack, television, active or quiet playing, story)
  Mood before nap or bedtime (wide awake, sleepy, happy, cranky)
  Which parent(s) participates in nap or bedtime rituals?
Nap and bedtime rituals
  Where is child allowed to fall asleep? (own bed or crib, couch, parent's bed, someone's lap, other)
  Is child helped to fall asleep? (rocked, walked, patted, given pacifier or bottle, placed in room with light, television, radio, or tape recorder on, other)
  Are patterns consistent each time or do they vary?
  Does child awake if sleep aids are changed or taken away? (placed in own bed, television turned off, other)
  Does child verbally insist that parents stay in room?
  Child's behaviors if refuses to go to sleep or stay in room
    If child complains of fears, how convincing are the fears?

Sleep environment
  Number of bedrooms
  Location of bedrooms, especially in relation to parent(s)' room
  Sensory features (light on, door open or closed, noise level, temperature)
Nightwakings
  Time, frequency, and duration
  Child's behavior (call out, cry, come out of room, appear frightened, confused, or upset)
  Parent(s)' responses (let child cry, go in immediately, take to own bed, feed, pick up, rock, give pacifier, talk, scold, threaten, other)
  Conditions that reestablish sleep
    Do they always work?
    How long do the interventions take to work?
    Which parents intervene?
    Do both parents use same or different approach?
Daytime sleepiness
  Occurrence of falling asleep at inappropriate times (circumstances, suddenness and irresistibility of onset, length of sleep, mood on awakening)
  Signs of fatigue (yawning, lying down, as well as overactivity, impulsivity, distractibility, irritability, temper tantrums)

Past sleep history

Sleep patterns since infancy, especially age when slept during the night, stopped daytime naps, later bedtime
Response to changes in sleep arrangements (crib to bed, different room or house, other)
Sleep behaviors (restlessness, snoring, sleepwalking, nightmares, partial wakings [young child may wake confused,

crying, and thrashing, but does not respond to parent; falls asleep with intervention if not excessively disturbed])
Parent(s)' perception of child's sleep habits (good or poor sleeper, light or deep sleeper, needs little sleep)
Family history of sleep problems (sibling behavior imitated by child; some sleep disorders, e.g. as narcolepsy and enuresis, tend to recur in families)

---

*Not all of these areas need to be assessed with every family. For example, if nightwakings are not a problem, this section of the interview can be eliminated.
†A convenient point to start the 24-hour history is the evening meal.
Adapted from Ferber R: Assessment procedures for diagnosis of sleep disorders in children. In Noshpitz J, editor: Sleep disorders for the clinician, London, 1987, Butterworths, pp 185-193.

TWO-WEEK SLEEP RECORD

PATIENT'S NAME _____   PARENT'S NAME _____

PATIENT'S DATE OF BIRTH _____   ADDRESS _____

DATE OF SLEEP RECORD: FROM ___ TO ___ TELEPHONE NUMBER _____

INSTRUCTIONS:

Leave blank the periods your child is awake.	Mark your child's bedtimes with downward-pointing arrows. ↓

Mon	sleep	nap	sleep
Tue	sleep	nap	sleep

Fill in the times your child is asleep with shaded boxes.	Mark the times your child gets up in the morning and after naps with arrows pointing upwards. ↑

	Midnight	_____ AM _____					Noon	_____ PM _____					Midnight
Day		2:00	4:00	6:00	8:00	10:00	Noon	2:00	4:00	6:00	8:00	10:00	

SPECIAL OBSERVATIONS AND NOTES: _____

_____

_____

_____

This section may be photocopied and distributed to families.

Modified from Ferber R: Solve Your Child's Sleep Problems, New York, Simon & Schuster, 1985.

GROWTH MEASUREMENTS

This section primarily includes reference data for evaluating and recording a child's growth. It begins with a comparison of the general trends in physical growth throughout childhood and a summary of pubertal sexual development. Included next is a chart illustrating the sequence of tooth eruption and shed-ding, which is another parameter of growth. The remainder of the section consists of tables and charts of height, weight, head circumference, triceps skinfold measurements, and midarm circumference for girls and boys at different ages.

General trends in physical growth during childhood

Age	Weight*	Height*
Infants		
Birth-6 months	Weekly gain: 140-200 g (5-7 ounces) Birth weight doubles by end of first 6 months†	Monthly gain: 2.5 cm (1 inch)
6-12 months	Weekly gain: 85-140 g (3-5 ounces) Birth weight triples by end of first year	Monthly gain: 1.25 cm (0.5 inch) Birth length increases by approximately 50% by end of first year
Toddlers	Birth weight quadruples by age 2½ years Yearly gain: 2-3 kg (4.4-6.6 pounds)	Height at 2 years is approximately 50% of eventual adult height Gain during second year: about 12 cm (4.8 inches) Gain during third year: about 6-8 cm (2.4-3.2 inches)
Preschoolers	Yearly gain: 2-3 kg (4.4-6.6 pounds)	Birth length doubles by 4 years of age Yearly gain: 6-8 cm (2.4-3.2 inches)
School-age children	Yearly gain: 2-3 kg (4.4-6.6 pounds)	Yearly gain after age 6 years: 5.0 cm (2 inches) Birth length triples by about 13 years of age
Pubertal growth spurt		
Females—between 10 and 14 years	Weight gain: 7-25 kg (15-55 pounds) Mean: 17.5 kg (38.1 pounds)	Height gain: 5-25 cm (2-10 inches); approximately 95% of mature height achieved by onset of menarche or skeletal age of 13 years Mean: 20.5 cm (8.2 inches)
Males—between 12 and 16 years	Weight gain: 7-30 kg (15-65 pounds) Mean: 23.7 kg (52.1 pounds)	Height gain: 10-30 cm (4-12 inches); approximately 95% of mature height achieved by skeletal age of 15 years Mean: 27.5 cm (11 inches)

*Yearly height and weight gains for each age group represent averaged estimates from a variety of sources.

†A study by Jung E and Czaijka-Narins DM: Birth weight doubling and tripling times: an updated look at the effects of birth weight, sex, race, and type of feeding, Am J Clin Nutr 42:182-189, 1985, has shown the mean doubling time for birth weight to be 4.7 months and mean tripling time to be 14.7 months.

Sexual development in adolescent males (Tanner stages)

Stage 1 (prepubertal)

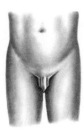

No pubic hair; essentially the same as during childhood; no distinction between hair on pubis and over the abdomen

Stage 2 (pubertal)

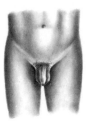

Fig. 1-39. Developmental stages of secondary sex characteristics and genital development in boys. Average age span is 12 to 16 years. (Modified from Marshall WA and Tanner JM: Arch Dis Child 45:13, 1970; Daniel WA and Paulshock BZ: Patient Care, May 13, 1979, pp. 122-124.)

Stage 3

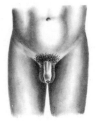

Initial enlargement of penis, mainly in length; testes and scrotum further enlarged; hair darker, coarser, and curly and spread sparsely over entire pubis

Stage 4

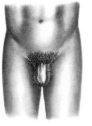

Increased size of penis with growth in diameter and development of glans; glans larger and broader; scrotum darker; pubic hair more abundant with curling but restricted to pubic area

Stage 5

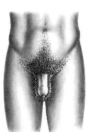

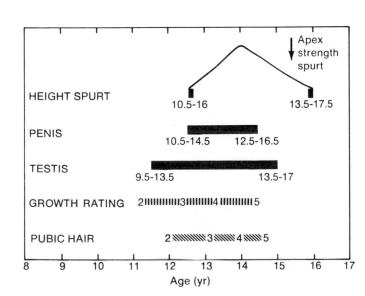

Fig. 1-40. Approximate timing of developmental changes in boys. Numbers across from growth rating and pubic hair indicate stages of development. Range of ages during which some of the changes occur is indicated by inclusive numbers. (From Marshall WA and Tanner JM: Arch Dis Child 45:13, 1970.)

Sexual development in adolescent females (Tanner stages)

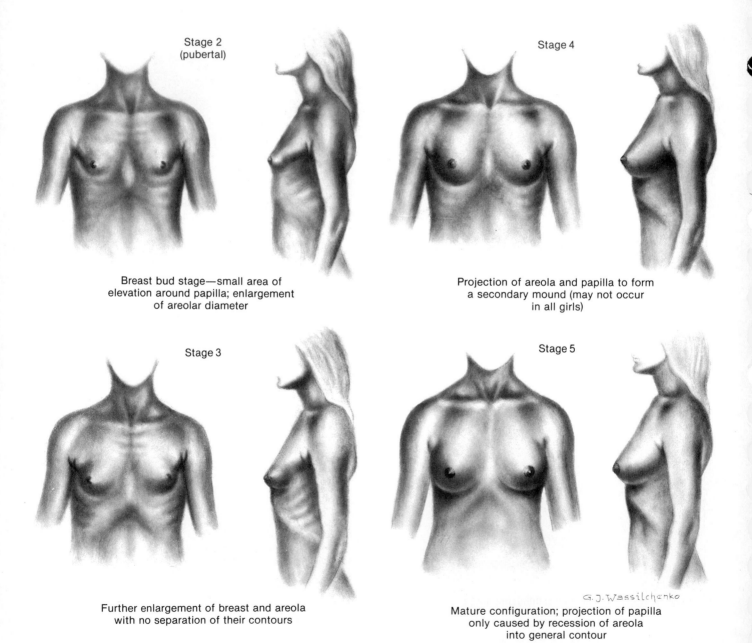

Stage 2
(pubertal)

Breast bud stage—small area of
elevation around papilla; enlargement
of areolar diameter

Stage 3

Further enlargement of breast and areola
with no separation of their contours

Stage 4

Projection of areola and papilla to form
a secondary mound (may not occur
in all girls)

Stage 5

Mature configuration; projection of papilla
only caused by recession of areola
into general contour

G.J.Wassilchenko

Fig. 1-41. Development of the breast in girls. Average age span is 11 to 13 years. Stage 1 (prepubertal—elevation of papilla only) is not shown. (Modified from Marshall WA and Tanner JM: Arch Dis Child 44:291, 1969; Daniel WA and Paulshock BZ: Patient Care, May 13, 1979, pp 122-124.)

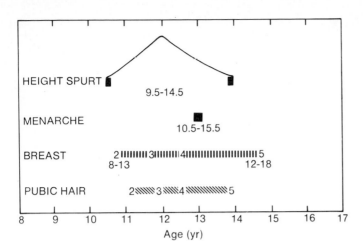

Fig. 1-42. Approximate timing of developmental changes in girls. Numbers across from breast and pubic hair indicate stages of development. Range of ages during which some of the changes occur is indicated by inclusive numbers. (From Marshall WA and Tanner JM: Arch Dis Child 45:13, 1970.)

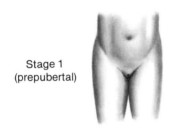

Stage 1
(prepubertal)

No pubic hair; essentially the same as during childhood; no distinction between hair on pubis and over the abdomen

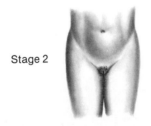

Stage 2

Sparse growth of long, straight, downy, and slightly pigmented hair extending along labia; between stages 2 and 3 begins to appear on pubis

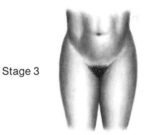

Stage 3

Hair darker, coarser, and curly and spread sparsely over entire pubis in the typical female triangle

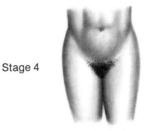

Stage 4

Pubic hair denser, curled, and adult in distribution but less abundant and restricted to the pubic area

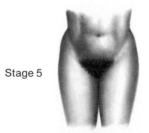

Stage 5

Hair adult in quantity, type, and pattern with spread to inner aspect of thighs

Fig. 1-43. Growth of pubic hair in girls. Average age span for stages 2 through 5 is 11 to 14 years. (Adapted from Marshall WA and Tanner JM: Arch Dis Child 44:291, 1969; Daniel WA and Paulshock BZ: Patient Care, May 13, 1979, pp 122-124.)

Unit 1

Sequence of tooth eruption and shedding

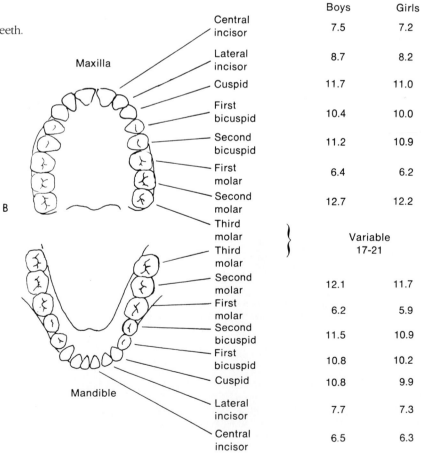

	Age of eruption (mo)			Average age of shedding (yr)
	Early	Average	Late	
Maxilla	6	9.6	12	7.5
	7	12.4	18	8
	11	18.3	24	11.5
	10	15.7	20	10.5
	13	26.2	31	10.5
Mandible	13	26.0	31	11
	10	15.1	30	10
	11	18.2	24	9.5
	7	11.5	15	7
	5	7.8	11	6

Fig. 1-44. A, Primary teeth. **B,** Secondary teeth.

	Average age of eruption (yr)	
	Boys	Girls
Central incisor	7.5	7.2
Lateral incisor	8.7	8.2
Cuspid	11.7	11.0
First bicuspid	10.4	10.0
Second bicuspid	11.2	10.9
First molar	6.4	6.2
Second molar	12.7	12.2
Third molar	Variable 17-21	
Third molar		
Second molar	12.1	11.7
First molar	6.2	5.9
Second bicuspid	11.5	10.9
First bicuspid	10.8	10.2
Cuspid	10.8	9.9
Lateral incisor	7.7	7.3
Central incisor	6.5	6.3

Growth standards of healthy Chinese children and adolescents (urban)*

Age (months or years)	Boys				Girls			
	Weight (kg)	Height (cm)	Head circumference (cm)	Chest circumference (cm)	Weight (kg)	Height (cm)	Head circumference (cm)	Chest circumference (cm)
Birth	3.27	50.6	34.3	32.8	3.17	50.0	33.7	32.6
1 mo	4.97	56.5	38.1	37.9	4.64	55.5	37.3	36.9
2 mo	5.95	59.6	39.7	40.0	5.49	58.4	38.7	38.9
3 mo	6.73	62.3	41.0	41.3	6.23	60.9	40.0	40.3
4 mo	7.32	64.4	42.0	42.3	6.69	62.9	41.0	41.1
5 mo	7.70	65.9	42.9	42.9	7.19	64.5	41.9	41.9
6 mo	8.22	68.1	43.9	43.8	7.62	66.7	42.8	42.7
8 mo	8.71	70.6	44.9	44.7	8.14	69.0	43.7	43.4
10 mo	9.14	72.9	45.7	45.4	8.57	71.4	44.5	44.2
12 mo	9.66	75.6	46.3	46.1	9.04	74.1	45.2	45.0
15 mo	10.15	78.3	46.8	46.8	9.54	76.9	45.6	45.8
18 mo	10.67	80.7	47.3	47.6	10.08	79.4	46.2	46.6
21 mo	11.18	83.0	47.8	48.3	10.56	81.7	46.7	47.3
24 mo	11.95	86.5	48.2	49.2	11.37	85.3	47.1	48.2
2½ yr	12.84	90.4	48.8	50.2	12.28	89.3	47.7	49.0
3 yr	13.63	93.8	49.1	50.8	13.1	92.8	48.1	49.8
3½ yr	14.45	97.2	49.4	51.5	14.00	96.3	48.5	50.5
4 yr	15.26	100.8	49.7	52.2	14.89	100.1	48.9	51.2
4¼ yr	16.07	103.9	50.0	53.0	15.63	103.1	49.1	51.8
5 yr	16.88	107.2	50.2	53.6	16.46	106.5	49.4	52.5
5½ yr	17.65	110.1	50.5	54.4	17.18	109.2	49.6	53.0
6 yr	19.25	114.7	50.8	55.6	18.67	113.9	50.0	54.2
7 yr	21.01	120.6	51.1	57.1	20.35	119.3	50.2	55.5
8 yr	23.08	125.3	51.4	58.8	22.43	124.6	50.6	57.1
9 yr	25.33	130.6	51.7	60.8	24.57	129.5	50.9	58.6
10 yr	27.15	134.4	51.9	62.0	27.05	134.8	51.3	60.7
11 yr	30.13	139.2	52.3	64.3	30.51	140.6	51.7	63.5
12 yr	33.05	144.2	52.7	66.5	34.82	146.6	52.3	67.2
13 yr	36.90	149.3	53.0	68.9	38.52	150.7	52.8	70.3
14 yr	42.03	156.5	53.5	72.4	42.26	153.7	53.1	73.3
15 yr	46.91	162.0	54.3	76.0	45.37	155.5	53.4	75.6
16 yr	50.90	165.6	54.9	78.8	47.43	156.8	53.8	76.6
17 yr	53.11	167.7	55.2	80.8	48.57	157.4	53.9	77.9

Adapted from Practical Pediatrics; edited by Peking Children Hospital, 1979.

*Measurements of rural Chinese children are slightly lower.

NOTE: A comparison of the average growth of American and Chinese children demonstrates that on the standard NCHS growth charts the mean height and weight for Chinese children falls on the 10th percentile, as compared to the mean growth measurements for American children, which comprise the 50th percentile.

Height and weight measurements for boys

Age*	Height by percentiles						Weight by percentiles					
	5		50		95		5		50		95	
	cm	inches	cm	inches	cm	inches	kg	lb	kg	lb	kg	lb
Birth	46.4	18¼	50.5	20	54.4	21½	2.54	5½	3.27	7¼	4.15	9¼
3 months	56.7	22¼	61.1	24	65.4	25¾	4.43	9¾	5.98	13¼	7.37	16¼
6 months	63.4	25	67.8	26¾	72.3	28½	6.20	13¾	7.85	17¼	9.46	20¾
9 months	68.0	26¾	72.3	28½	77.1	30¼	7.52	16½	9.18	20¼	10.93	24
1	71.7	28¼	76.1	30	81.2	32	8.43	18½	10.15	22½	11.99	26½
1½	77.5	30½	82.4	32½	88.1	34¾	9.59	21¼	11.47	25¼	13.44	29½
2†	82.5	32½	86.8	34¼	94.4	37¼	10.49	23¼	12.34	27¼	15.50	34¼
2½†	85.4	33½	90.4	35½	97.8	38½	11.27	24¾	13.52	29¾	16.61	36½
3	89.0	35	94.9	37¼	102.0	40¼	12.05	26½	14.62	32¼	17.77	39¼
3½	92.5	36½	99.1	39	106.1	41¾	12.84	28¼	15.68	34½	18.98	41¾
4	95.8	37¾	102.9	40½	109.9	43¼	13.64	30	16.69	36¾	20.27	44¾
4½	98.9	39	106.6	42	113.5	44¾	14.45	31¾	17.69	39	21.63	47¾
5	102.0	40¼	109.9	43¼	117.0	46	15.27	33¾	18.67	41¼	23.09	51
6	107.7	42½	116.1	45¾	123.5	48½	16.93	37¼	20.69	45½	26.34	58
7	113.0	44½	121.7	48	129.7	51	18.64	41	22.85	50¼	30.12	66½
8	118.1	46½	127.0	50	135.7	53½	20.40	45	25.30	55¾	34.51	76
9	122.9	48½	132.2	52	141.8	55¾	22.25	49	28.13	62	39.58	87¼
10	127.7	50¼	137.5	54¼	148.1	58¼	24.33	53¾	31.44	69¼	45.27	99¾
11	132.6	52¼	143.3	56½	154.9	61	26.80	59	35.30	77¾	51.47	113½
12	137.6	54¼	149.7	59	162.3	64	29.85	65¾	39.78	87¾	58.09	128
13	142.9	56¼	156.5	61½	169.8	66¾	33.64	74¼	44.95	99	65.02	143¼
14	148.8	58½	163.1	64¼	176.7	69½	38.22	84¼	50.77	112	72.13	159
15	155.2	61	169.0	66½	181.9	71½	43.11	95	56.71	125	79.12	174½
16	161.1	63½	173.5	68¼	185.4	73	47.74	105¼	62.10	137	85.62	188¾
17	164.9	65	176.2	69¼	187.3	73¾	51.50	113½	66.31	146¼	91.31	201¼
18	165.7	65¼	176.8	69½	187.6	73¾	53.97	119	68.88	151¾	95.76	211

Adapted from National Center for Health Statistics, Health Resources Administration, Department of Health, Education and Welfare, Hyattsville, Md. Values correspond with NCHS percentile curves (see Figs. 1-45 to 1-48). Conversion of metric data to approximate inches and pounds by Ross Laboratories.

*Years unless otherwise indicated.

†Height data include some recumbent length measurements, which make values slightly higher than if all measurements had been of stature (standing height).

Unit 1

Height and weight measurements for girls

	Height by percentiles						Weight by percentiles					
	5		50		95		5		50		95	
Age*	cm	inches	cm	inches	cm	inches	kg	lb	kg	lb	kg	lb
Birth	45.4	17¾	49.9	19¾	52.9	20¾	2.36	5¼	3.23	7	3.81	8½
3 months	55.4	21¾	59.5	23½	63.4	25	4.18	9¼	5.4	12	6.74	14¾
6 months	61.8	24¼	65.9	26	70.2	27¾	5.79	12¾	7.21	16	8.73	19¼
9 months	66.1	26	70.4	27¾	75.0	29½	7.0	15½	8.56	18¾	10.17	22½
1	69.8	27½	74.3	29¼	79.1	31¼	7.84	17¼	9.53	21	11.24	24¾
1½	76.0	30	80.9	31¾	86.1	34	8.92	19¾	10.82	23¾	12.76	28¼
2†	81.6	32¼	86.8	34¼	93.6	36¾	9.95	22	11.8	26	14.15	31¼
2½†	84.6	33¼	90.0	35½	96.6	38	10.8	23¾	13.03	28¾	15.76	34¾
3	88.3	34¾	94.1	37	100.6	39½	11.61	25½	14.1	31	17.22	38
3½	91.7	36	97.9	38½	104.5	41¼	12.37	27¼	15.07	33¼	18.59	41
4	95.0	37½	101.6	40	108.3	42¾	13.11	29	15.96	35¼	19.91	44
4½	98.1	38½	105.0	41¼	112.0	44	13.83	30½	16.81	37	21.24	46¾
5	101.1	39¾	108.4	42¾	115.6	45½	14.55	32	17.66	39	22.62	49¾
6	106.6	42	114.6	45	122.7	48¼	16.05	35½	19.52	43	25.75	56¾
7	111.8	44	120.6	47½	129.5	51	17.71	39	21.84	48¼	29.68	65½
8	116.9	46	126.4	49¾	136.2	53½	19.62	43¼	24.84	54¾	34.71	76½
9	122.1	48	132.2	52	142.9	56¼	21.82	48	28.46	62¾	40.64	89½
10	127.5	50¼	138.3	54½	149.5	58¾	24.36	53¾	32.55	71¾	47.17	104
11	133.5	52½	144.8	57	156.2	61½	27.24	60	36.95	81½	54.0	119
12	139.8	55	151.5	59¾	162.7	64	30.52	67¼	41.53	91½	60.81	134
13	145.2	57¼	157.1	61¾	168.1	66¼	34.14	75¼	46.1	101¾	67.3	148¼
14	148.7	58½	160.4	63¼	171.3	67½	37.76	83¼	50.28	110¾	73.08	161
15	150.5	59¼	161.8	63¾	172.8	68	40.99	90¼	53.68	118¼	77.78	171½
16	151.6	59¾	162.4	64	173.3	68¼	43.41	95¾	55.89	123¼	80.99	178½
17	152.7	60	163.1	64¼	173.5	68¼	44.74	98¾	56.69	125	82.46	181¾
18	153.6	60½	163.7	64½	173.6	68¼	45.26	99¾	56.62	124¾	82.47	181¾

Adapted from National Center for Health Statistics, Health Resources Administration, Department of Health, Education and Welfare, Hyattsville, Md. Values correspond with NCHS percentile curves (see Figs. 1-49 to 1-52). Conversion of metric data to approximate inches and pounds by Ross Laboratories.

*Years unless otherwise indicated.

†Height data include some recumbent length measurements, which make values slightly higher than if all measurements had been of stature (standing height).

NCHS growth percentiles

**BOYS: BIRTH TO AGE 36 MONTHS—PHYSICAL
GROWTH (LENGTH, WEIGHT), NCHS PERCENTILES**

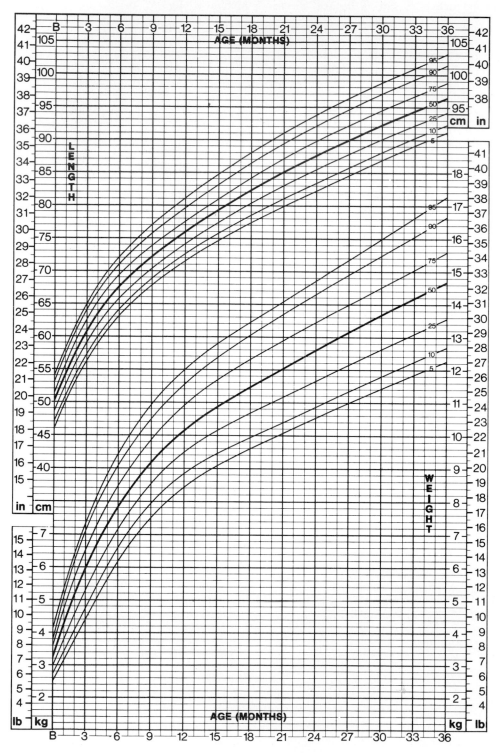

Fig. 1-45. Modified from Hamill PVV and others: Physical growth: National Center for Health Statistics percentiles, Am J Clin Nutr 32:607-629, 1979. (Data from the Fels Research Institute, Wright State University School of Medicine, Yellow Springs, Ohio. Provided as a service of Ross Laboratories, 1980.)

BOYS: BIRTH TO AGE 36 MONTHS—PHYSICAL GROWTH (HEAD CIRCUMFERENCE, LENGTH, WEIGHT), NCHS PERCENTILES

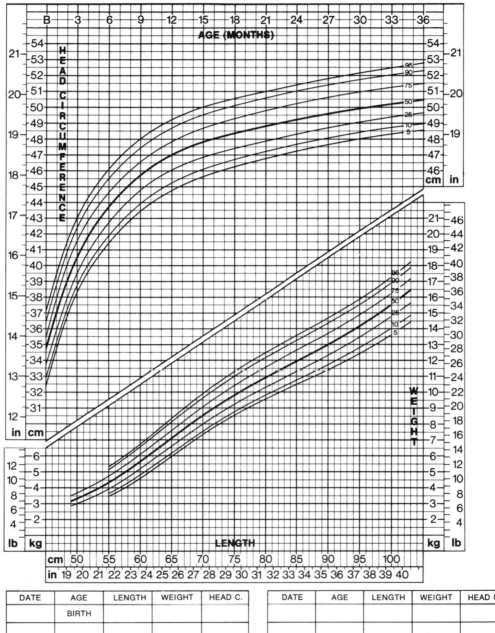

DATE	AGE	LENGTH	WEIGHT	HEAD C.
	BIRTH			

DATE	AGE	LENGTH	WEIGHT	HEAD C.

Fig. 1-46. Modified from Hamill PVV and others: Physical growth: National Center for Health Statistics percentiles, Am J Clin Nutr 32:607-629, 1979. (Data from the Fels Research Institute, Wright State University School of Medicine, Yellow Springs, Ohio. Provided as a service of Ross Laboratories, 1980.)

**BOYS: AGES 2 TO 18 YEARS—PHYSICAL GROWTH
(STATURE, WEIGHT), NCHS PERCENTILES**

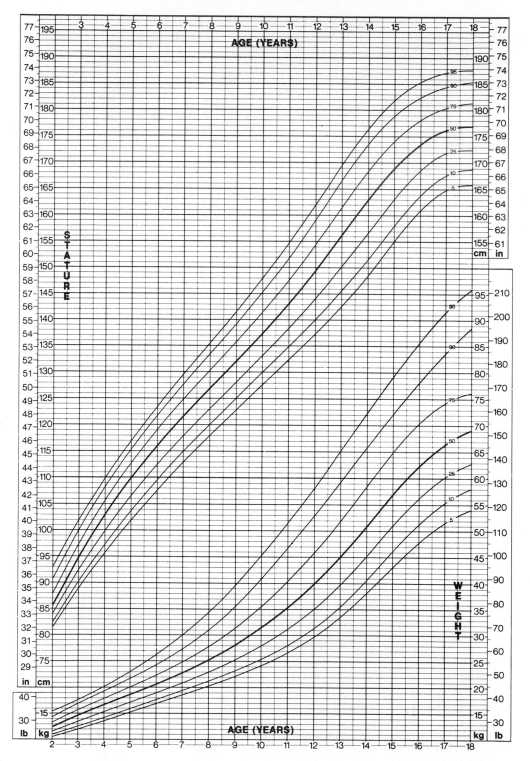

Fig. 1-47. Modified from Hamill PVV and others: Physical growth: National Center for Health Statistics percentiles, Am J Clin Nutr 32:607-629, 1979. (Data from the National Center for Health Statistics (NCHS), Hyattsville, Md. Provided as a service of Ross Laboratories, 1980.)

BOYS: PREPUBESCENT—PHYSICAL GROWTH (STATURE, WEIGHT), NCHS PERCENTILES

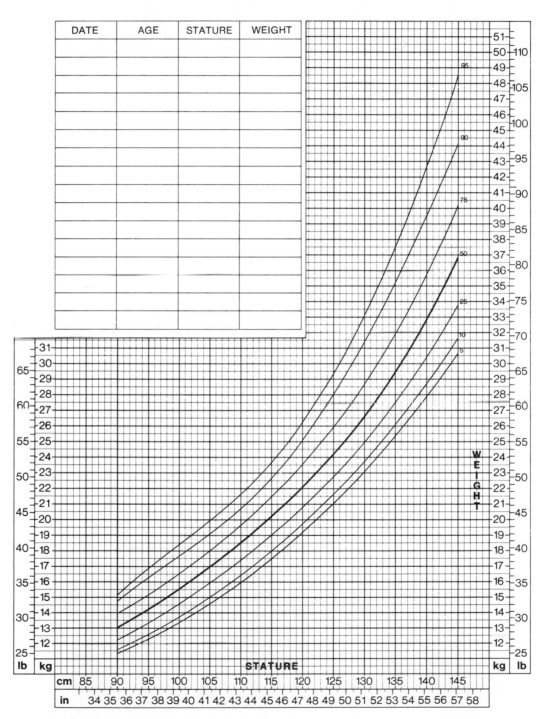

Fig. 1-48. Modified from Hamill PVV and others: Physical growth: National Center for Health Statistics percentiles, Am J Clin Nutr 32:607-629, 1979. (Data from the National Center for Health Statistics (NCHS), Hyattsville, Md. Provided as a service of Ross Laboratories, 1980.)

GIRLS: BIRTH TO AGE 36 MONTHS—PHYSICAL
GROWTH (LENGTH, WEIGHT), NCHS PERCENTILES

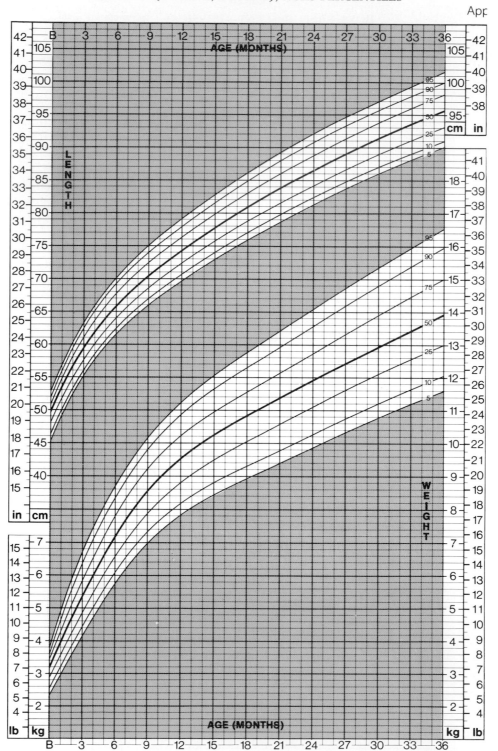

Fig. 1-49. Modified from Hamill PVV and others: Physical growth: National Center for Health Statistics percentiles, Am J Clin Nutr 32:607-629, 1979. (Data from Fels Research Institute, Wright State University School of Medicine, Yellow Springs, Ohio. Provided as a service of Ross Laboratories, 1980.)

GIRLS: BIRTH TO AGE 36 MONTHS—PHYSICAL GROWTH (HEAD CIRCUMFERENCE, LENGTH, WEIGHT), NCHS PERCENTILES

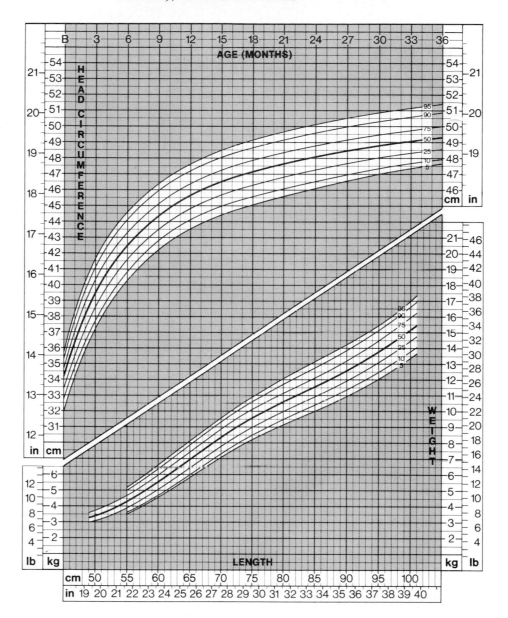

DATE	AGE	LENGTH	WEIGHT	HEAD C.
	BIRTH			

DATE	AGE	LENGTH	WEIGHT	HEAD C.

Fig. 1-50. Modified from Hamill PVV and others: Physical growth: National Center for Health Statistics percentiles, Am J Clin Nutr 32:607-629, 1979. (Data from Fels Research Institute, Wright State University School of Medicine, Yellow Springs, Ohio. Provided as a service of Ross Laboratories, 1980.)

GIRLS: AGES 2 TO 18 YEARS—PHYSICAL GROWTH (STATURE, WEIGHT), NCHS PERCENTILES

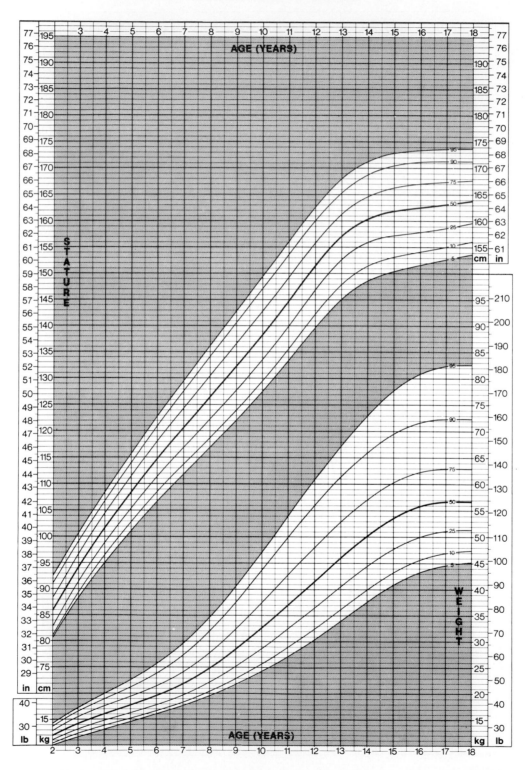

Fig. 1-51. Modified from Hamill PVV and others: Physical growth: National Center for Health Statistics percentiles, Am J Clin Nutr 32:607-629, 1979. (Data from the National Center for Health Statistics (NCHS) Hyattsville, Md. Provided as a service of Ross Laboratories, 1980.)

GIRLS: PREPUBESCENT—PHYSICAL GROWTH
(STATURE, WEIGHT), NCHS PERCENTILES

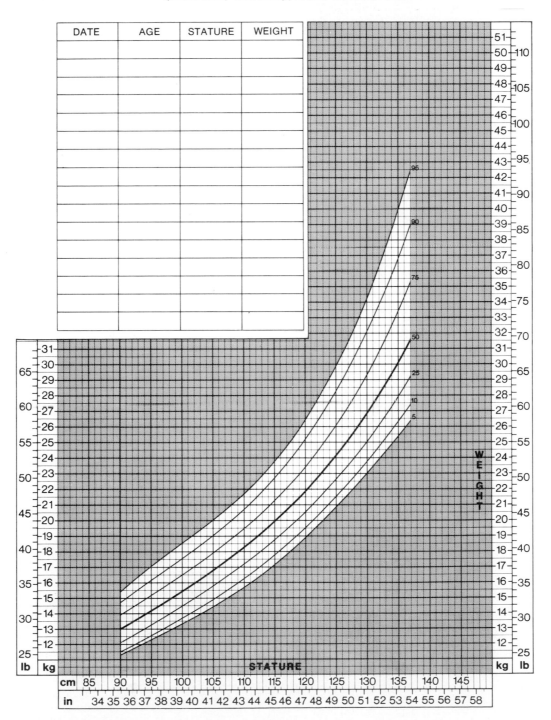

Fig. 1-52. Modified from Hamill PVV and others: Physical growth: National Center for Health Statistics percentiles, Am J Clin Nutr 32:607-629, 1979. (Data from the National Center for Health Statistics (NCHS) Hyattsville, Md. Provided as a service of Ross Laboratories, 1980.)

Head circumference charts

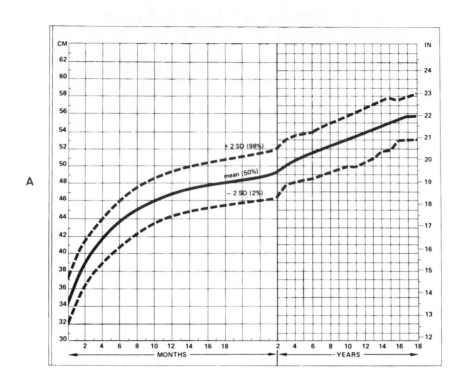

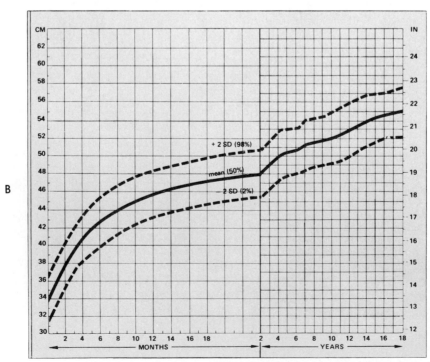

Fig. 1-53. A, Head circumference chart for boys. **B,** Head circumference chart for girls. (From Nellhaus G: Composite international and interracial graphs, Pediatrics 41:106, 1968. Reprinted by permission. Copyright American Academy of Pediatrics, 1968.)

Measurement of triceps skinfold thickness

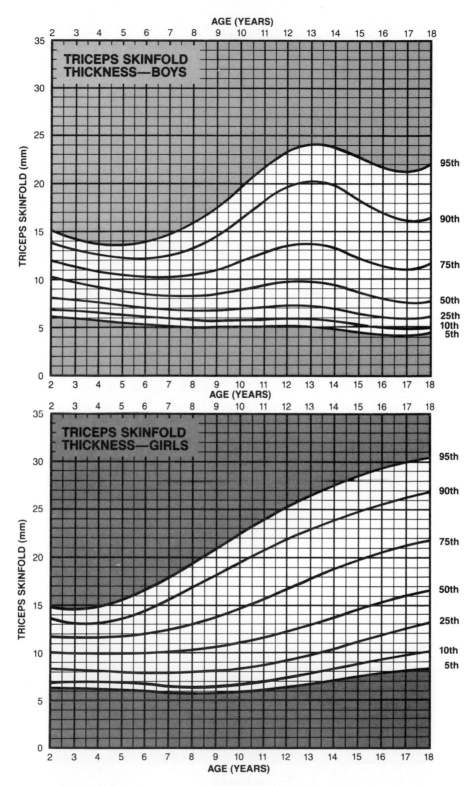

Fig. 1-54. Triceps skinfold. (Modified from Johnson CL, et al: Basic data on anthropometric measurements and angular measurements of the hip and knee joints for selected age groups, 1-74 years of age, United States, 1972-1975. Vital and Health Statistics Series 11, No. 219. DHHS Publication No. (PHS) 81-1669, 1981. Provided as a service of Ross Laboratories, Copyright 1983, Columbus, Ohio, 43216. May be copied for individual patient use.)

Measurement of midarm circumference

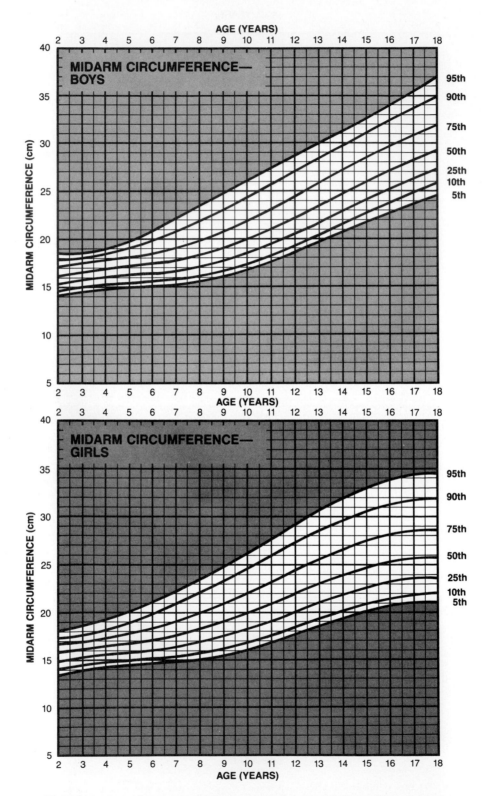

Fig. 1-55. Midarm circumference. (Modified from Johnson CL, et al: Basic data on anthropometric measurements and angular measurements of the hip and knee joints for selected age groups, 1-74 years of age, United States, 1971-1975. Vital Health Statistics Series 11, No. 219. DHHS Publication No. [PHS] 81-1669, 1981. Provided as a service of Ross Laboratories, Copyright 1983, Columbus, Ohio, 43216. May be copied for individual patient use.)

ASSESSMENT OF DEVELOPMENT
Revised Denver Prescreening Developmental Questionnaire*

The Revised Prescreening Developmental Questionnaire (R-PDQ) is a revision of the original PDQ. Advantages of the R-PDQ include the addition and arrangement of items to be more age-appropriate, simplified parent scoring, and easier comparison with Denver Developmental Screening Test (DDST) norms for professionals. The R-PDQ is a parent-answered prescreen consisting of 105 questions from the DDST, although only a subset of questions are asked for each age group. With less educated parents, the form may need to be read to the caregiver.

Preparation and scoring of the R-PDQ include the following:
1. Calculate the child's age as detailed in the DDST manual and choose the appropriate form* for the child: orange (0-9 months), purple (9-24 months), gold (2-4 years), white (4-6 years). (See sample of 0-9 month form, Fig. 1-56).
2. Give the appropriate form to the child's caregiver and have person note relationship to the child. Have the caregiver answer questions until: (1) 3 "NOs" are circled (they do not have to be consecutive); or (2) all of the questions on both sides of the form have been answered.
3. Check form to see that all appropriate questions have been answered.

---

*Forms and complete instructions are available from Denver Developmental Materials, Inc, PO Box 6919, Denver, CO 80206-0919 (303) 355-4729. A revised version of the R-PDQ based on the Denver II (see p. 118) should be available by midyear 1990.

†Suggested Denver Developmental Activities are available from Denver Developmental Materials, Inc.

4. Review "YES" and "NO" responses. Ensure that the child's caregiver understood each question and scored the items correctly. Give particular attention to the scoring of questions that require verbal responses by the child and that require the child to draw.
5. Identify "delays" (item passed by 90% of children at a younger age than the child being screened). Ages at which 90% of children in the DDST sample passed the items are indicated in parentheses in the "For Office Use" column. These ages are shown in months and weeks up to 24 months, and in years and months after 24 months. Highlight "delays" by circling the 90% age in parentheses to the right of the item that the child was not able to perform.
6. Children who have no "delays" are considered to be developing normally.
7. If a child has one "delay," give the caregiver age-appropriate developmental activities to pursue with the child,† and schedule the child for rescreening with the R-PDQ 1 month later. If on rescreening a month later the child has one or more "delays," schedule second-stage screening with the DDST as soon as possible.
8. If a child has two or more "delays" on the first-stage screening with the R-PDQ, schedule a second-stage screening with the DDST as soon as possible. If, on second-stage screening with the DDST, a child receives other than normal results, schedule the child for a diagnostic evaluation.

Denver Developmental Screening Test/Revised Denver Developmental Screening Test

The Denver Developmental Screening Test (DDST) and the Revised Denver Developmental Screening Test (DDST-R) (The major difference between the original DDST and the DDST-R is the arrangement of items on the form.) assess gross motor, language, fine motor, adaptive, and personal-social development in children from 1 month to 6 years (Fig. 1-57, *A* and *B*). They are accompanied by a detailed instruction manual.* Following are general guidelines for administering the DDST/DDST-R:
1. Draw a vertical line through the four sectors to represent the child's chronologic age in the DDST or mark the age line in the DDST-R. In children born prematurely, adjust the age by subtracting the number of months of prematurity from the chronologic age. (Instructions for calculating exact chronologic age are detailed in the manual.)
2. Explain to the parents that the DDST is not an intelligence test but a systematic appraisal of the child's present development. Stress that the child is not expected to perform each item.
3. Test the child for each item intersected by the age line, selecting initially items he is likely to pass. If the child is unable to perform these, select items to the left of the line until he performs them successfully. Each sector should

---

*To ensure that the Denver Developmental Screening Test is administered and interpreted in the prescribed manner, it is recommended that those intending to administer the DDST first take the proficiency test which can be obtained with the DDST forms and instructional manual from Denver Developmental Materials, PO Box 6919, Denver, CO 80206-0919 (303) 355-4729.

have at least three items that are passed and three items that are failed.
4. Mark each item with a "P" for passing.
5. Present the test as a game but lessen distraction by introducing only one testing object at a time. Choose a quiet, isolated area for testing.
6. Determine the score by counting the number of *delays,* defined as "failure to perform an item that is passed by 90% of children of the same age or any item that falls completely to the left of the age line." Possible scores are as follows:
   a. **Abnormal**—two or more sectors with two or more delays, or one sector with two or more delays plus one or more sectors with one delay and in the same sector no passes through the age line
   b. **Questionable**—one sector with two or more delays or one or more sectors with one delay and in that same sector, no passes through the age line
   c. **Untestable**—large number of refusals that if tested would yield questionable or abnormal results
   d. **Normal**—any score that does not meet the above three criteria
7. Ask the parent if the child's performance was typical. Explain the results of the test, emphasizing passes first, failures not scored as delays second, and delays last. Note the parent's response to abnormal or questionable results. Retest any child without a normal score.

Unit 1

REVISED DENVER PRESCREENING

0-9 MONTHS (R-PDQ)

Child's Name _____

Person Completing R-PDQ: _____

Relation to Child: _____

CONTINUE ANSWERING UNTIL 3 "NOs" ARE CIRCLED

			For Office Use

1. Equal Movements
When your baby is lying on his/her back, can (s)he move each of his/her arms as easily as the other and each of the legs as easily as the other? Answer No if your child makes jerky or uncoordinated movements with one or both of his/her arms or legs.

    Yes   No   (0) FMA

2. Stomach Lifts Head
When your baby is on his/her stomach on a flat surface, can (s)he lift his/her head off the surface?

    Yes   No   (0-3) GM

3. Regards Face
When your baby is lying on his/her back, can (s)he look at you and watch your face?

    Yes   No   (1) PS

4. Follows To Midline
When your child is on his/her back, can (s)he follow your movement by turning his/her head from one side to facing directly forward?

    Yes   No   (1-1) FMA

5. Responds To Bell
Does your child respond with eye movements, change in breathing or other change in activity to a bell or rattle sounded outside his/her line of vision?

    Yes   No   (1-2) L

6. Vocalizes Not Crying
Does your child make sounds other than crying, such as gurgling, cooing, or babbling?

    Yes   No   (1-3) L

7. Smiles Responsively
When you smile and talk to your baby, does (s)he smile back at you?

    Yes   No   (1-3) PS

DEVELOPMENTAL QUESTIONNAIRE

For Office Use

Today's Date:	_____ yr	_____ mo	_____ day
Child's Birthdate:	_____ yr	_____ mo	_____ day
Subtract to get Child's Exact Age:	_____ yr	_____ mo	_____ day
R-PDQ Age: ( )	_____ yr	_____ mo	_____ completed wks)

	For Office Use

8. Follows Past Midline
When your child is on his/her back, does (s)he follow your movement by turning his/her head from one side *almost all the way to the other side?*

    Yes   No   (2-2) FMA

9. Stomach, Head Up 45°
When your baby is on his/her stomach on a flat surface, can (s)he lift his/her head 45°?

    Yes   No   (2-2) GM

10. Stomach, Head Up 90°
When your baby is on his/her stomach on a flat surface, can (s)he lift his/her head 90°?

    Yes   No   (3) GM

11. Laughs
Does your baby laugh out loud without being tickled or touched?

    Yes   No   (3-1) L

12. Hands Together
Does your baby play with his/her hands by touching them together?

    Yes   No   (3-3) FMA

13. Follows 180°
When your child is on his/her back, does (s)he follow your movement from one side *all the way* to the other side?

    Yes   No   (4) FMA

14. Grasps Rattle
It is important that you follow instructions carefully. Do *not* place the pencil in the palm of your child's hand. When you touch the pencil to the back or tips of your baby's fingers, does your baby grasp the pencil for a few seconds?

  TRY THIS   NOT THIS

    Yes   No   (4) FMA

(Please turn page)

©Wm. K. Frankenburg, M.D., 1975, 1986

Fig. 1-56. Revised Prescreening Developmental Questionnaire. (The first page is reprinted with permission of William K. Frankenburg, MD. Copyright 1975, 1986, WK Frankenburg, MD.)

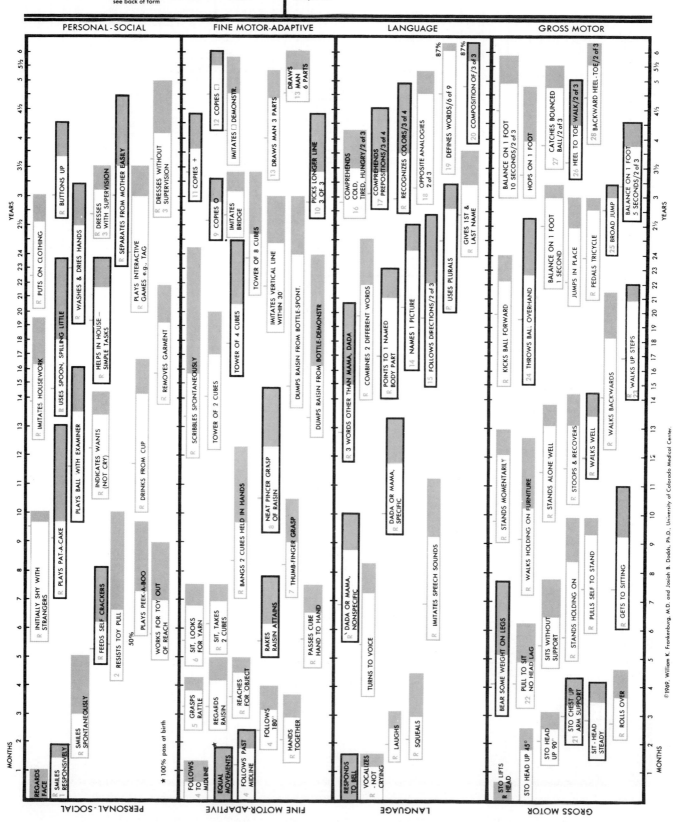

Fig. 1-57. A, Denver Developmental Screening Test. (From Frankenburg WK and Dodds JB, University of Colorado Medical Center, 1969.)

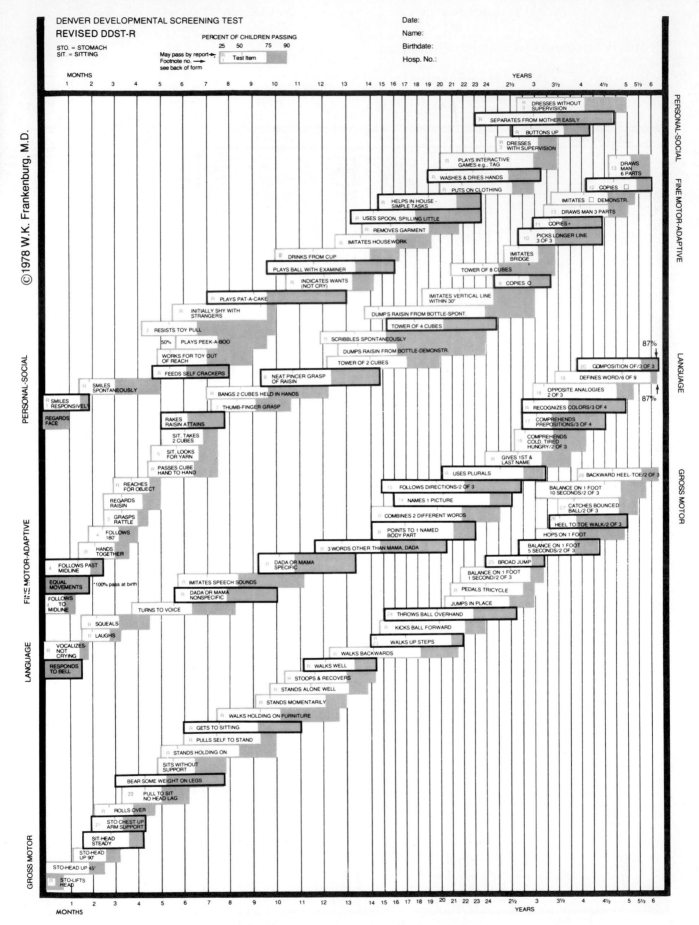

Fig. 1-57, cont'd. B, DDST revised (DDST-R). Resembling a growth curve, this form places items at lowest age level starting at bottom left and progresses upward to right with increasing age. (From Frankenburg WK, Sciarillo W, and Burgess D: The newly abbreviated and revised Denver Developmental Screening Test, J Pediatr 99(6):995-999, 1981.)

Unit 1

DATE:

NAME:

DIRECTIONS   BIRTHDATE:

HOSP. NO.:

1. Try to get child to smile by smiling, talking or waving to him. Do not touch him.
2. When child is playing with toy, pull it away from him. Pass if he resists.
3. Child does not have to be able to tie shoes or button in the back.
4. Move yarn slowly in an arc from one side to the other, about 6" above child's face. Pass if eyes follow 90° to midline. (Past midline; 180°)
5. Pass if child grasps rattle when it is touched to the backs or tips of fingers.
6. Pass if child continues to look where yarn disappeared or tries to see where it went. Yarn should be dropped quickly from sight from tester's hand without arm movement.
7. Pass if child picks up raisin with any part of thumb and a finger.
8. Pass if child picks up raisin with the ends of thumb and index finger using an over hand approach.

9. Pass any enclosed form. Fail continuous round motions.
10. Which line is longer? (Not bigger.) Turn paper upside down and repeat. (3/3 or 5/6)
11. Pass any crossing lines.
12. Have child copy first. If failed, demonstrate

When giving items 9, 11 and 12, do not name the forms. Do not demonstrate 9 and 11.

13. When scoring, each pair (2 arms, 2 legs, etc.) counts as one part.
14. Point to picture and have child name it. (No credit is given for sounds only.)

  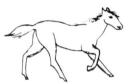 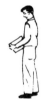

C

15. Tell child to: Give block to Mommie; put block on table; put block on floor. Pass 2 of 3. (Do not help child by pointing, moving head or eyes.)
16. Ask child: What do you do when you are cold? ..hungry? ..tired? Pass 2 of 3.
17. Tell child to: Put block on table; under table; in front of chair, behind chair. Pass 3 of 4. (Do not help child by pointing, moving head or eyes.)
18. Ask child: If fire is hot, ice is ?; Mother is a woman, Dad is a ?; a horse is big, a mouse is ?. Pass 2 of 3.
19. Ask child: What is a ball? ..lake? ..desk? ..house? ..banana? ..curtain? ..ceiling? ..hedge? ..pavement? Pass if defined in terms of use, shape, what it is made of or general category (such as banana is fruit, not just yellow). Pass 6 of 9.
20. Ask child: What is a spoon made of? ..a shoe made of? ..a door made of? (No other objects may be substituted.) Pass 3 of 3.
21. When placed on stomach, child lifts chest off table with support of forearms and/or hands.
22. When child is on back, grasp his hands and pull him to sitting. Pass if head does not hang back.
23. Child may use wall or rail only, not person. May not crawl.
24. Child must throw ball overhand 3 feet to within arm's reach of tester.
25. Child must perform standing broad jump over width of test sheet. (8-1/2 inches)
26. Tell child to walk forward, 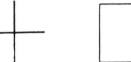 heel within 1 inch of toe. Tester may demonstrate. Child must walk 4 consecutive steps, 2 out of 3 trials.
27. Bounce ball to child who should stand 3 feet away from tester. Child must catch ball with hands, not arms, 2 out of 3 trials.
28. Tell child to walk backward, 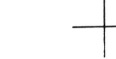 toe within 1 inch of heel. Tester may demonstrate. Child must walk 4 consecutive steps, 2 out of 3 trials.

DATE AND BEHAVIORAL OBSERVATIONS (how child feels at time of test, relation to tester, attention span, verbal behavior, self-confidence, etc,):

Fig. 1-57, cont'd. C, Directions for numbered items of testing form. (From Frankenburg WK and Dodds JB, University of Colorado Medical Center, 1969.)

Denver II*

The Denver II is a major revision and a restandardization of the DDST. It differs from the DDST in items included in the test, the test form, and the interpretation.

Item differences

The previous total of 105 items has been increased to 125, including an increase from 21 DDST to 39 Denver II language items.

Previous items that were difficult to administer and/or interpret have either been modified or eliminated. Many items that were previously tested by parental report now require observation by the examiner.

Each item was evaluated to determine if significant differences exist among sex, ethnic group, maternal education, and place of residence. Items for which clinically significant differences exist were replaced or, if retained, are discussed in the Technical Manual. When evaluating children delayed on one of these items, the diagnostician can look up norms for the subpopulations to determine if the delay may be due to sociocultural differences.

Test form differences

The age scale is similar to the American Academy of Pediatrics suggested periodicity schedule for health maintenance visits to facilitate use of the Denver II at these times.

In children born prematurely, the age is adjusted only until the child is 2 years old.

The items on the test form are arranged in the same format as the DDST-R.

The norms for the distribution bars were updated with the new standardization data but retain the 25th, 50th, 75th, and 90th percentile divisions.

The test form contains a place to rate the child's behavioral characteristics (compliance, interest in surroundings, fearfulness, and attention span).

Interpretation differences

To determine relative areas of advancement and areas of "delay," sufficient items should be administered to establish the basal and ceiling levels in each sector. By scoring appropriate items as "pass" or "fail" and relating such scores to the age of the child, each item can be interpreted as follows:

1. **Advanced**—Passed an item completely to the *right* of the age line (passed by less than 25% of children at an age older than the child.)
2. **OK**—Passed, failed, or refused an item intersected by the age line between the 25th and 75th percentile.
3. **Caution**—Failed or refused items intersected by the age line between the 75th and 90th percentile.
4. **Delay**—Failed an item completely to the *left* of the age line; refusals to the left of the age line may also be considered delays since the reason for the refusal may be inability to perform the task.

To screen solely for developmental delays, only the items located totally to the *left* of the child's age line are administered.

Scoring methods and criteria for referral are under investigation.

The Denver II is only recommended for interpretation of the

child's current developmental status for two reasons. First, as the child becomes older, more complex functions can be measured. Therefore, it is possible that a child is functioning normally at one age but that abnormalities in more complex functions are not recognizable until a later age. A second reason for not attempting to predict into the future is that the child's developmental status may change over time as a result of changes in his or her biological or environmental status. For these reasons it is recommended that the Denver II be readministered to the same child at repeated intervals much as growth is rechecked periodically.

*The Denver II will be available for distribution as of midyear 1990 from Denver Developmental Materials. For those currently administering the DDST or DDST/R, using the Denver II requires only three new testing materials (doll, feeding bottle, and cup), the new manual, and new forms. The authors suggest changing to the Denver II form after the examiner's current supply of DDST/DDST-R forms are exhausted, since the DDST is still a valid screen.

*Reference: Frankenburg WK: Personal communication, November 1989.

ASSESSMENT OF LANGUAGE AND SPEECH
Major developmental characteristics of language and speech

Age (years)	Normal language development	Normal speech development	Intelligibility
1	Says two to three words with meaning Imitates sounds of animals	Omits most final and some initial consonants Substitutes consonants "m," "w," "p," "b," "k," "g," "n," "t," "d," and "h" for more difficult sounds Height of unintelligible jargon at age 18 months	Usually no more than 25% intelligible to unfamiliar listener
2	Uses two- to three-word phrases Has vocabulary of about 300 words Uses "I," "me," "you"	Uses above consonants with vowels, but inconsistently and with much substitution Omission of final consonants Articulation lags behind vocabulary	At age 2 years, 65% intelligible in context
3	Says four- to five-word sentences Has vocabulary of about 900 words Uses "who," "what," and "where" in asking questions Uses plurals, pronouns, and prepositions	Masters "b," "t," "d," "k," and "g"; sounds "r" and "l" may still be unclear, omits or substitutes "w" Repetitions and hesitations common	At age 3 years, 70%-80% intelligible
4-5	Has vocabulary of 1500 to 2100 words Able to use most grammatic forms correctly such as past tense of verb with "yesterday" Uses complete sentences with nouns, verbs, prepositions, adjectives, adverbs, and conjunctions	Masters "f" and "v"; may still distort "r," "l," "s," "z," "sh," "ch," "y," and "th" Little or no omission of initial or last consonant	Speech is totally intelligible, although some sounds are still imperfect
5-6	Has vocabulary of 3000 words, comprehends "if," "because," and "why"	Masters "r," "l," and "th"; may still distort "s," "z," "sh," "ch," and "j" (usually mastered by age 7½ to 8 years)	

Assessment of communication impairment

Key questions for language disorders

1. How old was your child when he began to speak his first words?
2. How old was your child when he began to put words into sentences?
3. Does your child have difficulty in learning new vocabulary words?
4. Does your child omit words from sentences (i.e., do his sentences sound telegraphic?) or use short or incomplete sentences?
5. Does your child have trouble with grammar such as the verbs "is," "am," "are," "was," and "were"?
6. Can your child follow two to three directions given at once?
7. Do you have to repeat directions or questions?
8. Does your child respond appropriately to questions?
9. Does your child ask questions beginning with "who," "what," "where," and "why"?
10. Does it seem that your child has made little or no progress in speech and language in the last 6 to 12 months?

Key questions for speech impairment

1. Does your child ever stammer or repeat sounds or words?
2. Does your child seem anxious or frustrated when trying to express an idea?
3. Have you noticed behavior in your child such as blinking his eyes, jerking his head, or attempting to rephrase his thought with different words when he stammers?
4. What do you do when any of these occur?
5. Does your child omit sounds from his words?
6. Does it seem like your child uses "t," "d," "k," or "g" in place of most other consonants when he speaks?
7. Does your child omit sounds from his words or substitute the correct consonant with another one (such as "rabbit" with "wabbit")?
8. Do you have any difficulty in understanding his speech?
9. Has anyone else ever remarked about having difficulty in understanding him?
10. Has there been any recent change in the sound of his voice?

Clues for detecting communication impairment

Language disability

Assigning meaning to words

First words not uttered before second birthday

Vocabulary size reduced for age or fails to show steady increase

Difficulty in describing characteristics of objects, although may be able to name them

Infrequent use of modifier words (adjectives or adverbs)

Excessive use of jargon past 18 months

Organizing words into sentences

First sentences not uttered before third birthday

Short and incomplete sentences

Tendency to omit words (articles, prepositions)

Misuse of the "be," "do," and "can" verb forms

Difficulty understanding and producing questions

Plateaus at an early developmental level; uses easy speech patterns

Altering word forms

Omission of endings for plurals and tenses

Inappropriate use of plurals and tense endings

Inaccurate use of possession words

Speech impairment

Dysfluency (stuttering)

Noticeable repetition of sounds, words, or phrases after age 4 years

Obvious frustration when attempts to communicate

Demonstration of struggling behavior while talking (head jerks, eye blinks, retrials, or circumlocution)

Embarrassment about own speech

Articulation deficiency

Intelligibility of conversational speech absent by age 3 years

Omission of consonants at beginning of words by age 3 and at end of words by age 4

Persisting articulation faults after age 7

Omission of a sound where one should occur

Distortion of a sound

Substitution of an incorrect sound for a correct one

Voice disorders

Deviations in pitch (too high or too low, especially for age and sex); monotone

Deviations in loudness

Deviations in quality (hypernasality or hyponasality)

Guidelines for referral regarding communication impairment

Age	Assessment findings
2 years	Failure to speak any meaningful words spontaneously Consistent use of gestures rather than vocalizations Difficulty in following verbal directions Failure to respond consistently to sound
3 years	Speech is largely unintelligible Failure to use sentences of three or more words Frequent omission of initial consonants Use of vowels rather than consonants
5 years	Stutters, stammers, or has any other type of dysfluency Sentence structure noticeably impaired Substitutes easily produced sounds for more difficult ones Omits word endings (plurals, tenses of verbs, and so on)
School age	Poor voice quality (monontonous, loud, or barely audible) Vocal pitch inappropriate for age Any distortions, omissions, or substitutions of sounds after age 7 years Connected speech characterized by use of unusual confusions or reversals
General	Any child with signs that suggest a hearing impairment Any child who is embarrassed or disturbed by own speech Parents who are excessively concerned or who pressure the child to speak at a level above that appropriate for his age

Denver Articulation Screening Examination

The Denver Articulation Screening Examination (DASE) is designed to reliably discriminate between significant developmental delay and normal variations in the acquisition of speech sounds in children from 2½ to 6 years of age. It uses the *imitative* method for assessing speech sounds. A complete instructional manual is available.* General guidelines include the following:

1. Tell the child to say the word, such as "car," after you. Give child several examples to ensure understanding. Beginning with the first word "table," have the child repeat all 22 words after you. Score the child's pronunciation of the *underlined* sounds or blends in each word. (There are *30* articulated sound elements for testing.)
2. If the child is shy or hard to test, use the simple line drawings to illustrate each word.
3. To determine test results, match the raw score (number of correct sounds) line with the column denoting child's age. A child is considered to be the closest *previous* age shown on the percentile rank chart. The child's percentile rank is at the point where the line and column meet. Percentiles above the heavy line are *abnormal* and those below are *normal.*

4. Rate the child's spontaneous speech in terms of intelligibility:
   a. Easy to understand
   b. Understandable half the time
   c. Not understandable
   d. Can't evaluate (if the child does not speak in sentences or phrases during the interview)
5. Rate the child's total test results as follows:
   a. ***Normal***—normal on DASE *and* intelligibility
   b. ***Abnormal***—abnormal on DASE *and/or* intelligibility
6. Rescreen children with abnormal results within 2 weeks

*Available from Denver Developmental Materials, Inc, PO Box 6919, Denver CO 80206-0919; (303) 355-4729.

DENVER ARTICULATION SCREENING EXAM
for children 2 1/2 to 6 years of age

Instructions: Have child repeat each word after you. Circle the underlined sounds that he pronounces correctly. Total correct sounds is the Raw Score. Use charts on reverse side to score results.

NAME

HOSP. NO.

ADDRESS

Date: _____ Child's Age: _____ Examiner: _____ Raw Score: _____
Percentile: _____ Intelligibility: _____ Result: _____

1. table   6. zipper   11. sock   16. wagon   21. leaf
2. shirt   7. grapes   12. vacuum   17. gum   22. carrot
3. door   8. flag   13. yarn   18. house
4. trunk   9. thumb   14. mother   19. pencil
5. jumping   10. toothbrush 15. twinkle   20. fish

Intelligibility: (circle one)   1. Easy to understand   3. Not understandable
                                 2. Understandable 1/2   4. Can't evaluate
                                       the time.

Comments:

A

Date: _____ Child's Age: _____ Examiner: _____ Raw Score _____
Percentile: _____ Intelligibility: _____ Result: _____

1. table   6. zipper   11. sock   16. wagon   21. leaf
2. shirt   7. grapes   12. vacuum   17. gum   22. carrot
3. door   8. flag   13. yarn   18. house
4. trunk   9. thumb   14. mother   19. pencil
5. jumping   10. toothbrush 15. twinkle   20. fish

Intelligibility: (circle one)   1. Easy to understand   3. Not understandable
                                 2. Understandable 1/2   4. Can't evaluate
                                       the time.

Comments:

Date: _____ Child's Age: _____ Examiner: _____ Raw Score _____
Percentile: _____ Intelligibility: _____ Result: _____

1. table   6. zipper   11. sock   16. wagon   21. leaf
2. shirt   7. grapes   12. vacuum   17. gum   22. carrot
3. door   8. flag   13. yarn   18. house
4. trunk   9. thumb   14. mother   19. pencil
5. jumping   10. toothbrush 15. twinkle   20. fish

Intelligibility: (circle one)   1. Easy to understand   3. Not understandable
                                 2. Understandable 1/2   4. Can't evaluate
                                       the time.

Fig. 1-58. A, Denver Articulation Screening Examination for children 2½ to 6 years of age.

To score DASE words: Note Raw Score for child's performance. Match raw score line (extreme left of chart) with column representing child's age (to the closest previous age group). Where raw score line and age column meet number in that square denotes percentile rank of child's performance when compared to other children that age. Percentiles above heavy line are ABNORMAL percentiles, below heavy line are NORMAL.

PERCENTILE RANK

Raw Score	2.5 yr.	3.0	3.5	4.0	4.5	5.0	5.5	6 years
2	1							
3	2							
4	5							
5	9							
6	16							
7	23							
8	31	2						
9	37	4	1					
10	42	6	2					
11	48	7	4					
12	54	9	6	1	1			
13	58	12	9	2	3	1	1	
14	62	17	11	5	4	2	2	
15	68	23	15	9	5	3	2	
16	75	31	19	12	5	4	3	
17	79	38	25	15	6	6	4	
18	83	46	31	19	8	7	4	
19	86	51	38	24	10	9	5	1
20	89	58	45	30	12	11	7	3
21	92	65	52	36	15	15	9	4
22	94	72	58	43	18	19	12	5
23	96	77	63	50	22	24	15	7
24	97	82	70	58	29	29	20	15
25	99	87	78	66	36	34	26	17
26	99	91	84	75	46	43	34	24
27		94	89	82	57	54	44	34
28		96	94	88	70	68	59	47
29		98	98	94	84	84	77	68
30		100	100	100	100	100	100	100

To Score intelligibility:

	NORMAL	ABNORMAL
2 1/2 years	Understandable 1/2 the time, or, "easy"	Not Understandable
3 years and older	Easy to understand	Understandable 1/2 time Not understandable

Test Result: 1. NORMAL on Dase and Intelligibility = NORMAL

2. ABNORMAL on Dase and/or Intelligibility = ABNORMAL

* If abnormal on initial screening rescreen within 2 weeks. If abnormal again child should be referred for complete speech evaluation.

Fig. 1-58, cont'd. B, Percentile rank. (From Frankenburg WK, University of Colorado Medical Center, 1971.)

ASSESSMENT OF VISION
Major developmental characteristics of vision

Age (months)	Development
Birth	Visual acuity 20/100* Pupillary and corneal (blink) reflexes present Able to fixate on moving object in range of 45 degrees when held 8 to 10 inches away Cannot integrate head and eye movements well (doll's eye reflex—eyes lag behind if head is rotated to one side)
1	Can follow in range of 90 degrees Can watch parent intently as he or she speaks to infant Tear glands begin to function Visual acuity is hyperopic because infant has less spheric eyeball than adult
2-3	Has peripheral vision to 180 degrees Binocular vision begins at age 6 weeks and is well established by age 4 months Convergence on near objects begins by age 6 weeks and is well developed by age 3 months Doll's eye reflex disappears
4-5	Able to fixate on a ½-inch block Recognizes feeding bottle Looks at hand while sitting or lying on side Looks at mirror image Able to accommodate to near objects
5-7	Adjusts posture to see an object Able to rescue a dropped toy Develops color preferences for yellow and red Able to discriminate between simple geometric forms Prefers more complex visual stimuli Develops hand-eye coordination Pats image of self in mirror
7-11	Can fixate on very small objects Depth perception begins to develop Lack of binocular vision indicates strabismus
11-12	Visual acuity approaches 20/20* Visual loss may develop if strabismus is present Can follow rapidly moving objects
12-14	Able to identify geometric forms, for example, places round object into hole Displays intense and prolonged interest in pictures
18-24	Accommodation well-developed Able to fixate on small objects for up to 60 seconds
36-48	Able to copy geometric figures, for example, circle, cross Reading readiness may be present
48-60	Maximal potential for amblyopia Able to copy a square
60-72	Minimal potential for amblyopia Recognizes most colors Depth perception fully developed

Modified from Illingworth RS: The development of the infant and young child, New York, 1975, Churchill Livingstone, Inc.; and Chinn P and Leitch C: Child health maintenance: a guide to clinical assessment, ed 2, St Louis, 1979, The CV Mosby Co.
*Degree of visual acuity varies according to vision measurement procedures (see p 125).

Clues for detecting visual impairment

Cause	Behavior	Signs/symptoms
Congenital blindness	Does not follow a moving light; no orientation response to visual stimuli Does not initiate eye-to-eye contact with caregiver	Constant nystagmus Fixed pupils Marked strabismus Slow lateral movements
Refractive errors	Rubs eyes excessively Tilts head or thrusts head forward Has difficulty in reading or other close work Holds books close to eyes Writes or colors with head close to table Clumsy; walks into objects Blinks more than usual or is irritable when doing close work Is unable to see objects clearly Does poorly in school, especially in subjects that require demonstration, such as arithmetic	Dizziness Headache Nausea following close work
Strabismus	Squints eyelids together or frowns Has difficulty in focusing from one distance to another Inaccurate judgment in picking up objects Unable to see prints or moving objects clearly Closes one eye to see Tilts head to one side If combined with refractive errors, may see any of the above	Diplopia Photophobia Dizziness Headache Cross-eye
Glaucoma	Mostly seen in acquired types—Loses peripheral vision; may bump into objects that are not directly in front of him; sees halos around objects; may complain of mild pain or discomfort (severe pain, nausea, and vomiting if sudden rise in pressure)	Redness Excessive tearing (epiphora) Photophobia Spasmodic winking (blepharospasm) Corneal haziness Enlargement of the eyeball (buphthalmos)
Cataract	Gradually less able to see objects clearly May lose peripheral vision	Nystagmus (with complete blindness) Gray opacities of lens Strabismus

Special tests of visual acuity and estimated visual acuity at different ages

Test	Description	Birth	4 months	1 year	Age of 20/20 vision
Optokinetic nystagmus	A striped drum is rotated or a striped tape is moved in front of infant's eyes. Prseence of nystagmus indicates vision. Acuity is assessed by using progressively smaller stripes.	20/400	20/200	20/60	20-30 months
Forced choice preferential looking	Either a homogenous field or a striped field is presented to infant; an observer monitors the direction of the eyes during presentation of pattern. Acuity is assessed by using progressively smaller striped fields.	20/400	20/200	20/50	18-24 months
Visually evoked potentials	Eyes are stimulated with bright light or pattern, and electrical activity to visual cortex is recorded through scalp electrodes. Acuity is assessed by using progressively smaller patterns.	20/100 to 20/200	20/80	20/40	6-12 months

Data from Hoyt C, Nickel B, and Billson F: Ophthalmological examination of the infant: development aspects, Surv Ophthalmol 26:177-189, 1982.

Letter or symbol vision acuity tests

Test	Description	Comments*
Snellen Letter† (Fig. 1-60)	Uses letter of the English alphabet for testing at 20 feet	Suitable for most children above the second grade who are familiar with reading the alphabet
Snellen E†	Uses the capital letter E pointing in four directions; children "read" the chart by showing the direction of the letter E or using a large duplicate E to match the chart E at 20 feet	For illiterate or non-English speaking people and preschool children and grade 1
Preschool children often have difficulty with direction despite adequate vision
Home Eye Test for Preschoolers‡	Uses a large letter E for demonstration and an E chart for testing at 10 feet	Designed for use by parents for children 3 to 6 years
Blackbird Preschool Vision Screening System§	Uses a modified E to resemble a flying bird; children identify which way the bird is flying
Uses flash cards, story-telling, and disposable cardboard eyeglass occluders	Designed for children as young as 3 years
Blackbird Storybook Home Eye Test§	Similar to above	Designed for use by parents for children as young as 2½ years
HOTV or Matching Symbol†	Uses the four letters H, O, T, and V on a chart for testing at 10 or 20 feet
Child names the letters on the chart or matches them to a demonstration card	Suitable for children as young as 3 years
Avoids the problem with image reversal and eye-hand coordination which can occur with the letter E
Faye Symbol Chart†	Use pictures of a house, apple, and umbrella on a chart for testing at 10 feet	Suitable for children as young as 27 to 30 months
Denver Eye Screening Test (DEST)‖ (Fig. 1-59)	Uses single cards for the letter E, one for demonstration and one for testing at 15 feet
Also uses Allen Picture Cards (a tree, birthday cake, horse and rider, telephone, car, house, and teddy bear) for testing at 15 feet	Suitable for children 2½ years and older
May be reliably used with cooperative children from the age of 24 months
Dot Test†	Uses a series of different sized dots; child points to one of the nine dots randomly positioned on a disk	Suitable for children as young as 24 months

*Ages for testing are based on published reports. In actual practice only a small percentage of young children may be successfully screened with many of these tests.
†Available from Good-Lite Company, 1540 Hannah Ave., Forest Park, IL 60130 (312) 366-3860.
‡Available from the National Society to Prevent Blindness, 500 E. Remington Rd., Schaumburg, IL 60173; (800) 331-2020.
§Blackbird Vision Screening System, PO Box 277424, Sacramento, CA 95827, (916) 363-6884.
‖Available from Denver Developmental Materials, Inc, PO Box 6919, Denver, CO 80206-0919. (303) 355-4729.

Denver Eye Screening Test

The Denver Eye Screening Test (DEST) tests visual acuity in children 3 years or older by using a single card for the letter E (20/30) from a distance of 15 feet. A complete instructional manual is available. General guidelines include the following:

1. Mark a distance of 15 feet for testing.
2. Use the large E (20/100) to explain and demonstrate the testing procedure to the child. (See procedure for Snellen E, p. 129)
3. Use the small E for actual testing. Test each eye separately using the occluder.
4. Consider the results *abnormal* if the child fails to correctly identify the direction of the small E over three trials.
5. Test children from 2½ to 2¹¹/₁₂ years of age or those untestable with the letter E using the picture (Allen) cards. (Cooperative children as young as 2 years can also be tested.)
6. Show each card to the child at close range to make certain he can identify it.
7. Present the pictures at a distance of 15 feet for actual testing. Test each eye separately if possible.
8. Consider the results *abnormal* if the child fails to correctly name three of the seven cards in three to five trials.
9. Screen children from 6 to 30 months by testing for the following:
   a. Fixation (ability to follow a moving light source or spinning toy)
   b. Squinting (observation of the child's eyes or report by parent)
   c. Strabismus (report by parent and performance on cover and pupillary light reflex tests, p. 36)
10. Consider the results *abnormal* if failure to fixate, presence of a squint, and/or failing two of the three procedures for strabismus.
11. Retest all children with abnormal findings. Refer those with a repeat failure.

Unit 1

Lit. 217

DENVER EYE SCREENING TEST

Name
Hospital No.
Ward
Address

RESCREENING:DATE

Left Eye — Untestable: U U U | Abnormal: 3F 3F F yes | Normal: 3P 3P P P

Right Eye — Untestable: U U U | Abnormal: 3F 3F F yes | Normal: 3P 3P P P

Untestable: U U U
Abnormal: YES F F
Normal: NO P P

Normal
Abnormal
Untestable

Date:

1ST SCREENING:DATE

Left Eye — Untestable: U U U | Abnormal: 3F 3F F yes | Normal: 3P 3P P P

Right Eye — Untestable: U U U | Abnormal: 3F 3F yes F | Normal: 3P 3P P P

Untestable: U U U
Abnormal: YES F F
Normal: NO P P

Normal
Abnormal
Untestable

Date:

Vision Tests

1. "E" (3 years and above–3 to 5 trials) . . . . . .
2. Picture Card (2 1/2 – 2 11/12 yrs.–3 to 5 trials) . . . .
3. Fixation (6 months – 2 5/12 years) . . . .
4. Squinting . . . .

Tests for Non-Straight Eyes

1. Do your child's eyes turn in or out, or are they ever not straight? . . . .
2. Cover Test . . . .
3. Pupillary Light Reflex . . . . .

Total Test Rating (Both Eyes)

Normal (passed vision test plus no squint, plus passed 2/3 tests for non-straight eyes)

Abnormal (abnormal on any vision test, squinting or 2 of 3 procedures for non-straight eyes)

Untestable (untestable on any vision test or untestable on 2/3 tests for non-straight eyes)

Future Rescreening Appointment for Total Test Rating (Abnormal or Untestable)

Fig. 1-59. Denver Eye Screening Test. (From Frankenburg WK and Dodds JB, University of Colorado Medical Center, 1969.)

Snellen screening*

PREPARATION

1. Hang the Snellen chart on a light-colored wall so that the 20- to 30-foot lines are at eye level when children 6 to 12 years old are tested in the standing position.
2. Secure the chart to the wall with double-stick tape on the back side of all four corners. If the chart must be reversed for use of the letter or E chart, secure it at the top and bottom with tacks. Make sure that the chart does not swing when in place.
3. The illumination intensity on the chart should be 10 to 30 footcandles, without any glare from windows or light fixtures. The illumination should be checked with a light meter.
4. Mark an exact 20-foot distance from the chart. Mark the floor with a piece of tape or "footprints" positioned so that the heels touch the 20-foot line.

---

*Modified from recommendations of the National Society to Prevent Blindness: Guide to testing distance visual acuity, The Society, 1988, Schaumburg, IL.

PROCEDURE

1. Place the child at the 20-foot mark, with the heel edging the line if child is standing or with the back of the chair placed at the marker if the child is seated.
2. If the E chart is used, accustom the child to identifying which direction the "legs of the E" are pointing. Use a demonstration E card for this purpose.
3. Teach the child to use the occluder to cover one eye. Instruct child to keep both eyes open during the test. Provide a clean cover card for each child and then discard after use.
4. If the child wears glasses, test only with glasses on.
5. Test both eyes together, then right eye, then left eye.
6. Begin with the 40- or 30-foot line and proceed with test to include the 20-foot line.
7. With the child suspected of low vision, begin with the 200-foot line and proceed until the child can no longer correctly read three out of four or four out of six symbols on a line.
8. Use covers on the Snellen chart to expose only one symbol or one line at a time. When screening kindergarten or older children, expose one line but may use a pointer to point to one symbol at a time.

RECORDING AND REFERRAL

1. Record the last line the child read correctly (three out of four or four out of six symbols).
2. Record visual acuity as a fraction. The numerator represents the distance from the chart, and the denominator represents the last line read correctly. For example, 20/30 means that the child read the 30-foot line at a 20-foot distance.
3. Observe the child's eyes during testing and record any evidence of squinting, head tilting, thrusting the head forward, excessive blinking, tearing, or redness.
4. Only make referrals after a second screening has been made on children who are potential candidates for referral.
5. The following children should be referred for a complete eye examination:
   a. Three-year-old children with vision in either eye of 20/50 or less (inability to correctly identify one more than half the symbols on the 40-foot line) *or* a two-line difference in visual acuity between the eyes in the passing range; for example, 20/20 in one eye and 20/40 in the other
   b. All other ages and grades with vision in either eye of 20/40 or less (inability to correctly identify one more than half the symbols on the 30-foot line)
   c. All children who consistently show any of the signs of possible visual disturbances, regardless of visual acuity

Fig. 1-60. Snellen chart. **A,** Letter (alphabet) chart. **B,** Symbol E chart. (From National Society to Prevent Blindness, Inc. Schaumburg, IL.)

Unit 1

ASSESSMENT OF HEARING
Major developmental characteristics of hearing

Age (months)	Development
Birth	Responds to loud noise by startle reflex Responds to sound of human voice more readily than to any other sound Low-pitched sounds, such as lullaby, metronome, or heartbeat, have quieting effect
2-3	Turns head to side when sound is made at level of ear
3-4	Locates sound by turning head to side and looking in same direction
4-6	Can localize sounds made below ear, which is followed by localization of sound made above ear; will turn head to the side and then look up or down Begins to imitate sounds
6-8	Locates sounds by turning head in a curving arc Responds to own name
8-10	Localizes sounds by turning head diagonally and directly toward sound
10-12	Knows several words and their meaning, such as "no," and names of members of the family Learns to control and adjust own response to sound, such as listening for sound to occur again
18	Begins to discriminate between harshly dissimilar sounds, such as sound of doorbell and train
24	Refines gross discriminative skills
36	Begins to distinguish more subtle differences in speech sounds, such as between "e" and "er"
48	Begins to distinguish such similar sounds as "f" and "th" or between "f" and "s" Listening becomes considerably refined Able to be tested with an audiometer

Modified from Illingworth RS: The development of the infant and young child, New York, 1975, Churchill Livingstone, Inc.; and Weiss CE and Lillywhite HS: Communicative disorders: prevention and early intervention, ed 2, St Louis, 1981, The CV Mosby Co.

Assessment of child for hearing impairment

FAMILY HISTORY

Genetic disorders associated with hearing impairment
Family members, especially siblings, with hearing disorders

PRENATAL HISTORY

Miscarriages
Illnesses during pregnancy (rubella, syphilis, diabetes)
Drugs taken
Exposure to childhood diseases
Eclampsia

DELIVERY

Duration of labor, type of delivery
Fetal distress
Presentation (especially breech)
Drugs used
Blood incompatibility

BIRTH HISTORY

Birth weight < 1500 g
Hyperbilirubinemia at level exceeding indications for exchange transfusion
Severe asphyxia

Congenital perinatal infection (cytomegalovirus, rubella, herpes, syphilis, toxoplasmosis)
Congenital anomalies involving head and neck

PAST HEALTH HISTORY

Immunizations
Serious illness (e.g., bacterial meningitis)
Convulsions
High unexplained fevers
Ototoxic drugs
No history (adopted child)
Colds, ear infections, allergies
Treatment of ear problems
Visual difficulties
Exposure to excessive noise

HEARING

Parental concerns regarding hearing loss (what cues, at what age)
Response to name calling, loud noises, sounds of different frequencies (crinkling paper, whisper, bell, rattle)
Results of previous audiometric testing

SPEECH DEVELOPMENT

Age of babbling, first meaningful words, phrases
Intelligibility of speech
Present vocabulary

MOTOR DEVELOPMENT

Age of sitting, standing, walking
Level of independence in self-care, feeding, toileting, grooming

ADAPTIVE BEHAVIOR

Play activities
Socialization with other children
Behaviors: temper tantrums, stubbornness, self-vexation, vibratory stimulus
Educational achievement
Recent behavioral and/or personality changes

Clues for detecting hearing impairment

ORIENTATION RESPONSE

Lack of startle or blink reflex to a loud sound

Persistence of Moro reflex beyond 4 months of age (associated with mental retardation)

Failure to be awakened by loud environmental noises during early infancy

Failure to localize a source of sound by 6 months of age

General indifference to sound

Lack of response to the spoken word; failure to follow verbal directions

Response to loud noises as opposed to the voice

VOCALIZATIONS AND SOUND PRODUCTION

Monotone quality, unintelligible speech, lessened laughter

Normal quality in central auditory loss

Lessened experimental sound play and squealing

Normal use of jargon during early infancy in central auditory loss, with persistent use later on

Absence of babble or inflections in voice by age 7 months

Failure to develop intelligible speech by age 24 months

Vocal play, head banging, or foot stamping for vibratory sensation

Yelling or screeching to express pleasure, annoyance, or need

VISUAL ATTENTION

Augmented visual alertness and attentiveness

Responding more to facial expression than verbal explanation

Being alert to gestures and movement

Use of gestures rather than verbalization to express desires, especially after age 15 months

Marked imitativeness in play

SOCIAL RAPPORT AND ADAPTATIONS

Less interest and involvement in vocal nursery games

Intense preoccupation with things rather than persons

Avoidance of social interactions; often puzzled and unhappy in such situations

Inquiring, sometimes confused facial expression

Suspicious alertness, sometimes interpreted as paranoia, alternating with cooperation

Marked reactivity to praise, attention, and physical affection

Shows less interest than peers in casual conversation

Is often inattentive unless the environment is quiet and the speaker is close to the child

Is more responsive to movement than to sound

Intently observes the speaker's face, responding more to facial expression than verbalization

Often asks to have statements repeated

May not follow directions exactly

EMOTIONAL BEHAVIOR

Use of tantrums to call attention to self or needs

Frequently stubborn because of lack of comprehension

Irritable at not making self understood

Shy, timid, and withdrawn

Often appears "dreamy," "in a world of his own," or markedly inattentive

Selected hearing tests

Test	Description	Comments
Clinical hearing tests	In newborns, elicit the startle reflex and observe other neonatal responses to loud noises, such as facial grimaces, blinking, gross motor movement, quiet if crying or crying if quiet, opening the eyes, or ceasing sucking activity. During infancy note child's reaction to a noise: Stand about 18 inches away from infant, to the side, and out of child's peripheral field of vision. With the room silent and infant sitting in parent's lap, distracted by some object, make a voice sound such as PS or PHTH (high-pitched), or OO (low-pitched), ring a bell or a rattle, or rustle tissue paper.	An objective sign of alerting to sound may be an increase in heart rate or respiratory rate. Absence of alerting behaviors suggests hearing loss. Eliciting the startle reflex is used only in infants from birth to 4 months. Test is usually inadequate for children beyond infancy because of their tendency to ignore sounds or be distracted. Compare response of localizing sound to expected age response (see box on p. 130).
Crib-o-gram	Neonatal screening tool that analyzes hearing responses by comparing the infant's motor activity before, during, and after a sound is introduced. A motion-sensitive transducer is placed beneath the crib or Isolette mattress, and a microprocessor "reads" the infant's movements.	Both administration of the test and its scoring are totally automated. The test is repeated several times to increase reliability. A consistent change in activity that coincides with the test sound is scored as a pass. Neonates who are premature or ill may not respond to sound despite adequate hearing
Tympanometry	Measures tympanic membrane compliance (or mobility) and estimates middle ear air pressure. A soft rubber cuff is pressed over the external canal to produce an airtight seal; an automatic reading of air pressure registers on the machine.	Detects middle ear disease and abnormalities but does not indicate the degree of hearing loss or the interpretation of sound. Suitable for infants, young children, and those who are difficult to test by other methods because little cooperation is necessary, and the procedure is not painful. Requires special equipment although minimal training is necessary.
Conduction tests	**Rinne test**—Stem of tuning fork is placed against the mastoid bone until the sound ceases to be audible. Tuning fork is then moved so that the prongs are held near, but not touching, the auditory meatus. Child should again hear the sound *(Rinne positive)*. If sound is not again audible *(Rinne negative)*, some abnormality is interfering with the conduction of air through the external and middle chambers.	Requires the cooperation and ability of the child to signal when the sound is no longer audible and when it is again heard. Not useful for most children before preschool age.
	Weber test—Stem of tuning fork is held in the midline of the head. Child should hear the sound equally in both ears *(Weber positive)*. With air conductive loss child will hear the sound better in the affected ear *(Weber negative)*.	Frequently not suitable for young children because of their difficulty in discriminating between "better, more, or less."
Audiometry	Electrical audiometer measures the threshold of hearing for pure-tone frequencies and loudness. A sound is transmitted to the child's ear and reduced until child indicates the sound is no longer heard; this procedure is repeated for several sounds covering the range found in conversation. In an air conduction audiogram the sounds are transmitted through earphones. In a bone conduction audiogram the sounds are passed through a plaque placed over the mastoid bone.	Provides valuable information regarding the severity of the hearing loss, the sound cycles involved, and the possible location of the defect. Requires specialized training of personnel, expensive equipment, and cooperation from the child in terms of confirming the perception of sound. For children 24 months to about 5 years play audiometry can be used; it is based on behavior modification and involves reinforcement for correct response.
Brainstem-evoked auditory response (BEAR)	Through electrode wires attached to the infant's or child's scalp, electrical or brain wave potentials generated within the auditory system are transmitted to a computer for analysis. Following repetitive acoustic stimulation, the waveforms from a normal sleeping or quiet infant consist of several peaks and valleys that reflect activations of neural structures of the brain.	Requires specialized training of personnel and expensive equipment.

Any child who is suspected of a hearing loss because of poor performance using any of the first four screening tests is referred for special audiometric or BEAR testing.

SUMMARY OF GROWTH AND DEVELOPMENT

This summary of growth and development offers a broad overview of the significant physical, psychosocial, and mental achievements during childhood. It begins with a comparison of cognitive and personality development throughout the life span according to different theorists. Following are summaries of the specific developmental milestones associated with each major age group of children.

Personality, moral, and cognitive development

Stage/age	Radius of significant relationships (Sullivan)	Psychosexual stages (Freud)	Psychosocial stages (Erikson)	Cognitive stages (Piaget)	Moral judgment stages (Kohlberg)
I Infancy Birth to 1 year	Maternal person (uni-polar-bipolar)	Oral sensory	Trust vs mistrust	Sensorimotor (birth to 18 months)	
II Toddlerhood 1-3 years	Parental persons (tri-polar)	Anal-urethral	Autonomy vs shame and doubt	Preoperational thought, precon-ceptual phase (transductive rea-soning, for exam-ple, specific to specific) (2-4 years)	Preconventional (premoral) level Punishment and obedience ori-entation
III Early childhood 3-6 years	Basic family	Phallic-loco-motion	Initiative vs guilt	Preoperational thought, intuitive phase (transduc-tive reasoning) (4-7 years)	Preconventional (premoral) level Naive instrumental orientation
IV Middle childhood 6-12 years	Neighborhood, school	Latency	Industry vs infe-riority	Concrete operations (inductive rea-soning and begin-ning logic)	Conventional level Good-boy, nice-girl orientation Law and order ori entation
V Adolescence 13-18 years	Peer groups and out-groups Models of leadership Partners in friend-ship, sex, compe-tition, cooperation	Genitality	Identity and re-pudiation vs identity confu-sion	Formal operations (deductive and abstract reason-ing)	Postconventional or principled level Social-contract or-ientaton Universal ethical principle orien-tation (no longer included in re-vised theory)
VI Early adulthood	Divided labor and shared household		Intimacy and sol-idarity vs iso-lation		
VII Young and middle adulthood	Mankind "My kind"		Generativity vs self-absorption		
VIII Later adulthood			Ego integrity vs despair		

Unit 1

Growth and development during infancy

Age (months)	Physical	Gross motor	Fine motor
1	Weight gain of 150 to 210 g (5 to 7 ounces) weekly for first 6 months Height gain of 2.5 cm (1 inch) monthly for first 6 months Head circumference increases by 1.5 cm (½ inch) monthly for first 6 months Primitive reflexes present and strong Doll's eye reflex and dance reflex fading Obligatory nose breather (most infants)	■ Assumes flexed position with pelvis high, but knees not under abdomen when prone (at birth, knees flexed under abdomen) ■ Can turn head from side to side when prone, lifts head momentarily from bed Has marked head lag, especially when pulled from lying to sitting position Holds head momentarily parallel and in midline when suspended in prone position Assumes asymmetric tonic neck reflex position when supine Makes crawling movements when prone When held in standing position, body limp at knees and hips In sitting position back is uniformly rounded, absence of head control	Hands predominantly closed Grasp reflex strong Hand clenches on contact with rattle
2	Posterior fontanel closed Crawling reflex disappears	■ Assumes less flexed position when prone—hips flat, legs extended, arms flexed, head to side Less head lag when pulled to sitting position Can maintain head in same plane as rest of body when held prone and parallel to floor When prone, can lift head almost 45 degrees off table When held in sitting position, holds head up but head bobs forward Assumes asymmetric tonic neck reflex position intermittently	Hands frequently open Grasp reflex fading
3	Primitive reflexes fading	Able to hold head more erect when sitting, but still bobs forward Has only slight head lag when pulled to sitting Assumes symmetric body position Able to raise head and shoulders from prone position to a 45- to 90-degree angle from table; bears weight on forearms When held in standing position, able to bear slight fraction of weight on legs Regards own hand	■ Actively holds rattle but will not reach for it Grasp reflex absent Hands kept loosely open Clutches own hand, pulls at blankets and clothes
4	■ Moro, tonic neck, rooting, and Perez reflexes have disappeared Drooling begins	■ Has almost no head lag when pulled to sitting position ■ Balances head well in sitting position Back is less rounded, curved only in lumbar area Able to sit erect if propped up Able to raise head and chest off couch to angle of 90 degrees Assumes predominant symmetric position Rolls from back to side	■ Inspects and plays with hands, pulls clothing or blanket over face in play Tries to reach objects with hand but overshoots Grasps object with both hands Plays with rattle placed in hand, shakes it, but cannot pick it up if dropped Can carry objects to mouth

Milestones that represent essential integrative aspects of development that lay the foundation for the achievement of more advanced skills are indicated by a square.

Sensory	Vocalization	Socialization/cognition
Visual acuity approaches 20/100* ■ Able to fixate on moving object in range of 45 degrees when held at a distance of 20-25 cm (8-10 inches) Follows light to midline Quiets when hears a voice	Cries to express displeasure Makes small throaty sounds Makes comfort sounds during feeding	Is in sensorimotor phase—stage I, use of reflexes (birth-1 month) and stage II, primary circular reactions (1-4 months) Watches parent's face intently as she or he talks to infant
Binocular fixation and convergence to near objects beginning When supine, follows dangling toy from side to point beyond midline Visually searches to locate sounds Turns head to side when sound is made at level of ear	■ Vocalizes, distinct from crying Crying becomes differentiated Coos Vocalizes to familiar voice	■ Demonstrates social smile in response to various stimuli
■ Follows object to periphery (180 degrees) ■ Locates sound by turning head to side and looking in same direction Begins to have ability to coordinate stimuli from various sense organs	■ Squeals aloud to show pleasure Coos, babbles, chuckles Vocalizes when smiling "Talks" a great deal when spoken to Cries less during periods of wakefulness	Displays considerable interest in surroundings Ceases crying when parent enters room Can recognize familiar faces and objects, such as feeding bottle Shows awareness of strange situations
Able to accommodate to near objects Binocular vision well established Can focus on a 1.25 cm (½-inch) block Beginning eye-hand coordination	Makes consonant sounds n, k, g, p, b Laughs aloud Vocalization changes according to mood	Is in stage III, secondary circular reactions Demands attention by fussing; becomes bored if left alone Enjoys social interaction with people Anticipates feeding when sees bottle Shows excitement with whole body, squeals, breathes heavily Shows interest in strange stimuli Begins to show memory

*Degree of visual acuity varies according to vision measurement procedures (see p. 125).   *Continued.*

Growth and development during infancy—cont'd

Age (months)	Physical	Gross motor	Fine motor
5	Growth rate may begin to decline Beginning signs of tooth eruption	Has no head lag when pulled to sitting position When sitting, able to hold head erect and steady Able to sit for longer periods when back is well supported Back is straight When prone, assumes symmetric positioning with arms extended When held in standing position, able to bear most of weight Can turn over from abdomen to back When supine, puts feet to mouth	■ Able to grasp objects voluntarily Uses palmar grasp, bidextrous approach Plays with toes Takes objects directly to mouth Holds one cube while regarding a second
6	Birth weight doubled Weight gain of 90 to 150 g (3 to 5 ounces) weekly for next 6 months Height gain of 1.25 cm (½ inch) monthly for next 6 months Teething may begin with eruption of two lower central incisors ■ Chewing and biting occur Landau reflex appears—when infant is suspended in a horizontal prone position, the head is raised, legs and spine are extended	When prone, can lift chest and upper abdomen off table, bearing weight on hands When about to be pulled to a sitting position, lifts head Sits in high chair with back straight Rolls from back to abdomen When held in standing position, bears almost all of weight Hand regard is absent	Resecures a dropped object Drops one cube when another is given Grasps and manipulates small objects Holds bottle Grasps feet and pulls to mouth
7	Eruption of upper central incisors	■ When supine, spontaneously lifts head off table ■ Sits, leaning forward on both hands When prone, bears weight on one hand Sits erect momentarily Bears full weight on feet When held in standing position, bounces actively	■ Transfers objects from one hand to the other Has unidextrous approach and grasp Holds two cubes more than momentarily Bangs cube on table Rakes at a small object
8	Begins to show regular patterns in bladder and bowel elimination Parachute reflex appears When infant is suspended in a horizontal prone position and suddenly thrust downward, hands and fingers extend forward as if to protect self from falling	■ Sits steadily unsupported Readily bears weight on legs when supported, may stand holding on Adjusts posture to reach an object	Has beginning pincer grasp using the index, fourth, and fifth fingers against the lower part of the thumb Releases objects at will Rings bell purposely Retains two cubes while regarding the third cube Secures an object by pulling on a string Reaches persistently for toys out of reach

Sensory	Vocalization	Socialization/cognition
Visually pursues a dropped object Able to sustain visual inspection of an object Can localize sounds made below the ear	▪ Squeals Has vowel-like cooing sounds interspersed with consonantal sounds (for example, ah-goo)	Smiles at mirror image Pats bottle with both hands More enthusiastically playful, but may have rapid mood swings Able to discriminate strangers from family Vocalizes displeasure when object taken away Discovers parts of body
Visual acuity 20/60 to 20/40 Adjusts posture to see an object Prefers more complex visual stimuli Can localize sounds made above the ear Will turn head to the side, then look up or down	▪ Begins to imitate sounds ▪ Babbling resembles one-syllable utterances such as ma, mu, da, di, hi Vocalizes to toys, mirror image Laughs aloud Takes pleasure in hearing own sounds (self-reinforcement)	Recognizes parents; begins to fear strangers Holds arms out to be picked up Has definite likes and dislikes Beginning of imitation (cough, protrusion of tongue) Excites on hearing footsteps Laughs when head is hidden in a towel Has frequent mood swings—from crying to laughing with little or no provocation Briefly searches for a dropped object (object permanence beginning)
▪ Can fixate on very small objects Responds to own name Localizes sound by turning head in a curving arch Has beginning awareness of depth and space Has taste preferences	▪ Produces vowel sounds and chained syllables—baba, dada, kaka Vocalizes four distinct vowel sounds "Talks" when others are talking	▪ Is increasingly fearful of strangers, shows signs of fretfulness when parent disappears Imitates simple acts and noises Tries to attract attention by coughing or snorting Plays peekaboo Demonstrates dislike of food by keeping lips closed Exhibits oral aggressiveness in biting and mouthing Demonstrates expectation in response to repetition of stimuli ▪ Looks briefly for toy that disappears
	Makes consonant sounds t, d, and w Listens selectively to familiar words Utterances signal emphasis and emotion Combines syllables, such as dada, but does not ascribe meaning to them	Has increasing anxiety over loss of parent, particularly mother, and fear of strangers Responds to word "no" Dislikes dressing, diaper change

Continued.

Growth and development during infancy—cont'd

Age (months)	Physical	Gross motor	Fine motor
9	Eruption of upper lateral incisor may begin	Crawls, may progress backward at first Sits steadily on floor for prolonged time (10 minutes) Recovers balance when leans forward but cannot do so when leaning sideways Pulls self to standing position and stands holding onto furniture	▪ Uses thumb and index finger in crude pincer grasp Preference for use of dominant hand now evident Grasps third cube Compares two cubes by bringing them togther
10	Labyrinth-righting reflex is strongest—when infant is in prone or supine position, is able to raise head	Crawls by pulling self forward with hands Can change from prone to sitting position Pulls self to sitting position Stands while holding onto furniture, sits by falling down Recovers balance easily while sitting While standing, lifts one foot to take a step	Crude release of an object is beginning Grasps bell by handle
11	Eruption of lower lateral incisors may begin	▪ Creeps with abdomen off floor When sitting, pivots to reach toward back to pick up an object Cruises or walks holding onto furniture or with both hands held	Can hold crayon to make a mark on paper Explores objects more thoroughly (for example, clapper inside bell) Drops object deliberately for it to be picked up Puts one object after another into a container (sequential play) Able to manipulate an object to remove it from tight-fitting enclosure
12	Birth weight tripled Birth length increased by 50% Head and chest circumference equal (head circumference 46.5 cm [18½ inches]) Has total of six to eight deciduous teeth Anterior fontanel almost closed Landau reflex fading Babinski reflex disappears Lumbar curve develops, lordosis evident during walking	Walks with one hand held Cruises well May attempt to stand alone momentarily Can sit down from standing position without help	Has neat pincer grasp Releases cube in cup Attempts to build two-block tower but fails Tries to insert a pellet into a narrow-neck bottle but fails Can turn pages in a book, many at a time

Sensory	Vocalization	Socialization/cognition
Localizes sounds by turning head diagonally and directly toward sound Depth perception is increasing	Responds to simple verbal commands Comprehends "no-no"	Is in stage IV, coordination of secondary schemata Parent (mother) is increasingly important for own sake Increasing interest in pleasing parent Begins to show fears of going to bed and being left alone Puts arms in front of face to avoid having it washed ■ Searches for an object if sees it hidden
	■ Says dada, mama with meaning Comprehends "bye-bye" May say one word (for example, hi, bye, what, no)	Inhibits behavior to verbal command of "no-no" or own name Imitates facial expressions, waves bye-bye Extends toy to another person but will not release it Repeats actions that attract attention and are laughed at Pulls clothes of another to attract attention Plays interactive games such as pat-a-cake Reacts to adult anger, cries when scolded Demonstrates independence in dressing, feeding, locomotive skills, and testing of parents Looks at and follows pictures in a book Looks around a corner or under a pillow for an object
	Imitates definite speech sounds Uses jargon	Experiences joy and satisfaction when a task is mastered Reacts to restrictions with frustration Rolls ball to another on request Antipates body gestures when a familiar nursery rhyme or story is being told (for example, holds toes and feet in response to "This little piggy went to market") Plays game up-down, "so-big," or peekaboo by covering face
Discriminates simple geometric forms (for example, circle) Amblyopia may develop with lack of binocularity Can follow rapidly moving object Controls and adjusts response to sound; listens for sound to recur	■ Says two or more words besides dada, mama Comprehends meaning of several words (comprehension always precedes verbalization) Recognizes objects by name Imitates animal sounds Understands simple verbal commands (for example, "Give it to me," "Show me your eyes")	Shows emotions such as jealousy, affection (may give hug or kiss on request), anger, fear Enjoys familiar surroundings and explores away from parent Is fearful in strange situation, clings to parent May develop habit of "security blanket" or favorite toy Has unceasing determination to practice locomotor skills ■ Searches for an object even if has not seen it hidden, but searches only where object was last seen

Growth and development during toddler years

Age (months)	Physical	Gross motor	Fine motor
15	Steady growth in height and weight Head circumference 48 cm (19 inches) Weight 11 kg (24 pounds) Height 78.7 cm (31 inches)	Walks without help (usually since age 13 months) Creeps up stairs Kneels without support Cannot walk around corners or stop suddenly without losing balance Assumes standing position without support Cannot throw ball without falling	Constantly casts objects to floor Builds tower of two cubes Holds two cubes in one hand Releases a pellet into a narrow-necked bottle Scribbles spontaneously Uses cup well but rotates spoon
18	Physiologic anorexia from decreased growth needs Anterior fontanel closed Physiologically able to control sphincters	Runs clumsily, falls often Walks up stairs with one hand held Pulls and pushes toys Seats self on chair Throws ball overhand without falling	Builds tower of three to four cubes Release, prehension, and reach are well-developed Turns pages in a book two or three at a time In drawing, makes stroke imitatively Manages spoon without rotation, but some spilling
24	Head circumference 49 to 50 cm (19.6 to 20 inches) Chest circumference exceeds head circumference Lateral diameter of chest exceeds anteroposterior diameter Usual weight gain of 1.8 to 2.7 kg (4 to 6 pounds) Usual gain in height of 10 to 12.5 cm (4 to 5 inches) Adult height approximately double height at 2 years of age Physiologic systems, except for endocrine and reproductive, stable and mature May have achieved readiness for beginning daytime control of bowel and bladder Primary dentition of sixteen teeth	Goes up and down stairs alone with two feet on each step Runs fairly well, with wide stance Picks up object without falling Kicks ball forward without overbalancing	Builds tower of six to seven cubes Aligns two or more cubes like a train Turns pages of book one at a time In drawing, imitates vertical and circular strokes Turns doorknob; unscrews lid
30	Birth weight quadrupled Primary dentition (twenty teeth) completed May have daytime bowel and bladder control	Jumps with both feet Jumps from chair to step Stands on one foot momentarily Takes a few steps on tiptoe	Builds tower of eight cubes Adds chimney to train of cubes Has good hand-finger coordination; holds crayon with fingers rather than fist Can move fingers independently In drawing, imitates vertical and horizontal strokes; makes two or more strokes for cross

Sensory	Language	Socialization/cognition
Able to identify geometric forms; places round object into appropriate hole Displays an intense and prolonged interest in pictures	Uses expressive jargon Says four to six words, including names "Asks" for objects by pointing Understands simple commands May use head-shaking gesture to denote "no" Uses "no" even while agreeing to the request	Is in sensorimotor phase, stage V, tertiary circular reactions (13-18 months) Tolerates some separation from parent Less likely to fear strangers Beginning to imitate parents, such as cleaning house (sweeping, dusting, folding clothes) Feeds self using regular cup with little spilling May discard bottle Manages spoon but rotates it near mouth Kisses and hugs parents, may kiss pictures in a book Expresses emotions, has temper tantrums Can find hidden objects, but only in first location Able to insert a round object into a hole Fits smaller objects into each other (nesting) Realizes that "out of sight" is not out of reach; opens doors and drawers to find objects
	Says ten or more words Points to a common object, such as shoe or ball, and to two or three body parts	Is in stage VI, invention of new means through mental combinations Is great imitator ("domestic mimicry") Takes off gloves, socks, and shoes and unzips Temper tantrums may be more evident Beginning awareness of ownership ("my toy") May develop dependency on transitional objects, such as "security blanket" Searches for an object through several hiding places Will infer a cause by associating two or more experiences (such as candy missing, sister smiling) Follows directions and understands requests Uses words "up," "down," "come," and "go" with meaning Has some sense of time; waits in repsonse to "just a minute"; may use word "now"
Accommodation is well-developed In geometric discrimination, able to insert square block into oblong space	Has vocabulary of approximately 300 words Uses two- to three-word phrases Uses pronouns I, me, you Understands directional commands Gives first name; refers to self by name Verbalizes need for toileting, food, or drink Talks incessantly	Is in preconceptual stage (preoperational phase) and stage of parallel play Has sustained attention span Has fewer temper tantrums Pulls people to show them something Has increased independence from parent Dresses self in simple clothing Thinking is characterized by global organization of thought, transductive reasoning, concept of animism, and magical thinking
	Gives first and last name Refers to self by appropriate pronoun Uses plurals Names one color	Separates more easily from parent In play, helps put things away, can carry breakable objects, pushes with good steering Begins to notice sex differences; knows own sex May attend to toilet needs without help except for wiping

Growth and development during preschool years

Age (years)	Physical	Gross motor	Fine motor	Language
3	Usual weight gain of 1.8 to 2.7 kg (4 to 6 pounds) Usual gain in height of 7.5 cm (3 inches) May have achieved nighttime control of bowel and bladder	Rides tricycle Jumps off bottom step Stands on one foot for a few seconds Goes up stairs using alternate feet, may still come down using both feet on the step Broad jumps May try to dance, but balance may not be adequate	Builds tower of nine or ten cubes Builds bridge with three cubes Adeptly places small pellets in narrow-necked bottle In drawing, copies a circle, imitates a cross, names what he has drawn, cannot draw stickman but may make circle with facial features	Has vocabulary of about 900 words Uses primarily "telegraphic" speech Uses complete sentences of three to four words Talks incessantly regardless of whether anyone is paying attention Repeats sentence of six syllables Constantly asks questions
4	Pulse and respiration decrease slightly Growth rate is similar to that of previous year Length at birth is doubled Maximum potential for development of amblyopia	Skips and hops on one foot Catches ball reliably Throws ball overhand Walks down stairs using alternate footing	Imitates a gate with cubes Uses scissors successfully to cut out picture following outline Can lace shoes, but may not be able to tie bow In drawing, copies a square, traces a cross and diamond, adds three parts to stick figure	Has vocabulary of 1500 words or more Uses sentences of four to five words Questioning is at peak Tells exaggerated stories Knows simple songs May be mildly profane if associates with older children Obeys four prepositional phrases, such as "under," "on top of," "beside," "in back of" or "in front of" Names one or more colors Comprehends analogies, such as, "If ice is cold, fire is __" Repeats four digits Uses words liberally but frequently does not comprehend meaning

Socialization	Cognition	Family relationships
Dresses self almost completely if helped with back buttons and told which shoe is right or left	Is in preconceptual phase	Attempts to please parents and conform to their expectations
Buttons and unbuttons accessible buttons	Is egocentric in thought and behavior	Is less jealous of younger sibling; may be opportune time for birth of additional sibling
Pulls on shoes	Has beginning understanding of time; uses many time-oriented expressions, talks about past and future as much as about present, pretends to tell time	
Has increased attention span		Is aware of family relationships and sex role functions
Feeds self completely	Has improved concept of space as demonstrated in understanding of prepositions and ability to follow directional command	Boys tend to identify more with father or other male figure
Pours from a bottle or pitcher		
Can prepare simple meals, such as cold cereal and milk	Has beginning ability to view concepts from another perspective	Has increased ability to separate easily and comfortably from parents for short periods
Can help to set table, dry dishes without breaking any		
Likes to "help" entertain by passing around food		
May have fears, especially of dark and going to bed		
Knows own sex and appropriate sex of others		
Play is parallel and associative		
Begins to learn simple games and meaning of rules, but follows them according to self-interpretation		
Speaks to doll, animal, truck, and so on		
Begins to work out social interaction through play		
Able to share toys, although expresses idea of "mine" frequently		
Very independent	Is in phase of intuitive thought	Rebels if parents expect too much, such as perfect table manners
Tends to be selfish and impatient	Causality is still related to proximity of events	Takes aggression and frustration out on parents or siblings
Aggressive physically as well as verbally	Understands time better, especially in terms of sequence of daily events	Do's and don'ts become important
Takes pride in accomplishments	Is unable to conserve matter	May have rivalry with older or younger siblings, may resent older's privileges and younger's invasion of privacy and possessions
Has mood swings	Judges everything according to one dimension, such as height, width, or first	
Boasts and tattles	Immediate perceptual clues dominate judgment	
Shows off dramatically, enjoys entertaining others		May run away from home
Tells family tales to others with no restraint	Can choose longer of two lines or heavier of two objects	Identifies strongly with parent of opposite sex
Still has many fears	Is beginning to develop less egocentrism and more social awareness	Is able to run simple errands outside the home
Play is associative	May count correctly but has poor mathematic concept of numbers	
Imaginary playmates are common	Still believes that thoughts cause events	
Uses dramatic, imaginative, and imitative devices	Obeys because parents have set limits, not because of understanding of reason behind right or wrong	
Works through unresolved conflicts, such as jealousy toward sibling, anger toward parent, or unconquered fear in himself		
Sexual exploration and curiosity demonstrated through play, such as being "doctor" or "nurse"		

Continued.

Unit 1

Growth and development during preschool years—cont'd

Age (years)	Physical	Gross motor	Fine motor	Language
5	Pulse and respiration decrease slightly Eruption of permanent dentition may begin, especially if deciduous tooth eruption was early (before age 6 months) First permanent teeth to erupt are four molars, which come in behind the last temporary teeth (often mistaken for temporary molars) Handedness is established (about 90% are right-handed)	Skips and hops on alternate feet Throws and catches ball well Jumps rope Skates with good balance Walks backward with heel to toe Jumps from height of 12 inches, lands on toes Balances on alternate feet with eyes closed	Ties shoelaces Uses scissors, simple tools, or pencil very well In drawing, copies a diamond and triangle; adds seven to nine parts to stickman; prints a few letters, numbers, or words, such as first name	Has vocabulary of about 2100 words Uses sentences of six to eight words, with all parts of speech Names coins (nickel, dime, and so on) Names four or more colors Describes drawing or pictures with much comment and enumeration Asks meaning of words Asks inquisitive questions Can repeat sentence of ten syllables or more Knows names of days of week, months, and other time-associated words Defines words using action as well as description Knows composition of articles, such as, "A shoe is made of _____" Can follow three demands in succession

Socialization	Cognition	Family relationships
Is less rebellious and quarrelsome than at age 4 years	Begins to question what parents think by comparing them to age-mates and other adults	Gets along well with parents
Is more settled and eager to get down to business	May notice prejudice and bias in outside world	Does not try to run away from home
Is not as open and accessible in thoughts and behavior as in earlier years	Is more able to view other's perspective, but tolerates differences rather than understands them	May seek out parent more often than at age 4 years for reassurance and security, especially when entering school
Is independent but trustworthy, not foolhardy, more responsible	Tends to be matter-of-fact about differences in others	Is upset not to find parent, for example, when arriving home from school
Has fewer fears, relies on outer authority to control the world	May begin to show understanding of conservation of numbers through counting objects regardless of arrangement	Tolerates siblings, but finds 3-year-old children a special nuisance
Is eager to do things right and to please; tries to "live by the rules"	Uses time-oriented words with increased understanding	Begins to question parents' thinking and principles
Acts "manly" or "womanly"	Is very curious about factual information regarding the world	Strongly identifies with parent of same sex, especially boys with their fathers
Has fairly consistent and polished manners		Enjoys doing activities, such as sports, cooking, shopping, and so on, with parent of same sex
Cares for self totally, occasionally needing supervision in dress or hygiene		
May complain over minor injuries but tries to be brave for major pain		
Play is associative		
Likes rules and tries to follow them but may cheat to avoid losing		
Begins to notice group conformity and sense of belonging		
Is very industrious, tries to accomplish a goal and feels pride and satisfaction, as well as unhappiness and discontent		
May demand to watch television more now that understands programs better		
Is not ready for concentrated close work or small print because of slight farsightedness and still unrefined eye-hand coordination		
Imitative play mimics the portrayed adult like a mirror image		
Wants to use real objects during play, such as actual ingredients to make cookies rather than sand or mud		

Unit 1

Growth and development during school-age years

Age (years)	Physical and motor	Cognition	Adaptive	Socialization
6	Height and weight gain slower; 5 cm (2 inches) and 2.3 kg (5 pounds) Central mandibular incisors erupt Gradual increase in dexterity Active age; constant activity Often returns to finger feeding More aware of hand as a tool Likes to draw, print, and color	Attends first grade Counts 13 pennies Knows whether it is morning or afternoon Defines common objects such as fork and chair in terms of their use Obeys triple commands in succession Shows personal right hand and left ear Says which is pretty and which is ugly of a series of drawings of faces Describes the objects in a picture rather than simply enumerating them Reads from memory; enjoys oral spelling game Is in period of more tension, but is intellectually more stimulating	At table, uses knife to spread butter or jam on bread At play, cuts, folds, pastes paper toys, sews crudely if needle is threaded Cannot tie knot Enjoys making simple figures in clay Takes bath without supervision; performs bedtime activities alone Likes table games, checkers, simple card games Is more independent, probably influence of school Has own way of doing things Tries out own abilities	Can share and cooperate better Has great need for children of own age Often engages in rough play Is often jealous of younger brother or sister Does what child sees adults doing Often has temper tantrums Is a boaster Will cheat to win Has difficulty owning up to misdeeds Sometimes steals money or attractive items Giggles a lot Has increased socialization, such as tattling
7	Continues to grow 5 cm (2 inches) and 2.5 kg (5.5 pounds) a year Maxillary central incisors and lateral mandibular incisors erupt Gross motor actions are cautious but not fearful More cautious in approaches to new performances Repeats performances to master them Posture more tense and unstable; maintains one position longer	Attends second grade Notices that certain parts are missing from pictures Can copy a diamond Repeats three numbers backward Reads ordinary clock or watch correctly to nearest quarter hour; uses clock for practical purposes More mechanical in reading; often does not stop at the end of a sentence, skips words such as it, the, he, and so on	Uses table knife for cutting meat; may need help with tough or difficult pieces Brushes and combs hair acceptably without help or "going over"	Is becoming a real member of the family group Likes to help and have a choice Is less resistant and stubborn Spends a lot of time alone; does not require a lot of companionship Stealing may still be a problem Boys take part in group play with boys; girls prefer playing with girls

Age (years)	Physical and motor	Cognition	Adaptive	Socialization
8-9	Continues to grow at 5 cm (2 inches) and 3 kg (6.6 pounds) a year Movement fluid; often graceful and poised Always on the go; jumps, chases, skips Increased smoothness and speed in the motor control Dresses self completely Eyes and hands are well coordinated	Attends third and fourth grade Gives similarities and differences between two things from memory Counts backward from 20 to 1 Repeats days of the week and months in order; knows the date Describes common objects in detail, not merely their use Makes change out of a quarter Reads classic books but also enjoys comics Is more aware of time; can be relied on to get to school on time Is afraid of failing a grade; ashamed of bad grades	Makes use of common tools such as hammer, saw, or screwdriver Uses household and sewing utensils Helps with routine household tasks such as dusting, sweeping Assumes responsibility for share of household chores Looks after all of own needs at table Buys useful articles; exercises some choice in making purchases Goes about home and community freely, alone or with friends Runs useful errands Likes pictorial magazines Likes school; wants to answer all the questions Great reader; may plan to wake up early just to read Enjoys school Likely to overdo; hard to quiet down after recess	Easy to get along with at home; better behaved Likes the reward system Dramatizes Is more sociable Is better behaved Is interested in boy-girl relationships but will not admit it Likes to compete and play games More critical of self
10-12	Slow growth in height and rapid weight gain (6.25 cm [2.5 inches] and 4.5 kg [10 pounds]), may become obese in this period Posture is more similar to an adult's; will overcome lordosis Pubescent changes may begin to appear, especially in females Body lines soften and round out in females Rest of teeth will erupt and tend toward full development	Attends fifth to seventh grades Writes occasional short letters to friends or relatives on own initiative Uses telephone for practical purposes Responds to magazines, TV, or other advertising by mailing coupons Reads for practical information or own enjoyment stories or library books of adventure or romance, or animal stories	Does occasional or brief work on own initiative around home and neighborhood Is sometimes left alone at home or at work for short period Is successful in looking after own needs or those of other children left in own care Makes useful articles or does easy repair work Cooks or sews in small way Raises pets Writes brief stories Produces simple paintings or drawings Washes and dries own hair Is responsible for a thorough job of cleaning hair, but may need reminding to do so	Likes family; family really has meaning Likes mother and wants to please her in many ways Demonstrates affection Likes dad too; he is adored and idolized Respects parents Loves friends; talks about them constantly Chooses friends more selectively Loves conversation Has beginning interest in opposite sex Is more diplomatic

Growth and development during adolescence

Age (years)	Physical development and sexuality	Cognition and socialization	Personal/family relationships
Early adolescence	Maximum growth increase, especially in height; gain in height is abrupt at the onset and continues at a rapid rate the first 2 years, followed by a deceleration	Has limited ability for abstract thinking	Is most ambivalent
	Peak growth in height in males at 14 years and in females at 12 years	Is clumsy groping for new values and energies	Has wide mood swings
		Explores with new ability to think abstractly	Daydreams intensely
	Girls are generally 2 years ahead of boys in development at first	Tries out various roles	Expresses anger outwardly with moodiness, temper outbursts, verbal insults, and name-calling
	Beginning of menses (average age 12½ years)	Measures attractiveness by acceptance or rejection of peers	Attempts repeated separation from parents and concentrates on relationships with peers
	Boys experience nocturnal emissions	Conforms to group norms of dress, activity, and vocabulary	Is period of greatest parent-child conflict
	Bones increase in size; ossification speeds up	Develops close idealized friendships with members of the same sex	Takes instant exception to any opinion expressed by others
	Girls have more subcutaneous tissue so may be more obese	Uses girlfriend as girl's mother-substitute	Forms ego ideal of male (dad) through relationships with father
	Coordination improves until approximately 14 when it reaches a plateau, and child may then appear awkward	Struggle for mastery takes place within peer group	Has strong desire to remain dependent on parents while trying to detach
	Boys develop larger muscles	Differences are intolerable to the peer group; uniformity is the norm	
	Appears long-legged and gangling	Effectively uses humor to criticize family and friends	
	Girls become relatively broad-hipped about the age of 12	This is low point in sustained interest and creativity	
	Boys grow rapidly in shoulder breadth from about 13 years	Television is popular, since it appeals to fantasies of adventure	
	Has general anxiety about and intense occupation with developing body size and functioning, especially being too small	Talking to friends is a favorite activity; telephone is important link with peers	
	Gains mastery and control over increased physical capabilities	Discusses boys, clothes, makeup as girls congregate in bedrooms	
	Is very narcissistic	Boys' activities and interests center around sports; sports figures are heroes	
	Compares "normality" with peers of same sex	Group activities are valued by both sexes	
		Sports activities occupy much time	
		Pets are an important part in their lives; girls are especially interested in horses	
		Transistor radios are constant companions	

Age (years)	Physical development and sexuality	Cognition and socialization	Personal/family relationships
Middle adolescence	Attains physical maturity in female; growth in height ceases at 16 to 17 years Revival and resolution of oedipal conflict occurs Possible sexual experimentation with peers and homosexual episodes are possible Masturbation is a central concern	Develops capacity for abstract thinking Has ability to reason deductively from hypotheses Has ability to maintain an argument Under pressure may return to earlier cognitive level Gradually realizes that others' thoughts are not directed toward them Enjoys intellectual powers—Often in idealistic, altruistic terms Worries about school work Concerned with philosophic, political, and social problems; often has unrealistic ideals Uses defenses such as intellectualism and self-denial Invests love in another—Transferred from self; love object often resembles parent Acceptance by peers is extremely important—Has great fear of rejection Behavioral standards are set by peer group Turns toward heterosexuality (if is homosexual, knows by this time) Explores "sex appeal" May experience feeling of "being in love" Is most creative period More activities involve the opposite sex Appropriate behavior during date is a major concern Sports activities are still very important Has deep appreciation of beauty and nature Feels need for an automobile Has/wants outside jobs to earn money	Is very self-centered; increased narcissism Tends toward inner experience and self-discovery Struggles to define attractiveness as mediated through personal appearance Tends toward inner experiences; more introspective Tends to withdraw when upset or feelings are hurt Emotions vacillate in time and range Feelings of inadequacy are common; has difficulty in asking for help Low point in parent-child relationship occurs Greatest push for emancipation occurs Final and irreversible emotional detachment from parents occurs Has major conflicts over independence

Continued.

Growth and development during adolescence—cont'd

Age (years)	Physical development and sexuality	Cognition and socialization	Personal/family relationships
Late adolescence	Attains physical maturity in male; growth in height ceases at 18 to 20 years Comfortable with physical growth and attractiveness Sexual identity is irreversible Body image and gender role definition are nearly selected	Is capable of safeguarding the identity Has formal operational thought Able to view problems comprehensively Able to make stable relationships and form attachment to another Makes gains in social integration Importance of peer groups is lessening New depths in interpersonal relationships form Social roles are defined and articulated Creative imagination is fading Prefers purposeful action Life goals and tasks are assuming shape Pursues a career or vocation and decisions about lifestyle Is in a decisive turning point—a time of crisis Defines functional role in terms of life goals Relationships with opposite sex are no longer narcissistic	Has more constancy of emotion Anger is more apt to be concealed Is in phase of consolidation of identity Stability of self-esteem occurs Has growing capacity for mutuality and reciprocity Individual is preferred as dating partner Tests male-female relationships against possibility of permanent alliance Relationships are characterized by giving and sharing Has fewer conflicts with family Is independent from family Emancipation is nearly secured Is able to take or leave advice

REFERENCES

Caldwell B and Bradley R: Home Observation and Measurement of the Environment, revised edition, Little Rock, Ark., 1984, University of Arkansas.

Dunst C, Trivette C, and Deal A: Enabling and empowering families: principles and guidelines for practice, Cambridge, Mass., 1988, Brookline Books.

Feetham S and Humenick S: Feetham Family Functioning Survey. In Humenick S, (editor): Analysis of current assessment strategies in the health care of young children and childbearing families, Norwalk, Conn., 1982, Appleton-Century-Crofts.

Frankenburg W and Coons C: Home Screening Questionnaire: its validity in assessing home environment, J Pediatr 108(4):624-626, 1986.

Hartman A: Finding families: an ecological approach to family assessment in adoption, Beverly Hills, Calif., 1979, Sage Publications.

Hymovich D: Personal communication, 1989.

Roberts C and Feetham S: Assessing family functioning across three areas of relationship, Nurs Res 31(4):231-235, 1982.

Smilkstein G: The family APGAR: a proposal for a family function test and its use by physicians, J Fam Pract 6(6):1231-1239, 1978.

Thrower S, Bruce W, and Walton R: The Family Circle Method for integrating family systems concepts in family medicine, J Fam Pract 15(3):451-457, 1982.

2

Health Promotion

Symbol ■ indicates material that may be photocopied and distributed to families.

RECOMMENDATIONS FOR PREVENTIVE PEDIATRIC HEALTH CARE
Committee on Practice and Ambulatory Medicine

Each child and family is unique: therefore these **Recommendations for Preventive Pediatric Health Care** are designed for the care of children who are receiving competent parenting, have no manifestations of any important health problems, and are growing and developing in satisfactory fashion. **Additional visits may become necessary** if circumstances suggest variations from normal. These guidelines represent a consensus by the Committee on Practice and Ambulatory Medicine in consultation with the membership of the American Academy of Pediatrics through the Chapter Presidents. The Committee emphasizes the great importance of **continuity of care** in comprehensive health supervision and the need to avoid **fragmentation of care.**

A **prenatal visit** by the parents for anticipatory guidance and pertinent medical history is strongly recommended.

Health supervision should begin with medical care of the newborn in the hospital.

1. Adolescent related issues (e.g., psychosocial, emotional, substance usage, and reproductive health) may necessitate more frequent health supervision.
2. If a child comes under care for the first time at any point on the schedule, or if any items are not accomplished at the suggested age, the schedule should be brought up to date at the earliest possible time.
3. At these points, history may suffice: if problem suggested, a standard testing method should be employed.
4. By history and appropriate physical examination: if suspicious, by specific objective developmental testing.

5. At each visit, a complete physical examination is essential, with infant totally unclothed, older child undressed and suitably draped.
6. These may be modified, depending upon entry point into schedule and individual need.
7. Metabolic screening (e.g., thyroid, PKU, galactosemia) should be done according to state law.
8. Schedule(s) per Report of Committee on Infectious Disease, *1986 Red Book.**
9. For low risk groups, the Committee on Infectious Diseases recommends the following options: ① no routine testing or ② testing at three times—infancy, preschool, and adolescence. For high risk groups, annual TB skin testing is recommended.
10. Present medical evidence suggests the need for reevaluation of the frequency and timing of hemoglobin or hematocrit tests. One determination is therefore suggested during each time period. Performance of additional tests is left to the individual practice experience.
11. Present medical evidence suggests the need for reevaluation of the frequency and timing of urinalyses. One determination is therefore suggested during each time period. Performance of additional tests is left to the individual practice experience.
12. Appropriate discussion and counseling should be an integral part of each visit for care.
13. Subsequent examinations as prescribed by dentist.

N.B.: **Special chemical, immunologic, and endocrine testing** are usually carried out upon specific indications. Testing other than newborn (e.g., inborn errors of metabolism, sickle disease, lead) are discretionary with the physician.

From Committee on Psychosocial Aspects of Child and Family Health, 1985-1988: Guidelines for health supervision II, 1987, Elk Grove Village, IL, American Academy of Pediatrics.

*Author's note: For more current recommendations see p 176 and p 177.

	INFANCY						EARLY CHILDHOOD					LATE CHILDHOOD					ADOLESCENCE[1]			
AGE[2]	By 1 mo.	2 mos.	4 mos.	6 mos.	9 mos.	12 mos.	15 mos.	18 mos.	24 mos.	3 yrs.	4 yrs.	5 yrs.	6 yrs.	8 yrs.	10 yrs.	12 yrs.	14 yrs.	16 yrs.	18 yrs.	20+ yrs.
HISTORY Initial/Interval	•	•	•	•	•	•	•	•	•	•	•	•	•	•	•	•	•	•	•	•
MEASUREMENTS Height and Weight	•	•	•	•	•	•	•	•	•	•	•	•	•	•	•	•	•	•	•	•
Head Circumference	•	•	•	•	•	•														
Blood Pressure										•	•	•	•	•	•	•	•	•	•	•
SENSORY SCREENING Vision	S	S	S	S	S	S	S	S	S	S	○	○	○	○	S	○	○	S	○	○
Hearing	S	S	S	S	S	S	S	S	S	S	○	○	S[3]	S[3]	S[3]	○	S	S	○	S
DEVEL./BEHAV.[4] ASSESSMENT	•	•	•	•	•	•	•	•	•	•	•	•	•	•	•	•	•	•	•	•
PHYSICAL EXAMINATION[5]	•	•	•	•	•	•	•	•	•	•	•	•	•	•	•	•	•	•	•	•
PROCEDURES[6] Hered./Metabolic[7] Screening	•																			
Immunization[8]		•	•	•			•	•	•			•					•			
Tuberculin Test[9]						← → •			← → •				← →						← → •		
Hematocrit or Hemoglobin[10]					← → •			← → •					← →					← → •		
Urinalysis[11]				← → •				← → •					← →					← → •		
ANTICIPATORY[12] GUIDANCE	•	•	•	•	•	•	•	•	•	•	•	•	•	•	•	•	•	•	•	•
INITIAL DENTAL[13] REFERRAL										•										

NUTRITION
Vitamins and their nutritional significance

Physiologic functions/sources	Results of deficiency or excess	Nursing considerations

VITAMIN A (RETINOL)*

Functions

Necessary component in formation of pigment rhodopsin (visual purple)

Formation and maintenance of epithelial tissue

Normal bone growth and tooth development

Needed for growth and spermatogenesis

Involved in thyroxine formation

Sources

Natural form—liver, kidney, fish oils, milk and nonskimmed milk products, egg yolk

Provitamin A (carotene)—carrots, sweet potatoes, squash, apricots, spinach, collards, broccoli, cabbage, artichokes

Deficiency

Night blindness

Keratinization (hardening and scaling) of epithelium

Xerophthalmia (hardening and scaling of cornea and conjunctiva)

Phrynoderma (toadskin)

Drying of respiratory, gastrointestinal, and genitourinary tracts

Defective tooth enamel

Retarded growth

Impaired bone formation

Decreased thyroxine formation

Excess

Early signs—irritability, anorexia, pruritus, fissures at corners of nose and lips

Later signs—hepatomegaly, jaundice, retarded growth, poor weight gain, thickening of the cortex of long bones with pain and fragility, hard tender lumps in extremities and occiput of the skull

May cause birth defects from excessive maternal intake

NOTE: Overdose only results from ingestion of large quantities of the vitamin, not the provitamin; large amounts of carotene (carotenemia) cause yellow or orange discoloration of the skin (not the sclera, urine, or feces as in jaundice), but none of the above symptoms

Encourage foods rich in vitamin A, such as whole cow's milk

As milk consumption decreases, encourage foods rich in vitamin A

Emphasize correct use of vitamin supplements and potential hazards of excess

Investigate child's dietary habits to calculate approximate intake; if excessive, remove supplemental source

Advise parents of the benign nature of carotenemia; treatment is avoidance of excess pigmented fruits or vegetables, especially carrots; skin color returns to normal in 2 to 6 weeks

VITAMIN B_1 (THIAMIN)†

Functions

Coenzyme (with phosphorus) in carbohydrate metabolism

Needed for healthy nervous system

Sources

Pork, beef, liver, legumes, nuts, whole or enriched grains and cereals, green vegetables, fruits, milk

Deficiency

Beriberi

Gastrointestinal—anorexia, constipation, indigestion

Neurologic—apathy, fatigue, emotional instability, polyneuritis, tenderness of calf muscles, partial anesthesia, muscle weakness, paresthesia, hyperesthesia, decreased or absent tendon reflexes, convulsions, and coma (in infants)

Cardiovascular—palpitations, cardiac failure, peripheral vasodilation, edema

Excess

Headache   Rapid pulse
Irritability   Weakness
Insomnia

Vitamin B complex

Encourage foods rich in B vitamins

Stress proper cooking and storage techniques to preserve potency, such as minimal cooking of vegetables in small amount of liquid; storage of milk in opaque container

Advise against fad diets that severely restrict groups of food, such as vegetarianism

Explore need for vitamin supplements when dieting or when using goat milk exclusively for infant feeding (deficient in folic acid) or when the breast-feeding mother is a strict vegetarian (vitamin B_{12})

Emphasize correct use of vitamin supplements and potential hazards of excesses

*Fat soluble.
†Water soluble.

Vitamins and their nutritional significance—cont'd

Physiologic functions/sources	Results of deficiency or excess	Nursing considerations

VITAMIN B₂ (RIBOFLAVIN)†

Functions

Coenzyme (with phosphorus) in carbohydrate, protein, and fat metabolism

Maintains healthy skin especially around mouth, nose, and eye

Sources

Milk and its products, eggs, organ meat (liver, kidney, and heart), enriched cereals, some green leafy vegetables,‡ legumes

Deficiency

Ariboflavinosis

Lips—cheilosis (fissures at corners of lips), prelèche (inflammation at corners of lips)

Tongue—glossitis

Nose—irritation and cracks at nasal angle

Eyes—burning, itching, tearing, photophobia, corneal vascularization, cataracts

Skin—seborrheic dermatitis, delayed wound healing and tissue repair

Excess

Paresthesia, pruritus

Same as vitamin B complex

NIACIN (NICOTINIC ACID, NICOTINAMIDE)†

Functions

Coenzyme (with riboflavin) in protein and fat metabolism

Needed for healthy nervous system, skin, and normal digestion

Sources

Meat, poultry, fish, peanuts, beans, peas, whole or enriched grains except corn and rice

Milk and its products are sources of tryptophan (60 mg of tryptophan = 1 mg of niacin)

Deficiency

Pellagra

Oral—Stomatitis, glossitis

Cutaneous—scaly dermatitis on exposed areas

Gastrointestinal—anorexia, weight loss, diarrhea, fatigue

Neurologic—apathy, anxiety, confusion, depression, dementia

Death

Excess

Release of vasodilator, histamine (flushing, decreased blood pressure, increased cerebral blood flow; aggravates asthma)

Dermatologic problems (pruritus, rash, hyperkeratosis, acanthosis nigricans)

Increased gastric acidity (aggravates peptic ulcer disease)

Hepatotoxicity

Increased serum uric acid levels

Elevated plasma glucose levels

Certain cardiac arrhythmias

Same as vitamin B complex

VITAMIN B₆ (PYRIDOXINE)†

Functions

Coenzyme in protein and fat metabolism

Needed for formation of antibodies, hemoglobin

Needed for utilization of copper and iron

Aids in conversion of tryptophan to niacin

Sources

Meats, especially liver and kidney, cereal grains (wheat and corn), yeast, soybeans, peanuts, tuna, chicken, salmon

Deficiency

Scaly dermatitis, weight loss, anemia, retarded growth, irritability, convulsions, peripheral neuritis

Excess

Peripheral nervous system toxicity (unsteady gait, numb feet and hands, clumsiness of hands, sometimes perioral numbness)

May cause peptic ulcer disease or seizures

Same as vitamin B complex

Stress proper cooking and storing techniques to preserve potency

Cook food covered in small amount of water

Do not soak food in water

Store in light-resistant container

---

*Fat soluble.

†Water soluble.

‡Green leafy vegetables include spinach, broccoli, kale, turnip greens, mustard greens, collards, dandelion greens, and beet greens.

Physiologic functions/sources	Results of deficiency or excess	Nursing considerations

FOLIC ACID (FOLACIN; REDUCED FORM IS CALLED FOLINIC ACID OR CITROVORUM FACTOR)†

| **Functions**
Coenzyme for single-carbon transfer (purines, thymine, hemoglobin)
Necessary for formation of red blood cells

Sources
Green leafy vegetables, cabbage, asparagus, liver, kidney, nuts, eggs, whole grain cereals, legumes, bananas | **Deficiency**
Macrocytic anemia, bone marrow depression, glossitis, intestinal malabsorption

Excess
Rare because megadoses not available over the counter
May cause insomnia and irritability | Same as vitamin B complex
Stress proper cooking and storing techniques to preserve potency
Cook food covered in small amount of water
Do not soak food in water
Store in light-resistant container |

VITAMIN B₁₂ (COBALAMIN)†

| **Functions**
Coenzyme in protein synthesis; indirect effect on formation of red blood cells (particularly on formation of nucleic acids and folic and metabolism)
Needed for normal functioning of nervous tissue

Sources
Meat, liver, kidney, fish, shellfish, poultry, milk, eggs, cheese, nutritional yeast, sea vegetables | **Deficiency**
Pernicious anemia
(one form of deficiency from absence of intrinsic factor in gastric secretions)
General signs of severe anemia
Lemon yellow tinge to skin
Spinal cord degeneration

Excess
Excess is rare | Same as vitamin B complex |

BIOTIN

| Functions
Coenzyme in carbohydrate, protein, and fat metabolism
Interrelated with functions of other B vitamins

Sources
Liver, kidney, egg yolk, tomatoes, legumes, nuts | **Deficiency**
Deficiency is uncommon because synthesized by bacterial flora

Excess
Unknown | Same as vitamin B complex |

PANTOTHENIC ACID†

| **Functions**
Coenzyme in carbohydrate, protein, and fat metabolism
Synthesis of amino acids, fatty acids, and steroids

Sources
Liver, kidney, heart, salmon, eggs, vegetables, legumes, whole grains | **Deficiency**
Deficiency is uncommon because of its multiple food sources and synthesis by bacterial flora

Excess
Minimum toxicity (occasional diarrhea and water retention) | Same as vitamin B complex |

Continued.

Unit 2

NUTRITION
Vitamins and their nutritional significance—cont'd

Physiologic functions/sources	Results of deficiency or excess	Nursing considerations
VITAMIN C (ASCORBIC ACID)†		
Functions	**Deficiency**	
Essential for collagen formation	*Scurvy*	Encourage foods rich in vitamin C
Increases absorption of iron for hemoglobin formation	Skin—dry, rough, petechiae, perifollicular hyperkeratotic papules (raised areas around hair follicles)	Investigate infant's diet for sources of vitamin, especially when cow's milk is principal source of nutrition
Enhances conversion of folic to folinic acid	Musculoskeletal—bleeding muscles and joints, pseudoparalysis from pain, swelling of joints, costochondral beading (scorbutic rosary)	Stress proper cooking and storing techniques to preserve potency
Affects cholesterol synthesis and conversion of proline to hydroxyproline		Wash vegetables quickly; do not soak in water
Probably a coenzyme in metabolism of tyrosine and phenylalanine	Gums—spongy, friable, swollen, bleed easily, bluish red or black color, teeth loosen and fall out	Cook vegetables in covered pot with minimal water and for short time; avoid copper or cast iron cookware
May play role in hydroxylation of adrenal steroids	General disposition—irritable, anorexic, apprehensive, in pain, refuses to move, assumes semi-froglike position when supine (scorbutic pose)	Do not add baking soda to cooking water
May have stimulating effect on phagocytic activity of leukocytes and formation of antibodies		Use fresh fruits and vegetables as soon as possible; store in refrigerator
Antioxidant agent (spares other vitamins from oxidation)	Signs of anemia	Store juice in airtight opaque container
	Decreased wound healing	Wrap cut fruit or eat soon after exposing to air
	Increased susceptibility to infection	
Sources		In caring for child with scurvy:
Citrus fruits, strawberries, tomatoes, potatoes, melon, cabbage, broccoli, cauliflower, spinach, papaya, mango	**Excess**	Position for comfort and rest
	Diarrhea	Handle very gently and minimally
	Increased excretion of uric acid and acidification of urine (may cause urate precipitation and formation of oxalate stones)	Administer analgesics as needed
		Prevent infection
		Provide good oral care
	Hemolysis	Provide soft, bland diet
	Impaired leukocytosis activity	Emphasize rapid recovery when vitamin is replaced
	Damage to beta cells of pancreas and decreased insulin production	Emphasize correct use of vitamin supplement and potential hazards of excess
	Reproductive failure	Identify groups at risk for vitamin C supplements: those with thalassemia; those on anticoagulant or aminoglycoside antibiotic therapy
	"Rebound scurvy" from withdrawal of large amounts	
VITAMIN D₂ (ERGOCALCIFEROL) AND D₃ (CHOLECALCIFEROL)*		
Functions	**Deficiency**	
Absorption of calcium and phosphorus and decreased renal excretion of phosphorus	*Rickets*	Encourage foods rich in vitamin D, especially fortified cow's milk
	Head—craniotabes (softening of cranial bones, prominence of frontal bones), deformed shape (skull flat and depressed toward middle), delayed closure of fontanels	In breast-fed infants encourage use of vitamin D supplements if maternal diet inadequate or infant exposed to minimal sunlight
Sources		Emphasize importance of exposure to sun as source of vitamin
Direct sunlight		
Cod liver oil, herring, mackerel, salmon, tuna, sardines	Chest—rachitic rosary (enlargement of costochondral junction of ribs), Harrison groove (horizontal depression in lower portion of rib cage), pigeon chest (sharp protrusion of sternum)	In caring for child with rickets:
Enriched food sources—milk, milk products, cereals, margarine, breads, many breakfast drinks		Maintain good body alignment
		Reposition frequently to prevent decubiti and respiratory infection
	Spine—kyphosis, scoliosis, lordosis	Handle very gently and minimally
	Abdomen—potbelly, constipation	

*Fat soluble.
†Water soluble.

Physiologic functions/sources	Results of deficiency or excess	Nursing considerations
	Extremities—bowing of arms and legs, knock-knee, saber shins, instability of hip joints, pelvic deformity, enlargement of epiphysis at ends of long bones Teeth—delayed calcification, especially of permanent teeth Rachitic tetany—seizures	Prevent infection Institute seizure precautions Have 10% calcium gluconate available in case of tetany Observe for possibility of overdose from supplements If prescribed, supervise proper use of orthopedic splints or braces
	Excess Acute—vomiting, dehydration, fever, abdominal cramps, bone pain, convulsions, and coma Chronic—lassitude, mental slowness, anorexia, failure to thrive, thirst, urinary urgency, polyuria, vomiting, diarrhea, abdominal cramps, bone pain, pathologic fractures Calcification of soft tissue—kidneys, lungs, adrenal glands, vessels (hypertension), heart, gastric lining, tympanic membrane (deafness) Osteoporosis of long bones Elevated serum levels of calcium and phosphorus	Same as vitamin A; may include low-calcium diet during initial therapy

VITAMIN E (TOCOPHEROL)*

Functions

Production of red blood cells and protection from hemolysis
Muscle and liver integrity
Coenzyme factor in tissue respiration
Minimizes oxidation of polyunsaturated fatty acids and vitamins A and C in intestinal tract and tissues

Sources

Vegetable oils, wheat germ oil, milk, egg yolk, muscle meats, fish, whole grains, nuts, legumes, spinach, broccoli

Deficiency

Hemolytic anemia from hemolysis caused by shortened life of red blood cells, especially in premature infants, and focal necrosis of tissues
Causes infertility in rats, but not in humans (does *not* increase human male virility or potency)

Excess

Little is known: less toxic than other fat-soluble vitamins but excess of water-soluble preparations has been fatal in premature infants

Initiate early feeding in premature infants; may need supplementation

VITAMIN K*

Functions

Catalyst for production of prothrombin and blood clotting factors II, VII, IX, and X by the liver

Sources

Pork, liver, green leafy vegetables (spinach, kale, cabbage), tomatoes, egg yolk, cheese

Deficiency

Hemorrhage

Excess

Hyperbilirubinemia in infants
Hemolytic anemia in individuals who are deficient in glucose-6-phosphate dehydrogenase

Administer prophylactically to newborns
Other indications include intestinal disease, lack of bile, prolonged antibiotic therapy; may be used in management of blood-clotting time when anticoagulants such as warfarin (Coumadin), and dicumarol (bishydroxycoumarin), which are vitamin K antagonists, are used

Continued.

Minerals and their nutritional significance

Physiologic functions/sources	Results of deficiency or excess	Nursing considerations
CALCIUM*		
Functions	**Deficiency**	
Bone and tooth development and maintenance (in combination with phosphorus)	***Rickets*** Tetany Impaired growth, especially of bones and teeth	Encourage foods rich in calcium, especially dairy products Caution that oxalates in leafy vegetables (spinach) oxalates in chocolates, and a high phosphorus intake (especially from carbonated beverages) can decrease calcium absorption
Muscle contractions, especially the heart Blood clotting Absorption of vitamin B_{12} Enzyme activation Nerve conduction Integrity of intracellular cement substances and various membranes		Discourage use of whole cow's milk in newborns because the high phosphorus-to-calcium ratio favors excretion of calcium Advise against fad diets, especially those that restrict dairy products
Sources	**Excess**	
Dairy products, egg yolk, sardines, canned salmon with bones, dark-green leafy vegetables, soybeans, dried beans, and peas	Drowsiness, extreme lethargy Impaired absorption of other minerals (iron, zinc, manganese) Calcium deposits in tissues (renal failure)	Emphasize correct use of calcium supplement, especially the possible interaction between megadoses of calcium and resulting deficiency states of other minerals
CHLORIDE*		
Functions	**Deficiency**	
Acid-base and fluid balance Enzyme activation in saliva Component of hydrochloric acid in stomach	Acid-base disturbances (hypochloremic alkalosis, dehydration); occurs mostly in combination with sodium loss	Deficiency and excess are unusual; most diets supply adequate chloride (usually in combination with sodium) Disease states such as excessive vomiting can necessitate chloride replacement
Sources	**Excess**	
Salt, meat, eggs, dairy products, many prepared and preserved foods	Acid-base disturbance	
CHROMIUM†		
Functions	**Deficiency**	
Involved in glucose metabolism and energy production	Possible abnormal glucose metabolism	No specific recommendations are needed
Sources	**Excess**	
Meat, cheese, whole grain breads and cereals, legumes, peanuts, brewer's yeast, vegetable oils	Unknown	
COPPER†		
Functions	**Deficiency**	
Production of hemoglobin Essential component of several enzyme systems	Anemia, leukopenia, neutropenia	Deficiency from inadequate food sources is less likely than from excess intake of other minerals, especially zinc and possibly iron; therefore emphasize the correct use of any vitamin supplement
Sources	**Excess**	
Organ meats, oysters, nuts, seeds, legumes, corn oil margarine	Severe vomiting and diarrhea Hemolytic anemia	Caution against cooking acid foods in unlined copper pots, which can lead to chronic and toxic accumulation of copper

*Macrominerals—required intake >100 mg/day
†Microminerals or trace elements—required intake <100 mg/day

Physiologic functions/sources	Results of deficiency or excess	Nursing considerations
FLUORINE†		
Functions	**Deficiency**	
Formation of caries-resistant teeth Strong bone development	Increased susceptibility to tooth decay	In areas with optimally fluoridated water, encourage sufficient intake to supply recommended amount of fluoride (see p. 183)
Sources		In areas of unfluoridated water or when ready-to-use formula or breast milk are used, stress the importance of fluoride supplements
Fluoridated water and foods or beverages prepared with fluoridated water; fish, tea, commercially prepared chicken for infants	**Excess**	
	Fluorosis (mottling and/or pitting of enamel) Severe bone deformities	In areas with excess fluoride in the water consider the use of bottled water in drinking and possibly cooking to reduce the fluoride intake to safe levels Fluorine has the narrowest range of safe and adequate intake; therefore, stress the importance of storing supplements in a safe area
IODINE†		
Functions	**Deficiency**	
Production of thyroid hormone Normal reproduction	***Goiter*** (enlarged thyroid from decreased thyroxine formation)	Encourage use of iodized salt for individuals living far from the sea.
Sources	**Excess**	
Seafood, kelp, iodized salt, sea salt, enriched bread, milk (from dairy processing)	Unknown from food sources; may occur from ingestion of iodine preparations, such as saturated solutions of potassium iodide (SSKI)	If iodine preparations are in the home, stress the importance of safe storage
IRON†		
Functions	**Deficiency**	
Formation of hemoglobin and myoglobin Essential part of several enzymes and proteins	***Anemia*** (see p. 375)	Encourage foods rich in iron Discourage excessive milk consumption, especially more than 1 liter per day (milk is a very poor source of iron) If iron supplements are prescribed, teach parents factors that affect absorption (see box below)

FACTORS THAT AFFECT IRON ABSORPTION

Increase	Decrease
Acidity (low pH)—administer iron between meals (gastric hydrochloric acid) Ascorbic acid (vitamin C)—administer iron with juice, fruit, or multivitamin preparation Calcium Tissue need Meat, fish, poultry Cooking in cast iron pots	Alkalinity (high pH)—avoid any antacid preparation Phosphates—milk is unfavorable vehicle for iron administration Phytates—found in cereals Oxalates—found in many fruits and vegetables (plums, currants, green beans, spinach, sweet potatoes, tomatoes) Tannins—found in tea, coffee Tissue saturation Malabsorptive disorders Disturbances that cause diarrhea or steatorrhea Infection

Continued.

Minerals and their nutritional significance—cont'd

Physiologic functions/sources	Results of deficiency or excess	Nursing considerations
IRON—cont'd		
Sources	**Excess**	Stress the importance of storing iron supplements in a safe area
Liver, especially pork, followed by calf, beef, and chicken; kidney, red meat, poultry, shellfish, whole grains, iron-enriched infant formula and cereal, enriched cereals and bread, legumes, nuts, seeds, green leafy vegetables (except spinach), dried fruits, potatoes, molasses	Hemosiderosis (excess iron storage in various tissues of the body, especially the spleen, liver, lymph glands, heart, and pancreas) Hemochromatosis (excess iron storage with cellular damage)	
MAGNESIUM*		
Functions	**Deficiency**	Deficiency and excess are unusual, except in disease states such as prolonged vomiting or diarrhea or kidney dysfunction, where replacement may be needed
Bone and tooth formation Production of proteins Nerve conduction to muscles Activation of enzymes needed for carbohydrate and protein metabolism	Tremors, spasm Irregular heartbeat Muscular weakness Lower extremity cramps Convulsions, delirium	
Sources	**Excess**	
Whole grains, nuts, soybeans, meat, green leafy vegetables (uncooked), tea, cocoa, raisins	Nervous system disturbances due to imbalance in calcium-to-magnesium ratio	
MANGANESE†		
Functions	**Deficiency**	No specific recommendations are needed
Activation of enzymes involved in reproduction, growth, and fat metabolism Normal bone structure Nervous system functioning	Unknown **Excess** Unknown	
Sources		
Nuts, whole grains, legumes, green vegetables, fruit		
MOLYBDENUM†		
Functions	**Deficiency**	No specific recommendations are needed
Essential component of several oxidative enzymes	Very rare; diagnosed in patients on complete total parenteral alimentation	
Sources	**Excess**	
Legumes, whole grains, organ meats, some dark green vegetables	Produces secondary copper deficiency (growth failure, anemia, and disturbed bone development)	

*Macrominerals—required intake >100 mg/day.
†Microminerals or trace elements—required intake <100 mg/day.

Physiologic functions/sources	Results of deficiency or excess	Nursing considerations
PHOSPHORUS*		
Functions	**Deficiency**	
Bone and tooth development (in combination with calcium)	Weakness, anorexia, malaise, bone pain	Dietary deficiency is uncommon, although prolonged use of antacids can produce deficiency, in which case supplementation is recommended
Involved in numerous chemical reactions, including protein, carbohydrate, and fat metabolism	**Excess**	
Acid-base balance	Produces secondary calcium deficiency from disturbed calcium-to-phosphorus ratio	To preserve calcium-to-phosphorus ratio in newborns, discourage use of whole cow's milk
Sources		
Dairy products, eggs, meat, poultry, legumes, carbonated beverages		
POTASSIUM*		
Functions	**Deficiency**	
Acid-base and fluid balance (major extracellular fluid areas)	Cardiac arrhythmias	Dietary deficiency and excess are unlikely, although disease states such as prolonged nausea and vomiting, or the use of diuretics can result in hypokalemia; in such instances, encourage replacement with supplements of rich food sources, such as bananas
Nerve conduction	Muscular weakness	
Muscular contraction, especially the heart	Lethargy	
Release of energy	Kidney and respiratory failure	
	Heart failure	
	Excess	
Sources	Cardiac arrhythmias	
Bananas, citrus fruit, dried fruits, meat, fish, bran, legumes, peanut butter, potatoes, coffee, tea, cocoa	Respiratory failure	
	Mental confusion	
	Numbness of extremities	
SELENIUM†		
Functions	**Deficiency**	
Antioxidant, especially protective of vitamin E	Keshan disease—cardiomyopathy in children (found in China)	Deficiency and excess are uncommon in North America, although selenium deficiency can occur in patients on prolonged total parenteral alimentation; in these instances supplementation is required
Protects against toxicity of heavy metals	**Excess**	
Associated with fat metabolism	Eye, nose, and throat irritation	
Sources	Increased dental caries	
Seafood, organ meats, egg yolk, whole grain, chicken, meat, tomatoes, cabbage, garlic, mushrooms, milk	Liver and kidney degeneration	
SODIUM*		
Functions	**Deficiency**	
Acid-base and fluid balance (major extracellular fluid cation)	Dehydration	Deficiency intake is very rare, although losses secondary to nausea, vomiting, excessive sweating, and use of diuretics can occur and require replacement
Cell permeability; absorption of glucose	Hypotension	
Muscle contraction	Convulsions	
	Muscle cramps	
	Excess	
Sources	Edema	Encourage parents to limit excessive use of salt in preparing foods and commercial foods with high sodium content, such as smoked meats
Table salt, seafood, meat, poultry, numerous prepared foods	Hypertension	
	Intracranial hemorrhage	

Unit 2

Minerals and their nutritional significance—cont'd

Physiologic functions/sources	Results of deficiency or excess	Nursing considerations
SULFUR*		
Functions	**Deficiency**	
Essential component of cell protein, especially of hair and skin	Unknown	No specific recommendations are needed
Enzyme activation	**Excess**	
Associated with energy metabolism	Unknown	
Detoxification of certain chemical reactions		
Sources		
Dairy products, eggs, meat, fish, nuts, legumes		
ZINC†		
Functions	**Deficiency**	Encourage food sources rich in zinc, especially protein
Component of about 100 enzymes	Loss of appetite	Caution that fiber, phytates, oxalates, tannins (in tea or coffee), iron and calcium adversely affect zinc absorption
Synthesis of nucleic acids and protein in immune system and coagulation	Diminished taste sensation	
Release of vitamin A from liver	Delayed healing	
Improved wound healing with vitamin C	Skin lesions—erythematous, crusted lesions around body orifices	Recognize groups at risk for zinc deficiency, such as vegetarians and Mexican-Americans, whose diets may have restricted or low meat content and high fiber, phytate content; and patients with malabsorption syndromes
	Alopecia	
	Diarrhea	
Sources	Growth failure	
Seafood (especially oysters), meat, poultry, eggs, wheat, legumes	Retarded sexual maturity	
		Emphasize correct use of zinc supplements and the possible interaction with other minerals
	Excess	
	Vomiting and diarrhea	
	Malaise, dizziness	
	Anemia, gastric bleeding	
	Impaired absorption of calcium and copper	

*Macrominerals—required intake >100 mg/day.

†Microminerals or trace elements—required intake <100 mg/day.

Normal and special infant formulas

Formula (manufacturer)	Protein source	Carbohydrate source	Fat source	Indications for use	Comments (nutritional considerations)
HUMAN AND COW'S MILK FORMULAS					
Human breast milk	Mature human milk; whey/casein ratio: 60:40	Lactose	Mature human milk	For all full-term infants except those with galactosemia; may be used with low-birth-weight infants	Recommended sole form of feeding for the first 5 to 6 months; nutritionally complete except for fluoride
Evaporated cow's milk formulas Cow's milk	Milk protein; whey/casein ratio: 18:82	Lactose, sucrose	Butterfat	For full-term infants with no special nutritional requirements. Undiluted cow's milk after 6-12 months only	Supplement with iron and vitamin C; A and D if not fortified; fluoride if fluoridated water is not used for formula preparation
COMMERCIAL INFANT FORMULAS					
SMA (Wyeth)	Nonfat cow's milk, reduced mineral whey: whey/casein ratio: 60:40	Lactose	Oleo, coconut, oleic (safflower) and soy oils	For full-term and premature infants with no special nutritional requirements	Supplemented with iron, 12 mg/L
Enfamil (Mead Johnson)	Nonfat cow's milk, demineralized whey: whey/casein ratio: 60:40	Lactose	Soy, coconut oils	For full-term and premature infants with no special nutritional requirements	Available fortified with iron, 12 mg/L
Similac (Ross)	Nonfat cow's milk; whey/casein ratio: 18:82	Lactose	Soy and coconut oils, mono- and diglycerides	For full-term and premature infants with no special nutritional requirements	Available fortified with iron, 12 mg/L
Advance (Ross)	Nonfat cow's milk, soy protein isolate	Corn syrup	Corn and soy oils	For feeding of older infants	Lower-caloric content (16 cal/oz); fortified with iron, 12 mg/L
Good Start H.A. (Carnation)	Hydrolyzed whey	Lactose, maltodextrin	Palm, oleic, and coconut oils	For full-term infants	Manufacturer's claim regarding hypoallergenicity has been withdrawn
Good Nature (Carnation)	Nonfat cow's milk	Corn syrup solids	Palm, corn, and oleic oils	For feeding older infants	Contains more protein and calcium than "starter" formulas
Baby formula (Gerber)	Nonfat cow's milk; whey/casein ratio: 18:82	Lactose	Soy	For full-term and premature infants with no special nutritional requirements	Available fortified with iron, 11.5 mg/L

Modified from Kempe C, Silver H, O'Brien D, and Fulginiti V, editors: Current pediatric diagnosis and treatment, ed 9, Copyright 1987 by Lange Medical Publications, Los Altos, CA. Modifications based on product information from Carnation 1988; Loma Linda 1988; Mead Johnson Nutritionals, 1988; Ross Laboratories, 1988; Wyeth Laboratories, 1989. For the most current information, consult product labels or package enclosures.

Normal and special infant formulas—cont'd

Formula (manufacturer)	Protein source	Carbohydrate source	Fat source	Indications for use	Comments (nutritional considerations)
Similac Natural Care (Ross)	Nonfat cow's milk; whey protein concentrate	Hydrolyzed corn starch, lactose	MCT,* coconut, and soy oils	For low-birth-weight infants. Fed mixed with human milk or fed alternately with human milk. Improves vitamin/mineral content of human milk	Protein, 2.7 g/100 kcal. Osmolality, 24 cal/oz: 300 mOsm/kg water
Enfamil Human Milk Modifier (Mead Johnson)	Whey protein concentrate, casein	Corn syrup solids		For low-birth-weight infants. Fed mixed with human milk. Increases protein, calorie, calcium, phosphorus, and other nutrients	Used only as human milk fortifier, not as separate formula. One packet of powder supplies 3.5 kcal
FOR MILK PROTEIN–SENSITIVE INFANTS ("MILK ALLERGY")					
Prosobee (Mead Johnson)	Soy protein isolate	Corn syrup solids	Soy and coconut oils	With milk protein allergy, lactose intolerance, lactase deficiency, galactosemia	Hypoallergenic, zero band antigen. Lactose and sucrose free
Isomil (Ross)	Soy protein isolate	Corn syrup, sucrose	Soy and coconut oils	With milk protein allergy, lactose intolerance, lactase deficiency, galactosemia	Lactose free
Isomil SF (Ross)	Soy protein isolate	Hydrolyzed corn starch	Soy and coconut oils	With milk protein allergy or sucrose intolerance	Sucrose and lactose free
Nursoy (Wyeth)	Soy protein isolate	Sucrose (liquid formula) Corn syrup solids (powdered formula)	Oleo, coconut, oleic, and soy oils	With milk protein allergy, lactose intolerance, lactase deficiency, galactosemia	Lactose free
Soyalac (Loma Linda)	Soy bean solids	Sucrose, corn syrup	Soy oil	With milk protein allergy, lactose intolerance, lactase deficiency, galactosemia	Lactose free
I-Soyalac (Loma Linda)	Soy protein isolate	Sucrose, tapioca dextrin	Soy oil	With milk protein allergy, lactose intolerance, lactase deficiency, galactosemia	Lactose and corn free

*MCT, medium chain triglycerides.

Formula (manufacturer)	Protein source	Carbohydrate source	Fat source	Indications for use	Comments (nutritional considerations)
FOR INFANTS WITH MALABSORPTION SYNDROMES					
RCF (Ross Carbohydrate Free) (Ross)	Soy protein isolate		Soy and coconut oils	With carbohydrate intolerance	Carbohydrate is added according to amount infant will tolerate.
Portagen (Mead Johnson)	Sodium caseinate	Corn syrup solids, sucrose, lactose	MCT (coconut source) and corn oil	For impaired fat absorption secondary to pancreatic insufficiency, bile acid deficiency, intestinal resection, lymphatic anomalies.	Nutritionally complete.
Nutramigen (Mead Johnson)	Casein hydrolysate and L-amino acids*	Corn syrup solids, modified corn starch	Corn oil	For infants and children sensitive to food proteins. Use in galactosemic patients.	Nutritionally complete hypoallergenic formula. Lactose and sucrose free.
Pregestimil (Mead Johnson)	Casein hydrolysate and L-amino acids	Corn syrup solids, modified tapioca starch	Corn oil, MCT	Disaccharidase deficiencies, malabsorption syndromes, cystic fibrosis.	Nutritionally complete, easily digestible protein, carbohydrate, and fat. Lactose and sucrose free.
Alimentum (Ross)	Casein hydrolysate and L-amino acids	Sucrose, modified tapioca starch	MCT, oleic and soy oils	For infants and children sensitive to food proteins or with cystic fibrosis.	Nutritionally complete. Hypoallergenic formula. Lactose free.
SPECIALTY FORMULAS					
Lonalac (Mead Johnson) Powder	Casein	Lactose	Coconut	For children with congestive cardiac failure, who require reduced sodium intake.	For long-term management, additional sodium must be given. Supplement with vitamins C and D and iron. Na = 1 mEq/L
Similac PM 60/40 (Ross) Powder	Whey protein concentrate, sodium caseinate (60:40 ratio)	Lactose	Coconut, corn oils	For newborns predisposed to hypocalcemia and infants with impaired renal, digestive, and cardiovascular functions.	Low calcium, potassium, and phosphorus. Relatively low solute load. Na = 7 mEq/L
DIET MODIFIERS					
Polycose (Ross)		Glucose polymers (corn syrup solids)		Used to increase calorie intake, as in failure-to-thrive infants.	Carbohydrate only. A powdered or liquid calorie supplement. Powder 23 kcal/tbsp.
Moducal (Mead Johnson)		Hydrolyzed corn starch		Used to increase carbohydrate intake.	Carbohydrate only. A powdered calorie supplement: 30 kcal/tbsp.
Casec (Mead Johnson)	Calcium caseinate			Used to increase protein intake.	Protein only. Negligible fat and no carbohydrate.
MCT Oil (Mead Johnson)			90% MCT (coconut source)	Supplement in fat malabsorption conditions	Fat only. 8.3 kcal/g; 115 kcal/tbsp.

*L-amino acids include L-cystine, L-tyrosine, and L-tryptophan, which are reduced in hydrolyzed, charcoal-treated casein.

Unit 2

Normal and special infant formulas—cont'd

Formula (manufacturer)	Protein source	Carbohydrate source	Fat source	Indications for use	Comments (nutritional considerations)
FOR INFANTS WITH METABOLIC DEFECTS*					
Lofenalac (Mead Johnson)	Casein hydrolysate, L-amino acids	Corn syrup solids, modified tapioca starch	Corn oil	For infants and children with phenylketonuria.	111 mg phenylalanine per quart of formula (20 cal/qt). Must be supplemented with other foods to provide minimal phenylalanine.
Phenyl-free (Mead Johnson)	L-amino acids	Sucrose, corn syrup solids, modified tapioca starch	Corn oil, coconut oil	For children over 1 year of age with phenylketonuria.	Phenylalanine free. Permits increased supplementation with normal foods.
PKU 1 (Milupa)	L-amino acids	Sucrose		For infants with phenylketonuria. (Available as PKU 2 for children over 1 year of age.)	Phenylalanine- and fat-free. Contains vitamins, minerals, and trace elements. Must be supplemented with phenylalanine/protein, carbohydrate, and fat.
MSUD Diet (Mead Johnson)	L-amino acids	Corn syrup solids, modified tapioca starch	Corn oil	For children with branched-chain keto-aciduria (maple sugar urine disease)	Leucine-, isoleucine-, and valine-free; must be supplemented with these amino acids to maintain blood levels in normal range.
Protein-free diet powder (Powder 80056) (Mead Johnson)		Corn syrup solids, modified tapioca starch	Corn oil	In formulation of special diets.	Protein-free; carbohydrate, fat, vitamin, and mineral mix.
Low Phe/Tyr Diet Powder (Product 3200AB) (Mead Johnson)	Casein hydrolysate and L-amino acids	Corn syrup solids, modified tapioca starch	Corn oil	For infants with tyrosinemia.	Must be supplemented with tyrosine and phenylalanine.
Low Methionine Diet Powder (Product 3200K) (Mead Johnson)	Soy protein isolate with no added methionine	Corn syrup solids	Coconut and corn oil	For infants with homocystinuria	Nutritionally complete but requires monitoring of amino acid levels
Mono- and Di-saccharide-Free Diet Powder (Product 3232A) (Mead Johnson)	Casein hydrolysate with L-amino acids	Modified tapioca starch	MCT, corn oil	For infants with disaccharidase (lactase, sucrase, and maltase) deficiencies or impaired glucose transport.	Nutritionally complete

*Ross Laboratories manufactures several specialty formulas for metabolic disorders for infants over 1 year of age and children over 8 years of age.

Modified from Kempe C, Silver H, O'Brien D, and Fulginiti V, editors: Current pediatric diagnosis and treatment, ed 9, Copyright 1987 by Lange Medical Publications, Los Altos, CA. Modifications based on product information from Carnation 1988; Loma Linda 1988; Mead Johnson Nutritionals, 1988; Ross Laboratories, 1988; Wyeth Laboratories, 1989. For the most current information, consult product labels or package enclosures.

Age/type of feeding	Specific recommendations
BIRTH-6 MONTHS	
Breast-feeding	Most desirable complete diet for first half of year*
	Requires supplements of fluoride (0.25 mg), regardless of the fluoride content of the local water supply, and iron by 6 months of age
	Requires supplements of vitamin D (400 units) if mother's diet is inadequate or if infant is not exposed to sufficient sunlight
Formula	Iron-fortified commercial formula is a complete food for the first half of the year*
	Requires fluoride supplements (0.25 mg) when the concentration of fluoride in the drinking water is below 0.3 parts per million (ppm)
	Evaporated milk formula requires supplements of vitamin C, iron, and fluoride (in accordance with the fluoride content of the local water supply)
6-12 MONTHS	
Solid foods	May begin to add solids by 5 to 6 months of age; earlier introduction tends to contribute to overfeeding
	First foods are strained, pureed, or finely mashed
	"Finger foods" such as teething crackers, raw fruit, or vegetables can be introduced by 6 to 7 months
	Chopped table food or commercially prepared junior foods can be started by 9 to 12 months
	With the exception of cereal, the order of introducing foods is variable; a recommended sequence is weekly introduction of other foods, beginning with fruit, then vegetables, and then meat
	Breast-fed infants require more high-protein foods than formula-fed children
	As the quantity of solids increases, the amount of formula should be limited to approximately 900 ml (30 oz) daily
	METHOD OF INTRODUCTION
	Introduce solids when infant is hungry
	Begin spoon feeding by pushing food to back of tongue because of infant's natural tendency to thrust tongue forward
	Use small spoon with straight handle; begin with 1 or 2 teaspoons of food; gradually increase to 2 to 3 tablespoons per feeding
	Introduce one food at a time, usually at intervals of 4 to 7 days, identify food allergies
	As the amount of solid food increases, decrease the quantity of milk to prevent overfeeding
	Never introduce foods by mixing them with the formula in the bottle
Cereal	Introduce commercially prepared iron-fortified infant cereals and administer daily until 18 months
	Rice cereal is usually introduced first because of its low allergenic potential
	Can discontinue supplemental iron once cereal is given
Fruits and vegetables	Applesauce, bananas, and pears are usually well tolerated
	Avoid fruits and vegetables marketed in cans that are not specifically designed for infants because of variable and sometimes high lead content and addition of salt, sugar, and/or preservatives
	Offer fruit juice only from a cup, not a bottle, to reduce the development of "nursing bottle caries"
Meat, fish, and poultry	Avoid fatty meats
	Prepare by baking, broiling, steaming, or poaching
	Include organ meats such as liver, which has a high iron, vitamin A, and vitamin B complex content
	If soup is given, be sure all ingredients are familiar to child's diet
	Avoid commercial meat/vegetable combinations because protein is low
Eggs and cheese	Serve egg yolk hard boiled and mashed, soft cooked, or poached
	Introduce egg white in small quantities (1 tsp) toward end of first year to detect an allergy
	Use cheese as a substitute for meat and as "finger food"

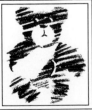

*The Academy of Pediatrics recommends breast-feeding or commercial formula feeding for up to 12 months of age. After 1 year whole cow's milk can be given.

Developmental milestones associated with feeding

Age (months)	Development
Birth	Has sucking, rooting, and swallowing reflexes Feels hunger and indicates desire for food by crying; expresses satiety by falling asleep
1	Has strong extrusion reflex
3-4	Extrusion reflex is fading Begins to develop hand-eye coordination
4-5	Can approximate lips to the rim of a cup
5-6	Can use fingers to feed self a cracker
6-7	Chews and bites May hold own bottle, but may not drink from it (prefers for it to be held)
7-9	Refuses food by keeping lips closed; has taste preferences Holds a spoon and plays with it during feeding May drink from a straw Drinks from a cup with assistance
9-12	Picks up small morsels of food (finger foods) and feeds self Holds own bottle and drinks from it Drinks from a household cup without assistance but spills some Uses a spoon with much spilling
12-18	Drools less Drinks well from a household cup, but may drop it when finished Holds cup with both hands
24	Can use a straw Chews food with mouth closed and shifts food in mouth Distinguishes between finger and spoon foods Holds small glass in one hand; replaces glass without dropping
36	Spills small amount from spoon Begins to use fork; holds it in fist Uses adult pattern of chewing, which involves rotary action of jaw
48	Rarely spills when using spoon Serves self finger foods Eats with fork held with fingers
54	Uses fork in preference to spoon
72	Spreads with knife
84	Cuts tender food with knife

Unit 2

Food group	Principal nutrients in group	Servings per day

Milk or equivalent (for calcium)
½ cup whole milk equals:
   ¾ ounce cheese
   ½ cup yogurt, milk pudding
   1 cup cottage cheese
	Protein
	Calcium
	Riboflavin (B_2)
		2-3 cups for child
		4 cups for adolescent
		Usual serving size:
		   Toddler and preschooler—½ to ¾ cup
		   School-age and older—1 cup

Meat, fish, poultry, or equivalent
1 ounce meat equals:
   1 egg
   1 ounce cheese
   2 tablespoons peanut butter
   ½ cup cooked legumes
	Protein
	Niacin
	Iron
	Thiamin (B_1)
		2 for child and adolescent
		Usual serving size:
		   Toddler and preschooler—1 egg, 1 to 2 ounces meat
		   School-age and older—1 egg, 3 ounces meat

Vegetables and fruits
Citrus equivalents:
   1 orange or tomato
   ½ cup orange or grapefruit juice
   ¾ cup strawberries
	Vitamin A
	Vitamin C
		4 for child and adolescent
		1 citrus daily; 1 yellow or dark green vegetable 3 to 4 times weekly
		Usual serving size
		   Toddler and preschooler—2 to 4 tablespoons to ¼ to ½ cup
		   School-age and older—½ cup

Breads and cereals
1 slice enriched bread equals:
   ¾ cup dry cereal
   ½ cup cooked pasta, rice, or cereal
   ½ hamburger bun
   1 small muffin or biscuit
	Carbohydrate
	Thiamin (B_1)
	Iron
	Niacin
		4 for child and adolescent
		Usual serving size:
		   Toddler and preschooler—½ slice bread, ¼ cup
		   School-age and older—1 slice bread, ½ cup

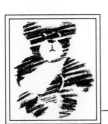

*Fats and carbohydrates should be served sparingly to meet caloric needs.

Toddler (2-3 yr)

Breakfast	⅓ cup dry, unsweetened cereal 4 oz lowfat milk ½ cup orange juice
Snack	½-1 whole banana
Lunch	1 tbsp peanut butter 1 slice whole wheat bread ½ apple 4-6 oz lowfat milk
Snack	1 graham cracker 4-6 oz lowfat milk
Dinner	1 chicken leg ¼ cup rice 2 tbsp green beans 4-6 oz lowfat milk

DAILY TOTAL:
Milk:	24 ounces
Meat:	2 ounces
Fruits/veg:	4 servings (½ piece or ¼ cup is a serving)
Breads/cereal:	4 servings (½ slice or ¼ cup is a serving)

Preschooler (3-6 yr)

Breakfast	½-1 cup dry, unsweetened cereal 4-6 oz lowfat milk ½ cup orange juice
Lunch	1 tbsp peanut butter 1-2 slices whole wheat bread 1 apple 6-8 oz lowfat milk
Snack	1 carton fruited yogurt 1 graham cracker
Dinner	1 broiled chicken leg ½ cup rice 2 tbsp-½ cup green beans 6-8 oz lowfat milk
Snack	1 banana

DAILY TOTAL:
Milk:	24 ounces or equivalent
Meat:	2-3 ounces
Fruits/veg:	4 servings (1 piece or ½ cup is a serving)
Breads/cereal:	4 servings (½ slice or ¼ cup is a serving)

School age (7-12 yr)

Breakfast	2 4-inch waffles 2 tbsp syrup ½ cup orange juice
Lunch	1 cheeseburger 1 medium soft drink
Snack	1 cup frozen yogurt OR 1 cup cereal with lowfat milk
Dinner	1 cup spaghetti with tomato sauce 1 piece garlic bread Green salad with romaine lettuce and dressing 1 banana 1 cup lowfat milk
Snack	2 cups plain popcorn

DAILY TOTAL:
Milk:	24 ounces
Meat:	4 ounces
Fruits/veg:	4 servings (1 piece or ½ cup is a serving)
Breads/cereal:	4 servings (1 slice or ½ cup cooked is a serving)

Adolescent (13-19 yr)

Breakfast	2 4-inch waffles ¼ cup syrup ½ cup orange juice 1 cup lowfat milk
Lunch	1 "quarter pounder" hamburger with cheese 1 small order french fries 1 medium soft drink
Snack	1 cup frozen yogurt with fruit and nut topping OR 1 peanut butter sandwich 1 cup lowfat milk
Dinner	1½ cups lasagna 1-2 pieces garlic bread Green salad with romaine lettuce and dressing 1 apple Iced tea
Snack	3-4 cookies 1 cup lowfat milk

DAILY TOTAL:
Milk:	32 ounces or equivalent
Meat:	4 ounces
Fruits/vegs:	4 servings (1 piece or ½ cup is a serving)
Breads/cereal:	4 servings (1 slice or ½ cup cooked is a serving)

*Prepared by Cecilia L. Davis, RD, LD, Nutrition Consultants of Tulsa, OK.
Fats and carbohydrates should be served sparingly to meet caloric needs.
Serving sizes are minimums for nutritional adequacy. Many children eat more.

TYPICAL SLEEP REQUIREMENTS IN INFANCY AND CHILDHOOD

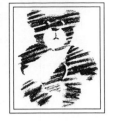

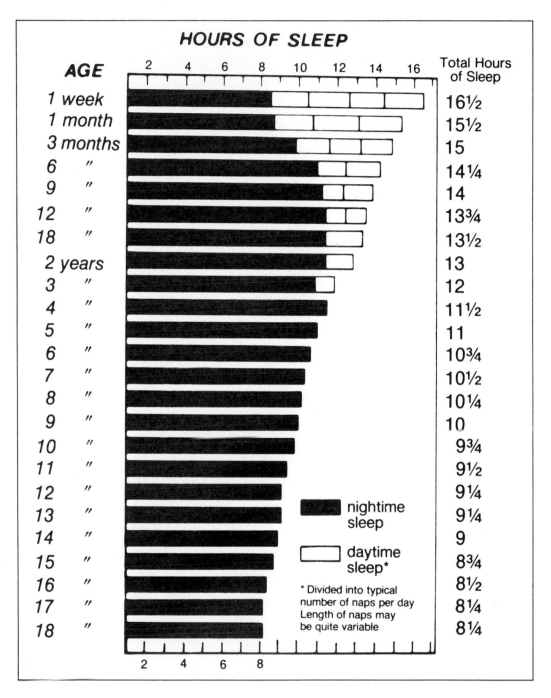

HOURS OF SLEEP

AGE	Total Hours of Sleep
1 week	16½
1 month	15½
3 months	15
6 "	14¼
9 "	14
12 "	13¾
18 "	13½
2 years	13
3 "	12
4 "	11½
5 "	11
6 "	10¾
7 "	10½
8 "	10¼
9 "	10
10 "	9¾
11 "	9½
12 "	9¼
13 "	9¼
14 "	9
15 "	8¾
16 "	8½
17 "	8¼
18 "	8¼

■ nightime sleep

□ daytime sleep*

* Divided into typical number of naps per day Length of naps may be quite variable

Selected sleep disturbances during infancy and childhood

Disorder/description	Management
NIGHTTIME FEEDING*	
Child has a prolonged need for middle-of-night bot-tle- or breast-feeding	Increase daytime feeding intervals to 4 hours or more (may need to be done gradually)
Child goes to sleep at the breast or with a bottle	Offer last feeding as late as possible at night; may need to gradually reduce amount of formula or length of breast-feeding
Awakenings are frequent (may be hourly)	Offer no bottles in bed
Child returns to sleep after feeding; other comfort measures (e.g., rocking or holding) are usually in-effective	Put to bed *awake*
	When child is crying, check at progressively longer intervals each night; reassure child but do not hold, rock, take to parent's bed, or give bottle or pacifier
DEVELOPMENTAL NIGHT CRYING	
Child aged 6-12 months with undisturbed nighttime sleep now awakes abruptly; may be accompanied by nightmares	Reassure parents that this is temporary phase
	Enter room immediately to check on child but keep reassurances *brief*
	Avoid feeding, rocking, taking to parent's bed, or any other routine that may initiate trained night crying
TRAINED NIGHT CRYING* **(INAPPROPRIATE SLEEP ASSOCIATIONS)**	
Child typically falls asleep in place other than own bed, e.g., rocking chair or parent's bed, and is brought to own bed while asleep; upon awakening, cries until usual routine is instituted, e.g., rocking	Put child in own bed when *awake*
	If possible, arrange separate sleeping area from other family members
	When child is crying, check at progressively longer intervals each night; reassure child but do not resume usual routine
REFUSAL TO GO TO SLEEP*	
Child resists bedtime and comes out of room re-peatedly	Evaluate if hour of sleep is too early (child may resist sleep if not tired)
Nighttime sleep may be continuous, but frequent awakenings and refusal to return to sleep may oc-cur and become a problem if parent allows child to deviate from usual sleep pattern	Assist parents in establishing consistent before-bedtime routine and en-forcing consistent limits regarding child's bedtime behavior
	If child persists in leaving bedroom, close door for progressively longer periods
	Use reward system with child to provide motivation
NIGHTTIME FEARS	
Child resists going to bed or wakes during the night because of fears	Evaluate if hour of sleep is too early (child may fantasize when nothing to do but think in dark room)
Child seeks parent's physical presence and with par-ent nearby, falls asleep easily, unless fear is over-whelming	Calmly reassure the frightened child; keeping a nightlight on may be helpful
	Use reward system with child to provide motivation to deal with fears
	Avoid patterns that can lead to additional problems, e.g., sleeping with child or taking child to parent's room
	If child's fear is overwhelming, consider desensitization, e.g., progressively spending longer periods of time alone; consult professional help for protracted fears
	Distinguish between nightmares and sleep terrors (confused partial arous-als) (see table on p. 173); best approach with sleep terrors is to remain uninvolved and allow child to stay asleep

Adapted from Ferber R: Behavioral "insomnia" in the child, Psychiatr Clin North Am 10(4):641-653, 1987.
*Guidelines for parents in dealing with these sleep problems are on pp. 173-175.

NIGHTMARES VS. SLEEP TERRORS*

	Nightmares	Sleep terrors
What is it?	A scary dream. It takes place within REM sleep and is followed by full waking	A partial arousal from very deep (stage IV, non-REM) non-dreaming sleep
When do you become aware your child had or is having one?	After the dream is over and he wakes and cries or calls. Not during the nightmare itself	During the terror itself, as he screams and thrashes. Afterwards he is calm
Time of occurrence	In the second half of the night, when dreams are most intense	Usually 1 to 4 hours after falling asleep, when nondreaming sleep is deepest
The child's appearance and behavior	Crying in younger children, fright in all. These persist even though the child is awake	Initially the child may sit up, thrash, or run in a bizarre manner, with eyes bulging, heart racing, and profuse sweating. He may cry, scream, talk, or moan. There is apparent fright, anger, and/or obvious confusion, which *disappears* when he is fully awake
Responsiveness	Child is aware of and reassured by your presence; he may be comforted by you and hold you tightly	Child is not very aware of your presence, is not comforted by you, and may push you away and scream and thrash more if you try to hold or restrain him
Return to sleep	May be considerably delayed because of persistent fear	Usually rapid
Description of a dream at the time or on waking in the morning	Yes (if old enough)	No memory of a dream or of yelling or thrashing

GUIDELINES FOR ELIMINATING EXTRA FEEDINGS AT SLEEP TIMES

Day	Ounces in each bottle or minutes nursing	Minimum hours between feedings
1	7	2.0
2	6	2.5
3	5	3.0
4	4	3.5
5	3	4.0
6	2	4.5
7	1	5.0
8	No more bottles or nursing at sleep times	

- The ounces and times in this chart are general guidelines. You will want to alter them to fit your own routines.
- If your child takes less than 8 ounces in the bottle, start with 1 ounce less than she usually takes and continue reducing from there.
- If you are breast-feeding, use the time spent nursing as an approximation of volume. Begin by nursing 1 or 2 minutes less than you usually nurse and continue decreasing the times from that point.
- If you prefer you may follow this chart but decrease every other day instead of every day. It will just take a little longer.

*This section may be photocopied and distributed to families.
From Ferber R: Solve your child's sleep problems, New York, 1985, Simon & Schuster, Inc. Used with permission.

GUIDELINES FOR HELPING YOUR CHILD LEARN TO FALL ASLEEP WITH THE PROPER ASSOCIATIONS—THE PROGRESSIVE APPROACH

NUMBER OF MINUTES TO WAIT BEFORE GOING IN TO YOUR CHILD BRIEFLY

Day	At first wait	If your child is still crying		
		Second wait	Third wait	Subsequent waits
1	5	10	15	15
2	10	15	20	20
3	15	20	25	25
4	20	25	30	30
5	25	30	35	35
6	30	35	40	40
7	35	40	45	45

1. This chart shows the number of minutes to wait before going in if your child is crying at bedtime or after nighttime wakings.
2. Each time you go in to your child, spend only 2 to 3 minutes. Remember, you are going in briefly to reassure him and yourself, not necessarily to help him stop crying and certainly not to help him fall asleep. The goal is for him to learn to fall asleep alone, without being held, rocked, nursed, or using a bottle or pacifier.
3. When you get to the maximum number of minutes to wait for that night, continue leaving for that amount of time until your child finally falls asleep during one of the periods you are out of the room.
4. If he wakes during the night, begin the waiting schedule at the minimum waiting time for that day and again work up to the maximum.
5. Continue this routine after all wakings until reaching a time in the morning (usually 5:30 to 7:30 A.M.) you have previously decided to be reasonable to start the day. If he wakes after that time, or if he is still awake then after waking earlier, get him up and begin the morning routines.
6. Use the same schedule for naps, but if your child has not fallen asleep after 1 hour, or if he is awake again and crying vigorously after getting some sleep, end that naptime period.
7. The number of minutes listed to wait are ones that most families find workable. If they seem too long for you, use the times shown on the chart on p. 175 (though without closing the door). In fact, any schedule will work as long as the times increase progressively.
8. Be sure to follow your schedule carefully and chart your child's sleep patterns daily) so you can monitor his progress accurately.*
9. By day 7 your child will most likely be sleeping very well, but if further work is necessary, just continue to add 5 minutes to each time on successive days.

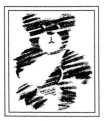

*A 2-week sleep record is on p. 93.
This section may be photocopied and distributed to families.
From Ferber R: Solve your child's sleep problems, New York, 1985, Simon & Schuster, Inc. Used with permission.

GUIDELINES FOR HELPING YOUR CHILD LEARN TO STAY IN BED

NUMBER OF MINUTES TO CLOSE THE DOOR IF YOUR CHILD WILL NOT STAY IN BED

Day	First closing	Second closing	If your child continues to get out of bed		
			Third closing	Fourth closing	Subsequent closings
1	1	2	3	5	5
2	2	4	6	8	8
3	3	5	7	10	10
4	5	7	10	15	15
5	7	10	15	20	20
6	10	15	20	25	25
7	15	20	25	30	30

1. This chart shows the number of minutes to close your child's door if he will not stay in bed at bedtime or after nighttime wakings.

2. When you get to the maximum number of minutes for that night, continue closing the door for that amount of time until he finally stays in bed.

3. Keep the door closed for the number of minutes listed, even if your child goes back to bed sooner. However, you may talk to him through the door and tell him how much time remains.

4. When you open the door, speak to him briefly if he is in bed, offer encouragement, and leave. If he is still out of bed, restate the rules, put him back in bed (if it can be done easily), and shut the door for the next amount of time listed. If he lets you put him back easily and you are convinced he will stay there, you may try leaving the door open, but if you are wrong, do not keep making the same mistake.

5. If your child wakes during the night and won't stay in bed, begin the door-closing schedule at the minimum time for that day and again work up to the maximum.

6. Continue this routine as necessary after all wakings until reaching a time in the morning (usually 5:30 to 7:00 A.M.) previously decided to be reasonable to start the day.

7. Use the same routine at naptimes, but if your child has not fallen asleep after 1 hour, or if he is awake again and out of bed after getting some sleep, end that naptime period.

8. If he wakes and calls or cries but does not get out of bed, switch to the progressive routine described in the chart on p. 174.

9. The number of minutes listed to close the door are ones that most families find workable. However, you may change the schedule as you think best as long as the times increase progressively.

10. Be sure to follow your schedule carefully and chart your child's sleep patterns daily so you can monitor his progress accurately.*

11. Remember, your goal is to help your child learn to sleep alone. You are using the door as a controlled way of enforcing this, not to scare or punish him. So reassure him by talking through the door; do not threaten or scream. By progressively increasing time of door closure, starting with short periods, your child does not have to be shut behind a closed door unsure of when it will be opened. He will learn that having the door open is entirely under his control.

12. By day 7 your child will most likely be staying in bed, but if further work is necessary, just continue to add 5 minutes to each time on successive days.

13. If you prefer you may use a gate instead of a closed door as long as your child can't open or climb over it. In this case you must be out of his view during the periods of gate closure, but you can still talk to him reassuringly from another room.

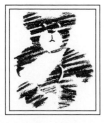

*A 2-week sleep record is on p. 93.
This section may be photocopied and distributed to families.
From Ferber R: Solve your child's sleep problems, New York, 1985, Simon & Schuster, Inc. Used with permission.

IMMUNIZATIONS
Recommended schedule for active immunization of normal infants and children*

Recommended age	Immunization(s)†	Comments
2 mo	DTP, OPV	Can be initiated as early as age 2 wk in areas of high endemicity or during epidemics
4 mo	DTP, OPV	2-mo interval desired for OPV to avoid interference from previous dose
6 mo	DTP	A third dose of OPV is not indicated in the U.S. but is desirable in geographic areas where polio is endemic
15 mo	Measles, mumps, rubella (MMR)	MMR preferred to individual vaccines; tuberculin testing may be done at the same visit
18 mo	DTP,‡§ OPV,‖ PRP-D	See footnotes
4-6 yr	DTP,¶ OPV	At or before school entry
14-16 yr	Td	Repeat every 10 yr throughout life

From Report of the Committee on Infectious Diseases, ed 21, Elk Grove Village, IL, 1988, American Academy of Pediatrics.

*For all products used, consult manufacturer's package insert for instructions for storage, handling, dosage, and administration. Biologics prepared by different manufacturers may vary, and package inserts of the same manufacturer may change from time to time. Therefore, the physician should be aware of the contents of the current package insert.

†DTP = diphtheria and tetanus toxoids with pertussis vaccine; OPV = oral poliovirus vaccine containing attenuated poliovirus types 1, 2, and 3; MMR = live measles, mumps, and rubella viruses in a combined vaccine (see text for discussion of single vaccines versus combination); PRP-D = *Haemophilus* b diphtheria toxid conjugate vaccine; Td = adult tetanus toxoid (full dose) and diphtheria toxoid (reduced dose) for adult use.

‡Should be given 6 to 12 months after the third dose.

§May be given simultaneously with MMR at age 15 months.

‖May be given simultaneously with MMR at 15 months of age or at any time between 12 and 24 months of age.

¶Up to the seventh birthday.

Author's note: Recent updates to these recommendations include:

(1) use of either PRP-D or the newly licensed HbOC (*Haemophilus* b conjugate vaccine [diphtheria CRM_{197} protein conjugate]) for immunization against *Haemophilus influenzae* type b (American Academy of Pediatrics, Committee on Infectious Diseases: *Haemophilus influenzae* type b conjugate vaccines: update, Pediatrics 84(2):386-387, 1989); and

(2) a second dose of MMR at entrance to middle or junior high school (American Academy of Pediatrics, Committee on Infectious Diseases: Measles: reassessment of the current immunization policy, Pediatrics 84(6):1110-1113, 1989).

Several exceptions to the schedules on pp. 176-177 and exist (i.e., in high-risk areas or during outbreaks of a disease) and changes in recommendations occur frequently. Nurses must update their information to keep abreast of specific circumstances warranting exceptions to these guidelines and new recommendations regarding childhood immunization.

Recommended immunization schedules for children not immunized in first year of life

Recommended time	Immunization(s)	Comments
Less than 7 years old		
First visit	DTP, OPV, MMR	MMR if child ≥ 15 mo old; tuberculin testing may be done at same visit
Interval after first visit:	PRP-D	For children aged 18-60 mo; can be given concurrently with DTP (at separate sites) and other vaccines*
1 mo		
2 mo	DTP, OPV	
4 mo	DTP	A third dose of OPV is not indicated in the U.S. but is desirable in geographic areas where polio is endemic
10-16 mo	DTP, OPV	OPV is not given if third dose was given earlier
4-6 yr (at or before school entry)	DTP, OPV	DTP is not necessary if the fourth dose was given after the fourth birthday; OPV is not necessary if recommended OPV dose at 10-16 mo following first vist was given after the fourth birthday
10 yr later	Td	Repeat every 10 yr throughout life
7 years old and older		
First vist	Td, OPV, MMR	
Interval after first visit:		
2 mo	Td, OPV	
8-14 mo	Td, OPV	
10 yr later	Td	Repeat every 10 yr throughout life

From Report of the Committee on Infectious Diseases, ed 21, 1988, Elk Grove Village, IL, American Academy of Pediatrics.

*The initial three doses of DTP can be given at 1- to 2-month intervals; so, for the child in whom immunization is initiated at age 24 months or older, one visit could be eliminated by giving DTP, OPV, and MMR at the first visit; DTP and PRP-D at the second visit (1 month later); and DTP and OPV at the third visit (2 months after the first visit). Subsequent DTP and OPV 10 to 16 months after the first visit are still indicated. PRP-D, MMR, DTP, and OPV can be given simultaneously at separate sites if return of vaccine recipient for future immunizations is doubtful.

Unit 2

Guide to tetanus prophylaxis in routine wound management

History of adsorbed tetanus toxoid (doses)	Clean, minor wounds		All other wounds*	
	Td†	TIG	Td†	TIG
Unknown or <3	Yes	No	Yes	Yes
3 or more	No‡	No	No§	No

*Such as, but not limited to, wounds contaminated with dirt, feces, soil, saliva, etc.; puncture wounds; avulsions; and wounds resulting from missiles, crushing, burns, and frostbite.

†For children less than 7 years old DTP (DT, if pertussis vaccine is contraindicated) is preferred to tetanus toxoid alone. For persons 7 years old and older, Td is preferred to tetanus toxoid alone.

‡Yes, if more than 10 years since last dose.

§Yes, if more than 5 years since last dose. (More frequent boosters are not needed and can accentuate side effects.)

From Report of the Committee on Infectious Diseases, ed 21, Elk Grove Village, IL, 1988, American Academy of Pediatrics.

Recommendations for selected nonmandated vaccines

Immunization	Description	Administration/precautions
Influenza virus vaccine	Affords protection against strains of influenza Recommended for children 6 months and older with chronic disorders of cardiovascular or pulmonary systems whose severity warranted regular medical care or hospitalization during preceding year. Other eligible children include those with diabetes mellitus, renal dysfunction, anemia, immunosuppression, human immunodeficiency virus (HIV) infection, or those on long-term aspirin therapy	Administered in fall, repeated yearly Intramuscular (preferred) or subcutaneous injection Associated with mild flulike symptoms for 1 to 2 days Contraindicated in persons with severe allergy to eggs Should not be given within 3 days of pertussis immunization (2 doses of split vaccine at least 4 weeks apart for children 12 years or younger; 1 dose of split or whole vaccine for children over 12 years)
Pneumococcal polysaccharide vaccine (Pneumovax; Pne-Immune)	Affords protection against 23 types of *Streptococcus pneumoniae* Recommended for children 2 years and older with sickle cell disease, functional or anatomic asplenia, nephrotic syndrome, human immunodeficiency virus (HIV) infection, and Hodgkin disease prior to beginning cytoreduction therapy	Subcutaneous or intramuscular injection Revaccination is not recommended Should be deferred during pregnancy
Meningococcal polysaccharide vaccine (Menomune)	Affords protection against *Neisseria meningitidis,* serogroups A, C, Y, and W-135 Recommended for children 2 years and older with terminal complement deficiencies and anatomic or functional asplenia	Subcutaneous injection Duration of protection unknown Safety during pregnancy not established
Hepatitis B vaccine (Heptavax-B)	Affords protection against hepatitis B virus (HBV) Recommended for several high-risk groups, especially adults at risk for infection from contaminated blood products; among children, infants born to mothers who are hepatitis B surface antigen (HBsAg) positive	Infants: combined hepatitis B immune globulin (HBIG) and HB vaccine Intramuscular injections at separate sites Administered at or soon after birth, with second and third doses given 1 and 6 months after the initial dose

Vaccines available in the United States and their routes of administration

Vaccine*	Type	Route
BCG	Live bacteria	Intradermal (preferred) or subcutaneous
Cholera	Inactivated bacteria	Subcutaneous, intramuscular, or intradermal†
DTP	Toxoids and inactivated bacteria	Intramuscular
Hepatitis B	Inactivated viral antigen	Intramuscular
	Yeast recombinant-derived antigen	Intramuscular
Haemophilus b	Polysaccharide	Subcutaneous, intramuscular
	Polysaccharide-protein conjugate (PRP-D)	Intramuscular
	Diphtheria CRM$_{197}$ protein conjugate (HbOC)	Intramuscular
Influenza	Inactivated virus	Intramuscular (preferred) or subcutaneous
Measles	Live virus	Subcutaneous
Meningococcal	Polysaccharide	Subcutaneous
MMR	Live viruses	Subcutaneous
Mumps	Live virus	Subcutaneous
Plague	Inactivated bacteria	Intramuscular
Pneumococcal	Polysaccharide	Intramuscular or subcutaneous
Poliomyelitis:		
OPV	Live virus	Oral
IPV	Inactivated	Subcutaneous
Rabies	Inactivated virus	Intramuscular
Rubella	Live virus	Subcutaneous
Tetanus and Td, DT	Toxoids	Intramuscular
Typhoid	Inactivated bacteria	Subcutaneous (boosters may be intradermal†)
Yellow fever	Live virus	Subcutaneous

From Report of the Committee on Infectious Diseases, ed 21, 1988, Elk Grove Village, IL, American Academy of Pediatrics.

*BCG = Bacillus Calmette-Guérin vaccine (tuberculosis); DTP = diphtheria and tetanus toxoids and pertussis vaccine; PRP-D = *Haemophilus* b diphtheria toxoid conjugate; IPV – inactivated poliovirus vaccine; MMR = measles, mumps, and rubella vaccine; OPV = oral poliovirus vaccine; Td = tetanus and diphtheria toxoid for adult (≥7 years old) use; DT = diphtheria and tetanus toxoids.

†The intradermal dose is different.

Contraindications to routine immunizations

Contraindications (exceptions)	Rationale	Nursing considerations
DIPHTHERIA, TETANUS, PERTUSSIS (DTP)		
Febrile illness (Minor, nonfebrile illness is not a contraindication)	Signs and symptoms associated with the illness may be erroneously attributed to the vaccine	Explain reason for postponement to family and reschedule immunization at earliest return visit
Immediate, severe, anaphylactic reaction to previous administration of one of these vaccines	Hypersensitivity to some component in the vaccine may result in a severe reaction during reimmunization	Take a careful history of reactions to previous vaccines or a component in the vaccine, e.g., the preservative, thimerosal
PERTUSSIS		
Neurologic disorder, e.g., infantile spasms, uncontrolled epilepsy, or progressive encephalopathy, characterized by progressive developmental delay or changing neurologic findings	Danger of serious reaction to pertussis vaccination is possibly increased if any of these conditions are present when receiving the vaccine and may result in confusion about causation of neurologic findings	Take a detailed neurologic history including past convulsions, fainting spells, tremors, and specific reactions to DTP; report any such findings to practitioner before administering the vaccine

From Report of the Committee on Infectious Diseases, ed 21, Elk Grove Village, IL, 1988, American Academy of Pediatrics. For more detailed information consult the Report, the vaccine manufacturers' package insert, and the child's health care practitioner.

Unit 2

Contraindications to routine immunizations—cont'd

Contraindications (exceptions)	Rationale	Nursing considerations
PERTUSSIS—cont'd		
Personal (not family) history of convulsions		
Have or suspected of having neurologic conditions, e.g., tuberous sclerosis, certain inherited metabolic or degenerative diseases, that predispose to seizures or neurologic deterioration		
Any of the following reactions *after* receiving pertussis vaccine:		
Encephalopathy within 7 days		
A convulsion, with or without fever, occurring within 3 days		
Persistent, inconsolable screaming or crying for 3 or more hours or an unusual high-pitched cry within 48 hours		
Collapse or shocklike state within 48 hours		
Temperature of 40.5° C (104.9° F) or greater, unexplained by another cause, within 48 hours		
An immediate severe or anaphylactic reaction to vaccine (extremely rare)		
MEASLES, MUMPS, AND RUBELLA (MMR); LIVE POLIO VIRUS (OPV)		
Febrile illness (Minor, nonfebrile or febrile illness is not a contraindication)	Signs and symptoms associated with the illness may be erroneously attributed to the vaccine	Explain reason for postponement to family and reschedule immunization at earliest return visit
Anaphylactic reaction to neomycin (Minor, delayed reaction of an erythematous pruritic papule after MMR inoculation is not a contraindication to a second dose)	Severe neomycin sensitivity can result in systemic anaphylactic reactions in allergic person receiving vaccine containing trace amounts of neomycin	Take a careful history of allergic reactions to neomycin Report positive findings to practitioner before administering vaccine
Pregnancy Live oral poliovirus vaccine may be given if substantial risk of exposure is present (inactivated polio virus [IPV] is preferred if immunization can be completed before anticipated exposure)	Theoretic risk to fetus	Take careful history of all women of childbearing age for possibility of pregnancy or conception within next 3 months
Congenital disorders of immune function Immunosuppressive therapy (except investigational varicella vaccine); may immunize 3 months after immunosuppressive therapy is discontinued	Depressed immune functions prevent antibody-response to vaccines; fatal vaccine-associated infections can occur	Emphasize to family need to avoid child's exposure to these viral infections Stress importance of regular immune globulin therapy to provide passive protection in selected children
Children on steroid therapy are evaluated for the risk of live virus vaccines	Duration and dosage of steroids affect immune system differently	Advise family that household contacts should not receive oral poliovirus vaccine because the virus can be transmitted to the immunocompromised child
Children with symptomatic or asymptomatic human immunodeficiency virus (HIV) infection should receive all routine vaccines except oral poliovirus vaccine (Inactivated polio virus [IPV] can be given although its effectiveness may be reduced)	Reports of severity of actual infection are thought to outweigh potential risks from vaccines	
MEASLES AND MUMPS		
Anaphylactic egg hypersensitivity (Milder forms of allergy to egg or chicken feathers are not a contraindication)	Severe egg hypersensitivity may result in systemic anaphylactic reactions in allergic person receiving vaccine containing trace amounts of egg antigens	Take a careful history of allergic reactions to egg Report positive findings to practitioner before administering vaccine

Possible side effects of recommended childhood immunizations and nursing responsibilities*

Immunization	Reaction	Nursing responsibilities†
Diphtheria	Fever usually within 24-48 hours Soreness, redness, and swelling at injection site	Instructions for DTP: advise parents of possible side effects
Tetanus	Same as for diphtheria but may include urticaria and malaise All may have delayed onset and last several days Lump at injection site may last for weeks, even months, but gradually disappears	May recommend prophylactic use of acetaminophen if fever occurred following previous DTP immunization Recommend use of antipyretics if fever occurs following present immunization Advise parents to notify physician *immediately* of any unusual side effects, such as those listed under pertussis
Pertussis	Same as for tetanus but may include loss of consciousness, convulsions, persistent inconsolable crying episodes, generalized or focal neurologic signs, fever (temperature at or above 40.5° C (10.5° F), systemic allergic reaction	Before administering next dose of DTP, inquire about reactions, especially those listed under pertussis on pp. 179-180
Poliovirus (TOPV)	Essentially no immediate side effects Vaccine-associated paralysis rarely occurs within 2 months of immunization (estimated risk 1:10 million doses)	Assess presence of family members at risk from TOPV because of immune deficiency states
Measles	Anorexia, malaise, rash, and fever may occur 7 to 10 days after immunization Rarely (estimated risk 1:1 million doses) encephalitis may occur	Advise parents of more common side effects and use of antipyretics for fever If a persistent fever with other obvious signs of illness occurs, have them notify physician immediately
Mumps	Essentially no side effects other than a brief, mild fever	See general comment to parents*
Rubella	Fever, lymphadenopathy, or mild rash that lasts 1 or 2 days within a few days after immunization Arthralgia, arthritis, or paresthesia of the hands and fingers may occur about 2 weeks after vaccination and is more common in older children and adults	Advise parents of side effects, especially of time delay before joint swelling and pain; assure them that these symptoms will disappear May recommend use of mild analgesics for pain
Haemophilus influenzae type B	Low-grade fever Mild local reactions at injection site Rarely fever above 40° C (105° F)	Advise parents of possible mild side effects

*General comment to parents regarding each immunization: the benefit of being protected by the immunization is believed to greatly outweigh the risk from the disease.

†The National Childhood Vaccine Injury Act of 1988 requires the following information for childhood mandated vaccines to be documented in the child's permanent medical record: (1) type, manufacturer, and lot number of the vaccine; (2) date of administration; and (3) name, address, and title of the person administering the vaccine. Other suggested information to record is the site and route of administration and the expiration date of the vaccine.

Unit 2

GUIDELINES FOR CHILDREN'S DENTAL CARE

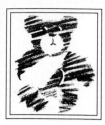

Begin regular visits to the dentist soon after the first teeth erupt and no later than when the child is 2½ years old.

Plan the first examination to be a "friendly visit"—meeting the dentist, seeing the room and equipment, and sitting in the chair.

BRUSHING AND FLOSSING

Begin cleaning the teeth as soon as the first tooth erupts. This is done by wiping it with a cloth.

Begin regular brushing and flossing soon after several "baby" teeth have erupted. Make mouth care pleasant by talking or singing to child.

Use a small toothbrush with soft, rounded, multitufted nylon bristles that are short and even. Change the toothbrush *often*, as soon as the bristles are bent or frayed.

For young children, place the tips of the bristles firmly at a 45-degree angle against the teeth and gums and move them back and forth in a vibratory motion. Do not move the ends of the bristles forcefully back and forth because this can damage the gums and enamel.

For children whose permanent teeth have erupted, place the sides of the bristles firmly against the gums and brush the gums and teeth in the direction the teeth grow, using a rolling action.

Clean all surfaces of the teeth in this manner except the inner surfaces of the front teeth. To clean these areas, place the toothbrush vertical to the teeth and move it up and down.

Brush only a few teeth at one time, using six to eight strokes for each section.

Use a systematic approach so that all surfaces are thoroughly cleaned.

In brushing young children's teeth, use any of these positions:

Stand with the child's back toward you.

Sit on a couch or bed with the child's head in your lap.

Sit on a floor or stool with the child's head resting between your thighs.

Use one hand to cup the chin and the other hand to brush the teeth.

When child wants to begin brushing his own teeth, let him "help" by brushing before or after.

Floss the teeth after brushing. Wrap a piece of dental floss (about 18 inches long) around the middle finger and grasp it between the index finger and thumb of both hands. With about 1 inch of floss held firmly between the thumbs, insert the floss between two teeth and wrap it around the base of the tooth and below the gum in a C shape. Move the floss toward the top of the tooth in a sweeping motion. Repeat this a few times on every tooth, using a clean piece of floss. Children may find it easier to tie the floss in a circle, rather than wrapping it around the middle finger.

Check the thoroughness of the cleaning by having the child chew a special dental disclosing tablet (available commercially or from dentists) that stains any remaining plaque red. Rebrush any colored areas.

Form the habit of cleaning the teeth after each meal and especially before bedtime. Give the child nothing to eat or drink (except water) after the night brushing.

Use the "swish and swallow" method of cleaning the mouth at times when brushing is impractical. Have child rinse mouth with water and swallow, repeating this three to four times.

FLUORIDE

Use a fluoridated toothpaste, but supervise the amount used by the child. Use only a "pea-sized" amount on the brush and teach child not to eat toothpaste.

Use a fluoridated mouthrinse if the child is older than 6 years and can safely rinse and spit out without swallowing the rinse. Use only the recommended amount; time the 1-minute rinse with a clock. Give the child nothing to eat or drink for 30 minutes afterward.

If the local water supply is fluoridated, make sure that the child is drinking the water—plain, in juices, soups, or other foods prepared with tap water.

If the local water supply is not fluoridated or if the infant is breast-fed or given commercial ready-to-feed formula, make sure fluoride supplements are prescribed by a health professional.

When supplemental fluoride is prescribed:

- Place the drops directly on the tongue to allow them to mix with saliva and come in contact with the teeth.
- Encourage older children to chew the tablet and swish it around the teeth for 30 seconds before swallowing.
- Give the child nothing to eat or drink for 30 minutes afterward.
- Store fluoride supplements and fluoridated toothpaste and mouthrinse in a safe place away from small children.

DIET

Keep sweet foods to a minimum, especially sticky or chewy candy and dried fruits (raisins, "fruit rolls," chewing gum) and hard candy (lollipops, "lifesavers"). Read labels on packaged foods (e.g., dry cereals) for hidden sources of sugar, including honey, molasses, and corn syrup.

Remember: *It is how often children eat sweets, rather than the amount of sweets eaten at one time,* that is most important. Plan sweets to follow a meal when the child is likely to brush immediately afterward. Discourage frequent snacking with sweets.

Encourage snacks that are less likely to cause cavities (caries), such as cheese, fresh fruit, raw vegetables, crackers, pretzels, potato or corn chips, popcorn, peanuts, and artificially sweetened candy, gum, and soda. When choosing these snacks, avoid foods, such as grapes, popcorn, or nuts, that can choke young children.

If the child takes a bottle to bed, fill it only with water, *never* formula, breast milk, cow's milk, or juice. Avoid frequent or prolonged breast-feeding during sleep.

If the child routinely takes any medicine in sweetened liquid or chewable tablet form, clean the teeth immediately afterward or at least have the child drink water to rinse the mouth.

Guidelines for a systemic fluoride regimen for children*

I. Children living in an unfluoridated community
  1. Know the fluoride (Fl) content of the drinking water before recommending Fl supplements (see below). If the family uses well water, have the Fl content analyzed.
  2. Recommend liquid Fl preparations for infants and young children. Place the drops directly on the tongue to allow it to mix with saliva and contact any teeth.
  3. Recommend Fl tablets for older children. Encourage them to chew the tablet and swish it in the mouth for 30 seconds before swallowing. Give nothing to eat or drink afterward for 30 minutes.
  4. Administer Fl supplements on an empty stomach without calcium-rich products, such as milk.
  5. Advise parents to store the Fl supplements in a safe place away from small children and to keep no more than a 4-month supply in the home.
  6. If the child spends extended periods of time in areas where the water is fluoridated (for example, school or summer vacation), assess the child's drinking habits, and consider temporarily discontinuing the supplement until unfluoridated water consumption is resumed.
  7. Encourage parents to supervise the toothbrushing habits of young children, especially those under 4 years, and use a pea-sized amount of fluoridated toothpaste to minimize the amount ingested. If this is impractical, suggest the use of a nonfluoridated toothpaste.
  8. Recommend the daily use of a fluoridated mouthrinse in children 4 years and older. Instruct parents regarding proper technique: use only the recommended amount; time the 1-minute rinse with a clock; expectorate the solution; and avoid food or fluid immediately afterward.
  9. Advise parents to store fluoridated dentifrice and mouthrinse in a safe place away from small children and teach children not to eat toothpaste.

*Modified from "Fluoride: Too Much or Too Little?" by Caryn S Hess, et al, 1984, *Pediatric Nursing*, 10, p 401. Copyright 1984 by Anthony J Jannetti, Inc. Reprinted by permission.

II. Children living in a fluoridated community
  1. Determine if the Fl content of the drinking water contains optimal levels of fluoride (0.7-1.2 ppm).
    a. Contact local water or health department for water fluoride content.
    b. If the family uses well water, have the Fl content analyzed.
    c. If the water contains excessive amounts of Fl, consider advising the family to use bottled water, and alert them to sources of additional Fl intake, such as tea and fluoridated toothpaste.
  2. Take a diet history to assess the infant's and child's drinking and eating habits.
    a. *Infants.* Assess the method of formula preparation; if ready-to-serve formula or breast milk is used and little or no water is offered, recommend a Fl supplement until sufficient tap water is added to the diet.
    b. *Children.* Assess the types of liquid consumed, especially tap water and tea, which has a high fluoride content. If little tap water is ingested, advise parents to prepare frozen-concentrated juice, powdered drinks, soup, Jell-O, or other foods with fluoridated water. If this is impractical and the child ordinarily drinks little tap water, consider a Fl supplement.
  3. Retake the diet history as the climate changes since children are likely to drink more in warmer weather, thus increasing their Fl intake.
  4. Encourage parents to supervise the young child's tooth brushing habits and use a pea-sized amount of fluoridated toothpaste to minimize the amount swallowed. If this is impractical, suggest the use of a nonfluoridated toothpaste.
  5. Recommend the daily use of a fluoridated mouthrinse in children 6 years and older. Instruct parents regarding proper technique: use only the recommended amount; time the 1-minute rinse with a clock; expectorate the solution; and avoid food or fluid immediately afterward.
  6. Advise parents to store fluoridated toothpaste and mouthrinse in a safe place away from small children, and to teach children not to eat toothpaste.

Supplemental fluoride dosage schedule (mg/day*)

Age	Concentration of fluoride in drinking water (ppm)		
	<0.3	0.3-0.7	>0.7
2 weeks-2 years	0.25	0	0
2-3 years	0.50	0.25	0
3-16 years	1.00	0.50	0

From American Academy of Pediatrics Committee on Nutrition: Fluoride supplementation: revised dosage schedule, Pediatrics 63:150, 1979.
*2.2 mg sodium fluoride contains 1 mg fluoride.

CHILD SAFETY HOME CHECKLIST

SAFETY: FIRE, ELECTRICAL, BURNS

- Guards in front of or around any heating appliance, fireplace, or furnace (including floor furnace)*
- Electrical wires hidden or out of reach*
- No frayed or broken wires
- No overloaded sockets
- Plastic guards or caps over electrical outlets, furniture in front of outlets*
- Hanging tablecloths out of reach and away from open fires*
- Smoke detectors tested and operating properly
- Kitchen matches stored out of child's reach*
- Large, deep ashtrays throughout house (if used)
- Small stoves, heaters, and other hot objects (cigarettes, candles, coffee pots, slow cookers) placed where they cannot be tipped over or reached by children
- Hot water heater set 49° C (120° F) or lower
- Pot handles turned toward back of stove
- No loose clothing worn near stove
- No cooking or eating hot foods or liquids with child standing nearby or sitting in lap
- All small appliances, such as iron, turned off, disconnected, and placed out of reach when not in use
- Cool, not hot, mist vaporizer used
- Fire extinguisher available on each floor and checked periodically
- Electrical fuse box and gas outlet accessible
- Family escape plan in case of a fire and practiced periodically; fire escape ladder available on upper level floors
- Telephone number of fire or rescue squad and address of home with nearest cross street posted near phone

SAFETY: POISONING

- Toxic substances placed on a high shelf and preferably in locked cabinet
- Toxic plants hung or placed on high surface rather than on floor*
- Excess quantities of cleaning fluid, paints, pesticides, drugs, and other toxic substances not stored in home
- Used containers of poisonous substances discarded where child cannot obtain access
- Telephone number of local poison control center and address of home with nearest cross street posted near phone
- Syrup of ipecac in home with 2 doses per child
- Medicines clearly labeled in childproof containers and stored out of reach
- Household cleaners, disinfectants, and insecticides kept in their original containers, separate from food and out of reach

SAFETY: FALLS

- Non-skid mats, abrasive strips, or textured surfaces in tubs and showers
- Exits, halls, and passageways in rooms kept clear of toys, furniture, boxes, or other items that could be obstructive
- Stairs and halls well lighted, with switches at both top and bottom
- Sturdy handrails for all steps and stairways
- Nothing stored on stairways
- Treads, risers, and carpeting in good repair
- Glass doors and walls marked with decals
- Safety glass used in doors, windows, and walls
- Gates on top and bottom of staircases and elevated areas, such as porch, fire escape*
- Guardrails on upstairs windows with locks that limit height of window opening and access to areas, such as fire escape*
- Crib side rails raised to full height; mattress lowered as child grows*
- Restraints used in high chairs, walkers, or other baby furniture; walkers not used near stairs*
- Scatter rugs secured in place or used with nonskid backing
- Walks, patios, and driveways in good repair

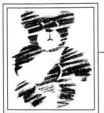

*Safety measures are specific for homes with young children. All safety measures should be implemented in homes where children reside and visit frequently, such as those of grandparents or babysitters.

†Federal regulations available from U.S. Consumer Product Safety Commission 1-800-638-CPSC; teletypewriter service for the hearing impaired is available at 1-800-638-8270 (in Maryland, 1-800-492-8104).

‡Home care instructions for infant cardiopulmonary resuscitation and infant/child choking are in Unit 5.

This checklist may be photocopied and distributed to families either alone or with the Injury Prevention handouts on pp 186-194. From Wong D and Whaley L: Clinical manual of pediatric nursing, ed 3. Copyright 1990, The CV Mosby Co, St Louis.

SAFETY: SUFFOCATION AND ASPIRATION

- Small objects stored out of reach*
- Toys inspected for small removable parts or long strings*
- Hanging crib toys and mobiles placed out of child's reach*
- Plastic bags stored away from young child's reach; large plastic garment bags discarded after tying in knots*
- Mattress or pillow not covered with plastic or in manner accessible to child*
- Crib design according to federal regulations with snug-fitting mattress*†
- Crib positioned away from other furniture or windows*
- Portable playpen gates up at all times while in use*
- Accordion-style gates not used*
- Button-size batteries stored safely and discarded properly, where child will not have access*
- Bathroom doors kept closed and toilet seats down*
- Faucets turned off firmly*
- Pool fenced with locked gate
- Proper safety equipment at poolside
- Electric garage door openers stored safely and adjusted to raise when door strikes object
- Doors of ovens, trunks, dishwashers, refrigerators, and front-loading clothes washers and dryers closed at all times*
- Unused appliance, such as a refrigerator, securely closed with lock or doors removed*
- Food served in small noncylindric pieces to young children*
- Toy chests without lids or with lids that securely lock in open position*
- Pails, buckets, and wading pools kept empty when not in use*
- Clothesline above head level
- At least one member of household trained in basic life support (CPR), including first aid for choking‡

SAFETY: BODILY INJURY

- Knives, power tools, and unloaded firearms stored safely or placed in locked cabinet
- Garden tools returned to storage racks after use
- Pets properly restrained and immunized for rabies
- Swings, slides, and other outdoor play equipment kept in safe condition
- Yard clear of broken glass, nail-studded boards, and other litter
- Cement birdbaths placed where young child cannot tip them over*
- Telephone number of ambulance or rescue squad and address of home with nearest cross street posted near phone

Age (months)	Developmental abilities related to risk of injury	Injury prevention
BIRTH-4	Involuntary reflexes, such as the crawling reflex, may propel infant forward May roll over Increasing eye-hand coordination and voluntary grasp reflex	**CHOKING** Not as great a danger to this age-group but should begin practicing safeguards early (see under 4-7 months) Know emergency procedures for choking* Never shake baby powder directly on infant; place powder in hand and then on infant's skin; store container closed and out of infant's reach Hold infant for feeding; do not prop bottle **SUFFOCATION** Keep all plastic bags stored away from infant's reach; discard large plastic garment bags after tying knots Do not cover mattress or pillows with plastic Use a firm mattress, no pillows, and loose blankets Make sure crib design follows federal regulations (distance between crib slats no more than 2 3/8 inches) and mattress fits snugly† Position crib away from other furniture Avoid sleeping in bed with infant Use pacifier with safe design of one-piece construction with loop handle; do not use stuffed bottle nipple for pacifier Do not tie pacifier on a string around infant's neck Remove bibs at bedtime Drowning—never leave infant alone in bath Keep playpen sides up **FALLS** Always raise crib rails Never leave infant on a raised, unguarded surface When in doubt where to place child, use the floor Restrain child in the infant seat and never leave him unattended while the seat is resting on a raised surface Use high chair when child is old enough to sit well Hold rail when carrying infant downstairs **POISONING** Not as great a danger to this age-group but should begin practicing safeguarding early (see under 4-7 months) **BURNS** Have fire extinguisher in home Install smoke detectors in home on each floor near bedrooms Avoid or use caution when warming formula in microwave oven; always check temperature of liquid before feeding Always check bath water; adjust hot-water heater temperature to 120° F Do not pour or drink hot liquids when infant is close by, such as sitting on lap Do not smoke near infant Do not leave infant in the sun for more than a few minutes; use sunscreen when in sun Use flame-retardant sleepwear and wash according to label directions Use cool mist vaporizers Do not keep child in parked car (risk of overheating) Check surface heat of car restraint before placing child in seat

*Instructions for care of the choking infant are in Unit 5.
†Information is available from U.S. Consumer Product Safety Commission, 1-800-638-CPSC.

Age (months)	Developmental abilities related to risk of injury	Injury prevention
BIRTH-4— cont'd		**MOTOR VEHICLES** Transport infant in federally approved rearward-facing car seat* Do not place infant on the seat or in one's lap Do not place a child in a carriage or stroller behind a parked car **BODILY DAMAGE** Avoid sharp, jagged-edged objects Keep diaper pins closed and away from infant Protect infant from young children and animals, especially dogs
4-7	Rolls over Sits alone momentarily May stand while holding on to support Grasps and manipulates small objects Resecures a dropped object Has well-developed eye-hand coordination Can focus on and locate very small objects Mouthing very prominent	**CHOKING** Keep buttons, beads, and other small objects out of infant's reach, including sibling's small toys Use pacifier with one-piece construction and loop handle Keep floor and carpet free of any small objects Do not feed infant hard candy, nuts, food with pits or seeds, whole hot dogs or grapes, or other large pieces of food Do not feed infant while child is lying down Inspect toys for removable parts Avoid balloons as playthings Discard used button-size batteries; store new batteries in safe area Keep baby powder, if used, out of reach **SUFFOCATION** May begin to teach swimming as part of water safety Do not tie toys across crib or playpen **FALLS** Use lap/crotch belt to restrain in a high chair Keep crib rails raised to full height Remove bumper pads when child can stand in crib **POISONING** Make sure that paint for furniture or toys does not contain lead Place toxic substances on a high shelf and/or in locked cabinet Hang plants or place on high surface rather than on floor Avoid storing large quantities of cleaning fluid, paints, pesticides, and other toxic substances Discard used containers of poisonous substances Do not store toxic substances in food containers Know telephone number of local poison control center (usually listed in front of telephone directory) Keep syrup of ipecac in home; use only if advised **BURNS** Always check bath water; adjust hot-water heater temperature to 49° C (120° F) or lower Keep faucets out of reach Cover tub spout or run cold water after using hot water Place hot objects (cigarettes, candles, incense) and liquids on high surface; do not drink hot liquids or smoke near infant **MOTOR VEHICLES** (See under Birth-4 months)

*See pp. 195-197 for car safety instructions for families.

Continued

Age (months)	Developmental abilities related to risk of injury	Injury prevention
4-7—cont'd		**BODILY DAMAGE** Give toys that are smooth and rounded, preferably made of wood or plastic Avoid long, pointed objects as toys Keep sharp objects out of infant's reach
8-12	Crawls Stands, holding onto furniture Stands alone Cruises around furniture Walks Climbs Pulls on objects Throws objects Able to pick up small objects Explores by putting objects in mouth Dislikes being restrained Explores away from parent Increasing understanding of simple commands and phrases Helpless in water	**CHOKING** (See under 4-7 months) **SUFFOCATION** Keep doors of ovens, dishwashers, refrigerators, and frontloading clothes washers and dryers closed at all times If storing an unused appliance, such as a refrigerator, remove the door Fence swimming pools Always supervise when near any source of water, such as cleaning buckets, drainage areas Eliminate unnecessary pools of water Keep bathroom doors closed **FALLS** Place gates at top and bottom of stairs if child has access to either end Dress in safe shoes and clothing (soles that do not "catch" on floor, tied shoelaces, pant legs that do not hang on floor) Keep large toys and bumper pads out of crib or playpen (child can use these as "stairs" to climb out) Avoid using walkers, especially near stairs **POISONING** Administer medications as a drug, not as a candy Do not administer medications unless so prescribed by a physician Replace medications and poisons immediately after use Replace child-protector cap properly Have syrup of ipecac in home; use only if advised **BURNS** Place guards in front of or around any heating appliance, fireplace, or furnace Keep electrical wires hidden or out of reach Place plastic guards over electrical outlets; place furniture in front of outlets Keep hanging tablecloths out of reach Do not allow infant to play with electrical appliance, cigarette lighter Apply a sunscreen when infant is exposed to sunlight **MOTOR VEHICLES** Transport infant over 17 to 20 lbs in federally approved forward-facing car seat Do not allow to crawl behind a parked car If infant plays in a yard, have the yard fenced or use a playpen **BODILY DAMAGE** Do not allow infant to use a fork for self-feeding Use plastic cups or dishes Check safety of toys and toy box Protect from young children and animals, especially dogs

---

Toy safety

Use toys recommended for child's age.

Avoid toys with sharp edges that can cut or sharp points either inside or outside that can puncture if the toy is broken.

Select toys that are durable enough to survive rough play.

Avoid toys with any small parts that can be swallowed or inhaled in children under 3 years.

Avoid toys with any shooting or throwing objects that can injure eyes or toys that make loud noises that could damage a child's hearing.

Keep cords and strings on toys less than 12 inches long.

Select toy box or chest without heavy, hinged lid.

Check all toys periodically for breakage and other potential hazards.

Repair broken toys or discard them.

Use only paint labeled "nontoxic" to repaint toys, toy boxes, or children's furniture.

Examine all outdoor toys regularly for rust or weak or sharp parts that could become dangerous.

Developmental abilities related to risk of injury	Injury prevention

Walks, runs, and climbs
Able to open doors and gates
Can ride tricycle
Can throw ball and other objects
	MOTOR VEHICLES
	Use federally approved car restraint; if restraint is not available, use lap belt*
	Supervise children while playing outside
	Do not allow to play on curb or behind a parked car
	Do not permit to play in pile of leaves, snow, or large cardboard container in trafficked area
	Supervise tricycle riding
	Lock fences and doors if not directly supervising children
	Teach children to obey pedestrian safety rules
	    Obey traffic regulations; cross only at crosswalks and only when the traffic signal indicates it is safe to cross
	    Stand back a step from the curb until it's time to cross
	    Look left, right, and left again and check for turning cars before crossing the street
	    Use sidewalks; when there is no sidewalk, walk on the left, facing the traffic
	    Wear light colors at night, and attach fluorescent material to clothing

Able to explore if left unsupervised Has great curiosity Helpless in water; unaware of its danger; depth of water has no significance	**DROWNING** Supervise closely when near any source of water Keep bathroom doors closed Have fence around swimming pool and lock gate Teach swimming and water safety
Able to reach heights by climbing, stretching, and standing on toes Pulls objects Explores any holes or opening Can open drawers and closets Unaware of potential sources of heat or fire Plays with mechanical objects	**BURNS** Turn pot handles toward back of stove Place electric appliances, such as coffee maker and popcorn machine, toward back of counter Place guardrails in front of radiators, fireplaces, or other heating elements Store matches and cigarette lighters in locked or inaccessible area; discard carefully Place burning candles, incense, hot foods, and cigarettes out of reach Do not let tablecloth hang within child's reach Do not let electric cord from iron or other appliance hang within child's reach Cover electrical outlets with protective plastic caps Keep electrical wires hidden or out of reach Do not allow child to play with electrical appliance, wires, or lighters Stress danger of open flames; teach what "hot" means Always check bath water temperature; adjust hot-water heater temperature to 120° F or lower; do not allow to play with faucets Apply a sunscreen when child exposed to sunlight

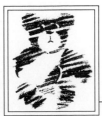

*See pp. 195-197 for car safety instructions for parents.

Continued.

Developmental abilities related to risk of injury	Injury prevention
Explores by putting objects in mouth Can open drawers, closets, and most containers Climbs Cannot read labels Does not know safe dose or amount	**POISONING** Place all potentially toxic agents out of reach or in a locked cabinet Caution against eating nonedible items, such as plants Replace medications and poisons immediately; replace child-protector caps properly Administer medications as a drug, not as a candy Do not store large surplus of toxic agents Promptly discard empty poison containers; never reuse to store a food item or other poison Teach child not to play in trash containers Never remove labels from containers of toxic substances Have syrup of ipecac in home; use only if advised Know number and location of nearest poison control center (usually listed in front of telephone directory)
Able to open doors and some windows Goes up and down stairs Depth perception unrefined	**FALLS** Keep screen in window, nail securely, and use guardrail Place gates at top and bottom of stairs Keep doors locked or use child-proof doorknob covers at entry to stairs, high porch, or other elevated area Remove unsecured or scatter rugs Apply nonskid decals in bathtub or shower Keep crib rails fully raised and mattress at lowest level Place carpeting under crib and in bathroom Keep large toys and bumper pads out of crib or playpen (child can use these as "stairs" to climb out), then move to youth bed when child is able to crawl out of crib Avoid using walkers, especially near stairs Dress in safe clothing (soles that do not "catch" on floor, tied shoelaces, pant legs that do not hang on floor) Keep child restrained in vehicles; never leave unattended in shopping cart Supervise at playgrounds; select safe play areas with soft ground cover
Puts things in mouth May swallow hard or nonedible pieces of food	**CHOKING AND SUFFOCATION** Avoid large round chunks of meat, such as whole hot dogs (slice lengthwise into short pieces) Avoid fruit with pits, fish with bones, dried beans, hard candy, chewing gum, nuts, popcorn, grapes Choose large sturdy toys without sharp edges or small removable parts Discard old refrigerators, ovens, and so on If storing an old appliance, remove the doors Keep automatic garage door transmitter in inaccessible place Select safe toy boxes or chests without heavy, hinged lids

Developmental abilities related to risk of injury	Injury prevention

Still clumsy in many skills
Easily distracted from tasks
Unaware of potential danger from strangers or other people
	BODILY DAMAGE
	Avoid giving sharp or pointed objects—such as knives, scissors, or toothpicks—especially when walking or running
	Do not allow lollipops or similar objects in mouth when walking or running
	Teach safety precautions, for example, to carry knife or scissors with pointed end away from face
	Store all dangerous tools, garden equipment, and firearms in locked cabinet
	Be alert to danger of supervised animals and household pets
	Use safety glass and decals on large glassed areas, such as sliding glass doors
	Teach name, address, and phone number and to ask for help from appropriate people (cashier, security guard, policeman) if lost; have identification on child (shown in clothes, inside shoe)
	Teach stranger safety:
	  Avoid personalized clothing in public places
	  Never go with a stranger
	  Tell parents if anyone makes child feel uncomfortable in any way
	  Always listen to child's concerns regarding others' behavior
	  Teach child to say "no" when confronted with uncomfortable situations

Developmental abilities related to risk of injury	Injury prevention
Is developing increasing independence	**MOTOR VEHICLES** Educate regarding proper use of seat belts while a passenger in a vehicle

Has increased physical skills
Needs strenuous physical activity
Is interested in acquiring new skills and perfecting attained skills
Is daring and adventurous, especially with peers
Frequently plays in hazardous places
Confidence often exceeds physical capacity
Desires group loyalty and has strong need for friends' approval
Attempts hazardous feats
Accompanies friends to potentially hazardous facilities
Delights in physical activity
Is likely to overdo
Growth in height exceeds muscular growth and coordination
	Maintain discipline while a passenger in a vehicle, for example, keep arms inside, do not lean against doors or interfere with driver
	Emphasize safe pedestrian behavior
	Teach safety and maintenance of two-wheeled vehicles, such as bicycles (see box)
	Insist on wearing of safety apparel (e.g., helmet) where applicable, such as riding motorcycle
	
	DROWNING
	Teach to swim
	Teach basic rules of water safety
	  Select safe and supervised places to swim
	  Check sufficient water depth for diving
	  Swim with a companion
	  Use an approved flotation device in water or boat
	
	BURNS
	Instruct in behavior in the areas involving contact with potential burn hazards, for example, gasoline, matches, bonfires or barbecues, lighter fluid, firecrackers, cigarette lighters, cooking utensils, chemistry sets; avoid climbing or flying kites around high-tension wires
	Instruct in proper behavior in the event of fire (e.g., fire drills at home, school, and so on)
	Teach "stop, drop, and roll" if clothing becomes ignited
	Advise regarding excessive exposure to sunlight (ultraviolet burn); encourage use of sunscreens
	Teach safe cooking (use low heat, avoid any frying, be careful of steam burns especially from microwaving)
	
	POISONING
	Educate regarding hazards of taking nonprescription drugs and chemicals, including aspirin and alcohol
	Teach child to say "no" if offered illegal or dangerous drugs, alcohol
	Keep potentially dangerous products in properly labeled receptacles—preferably out of reach

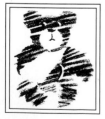

Developmental abilities related to risk of injury	Injury prevention
	FALLS
	Discourage climbing or walking up or on high structures, such as trees, utility poles, walls, fences
	Instruct in proper use of playground equipment
	Instruct in proper use and care of sports equipment, especially the more hazardous devices (skateboards, trampolines, skis, and motorized vehicles)
	Emphasize use of protective equipment and safe practices when engaged in activities such as skateboarding, cycling, soccer, hockey, and football

Bicycle safety

Ride bicycles with traffic and away from parked cars

Ride single file

Walk bicycles through busy intersections only at crosswalks

Give hand signals well in advance of turning or stopping

Keep as close to the curb as practical

Watch for drain grates, potholes, soft shoulders, and loose dirt or gravel

Keep both hands on handlebars, except when signaling

Never ride double on a bicycle

Do not carry packages that interfere with vision or control; do not drag objects behind bike

Watch for and yield to pedestrians

Watch for cars backing up or pulling out of driveways; be especially careful at intersections

Look left, right, then left before turning into traffic or roadway

Never hitch a ride on a truck or other vehicle

Learn rules of the road and respect for traffic officers

Obey all local ordinances

Wear well-fitted helmet

Wear shoes while riding

Wear light colors at night and attach fluorescent material to clothing and bicycle

Be certain the bicycle is the correct size for rider

Equip bicycle with proper lights and reflectors

Have the bicycle inspected to ensure good mechanical condition

BODILY DAMAGE

Help provide facilities for supervised activities

Encourage playing in safe places

Keep firearms safely locked up except during adult supervision

Teach proper care of, use of, and respect for devices with potential danger (power tools, firecrackers, and so on)

Stress eye protection when using potentially hazardous objects or devices or when engaged in potentially hazardous sports

Teach safety regarding use of corrective devices (glasses); if child wears contact lenses, monitor duration of wear to prevent corneal damage

Stress careful selection and maintenance of sport and recreation equipment

Emphasize proper conditioning, safe practices, and use of safety equipment for sports or recreational activities

Caution against engaging in hazardous sports, such as those involving trampolines

Use safety glass and decals on large glassed areas, such as sliding glass doors

Teach name, address, and phone number and to ask for help from appropriate people (cashier, security guard, policeman) if lost; have identification on child (sewn in clothes, inside shoe)

Teach stranger safety:

Avoid personalized clothing in public places

Never go with a stranger

Tell parents if anyone makes child feel uncomfortable in any way

Always listen to child's concerns regarding others' behavior

Teach child to say "no" when confronted with uncomfortable situations

Developmental abilities related to risk of injury	Injury prevention

Need for independence and freedom
Testing independence
Tendency toward risk-taking, especially with peers
Feeling of indestructibility
Age permitted to drive a motor vehicle (varies)
Need for discharging energy, often at expense of logical thinking and other control mechanisms
Peak incidence for practice and participation in sports
Strong need for peer approval; may attempt hazardous feats
Access to more complex tools, objects, and locations
Can assume responsibility for own actions
	MOTOR VEHICLES
	Pedestrian—emphasize and encourage safe pedestrian behavior
	Passenger—promote appropriate behavior while riding in a motor vehicle
	Driver—provide competent driver education; encourage judicious use of vehicle, discourage drag racing or "chicken;" maintain vehicle in proper condition (e.g., brakes, tires)
	Stress the necessity of using car restraint system at *all* times
	Teach and promote safety and maintenance of two-wheeled vehicles
	Promote and encourage wearing of safety apparel such as helmet, long trousers
	Reinforce the dangers of drugs (including alcohol) when operating a motor vehicle
	
	DROWNING
	Teach to swim (if unable to do so)
	Teach basic rules of water safety
	    Select safe, and preferably supervised, places to swim
	    Check sufficient water depth for diving
	    Swim with companion
	    Use an approved flotation device in water or boat
	
	BURNS
	Reinforce proper behavior in areas involving contact with burn hazards (e.g., gasoline, electric wires, fires)
	Advise regarding excessive exposure to sunlight (ultraviolet burn), including indoor tanning
	Encourage use of sunscreens
	
	POISONING
	Educate in hazards of drug use, including alcohol
	Avoid storing large quantities of drugs
	
	FALLS
	Teach and encourage general safety measures in all activities
	
	BODILY DAMAGE
	Encourage proper instruction in sports and use of sports equipment
	Promote use of appropriate arena for sports activities
	Instruct in safe use of and respect for firearms and other devices with potential danger (power tools or firecrackers)
	Provide and encourage use of protective equipment when using potentially hazardous devices
	Promote access to and/or provision of safe sports and recreational facilities
	Be alert for signs of depression (potential suicide)
	Discourage use of and/or availability of hazardous sports equipment (e.g., trampoline, surfboards)
	Instruct regarding proper use of corrective devices such as glasses, contact lenses, hearing aids
	Encourage the practice of safety principles and prevention
	Encourage considering consequences of behavior *before* acting

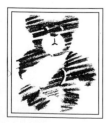

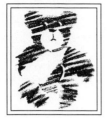

This important information is given to you because car accidents are the number one killer of infants and young children that can be prevented. All states now have laws that require children to be buckled up in cars. For more information about your state law, contact your state Highway Safety Office.

Remember that the most dangerous place for an infant or child to ride is in the arms of another person.

SEAT SELECTION

If you are buying or borrowing a used safety seat, make sure that the seat meets Federal Motor Vehicle Safety Standard 213; a manufacture date after January 1, 1981, should be stamped on the seat. Problems with a used safety seat include the possibility of missing parts and instructions, or that the seat may have been in a crash. *Be cautious: buy or borrow a used seat only if you are sure it's safe.*

Make sure that the safety seat can be used with your make of car and type of seat belts. Some safety seats are too large for compact cars. Choose a seat that is simple to use. Practice with harness straps, shield, or other seat features. Ask yourself: "How many steps are involved in using the safety seat? Will it be easy to get the child into and out of the seat?" Try the seat before you buy it, or make certain that you can return the seat if it does not fit or is not easy to use in your car.

Shop around: there are many safety seats for sale and costs vary. Watch for sales.†

Some towns have low-cost rental or loan programs that are worth checking.

*Prepared by Kristie S Nix, EdD, RN, Associate Professor, University of Tulsa, Tulsa, OK.
†Shopping guide for different models of seats may be obtained from: American Academy of Pediatrics, Division of Public Education, 141 Northwest Point Blvd., PO Box 927, Elk Grove, IL 60007 (free; send a self-addressed, stamped envelope with request).

Possible places to check for these services are local and state health departments, hospitals, American Red Cross, or library reference desks.

SAFETY SEATS FOR NEWBORNS AND INFANTS

Look into the seats and choose one before the birth of an infant (a gift certificate for a safety seat is a good idea for a baby gift as it lets parents choose a seat that works well with their car). Take the seat and its instructions to the hospital. Before the baby is discharged, practice putting the infant into the seat and adjust the straps. Adjust straps snugly so that only two fingers fit between strap and child. *Use the seat starting with the first ride home from the hospital.*

You can choose from infant-only seats (Fig. 1), which are for babies from birth to about 17 to 20 pounds (or 26 inches) and only face rearward, or from convertible seats, which may be faced rearward for infants, then faced forward (Figs. 2 and 3) as the child reaches 9 months or 20 pounds and is able to sit upright. Advantages of infant-only seats include their size suitability for the infants (particularly during the first 3 months) and their ease of

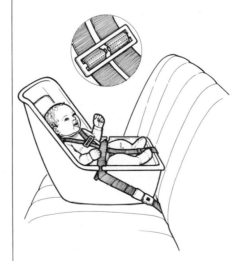

Fig. 1. Rear-facing infant-only safety seat. Inset: harness retainer (clip).

use in and out of the car. While convertible seats cost more than infant seats, they may be used from birth until the child outgrows it, usually about 4 years.

Dress the infant comfortably. Some types of clothing, such as buntings, do not let the buckle go between the infant's legs and should not be used. If blankets are needed, place them over the infant after the harness is buckled.

Although some safety seats may double as infant carriers, remember that lightweight household infant carriers and beds do not provide the protection given by a safety seat, which meets federal standards. These seats and beds are unsafe if used as a car restraint.

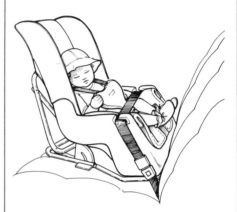

Fig. 2. Convertible seat in rear-facing position for use with infants.

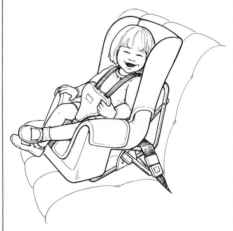

Fig. 3. Convertible seat in forward-facing position for older infants and children.

Continued

SAFETY SEATS FOR TODDLERS AND YOUNG CHILDREN

A child who can sit alone well, weighs 17 to 20 pounds, and is about 9 months old can use a forward-facing seat. Appropriate safety seats include the convertible models (mentioned above) and seats that are for use in a forward-facing position only. These models can be adjusted (semireclining to upright) so the child is comfortable for napping. Follow the manufacturer's instructions for safe travel positions and for adjusting the harness system as a child grows.

The safety seat should be used until the child outgrows it, at about 40 pounds, 40 inches tall, or 4 years of age. Then the child should use the lap/shoulder belt alone or in combination with a booster seat (Fig. 4). A booster safety seat may be preferred because it allows the child to see out of the car more easily. Use the shoulder belt *only* if it does not cross the child's face or neck. To avoid the head and neck, try moving the child more inboard, toward the buckle. If the shoulder belt still cannot be positioned properly over the shoulder and chest, use the lap belt alone, placing the shoulder belt behind the child. Never tuck the shoulder belt under the child's arm. The lap belt should go across the lap below the hip bones, as low as possible, and should fit snugly.

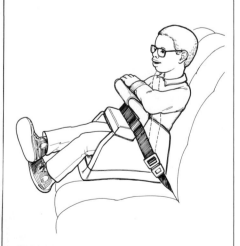

Fig. 4. Automobile booster seat. Dashed lines indicate placement of shoulder strap.

Although a booster seat can be used for a young child, it lacks side protection offered by toddler seats. While some booster models are sold for children who weigh 20 pounds, the recommended minimum weight is 30 pounds. A child who weighs less than 30 pounds is too young or too small for a booster seat. Most booster seats will accommodate a child up to 60 pounds. For all booster seats, the center of the child's head must not be higher than the back of the seat. If this happens, the child is too big for the booster seat.

RESTRAINING THE INFANT OR CHILD IN THE SEAT

Always follow the manufacturer's instructions for the seat about how to harness the child and thread the seat belt. Seat models manufactured since 1981 have instructions attached to the seat. Refer also to the car owner's guide for placement of or special changes required for seat belts with safety seats.

Apply all harness straps snugly so that only two fingers fit between strap and child. Many models have a harness retainer (clip) that keeps shoulder straps from slipping off the child's shoulders (See inset, Fig. 1). The clip should be placed at the middle of the child's chest and not near the neck or stomach.

Anchor all safety seats with the car's standard seat belt so that the safety seat cannot be moved. The seat belt is placed through the frame or shell, or across the front of the safety seat (follow the manufacturer's instructions). The belt is then pulled tight so that the safety seat is securely fastened and cannot be moved. If it can be moved, the safety seat cannot be used with the seat belt. Try another seat belt location within the car; in some cases, the seat belts must be replaced for the safety seat to be buckled in properly. If the car is equipped with automatic seat belts, it may be necessary for the dealer to install special equipment to properly secure the safety seat. For information regarding your car, refer to the car manufacturer's instruction booklet.

Inertia-type seat belt systems allow the passenger freedom of movement but lock into place upon braking or impacts. With this system, a safety seat may seem loose or slide around after it has been buckled in. Inertia-type belts that have a "sliding tongue" require use of a locking clip to prevent this movement (Fig. 5). Locking clips are packaged with new safety seats or are available through safety seat manufacturers, car dealers' parts departments, or retailers of safety seats.

When a rearward-facing seat is secured against a soft car seat, the safety seat may tilt into the car seat, causing the infant to slump forward. To correct this forward tilt, roll a small blanket or towel and place it beneath the safety seat base until the safety seat is level.

The safest place for the car seat is in the middle of the back seat; however, this position may not be practical when the driver needs to tend the infant/child and should not take his eyes from the road. In this case placing the safety seat in the front passenger seat may be preferred.

Some safety seats for children with disabilities* and selected older models require the use of a tether (anchor) strap that must be bolted to a sturdy metal panel of the car (Fig. 6). Optional tethers may be added to some seat models as an extra measure of protection for the child's head. If using a tethered seat in more than one car, keep in mind that a tether strap

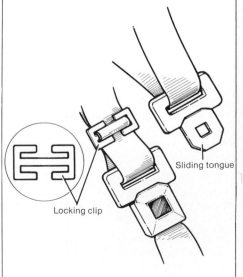

Fig. 5. Use of a locking clip.

and bolt system must be in place in each car in order to use the seat properly. The car dealer service department or a knowledgeable mechanic can install a tether. Choose a different seat if you cannot anchor it on every ride.

While a safety seat should be used every ride, there may be a time when no safety seat is available. Experts believe that there is no safe alternative to safety seats for infants. However, toddlers or older children may be buckled with the car's standard lap belt. Make sure that the lap belt is placed below the child's waist, over the hip bones and not over the stomach. Use the shoulder belt only if it does not cross the head or throat. Never buckle the child in someone's lap. In the event of an accident, that person's weight could crush the child.

Make it a rule: Do not start the car until everyone is buckled up.

---

*For information on safety seats for children with special needs, contact the Automobile Safety for Children Program, James Whitcomb Riley Hospital for Children, Indiana School of Medicine, 702 Barnhill Drive, S-139, Indianapolis, IN 46223, Phone: (317) 274-2977; in Indiana: (800) KID-N-CAR.

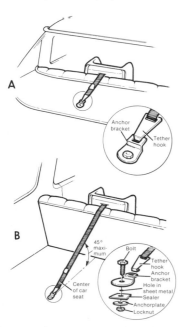

Fig. 6. Tether straps. **A,** Rear window shelf installation for sedans. **B,** Floor mount installation for hatchback or station wagon.

GENERAL TIPS

Seats with vinyl covering and metal pieces can become very hot and burn a child's skin. Place a cloth cover over the seat; a "homemade" cover, such as a towel or blanket, with slip openings for harness straps works just as well as those that can be bought. Cool metal pieces before use (a damp cloth works well).

When two parents transport the child, having a safety seat for each car is more convenient than having to move one safety seat between cars.

Always keep the safety seat buckled properly in the car when it is not being used to transport a child. In a quick stop or accident, the seat can become a deadly object inside the car. For the same reason, avoid "loose" objects in the car, such as toys or groceries, and use the trunk for these whenever possible.

If the safety seat is involved in an accident, it must be replaced. Even low mile-per-hour accidents can damage seat belts. Check harness straps for wear. Some manufacturers will replace seats free in order to study their products. Check with your insurance agent regarding replacement of a safety seat involved in an accident since most policies cover this loss.

TIPS FOR GOOD BEHAVIOR

Besides safety, another benefit of always using safety seats is that children who ride buckled up behave better and are less likely to distract the driver. To make safety seats a habit, try the following tips:

- Praise children often for good behavior while riding in the seat.
- Insist that others who transport children (baby-sitters, grandparents) also follow safety rules.
- Never allow children to ride unbuckled or to climb out of their seats. If this happens, stop the car and say, "You must put on your seat belt." Be firm.

To help a young child use a safety seat when he has not previously been required to do so, follow these hints:

- Give the seat as a special present.
- Let the child help put the seat in the

car, then try it out for a ride around the block.
- Let the child personalize the seat with stickers.
- Help the child pretend being an astronaut, pilot, or fireman while in the seat.
- Be firm and patient when teaching a child this new seat habit.

Remember: a good example helps children learn—buckle your seat belt.

TRIP TIPS

Expect that infants and young children will need to stop more often for feeding, changing, stretching, and play. Plan frequent travel breaks.

Dress the child comfortably and for convenience. Take along disposables: diapers, wash cloths, tissues.

Plan ahead to have activities ready: for infants, secure pictures and toys to the seat with Velcro or tape for the child to look at. Small, soft teething toys, stuffed animals, and pacifiers are helpful. For young children, books, toys (new ones provide greater diversion and interest), and games (counting, finding numbers or colors in the scenery) ease the restlessness of long trips.

One way to decrease boredom on long trips is to allow the child to change positions in the car by moving the safety seat. Be sure to buckle the seat securely in its new place.

Sing or listen to stories on a tape recorder. The child will enjoy recording and listening to his own sounds.

Prepare small snacks (cereal, raisins, carrots, crackers, fresh fruit) and drinks (cups with lids are handy). Avoid hard candies or candy on sticks, which could cause injury in case of quick stops.

When making an airline trip, check the safety seat as baggage so that it will be available at your destination, or make plans to rent a seat. The safety seat label will indicate if the seat may be used in-flight for air travel, but some airlines may not allow use of safety seats and may charge a fare for children under 2 who occupy a seat. Check with the airline company or a travel agent regarding their policies.

PARENTAL GUIDANCE
Guidance during infancy

Age (months)	Guidance	Age (months)	Guidance
BIRTH-6	Understand each parent's adjustment to newborn, especially mother's postpartal emotional needs Teach care of infant and assist parents to understand child's individual needs and temperament and that wants are expressed through crying Reassure that infant cannot be spoiled by too much attention during the first 4 to 6 months Encourage parents to establish a schedule that meets needs of child and themselves Help parents understand infant's need for stimulation in environment Support parents' pleasure in seeing child's growing friendliness and social response, especially smiling Plan anticipatory guidance for safety Stress need for artificial immunization Prepare for introduction of solid foods	6-12	Prepare parents for child's "stranger anxiety" Encourage parents to allow child to cling to mother or father and avoid long separation from either Teach dental care of new teeth and discourage giving a bottle to infant at sleep times Guide parents concerning limit setting because of infant's increasing mobility Encourage use of negative voice and eye contact rather than physical punishment as a means of discipline; if unsuccessful, use one slap on the hand Encourage showing most attention when infant is behaving well, rather than when crying Teach injury prevention because of child's advancing motor skills and curiosity (see p. 186) Encourage parents to leave child with suitable caregiver to allow some free time Discuss readiness for weaning Explore parents' feelings regarding infant's sleep patterns

Unit 2

Guidance during toddler years

Age (months)	Guidance	Age (months)	Guidance
12-18	Prepare parents for expected behavioral changes of toddler, especially negativism and ritualism	**18-24**	Stress importance of peer companionship in play
	Assess present feeding habits and encourage gradual weaning from bottle and increased intake of solid foods		Explore need for preparation for additional sibling; stress importance of preparing child for new experiences
	Stress expected feeding changes of physiologic anorexia, presence of food fads and strong taste preferences, need for scheduled routine at mealtimes, inability to sit through an entire meal, and lack of table manners		Discuss present discipline methods, their effectiveness, and parents' feelings about child's negativism; stress that negativism is important aspect of developing self-assertion and independence and is not a sign of spoiling
	Assess sleep patterns at night, particularly habit of a bedtime bottle, which is a major cause of dental caries, and procrastination behaviors that delay hour of sleep		Discuss signs of readiness for toilet training; emphasize importance of waiting for physical and psychologic readiness
	Prepare parents for potential dangers of the home, particularly motor vehicular, poisoning, and falling injuries; give appropriate suggestions for safeproofing the home (see p. 184)		Discuss development of fears, such as darkness or loud noises, and of habits, such as security blanket or thumb-sucking; stress normalcy of these transient behaviors
	Discuss need for firm but gentle discipline and ways in which to deal with negativism and temper tantrums; stress positive benefits of appropriate discipline		Prepare parents for signs of regression in time of stress
	Emphasize importance for both child and parents of brief, periodic separations		Assess child's ability to separate easily from parents for brief periods of separation under familiar circumstances
	Discuss new toys that use developing gross and fine motor, language, cognitive, and social skills		Allow parents opportunity to express their feelings of weariness, frustration, and exasperation; be aware that it is often difficult to love toddlers at times when they are not asleep!
	Emphasize need for dental supervision, types of basic dental hygiene at home, and food habits that predispose to caries; stress importance of supplemental fluoride		Point out some of the expected changes of the next year, such as longer attention span, somewhat less negativism, and increased concern for pleasing others
		24-36	Discuss importance of imitation and domestic mimicry and need to include child in activities
			Discuss approaches toward toilet training, particularly realistic expectations and attitude toward accidents
			Stress uniqueness of toddlers' thought processes, especially through their use of language, poor understanding of time, casual relationships in terms of proximity vents, and inability to see events from another's perspective
			Stress that discipline still must be quite structured and concrete and that relying solely on verbal reasoning and explanation leads to injuries, confusion, and misunderstanding
			Discuss investigation of nursery school or day-care center toward completion of second year

Unit 2

Guidance during preschool years

Age (years)	Guidance	Age (years)	Guidance
3	Prepare parents for child's increasing interest in widening relationships Encourage enrollment in nursery school Emphasize importance of setting limits Prepare parents to expect exaggerated tension-reduction behaviors, such as need for "security blanket" Encourage parents to offer the child choices when the child vacillates Expect marked changes at 3½ years when the child becomes less coordinated (motor and emotional), becomes insecure, exhibits emotional extremes, and develops behaviors such as stuttering Prepare parents to expect extra demands on their attention as a reflection of the child's emotional insecurity and fear of loss of love Warn parents that the equilibrium of the 3-year-old will change to the aggressive out-of-bounds behavior of the 4-year-old Anticipate a more stable appetite with more expansive food selection Stress need for protection and education of child to prevent injury (see p. 189)	4 5	Prepare for more aggressive behavior including motor activity and shocking language Expect resistance to parental authority Explore parental feelings regarding child's behavior Suggest some kind of respite for primary caregiver such as placing the child in nursery school for part of the day Prepare for increasing sexual curiosity Emphasize importance of realistic limit setting on behavior and appropriate discipline techniques Prepare parents for the highly imaginary 4-year-old who indulges in "tall tales" (to be differentiated from lies) and for the child's acquisition of imaginary playmates Suggest swimming lessons if not begun earlier Expect nightmares or an increase in them and suggest they make certain the child is fully awakened from a frightening dream Provide reassurance that a period of calm begins at 5 years of age Expect a tranquil period at 5 years Prepare and assist child through initial entrance into school environment Make certain immunizations are up to date before entering school

Guidance during school-age years

Age (years)	Guidance	Age (years)	Guidance
6 7-10	Expect strong food preferences and frequent refusals of specific food items Expect increasingly ravenous appetite Prepare parents for emotionality as child experiences erratic mood changes Anticipate increase in susceptibility to illness and more sickness than at previous ages Teach injury prevention and safety, especially bicycle safety (see p. 200) Respect the child's need for privacy; provide own room if possible Prepare for increasing interests outside the home Encourage interaction with peers Expect improvement in health with fewer illnesses; however, allergies may increase or become apparent Prepare for increase in minor injuries Emphasize caution in selection and maintenance of sports equipment and re-emphasize teaching safety	7-10—cont'd 11-12	Expect increased involvement with peers and interest in activities outside the home Encourage independence but maintain limit-setting and discipline Expect more demands upon mother at 8 years Expect increasing admiration for father at 10 years; encourage father-child activities Prepare for prepubescent changes in girls Prepare child for body changes of pubescence Expect a growth spurt in girls Make certain the child's sex education is adequate with accurate information Expect energetic but stormy behavior at 11 to become more even-tempered at 12 Encourage child's desire to "grow up" but allow regressive behavior when needed Expect an increase in sexual behavior, e.g., masturbation and sexual interest Child may need increased amount of rest Educate child regarding experimentation with potentially harmful activities

Guidance during adolescence

Age (years)	Guidance	Age (years)	Guidance
12-15	Support and reassure the adolescent	**15-18**	Help the adolescent prepare for the adult role
	Be available to the adolescent when needed but avoid pressing him too far		Assist in selection of career goals
	Explain that rejecting behavior is a manifestation of the struggle for independence		Help parents have realistic expectations of the adolescent and avoid "pushing" them in a direction unsuited to their capabilities
	Provide undemanding love		Help parents recognize that present times are different from those of their youth
	Allow increasing independence but maintain suitable limit-setting for the adolescent's safety and well-being		Help parents cope with the multiple and diversified problems of relationships with adolescents
	Suggest parents acquire outside interests for themselves		Provide support and reassurance
	Allow parents to express feelings regarding the sometimes frustrating experience of coping with an adolescent		
	Emphasize the need for safety education (see p. 201)		

Be aware that:

Adolescent is subject to turbulent, unpredictable behavior

Adolescent is struggling for independence

Adolescent is extraordinarily sensitive to feelings and behavior that affect him or her

Message given to adolescent may not be message received

Friends are extremely important to adolescent

Adolescent has a strong need "to belong"

Adolescent sees things in black or white, good or bad

Unit 2

PLAY
Functions of play

SENSORIMOTOR DEVELOPMENT

Improves fine and gross motor skill and coordination
Enhances development of all the senses
Encourages exploration of the physical nature of the world
Provides for release of surplus energy

INTELLECTUAL DEVELOPMENT

Provides multiple sources of learning:
  Exploration and manipulation of shapes, sizes, texures, colors
  Experience with numbers, spatial relationships, abstract concepts
  Opportunity to practice and expand language skills
Provides opportunity to rehearse past experiences to assimilate them into new perceptions and relationships
Helps children to comprehend the world in which they live and to distinguish between fantasy and reality

SOCIALIZATION AND MORAL DEVELOPMENT

Teaches adult roles, including sex role behavior
Provides opportunities for testing relationships
Develops social skills
Encourages interaction and development of positive attitudes toward others
Reinforces approved patterns of behavior and moral standards

CREATIVITY

Provides an expressive outlet for creative ideas and interests
Allows for fantasy and imagination
Enhances development of special talents and interests

SELF-AWARENESS

Facilitates the development of self-identity
Encourages regulation of own behavior
Allows for testing of own abilities (self-mastery)
Provides for comparison of own abilities with those of others
Allows for opportunity to learn how own behavior affects others

THERAPEUTIC VALUE

Provides for release from tension and stress
Allows for expression of emotions and release of unacceptable impulses in a socially acceptable fashion
Encourages experimentation and testing of fearful situations in a safe manner
Facilitates nonverbal and indirect verbal communication of needs, fears, and desires

General trends during childhood

Age	Social character of play	Content of play	Most prevalent type of play	Characteristics of spontaneous activity	Purpose of dramatic play	Development of ethical sense
Infant	Solitary	Social-affective	Sensorimotor	Sense-pleasure	Self-identity	—
Toddler	Parallel	Imitative	Body movement	Intuitive judgment	Learning gender role	Beginning of moral values
Preschool	Associative	Imaginative	Fantasy Informal games	Concept formation Reasonably constant ideas	Imitating social life Learning social roles	Developing concern for playmates Learning to share and cooperate
School-age	Cooperative	Competitive games and contests Fantasy	Physical activity Gang activities Formal games Play acting	Testing concrete situations and problem solving Adding fresh information	Vicarious mastery	Peer loyalty Playing by the rules Hero worship
Adolescent	Cooperative	Competitive games and contests Daydreaming	Social interaction	Abstract problem solving	Presenting ideas	Causes and projects

Select toys that suit the skills, abilities, and interests of the child.

Select toys that are safe for the specific child; look for a label that indicates the intended age-group. Toys that are safe at one age may not be safe for another.

Make certain all parts are present and directions for use are clear and appropriate to the child.

Check for safety labels such as "flame retardant" or "flame resistant."

Select toys durable enough to survive rough play.

Select toys light enough that they will not cause harm if one falls on a child.

Look for toys with smooth, rounded edges. Avoid toys with sharp edges that can cut or sharp points. Points on the inside of the toy can puncture if the toy is broken.

Avoid toys with any small parts that can be swallowed or aspirated, especially for children under 3 years of age.

Avoid toys with any shooting or throwing objects that can injure eyes. This includes toys into which other missiles, such as sticks or pebbles, might be used as substitutes for the intended projectiles. Arrows and darts used by children should have blunt tips and be manufactured from resilient materials; make certain tips are securely attached.

Avoid toys that make loud noises that might be damaging to a child's hearing. Even some squeaking toys are too loud when held close to the ear.

Remove and discard plastic wrapping from toys that could suffocate a child.

Make certain an older child understands that a toy inappropriate for smaller children should be kept out of the hands of younger brothers and sisters.

Teach the child the proper way to unplug an electric toy—pull on the plug, not the cord.

Teach the child the safe use of utensils that under certain circumstances can cause injury—scissors, knives, needles, heating elements, or loops, long string, or cord (a potential for strangulation in very young children).

Teach chidren to beware of electrical appliances and even electrically operated playthings. Children are unfamiliar with the hazards of electricity in association with water.

Provide a safe place for the child to store toys.

Select a toy chest or toy box that is ventilated, is free of self-locking devices that could trap a child inside, and has a lid designed not to pinch a child's fingers or fall on a child's head.

Teach the child to store toys safely in order to prevent accidental injury from stepping or falling on a toy.

Check all toys periodically for breakage, loose parts, and other potential hazards.

Check movable parts to make certain they are attached securely to the toy. Sometimes pieces that are safe when attached to the toy become a danger when detached.

Repair or discard broken toys.

Make certain that materials in toys are nontoxic and repaired with nontoxic materials, and use only paint labeled "nontoxic" to repaint toys, toy boxes, or children's furniture.

Sand sharp wooden toys or splintered surfaces smooth.

Examine all outdoor toys regularly for rust and weak or sharp parts that could become a danger to a child.

Maintain toys in good repair, without signs of possible hazards such as sharp edges, splinters, weak seams, rust; keep electrical cords and plugs in good condition.

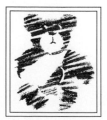

Age (months)	Visual stimulation	Auditory stimulation	Tactile stimulation	Kinetic stimulation
SUGGESTED ACTIVITIES				
Birth-1	Look at infant within close range Hang bright, shiny object within 20-25 cm (8-10 inches) of infant's face and in midline	Talk to infant, sing in soft voice Play music box, radio, television Have ticking clock or metronome nearby	Hold, caress, cuddle Keep infant warm May like to be swaddled	Rock infant, place in cradle Use carriage for walks
2-3	Provide bright objects Make room bright with pictures or mirrors on walls Take infant to various rooms while doing chores Place infant in infant seat for vertical view of environment	Talk to infant Include in family gatherings Expose to various environmental noises other than those of home Use rattles, wind chimes	Caress infant while bathing, at diaper change Comb hair with a soft brush	Use cradle gym or swing Take in car for rides Exercise body by moving extremities in swimming motion
4-6	Place infant in front of mirror Place in front of television with family Give brightly colored toys to hold (small enough to grasp)	Talk to infant, repeat sounds infant makes Laugh when infant laughs Call infant by name Crinkle different papers by infant's ear Place rattle or bell in hand, show how to shake them	Give infant soft squeeze toys of various textures Allow to splash in bath Place nude on soft furry rug and move extremities	Use swing or stroller Bounce infant in lap while holding in standing position Help infant roll over Support infant in sitting position, let lean forward to balance self Put infant in an open box and tilt gently
SUGGESTED TOYS				
Birth-6	Nursery mobiles Unbreakable mirrors See-through crib bumpers Contrasting-colored sheets Tracking tube* Visual panels*	Music boxes Musical mobiles Crib dangle bells Small-handled clear rattle Spin-a-round*	Stuffed animals Soft clothes Soft or furry quilt Soft mobiles	Rocking crib/cradle Weighted or suction toy

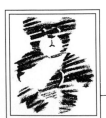

*These toys are from a specially designed series called Child Development Toys produced as part of the Johnson & Johnson Baby Products Child Development Program. They are available for purchase; information can be obtained by calling 1-800-678-2686.

This section may be photocopied and distributed to families.
From Wong D and Whaley L: Clinical manual of pediatric nursing, ed 3. Copyright © 1990, The CV Mosby Co, St Louis.

Age (months)	Visual stimulation	Auditory stimulation	Tactile stimulation	Kinetic stimulation
SUGGESTED ACTIVITIES				
6-9	Give infant large toys with bright colors, movable parts, and noisemakers Play peekaboo, especially hiding face in a towel Make funny faces to encourage imitation Give paper to tear, crumble Give ball of yarn or string to pull apart	Call infant by name Repeat simple words such as "dada, mama, bye-bye" Speak clearly Name parts of body, people, and foods Tell infant what you are doing Use word "no" only when necessary Give simple commands Show infant how to clap hands, bang a drum	Let infant play with various textures of fabric Have bowl with foods of different size and textures to feel Let infant "catch" running water Encourage "swimming" in large bathtub or shallow pool Give wad of sticky tape to manipulate	Place infant on floor to crawl, roll over, sit Hold upright to bear weight and bounce Pick up—say "up" Put down—say "down" Place toys out of reach; encourage infant to get them Play pat-a-cake
9-12	Show infant large pictures in books Take infant to places where there are animals, many people, different objects (shopping center) Play ball by rolling it to child, demonstrate "throwing" it back Demonstrate building a two-block tower	Read infant simple nursery rhymes Point to body parts and name each one Imitate sounds of animals	Give infant finger foods of different textures Let infant mess and squash food Let infant feel cold (ice cube) or warm objects, say what temperature each is Let infant feel a breeze (fan blowing)	Give large push-pull toys to encourage walking Place furniture in a circle to encourage cruising Encourage "roughhouse" play; turn infant in different positions
SUGGESTED TOYS				
6-12	Various colored blocks Nested boxes or cups Books with rhymes and bright pictures Strings of big beads and snap beads Simple take-apart toys Large ball Cup and spoon Fitting forms* Large puzzles	Rattles of different sizes, shapes, tones, and bright colors Squeaky animals and dolls Records with light, rhythmic music Balls in a bowl*	Soft, different textured animals and dolls Sponge toys, floating toys Squeeze toys Teething toys Books with textures/objects, such as fur and zipper	Activity box for crib Push-pull toys Swing

PLAY DURING CHILDHOOD

Age	Physical development	Social development	Mental development and creativity
SUGGESTED ACTIVITIES			
Toddler	Provide space in which to encourage physical activity Provide sandbox, swing, and other scaled-down playground equipment	Provide replicas of adult tools and equipment for imitative play Permit child to "help" with adult tasks Encourage imitative play Provide toys and activities that allow for expression of feelings Allow child to play with some actual items used in the adult world, for example, let help wash dishes or play with pots and pans and other utensils (check for safety)	Provide for water play Encourage building, drawing, and coloring Provide various textures in objects for play Provide large boxes and other safe containers for imaginative play Read stories appropriate to age Monitor television viewing
Preschool	Provide space for the child to run, jump, and climb Teach child to swim Teach simple sports and activities	Encourage interaction with neighborhood children Intervene when children become destructive Enroll in nursery school	Encourage creative efforts with raw materials Read stories Monitor television viewing Attend theater and other cultural events appropriate to the child's age Take short excursions to park, seashore, museums
School-age	Provide play equipment appropriate to skill and interests Provide professional instruction where feasible	Encourage peer interaction Permit group projects and activities	Encourage collections Provide access to raw materials for creative efforts Encourage musical inclinations Monitor television viewing and movies
Adolescent	Provide play equipment appropriate to skill and interests Provide for professional instruction where interest and feasibility allow	Do not discourage peer interaction Attempt to encourage selection of friends with positive influence	Encourage in stimulating activities and interests safe and appropriate to child's capabilities Monitor television viewing and movies
SUGGESTED TOYS			
Toddler	Push-pull toys Rocking horse, stick horse Blocks (unpainted) Pounding board Low gym and slide Pail and shovel Containers Play dough	Music and a phonograph Purse Housekeeping toys (broom, dishes) Toy telephone Dishes, stove, table and chairs Mirror (unbreakable)	Wooden puzzles Cloth picture books Paper, finger paint, thick crayons Blocks Large beads to string Wooden shoe for lacing Appropriate TV programs

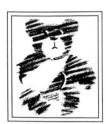

Age	Physical development	Social development	Mental development and creativity
SUGGESTED TOYS—cont'd			
Preschool	Seesaw	Sailboat	Books
	Medium-height slide	Cash register, toy typewriter	Jigsaw puzzles
	Adjustable swing	Child-size playhouse	Musical toys (xylophone, toy piano, drum, horns)
	Vehicles to ride in	Dolls and stuffed toys	
	Tricycle	Dishes, table	Picture games
	Wading pool	Play ironing board and iron	Blunt scissors, paper, paste
	Wheelbarrow	Trucks, cars, trains, airplanes	Newsprint, crayons, poster paint, large brushes, easel, finger paint
	Sled	Play clothes for dress-up	
	Wagon	Doll carriage, bed, high chair	Musical and rhythmic toys
	Roller skates, speed-graded to skill	Doctor and nurse kits	Flannel board and pieces of felt in colors and shapes
		Nails, hammer, saw	
		Grooming aids and makeup or shaving kits	Pregummed geometric shapes (colored)
			Records or tapes
			Blackboard and chalk (colored and white)
			Wooden and plastic construction sets
			Magnifying glass, magnet
School-age	Sports equipment	Games that involve more than one person	Games of skill, puzzles, riddles
	Bicycle		Books to read
	Yo-yo	Cooking set	Paper, drawing and painting supplies
	Jacks and marbles	Play camping tent	Camera
	Playground equipment	Raw materials for building club-houses	Scrapbooks, collection books
	Roller skates		Looms, beads
		Realistic cars	Simple wind instruments (harmonica, ocarina)
		Cosmetic kit	Erector sets
		Action dolls	Microscope
		Paper dolls	Craft materials
		Fashion dolls	Electronic (computer) games
Adolescent	Sports equipment	Games that involve more than one player (board games, chess, checkers, dominoes)	Games of skill such as chess, puzzles, mental games
			Craft materials
		Automobile (individual evaluation)	Raw materials for creativity (paint, paper or canvas, crayons)
		Tape recorder, stereo	Piano and/or other musical instrument
			Tape recorder, records, radio
			Sewing machine
			Shop tools
			Chemistry set
			Books and magazines
			Computer

3

Pediatric Variations of Nursing Interventions

For additional procedures or skills, see:

Measuring height, weight, and head circumference
(Unit 1)

Measuring triceps skinfold thickness and midarm circumference (Unit 1)

Measuring vital signs (Unit 1)

Nursing care plan: The child in pain (Unit 4)

Nursing care plan: The child at risk for infection
(Unit 4)

Nursing care plan: The child with special nutritional
needs (Unit 4)

Nursing care plan: The child undergoing surgery
(Unit 4)

Home Care Instructions (Unit 5)

Unit 3

GUIDELINES FOR SELECTING NONTHREATENING WORDS OR PHRASES

Words to avoid	Suggested substitutions
Shot, bee sting, stick	Medicine under the skin
Organ	Special place in body
Test	See how ___ is working
Incision	Special opening
Fissure	Opening
Stretcher, gurney	Rolling bed
Stool	Child's usual term
Dye	Special medicine
Pain	Hurt, discomfort, "owie," "boo-boo"
Deaden	Numb, make sleepy
Cut, fix	Make better
Take (e.g., temperature)	See how warm you are
Put to sleep, anesthesia	Special sleep
Catheter	Tube
Monitor	TV screen
Specimen	Sample

GUIDELINES FOR PREPARING CHILDREN FOR PROCEDURES
General guidelines

Determine the details of the exact procedure to be performed.

Review the parents' and child's present level of understanding.

Plan the actual teaching based on the child's developmental age and existing level of knowledge.

Incorporate parents in the teaching if they desire and especially if they plan to participate in the care.

Inform parents of their role during procedure, such as stand near child's head or in line of vision and talk softly to child.

While preparing the child and family, allow for ample discussion to prevent information overload and ensure adequate feedback.

Use concrete, not abstract, terms and visual aids to describe the procedure. For example, use a simple line drawing of a boy or girl (Figs. 3-1 and 3-2), and mark the body part that will be involved in the procedure.

Emphasize that no other body part will be involved.

If the body part is associated with a specific function, stress the change or noninvolvement of that ability, for example, following tonsillectomy, the child can still speak.

Use words appropriate to the child's level of understanding (a rule of thumb for number of words is the age in years plus 1).

Avoid words/phrases with dual meanings (see box on p. 210) unless the child understands such words.

Clarify all unfamiliar words, such as "anesthesia is a *special* sleep."

Emphasize the sensory aspects of the procedure—what the child will feel, see, smell, and touch and what he can do during the procedure, such as lie still, count out loud, squeeze a hand, or hug a doll.

Allow the child to practice those procedures that will require cooperation, such as turning, deep breathing, using an incentive spirometer or mask, or breathing on an intermittent positive pressure (IPPB) machine.

Introduce anxiety-laden information last, such as the preoperative injection.

Be honest with the child about the unpleasant aspects of a procedure but avoid creating undue concern. When discussing that a procedure may be uncomfortable, state that it feels differently to different people and have the child describe how it felt.

Emphasize the end of the procedure and any pleasurable events afterward, such as going home or seeing the parent. Stress the positive benefits of the procedure, for example, "After your tonsils are fixed, you won't have as many sore throats."

Unit 3

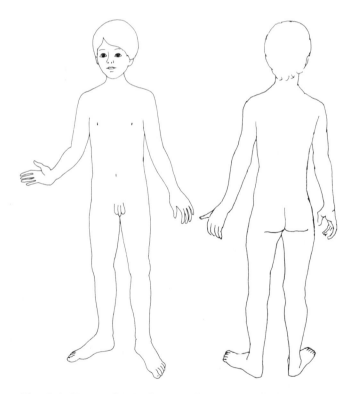

Fig. 3-1. Human figure drawing (boy) for preparing children for procedures and for assessing pain.

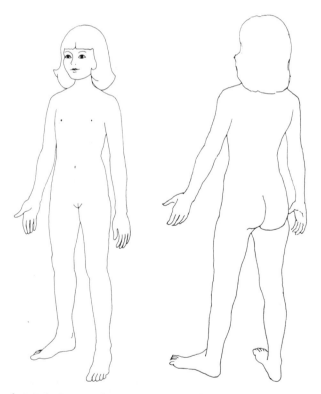

Fig. 3-2. Human figure drawing (girl) for preparing children for procedures and for assessing pain.

Figures 3-1 and 3-2 may be photocopied and distributed to staff for their use. From Wong D and Whaley L: Clinical manual of pediatric nursing ed. 3, 1990, The CV Mosby Co, St. Louis.

Age-specific guidelines

Developmental characteristics	Responsibilities
INFANCY: DEVELOPING A SENSE OF TRUST	
Attachment to parent	*Involve parent in procedure if desired Keep parent in infant's line of vision If patient is unable to be with infant, place familiar object with infant, such as stuffed toy
Stranger anxiety	*Have usual caregivers perform or assist with procedure Make advances slowly and in nonthreatening manner *Limit number of strangers entering room during procedure
Sensorimotor phase of learning	During procedure use sensory soothing measures (e.g., stroking skin, talking softly, giving pacifier) *Use analgesics (e.g., local anesthetic, intravenous narcotic) to control discomfort Cuddle and hug child after stressful procedure; encourage parent to comfort child
Increased muscle control	Expect older infants to resist Restrain adequately Keep harmful objects out of reach
Memory for past experiences	Realize that older infants may associate objects or persons with prior painful experiences Keep in mind that older infants will cry and resist at sight of objects or persons that inflict pain *Keep frightening objects out of view *Perform painful procedures in a separate room, not in crib (or bed)
Imitation of gestures	Model desired behavior (e.g., opening mouth)
TODDLER: DEVELOPING A SENSE OF AUTONOMY	
	Use same approaches as above in addition to following:
Egocentric	Explain procedure in relation to what child will see, hear, taste, smell, and feel Emphasize those aspects of procedure that require cooperation, such as lying still Tell child it's okay to cry, yell, or use other means to verbally express discomfort
Negative behavior	Expect treatments to be resisted; child may try to run away Use firm, direct approach Ignore temper tantrums Use distraction techniques Restrain adequately
Limited language skills	Communicate using behaviors Use few and simple terms that are familiar to child Give one direction at a time, such as "Lie down" and then "Hold my hand" Use small replicas of equipment; allow child to handle equipment Use play; demonstrate on doll but avoid child's favorite doll as child may think doll is really "feeling" procedure Prepare parents separately to avoid child's misinterpreting words
Limited concept of time	Prepare child shortly or immediately before procedure Keeping teaching sessions short (about 5 to 10 minutes) Have preparations completed before involving child in procedure Have extra equipment nearby (e.g., alcohol swabs, new needle, or Band-Aids) to avoid delays Tell child when procedure is completed
Striving for independence	Allow choices whenever possible but realize that child may still be resistant and negative Allow child to participate in care and to help whenever possible (e.g., drink medicine from a cup, hold a dressing)
PRESCHOOLER: DEVELOPING A SENSE OF INITIATIVE	
Preoperational thought: egocentric	Explain procedure in simple terms and in relation to how it affects child (as with toddler, stress sensory aspects) Demonstrate use of equipment Allow child to play with miniature or actual equipment Encourage "playing out" experience on a doll both before and after procedure to clarify misconceptions Use neutral words to describe the procedure (see box on p. 210)
Increased language skills	Use verbal explanation but avoid overestimating child's comprehension of words Encourage child to verbalize ideas and feelings

*Applies to any age.

Developmental characteristics	Responsibilities
Concept of time and frustration tolerance still limited	Implement same approaches as for toddler but may plan longer teaching session (10 to 15 minutes); may divide information into more than one session
Illness and hospitalization often viewed as punishment	Clarify why all procedures are performed, such as "This medicine will make you feel better" Ask child his thoughts regarding why a procedure is performed State directly that procedures are never a form of punishment
Fears of bodily harm, intrusion, and castration	Point out on drawing, doll, or child where procedure is performed Emphasize that no other body part will be involved Use nonintrusive procedures whenever possible (e.g., axillary temperatures, oral medication) Apply a Band-Aid over puncture site Realize that procedures involving genitals provoke anxiety Allow child to wear underpants with gown Explain unfamiliar situations, especially noises or lights
Striving for initiative	Involve child in care whenever possible (e.g., hold equipment, remove dressing) Give choices whenever possible but avoid excessive delays Praise child for helping and cooperating; never shame child for lack of cooperation

SCHOOL-AGE: DEVELOPING A SENSE OF INDUSTRY

Increased language skills; interest in acquiring knowledge	Explain procedures using correct scientific/medical terminology Explain reason for procedure using simple diagrams of anatomy and physiology Explain functioning and mechanism of equipment in concrete terms Allow child to manipulate equipment; use doll or another person as model to practice using equipment whenever possible (doll play may be considered "childish" by older school-age child) Allow time before and after procedure for questions and discussion
Improved concept of time	Plan for longer teaching sessions (about 20 minutes) Prepare in advance of procedure
Increased self-control	Gain child's cooperation Tell child what is expected Suggest ways of maintaining control (e.g., deep breathing, relaxation, counting)
Striving for industry	Allow responsibility for simple tasks, such as collecting specimens Include in decision making, such as time of day to perform procedure, preferred site Encourage active participation, such as removing dressings, handling equipment, opening packages
Developing relationships with peers	May prepare two or more children for same procedure or encourage one to help prepare another peer Provide privacy from peers during procedure to maintain self-esteem

ADOLESCENTS: DEVELOPING A SENSE OF IDENTITY

Increasingly capable of abstract thought and reasoning	Supplement explanations with reasons why procedure is necessary or beneficial Explain long-term consequences of procedures Realize that adolescent may fear death, disability, or other potential risks Encourage questioning regarding fears, options, and alternatives
Conscious of appearance	Provide privacy Discuss how procedure may affect appearance, such as scar, and what can be done to minimize it Emphasize any physical benefits of procedure
Concerned more with present than future	Realize that immediate effects of procedure are more significant than future benefits
Striving for independence	Involve in decision making and planning, for example, choice of time, place, individuals present during procedure (such as parents), clothing to wear Impose as few restrictions as possible Suggest methods of maintaining control Accept regression to more childish methods of coping Realize that adolescent may have difficulty in accepting new authority figures and may resist complying with procedures
Developing peer relationships and group identity	Same as for school-age child but assumes even greater significance

Unit 3

PLAY DURING HOSPITALIZATION
Functions of play in the hospital

Facilitates mastery over an unfamiliar situation

Provides opportunity to learn about parts of body, their functions, and own disease/disability

Corrects misconceptions about the use and purpose of medical equipment and procedures

Provides diversion and brings about relaxation

Helps the child feel more secure in a strange environment

Helps to lessen homesickness

Provides a means for release of tension and expression of feelings

Encourages interaction and development of positive attitudes toward others

Provides an expressive outlet for creative ideas and interests

Provides a means for accomplishing therapeutic goals

Using play in procedures
Projects involving hospital routines and environment

Language games

State or list nouns found in the hospital and what they do or how they are used; recognize pictures and words of hospital equipment and/or match them

Sort hospital nouns (words on cards) into people, places, and things

List on board the equipment found in hospital. One child gives description of its use—other children guess which equipment is being described

Have children write, illustrate stories: "sounds at night," "advice to doctors," "hospitals in the future," "things I like and don't like in the hospital"

Ongoing journals with pictures (captioned only or with stories), "Me in the Hospital," "The Part of Me That is Sick," "My Doctor," "My Nurse," "My Room," "Me at Home With My Family," "My Roommate," "Before I Got Sick," "After I Got Sick"

Science

Learn about body systems. List, put in alphabetical order, draw pictures, make organs out of clay or playdough, have children identify which of their body systems is involved in medical problem

Learn about nutrition in general and reasons for special diets

Discuss how medicines, traction, and cast work, how healing takes place

Mathematics

Use hospital material to discuss metric system and become familiar with weights, lengths, and volumes. Measure in appropriate units routine and hospital objects

Hospital word problems: use hospital situations (if each nurse works 8 hour shifts and you need six nurses on each shift, how many nurses do you need for 1 day)

Social sciences

How many different jobs are there in a hospital? Older children can be more detailed about skills and education required for each job

Talk about each child's neighborhood attractions

Geography

Make map of unit or of hospital

Map of what is seen from hospital windows—locate on map of the city/county/state

History

Research the hospital's history, the history of a branch of medical science or a medical profession, find out more about famous people in medicine's history (Hippocrates, Florence Nightingale, Clara Barton, Roentgen) or of medical discoveries and progress (the first lenses, discovery of penicillin)

Interaction with hospital departments and personnel

Take field trips to cafeteria, kitchen, animal labs, historical places within the hospital, offices (medical records, etc.)

Have personnel talk about their professions (electrical engineering, security guards, housekeeping, nurses, doctors, technicians, public relations, social workers, pharmacists, occupational and physical therapists)

Have staff teach part of lesson (nurse or doctor discuss how medicine works, technician explain X-rays, dieticians about an aspect of nutrition)

*From Ideas for activities with hospitalized children, Washington DC, 1982, The Association for the Care of Children's Health.

PLAY ACTIVITIES FOR SPECIFIC PROCEDURES

Fluid intake

Make freezer pops using child's favorite juice

Cut Jell-O into fun shapes

Makes game of taking sip when turning page of book or in games like "Simon Says"

Use small medicine cups; decorate the cups

olor water with food coloring or Kool Aid

Have tea party; pour at small table

Let child fill a syringe and squirt it into his mouth or use it to fill small decorated cups

Cut straws in half and place in small container (much easier for child to suck liquid)

Decorate straw—cut out small design with two holes and pass straw through; place small sticker on straw

Use a "crazy" straw

Make a "progress poster"; give rewards for drinking a predetermined quantity

DEEP BREATHING

Blow bubbles with bubble blower

Blow bubbles with straw (no soap)

Blow on pinwheel, feathers, whistle, harmonica, balloons, toy horns

Practice band instruments

Draw face on rubber glove to expand when blown up

Have blowing contest using balloons, boats, cotton balls, feathers, marbles, Ping-Pong balls, pieces of paper; blow such objects on a tabletop over a goal line, over water, through an obstacle course, up in the air, against an opponent, or up and down a string

Suck paper or cloth from one container to another using a straw

Use blow bottles with colored water to transfer water from one side to the other

Dramatize stories, as "I'll huff and puff and blow your house down" from the Three Little Pigs

Do straw blowing painting

Take a deep breath and "blow out the candles" on a birthday cake

Use a little paint brush to "paint" nails with water and blow nails dry

RANGE OF MOTION AND USE OF EXTREMITIES

Throw bean bags at fixed or movable target, wadded paper into wastebasket

Touch or kick Mylar balloons held or hung in different positions (if child is in traction, hang balloon from trapeze)

Play "tickle toes"; wiggle them on request

Play Twister game or "Simon Says"

Play pretend and guess games, such as imitate a bird, butterfly, horse

Have tricycle or wheelchair races in safe area

Play kick or throw ball with soft foam ball in safe area

Position bed so that child must turn to view television or doorway

Climb wall like "spider"

Pretend to teach "aerobic" dancing or exercises; encourage parents to participate

Encourage swimming, if feasible

Play video games or pinball (fine motor movement)

Play "hide and seek" game—hide toy somewhere in bed (or room, if ambulatory) and have child find using specified hand or foot

Provide clay to mold with fingers

Paint or draw on large sheets of paper placed on floor or wall

Encourage combing own hair; play "beauty shop" with "customer" in different positions

SOAKS

Play with small toys or objects (cups, syringes, soap dishes) in water

Wash dolls or toys

Bubbles may be added to bath water if permissible; move bubbles to create shapes or "monsters"

Pick up marbles, pennies* from bottom of bath container

Make designs with coins on bottom of container

Pretend to make a boat or submarine by keeping it immersed

Have "Instant Products"† (a capsule filled with a design that when immersed in warm water dissolves and foam rubber animals or other surprises appear) for child over age 3 years

Read to child during soaks, sing with child, or play game, such as cards, checkers, or other board game (if both hands are immersed, move the board pieces for the child)

Sitz bath—give child something to listen to (music, stories) or look at (Viewmaster, book, etc.)

INJECTIONS

Let child handle syringe, vial, alcohol swab and give an injection to doll or stuffed animal

Use syringes to decorate cookies with frosting, squirt paint, or target shoot into a container

Draw a "magic circle" on area before injection; draw smiling face in circle after injection

Allow child to have a "collection" of syringes (without needles); make "wild" creative objects with syringes

If multiple injections or venipunctures, make a "progress poster", give rewards for predetermined number of injections

AMBULATION

Give child someting to push

    Toddler—push-pull toy

    School age—wagon or decorated IV

    Teenage—a baby in a stroller or wheelchair

Have a parade—make hats, drums, etc.

EXTENDING ENVIRONMENT (PATIENTS IN TRACTION, ETC.)

Make bed into a pirate ship or airplane with decorations

Put up mirrors so patient can see around room

Move patient's bed frequently, especially to playroom, hallway, or outside

Remind older children to brush and floss.

Provide a toothbrush or toothpaste for those children who do not have their own, or ask parents to bring it from home.

See p. 182 for specific oral hygiene techniques.

---

*Small objects such as marbles or coins are unsafe for young children.
†Instant Products, Inc, PO Box 33068, Louisville, KY 40232.

INFORMED CONSENT TO TREAT CHILD

Children are considered minors and, except under special circumstances, the parent or the person designated as legal guardian for the child is required to give informed consent before medical treatment is implemented or any procedure is performed on the child.

Separate permission is also required for the following:

Major surgery

Minor surgery, for example, cutdown, biopsy, dental extraction, suturing a laceration (especially one that may have a cosmetic effect), removal of a cyst, and closed reduction of a fracture

Diagnostic tests with an element of risk, for example, bronchoscopy, needle biopsy, angiography, electroencephalogram, lumbar puncture, cardiac catheterization, ventriculography, and bone marrow aspiration

Medical treatments with an element of risk, for example, blood transfusion, thoracentesis or paracentesis, radiation therapy, and shock therapies

Other hospital situations that require written parental permission include:

Taking photographs for medical, educational, or other public use

Removal of the child from the hospital against the advice of the physician

Postmortem examinations except in unexplained deaths, such as sudden infant death, violent death, or suspected suicide

Examination of medical records by unauthorized persons, such as attorneys, insurance representatives, etc.

Following are exceptions to the previously mentioned regulations:

Informed consent of persons other than parents or guardian in loco parentis (in place of the parent); permission granted by person responsible for the child during parents' absence

Oral informed consent: telephone consent or oral consent from parent who is unable to sign permit

Mature or emancipated minors: person who is legally underage but who is recognized as having the legal capacity of an adult such as the unmarried pregnant minor, the minor who is married, or the minor who lives apart from the parents and is self-supporting

Treatment without parental consent: situations in which children need prompt medical or surgical treatment and a parent is not readily available to give consent

Parental negligence: when children need protection from their parents such as parents who neglect or impose improper punishment on a child or refuse needed treatment, or when refusal is a direct violation of the law

GENERAL HYGIENE AND CARE
Bathing

Unless contraindicated, bathe infant or child in a tub at the bedside, on the bed, or in a standard bathtub.

Never leave infant or small child unattended in a bathtub.

Hold infant who is unable to sit alone.

Support infant's head securely with one hand or grasp the infant's farther arm firmly and rest the head comfortably on the wrist.

Closely supervise the infant or child who is able to sit without assistance.

Place a pad in the bottom of the tub to prevent slipping and loss of balance.

Offer older children the option of a shower if available.

Use judgment regarding the amount of supervision older children require.

Retarded children, those with physical limitations such as severe anemia or leg deformities, and suicidal or psychotic children (who may commit bodily harm) require close supervision.

Clean the ears, between skinfolds, the neck, the back, and the genital area carefully.

Retract the foreskin of uncircumcised boys gently, clean the exposed surfaces, and replace the foreskin. Never forcefully retract the foreskin.

Provide more extensive assistance with bathing and other aspects of hygienic care to children who are ill or debilitated

Encourage them to perform as much as they are capable of without overtaxing their energies.

Expect increasing involvement with improved strength and endurance.

Hair care

Brush and comb hair or help children with hair care at least once daily.

Style hair for comfort and in a manner pleasing to the child and parents.

Do not cut hair without parental permission, although shaving hair to provide access to scalp vein for intravenous needle insertion is permissible.

Wash the hair of the newborn daily as part of the bath if this is the institution's policy.

Wash the hair and scalp once or twice weekly in later infancy and childhood.

Teenagers may need more frequent hair care and shampoos.

Shampoo the hair in the tub or shower or transport the child by gurney to an accessible sink or washbasin.

If the child is unable to be transported, shampoo in the bed with adequate protection and/or with specially adapted equipment or positioning.

Use commercial "dry shampoo" products on a short-term basis.

Provide special hair care for black children:

Avoid using most standard combs, which cause hair breakage and discomfort.

Use a special comb with widely spaced teeth.

Combing hair wet causes less breakage.

Remind the parent to bring a comb (if possible) if it is not available on the unit.

Apply special hair dressing or pomade.

Consult the child's parents regarding the preparation they wish to be used and ask if they can provide some.

Do not use petroleum jelly.

Rub the preparation on the hair to make it more pliable and manageable.

Mouth care

Perform mouth care for infants and debilitated children.

Assist small children to brush teeth, although many can manage a toothbrush satisfactorily and are encouraged to use it.

Remind older children to brush and floss.

Provide a toothbrush or toothpaste for those children who do not have their own, or ask parents to bring it from home.

See p. 182 for specific oral hygiene techniques.

PROCEDURES RELATED TO MAINTAINING SAFETY

Ensure that environmental safety measures are in operation, such as:

Good illumination

Floors clear of fluid or other objects that might contribute to falls

Nonskid surfaces in showers and tubs

Electrical equipment maintained in good working order, used only by personnel familiar with its use, and not in contact with moisture or near tubs

Beds of ambulatory patients locked in place and at a height that allows easy access to the floor

Proper care and disposal of small breakable items, such as thermometers and bottles

A well-organized fire plan known to all staff members

All windows securely screened

Electrical outlets covered to prevent burns.

Be sure the child is wearing proper identification band

Check bath water carefully before placing the child in the bath.

Use furniture that is scaled to the child's proportions, sturdy and well balanced to prevent tipping over.

Strap infants and small children into infant seats, feeding chairs, and strollers securely.

Do not leave infants, young children, and youngsters who are agitated or mentally retarded unattended on treatment tables, on scales, or in treatment areas.

Keep portholes in Isolettes securely fastened when not attending the infant.

Keep crib sides up and fastened securely unless an adult is at the bedside.

Leave crib sides up even when the crib is unoccupied to remove the temptation for the child to climb in.

Never turn away from an infant or small child in a crib that has the sides down without maintaining contact on the child's back or abdomen to protect from rolling, crawling, or jumping from the open crib.

Place the child who may climb over the side of the crib in a specially constructed crib with a cover or one that has a safety net placed over the top.

Tie net to the frame in such a manner that there is ready access to the child in case of emergency.

Never tie nets to the movable crib sides, or use knots that do not permit quick release.

Do not place cribs within reach of heating units, appliances, dangling cords, or other objects that can be reached by curious hands.

Assess the safety of toys brought to the hospital by well-meaning parents and determine whether they are appropriate to the child's age and condition.

Inspect to make certain toys are allergy-free, washable, and unbreakable and that they have no small, removable parts that can be aspirated or swallowed.

Set limits for the child's safety.

Make sure children understand where they are permitted to go and what they are permitted to do in the hospital.

Enforce the limitations consistently and repeat as frequently as necessary to make certain that they are understood.

Transporting

Carry infants and small children for short distances within the unit.

In the horizontal position, hold or carry small infants with the back supported and the thigh grasped firmly by the carrying arm.

In the football hold, support the infant on nurse's arm with the head supported by the hand and the body held securely between the body and elbow.

In the upright position, hold the infant with the buttocks on nurse's forearm and the front of the body resting against the chest. Support the infant's head and shoulders with other arm to allow for any sudden movement by the infant.

For more extended trips use a suitable conveyance.

Determine the method of transporting chidlren by their age, condition, and destination.

Use appropriate safety belts and/or raised sides to secure child.

Transport infants in their Isolettes, cribs, baby buggies, strollers, wheeled feeding chairs, or tables or in wagons with raised sides.

Use wheelchairs or gurneys for older children.

Restraining methods
General guidelines

Understand the purpose of restraints.
   Provide safety.
   Maintain desired position.
   Facilitate examination.
   Aid in performing diagnostic tests and therapeutic procedures
Never use restraining devices as a punishment or as a substitute for observation
Assess restraining devices frequently for the following:
   Correctly applied.
   Accomplishing the purpose for which applied.
   Do not impair circulation or cause damage to nerves or tissues.
Make certain that all restraints allow for easy access to the child in case of emergency.
   Restraints with ties are secured to bed or crib frame, not side rails. They do not interfere with raising and lowering crib sides or bedrails.
   They are tied with a slipknot for easy removal.

Pad rigid or constricting devices for comfort and to reduce possibility of injury.
Prepare child for needed restraints.
   Explain the restraint and the reason for the restraint.
   Repeat information as often as needed to gain cooperation.
   Explain how the child can help.
   Reassure child that the restraint is not a punishment.
Explain restraints and their purpose to parents.
   Explain purpose and function of restraints.
   Show parents how to remove and reapply them (if feasible).
   Teach signs of complications.
   Explain ways in which they can help to ensure maximal benefit and minimal stress.
Release long-term restraints periodically to allow the child to move extremities when this practice does not interfere with therapy.

Types of restraints

Type	Function	Description
Jacket restraint	To prevent child from climbing out of crib or bed	Waist-length, sleeveless jacket with back closure fastened with ties Long ties on bottom of jacket secure child to crib, chair, or bed

Mummy restraint	To control child's movements
	To immobilize extremities
	To provide temporary restraining device for short procedures
		Place opened sheet or blanket on flat surface with one corner folded to the center
		Place infant on blanket with shoulders at blanket fold and feet toward opposite corner
		Place infant's right arm straight against side of body
		Pull side of blanket on right side firmly across right shoulder and chest
		Secure beneath left side of body
		Place left arm straight against side
		Bring remaining side of blanket across left shoulder and chest
		Secure beneath body
		Fold lower corner and bring up to shoulders and secure ends beneath body
		Fasten in place with safety pins or tape
		Modification for chest examination
		   Left and right corners are brought over arms only to, but not including, chest and secured under body
		   Bottom corner is secured at waist rather than at shoulders

Arm and leg restraints	To immobilize one or more extremities
	  1. For treatments
	  2. For procedures
	  3. To facilitate healing
		Soft, padded commercial restraints
		Clove-hitch restraint
		Folded towel, pinned around extremity
		Gauze or cotton bandage, padded well

Elbow restraint	To prevent child from bending elbow To prevent child from reaching head, face, neck, or chest	Muslin square with vertical pockets to contain tongue depressors to supply vertical rigidity and horizontal flexibility; ties secure the device around the arm Padded large-diameter towel roller Tubular plastic container with top and bottom removed and suitably padded for comfort and safety

Unit 3

POSITIONING FOR PROCEDURES

Extremity venipuncture

Place child supine.
Have operator on one side of bed, stabilizing arm used for venipuncture.
Have assistant on other side of bed, leaning across child's upper body to apply restraint and using arm closest to operator to help restrain venipuncture site.

or

Place child sitting in assistant's (or parent's) lap.
Have operator in front or on one side of child, stabilizing arm used for venipuncture.
Have assistant use arms to hug and restrain child's upper body; if needed place child's legs between assistant's legs to restrain lower body.

Jugular venipuncture

Place child in mummy restraint.
Alternate procedure may be used.
   An infant or small child's arm and legs can be restrained with the nurse's forearms at the same time the child's head is positioned and restrained.
   Facing the child, position child with head and shoulders extended over the edge of a table or small pillow with neck extended and turned sharply to the side.
   Take care that excessive pressure does not compromise circulation or breathing and that the nose and mouth are not covered by the restrainer's hand.

Femoral venipuncture

Place infant supine with legs in frog position to provide extensive exposure of the groin.
Restrain legs in frog position with hands while controlling the child's arm and body movements with downward and inward pressure of forearms.
Cover genitalia to protect the operator and the venipuncture site from contamination if the child urinates during the procedures

Lumbar puncture

Infant
   Place infant in sitting position with buttocks extended over the edge of the table and head flexed on chest.
   Immobilize arms and legs with nurse's hands.
   Observe child for difficulty in breathing.

Child
   Place child on side with back close to or extended over the edge of examining table, head flexed, and knees drawn up toward the chest.
   Reach over the top of the child and place one arm behind child's neck and the other behind the knees.
   Stabilize this position by clasping own hands in front of the child's abdomen.
Older infant or young child
   While standing, hold child upright against the nurse's (or parent's) chest with child's legs wrapped around the adult's waist.
   Use arms to hug and restrain child.
   Place a small pillow or folded towel between child's abdomen and adult to help arch the child's back.

Bone marrow examination

For posterior iliac site
   Position child prone.
   Place a small pillow or folded towel under the hips to raise them slightly.
   Apply restraint at upper body and lower extremities, preferably with two persons.
For anterior iliac site or tibia
   Position child supine.
   Apply restraint at upper body and lower extremities, preferably with two persons.

Subdural puncture (through fontanel or bur holes)

Place infant in mummy restraint.
Position supine with head accessible to examiner.
Control head movement with firm hold on each side of the head.

Nose and/or throat access

Control head as for subdural puncture.
Alternate procedure may be used; control head and arms by holding child's extended arms over and close to the head, thus immobilizing both head and arms.

COLLECTION OF SPECIMENS
Urine*

Non–toilet-trained child

Obtain urine from wet diaper.
  Use a syringe without needle to aspirate urine directly from the diaper.
  Place cotton balls or small gauze pad in diaper to collect urine and aspirate urine with syringe or with gloved hand squeeze urine into container.
  With some brands of diaper, it may be necessary to place some of the absorbent lining into the barrel of a syringe and with the plunger, squeeze the lining to extract urine.
                or
Apply a urine collection bag.†
Cut a small slit in the diaper and pull the bag through to allow room for urine to collect and to check on contents.
Check bag frequently and remove as soon as specimen is available.
  Urine collected for culture should be tested within 2 hours of collection or refrigerated at 4° C for up to 24 hours before being cultured.

Toilet-trained young child

May not be able to urinate on request.
May be more successful if potty-chair or bedpan is placed on the toilet.
Use familiar terms, such as "pee pee," "wee wee," or "tinkle."
Enlist parent's assistance.

Toilet-trained older child

Cooperative but appreciates explanation of what specimen is for.
Provide a receptacle, preferably with some means of concealing it such as a paper bag, and privacy.

---

*NOTE: Traditionally urine for culture has been collected after meatal cleansing and in toilet-trained patients from a midstream specimen (known as clean-catch midstream specimen). However, research has shown that these procedures do not significantly reduce bacterial contamination of the specimen. (MacDonald N and others: Efficacy of chlorhexidine cleansing in reducing contamination of bagged urine specimens, Can Med Assoc J 133:1211-1213, 1985; Lohr J, Donowitz L, and Dudley S: Bacterial contamination rates in voided urine collection in girls, J Pediatr 114(1):91-93, 1989; and Saez-Llorens X, Umana M, Odio C, and Lohr J: Bacterial contamination rates for non-clean-catch and clean-catch midstream urine collection in uncircumcised boys, J Pediatr 114(1):93-95, 1989.)
†See Home Care Instructions, p. 536.

Twenty-four-hour urine collection

Begin and end collection with an empty bladder.
  At time collection begins, instruct child to void and discard specimen.
  Twenty-four hours after specimen was discarded instruct child to void for last specimen.
Save all voided urine during the 24 hours in a refrigerated container marked with date, total time, and child's name.
Non–toilet-trained child
  Prepare skin with thin coating of skin sealant and apply a urine collection bag with a collection tube that allows urine to drain into a large receptacle.†
  If a collection tube is not available, insert a small feeding tube through a puncture hole at the top of the bag; use a syringe without needle to aspirate urine through the feeding tube.

Stool

Collect stool without urine contamination, if possible.

Non–toilet-trained child

Apply a urine collecting bag.
Apply diaper over bag.
After bowel movement, use tongue blade to collect stool.
Place specimen in appropriate covered container.

Toilet-trained child

Have child urinate, then flush toilet.
Have child defecate into bedpan or toilet.
To facilitate collecting specimen, place a sheet of plastic wrap over toilet seat.
After bowel movement, use tongue blade to collect stool.
Place in appropriate covered container.

Nasal secretions

To obtain nasal secretions, using a nasal washing:
  Place child supine.
  Instill 1 to 3 cc sterile normal saline with a sterile syringe (without needle) into one nostril.
  Aspirate contents with a small, sterile bulb syringe.
  Place in sterile container.

Sputum

Older children and adolescents are able to cough as directed and supply specimens when given proper direction.
Specimens can sometimes be collected from infants and young children by means of a tracheal aspiration with a mucous trap or suction apparatus.

Unit 3

PROCEDURES RELATED TO ADMINISTRATION OF MEDICATIONS
General guidelines

ESTIMATING DRUG DOSAGE

Body surface area as a basis: estimated from height and weight by use of West nomogram (Fig. 3-3)

Body surface area related to adult dose:

$$\frac{\text{Body surface area of child}}{\text{Mean body surface area of adult}} \times \frac{\text{Average}}{\text{adult dose}} = \frac{\text{Estimated}}{\text{child's dose}}$$

Body surface area related to average dose per square meter (m^2):

$$\text{Surface area of child } (m^2) \times \text{Dose}/m^2 = \text{Estimated child's dose}$$

WEST NOMOGRAM

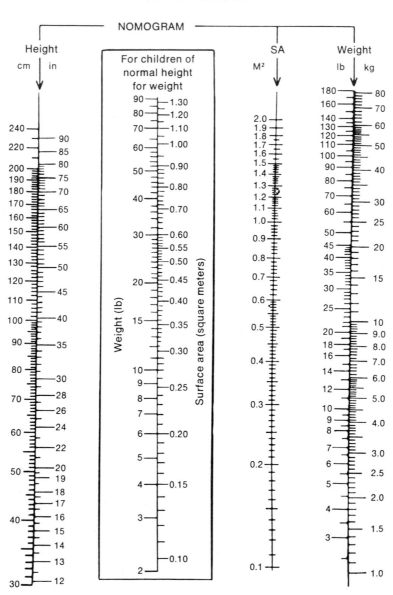

Fig. 3-3. West nomogram (for estimation of surface areas). The surface area is indicated where a straight line connecting the height and weight intersects the surface area (SA) column or, if the patient is roughly of normal proportion, from the weight alone (enclosed area). (Nomogram modified from data of E Boyd by CD West. In Behrman RE and Vaughan VC, editors: Nelson textbook of pediatrics, ed 13, Philadelphia, 1987, WB Saunders Co., p. 1521.)

APPROACHES TO PEDIATRIC PATIENTS

Children's reactions to treatments are affected by the following:
 Developmental characteristics, such as physical abilities and
  cognitive capabilities
 Environmental influences
 Past experiences
 Current relationship with the nurse
 Perception of the present situation

SPECIFIC GUIDELINES (see also p. 211)

Expect success; use a positive approach
Provide an explanation appropriate to the developmental level
 of the child.
Allow the child choices whenever possible.
Be honest with the child.
Involve the child in order to gain cooperation.
Provide distraction for a frightened or uncooperative child.
Allow the child the opportunity to express feelings.
Praise the child for doing his/her best.
Spend some time with the child after administering the medi-
 cation.
Let the child know he/she is accepted as a person of value.

SAFETY PRECAUTIONS

Take a drug allergy history
 Check the following 5 "Rs" for correctness:
  Right drug
  Right dosage
  Right time
  Right route
  Right child (identification band)
 Double-check drug and dosage with another nurse.
  Always double-check the following:
   Digoxin
   Insulin
   Heparin
   Blood
  May also double-check the following:
   Epinephrine
   Narcotics
   Sedatives
Be aware of drug-drug or drug-food interactions.
Document all drugs administered.

Teaching family to administer medication

Family needs to know the following:
 The name of the drug
 The purpose for which the drug is given
 The amount of the drug to be given
 The frequency with which it will be given
 The length of time to be administered
 The anticipated effects of the drug
 Signs that might indicate an adverse reaction to the drug
Assess the family's level of understanding.
Explain the administration procedure. Instruction needed varies
 markedly with the intellectual level of the learner and the
 type and route of medication to be administered.

Demonstrate and have family return the demonstration (if appropriate).
Give written instructions. (See Home Care Instructions related
 to administering medication on pp. 542 to 558.)
Assist family in scheduling the time for administration around
 the family routine.
Be certain family knows what to do and whom to contact if any
 untoward signs are observed.

Oral administration*

1. Follow safety precautions for administration.
2. Select appropriate vehicle, for example, cup, measuring
   spoon, syringe, dropper, nipple.
3. Prepare medication.
   Measure into appropriate vehicle.
   Crush tablets for children who will have difficulty swallowing;
    mix with syrup, juice, and so on.
   Avoid mixing medications with essential food items such as
    milk, formula, and so on.
4. Administer the medication employing safety precautions in
   identification and administration.
   Infants
    Hold in semireclining position.
    Place syringe, measuring spoon, or dropper with medi-
     cation in mouth well back on the tongue or to the side
     of the tongue.

Administer slowly to reduce likelihood of choking or as-
 piration.
Allow infant to suck medication placed in a nipple.
Older infant or toddler
 Offer medication in cup or spoon.
 Administer with syringe, measuring spoon, or dropper as
  with infants.
 Use mild or partial restraint with reluctant children.
 Do not force actively resistive children because of danger
  of aspiration; postpone 20 to 30 minutes and offer med-
  ication again.
Preschool children
 Use straightforward presentation.
 For reluctant children use the following:
  Simple persuasion
  Innovative containers
  Reinforcement, such as stars, stickers, or other tangible
   rewards for compliance

*See Home Care Instructions, pp. 542 and 543.

Intramuscular administration*

1. Use safety precautions in administering medications.
2. Prepare medication.
   Select needle and syringe appropriate to the following:
   Amount of fluid to be administered (syringe size)
   Viscosity of fluid to be administered (needle gauge)
   Amount of tissue to be penetrated (needle length)
   Maximum volume to be administered in a single site is 1 ml for older infants and small children.
3. Determine the site of injection (pp. 226-227); make certain muscle is large enough to accommodate volume and type of medication.
   Older children—select site as with the adult patient; allow child some choice of site, if feasible.
   Following are acceptable sites for infants and small or debilitated children:
   Vastus lateralis muscle
   Ventrogluteal muscle
   Dorsogluteal muscle is insufficiently developed to be a safe site for infants and small children.
4. Administer the medication.
   Provide for sufficient help in restraining the child; children are often uncooperative, and their behavior is usually unpredictable.
   Explain briefly what is to be done and, if appropriate, what the child can do to help.
   Expose injection area for unobstructed view of landmarks.
   Select a site where the skin is free of irritation and danger of infection; palpate for and avoid sensitive or hardened areas. With multiple injections, rotate sites.
   Place the child in a lying or sitting position; the child is not allowed to stand because:
   Landmarks are more difficult to assess.
   Restraint is more difficult.
   The child may faint and fall.
   Use a new sharp needle with the smallest diameter that permits free flow of the medication.
   Grasp the muscle firmly between the thumb and fingers to isolate and stabilize the muscle for deposition of the drug in its deepest part; in obese children spread the skin with the thumb and index finger to displace subcutaneous tissue and grasp the muscle deeply on each side.
   Allow the skin preparation to dry completely before the skin is penetrated.

---

*See Home Care Instructions, p. 545 for intramuscular injection and p. 547 for subcutaneous injection.

Have the medication at room temperature.
Decrease the perception of pain:
   Distract the child with conversation.
   Give the child something on which to concentrate, such as squeezing a hand or bed rail, pinching own nose, humming, or yelling "ouch."
   Place a wrapped ice cube on the site about a minute before the injection or apply cold to contralateral site.
   Say to the child, "If you feel this, tell me to take it out please."
Insert the needle quickly, using a dartlike motion.
Aspirate for blood.
   If blood is found, remove syringe from site, change needle, and reinsert into new location.
   If no blood is found, inject into a relaxed muscle:
      Dorsogluteal—place child on abdomen with legs and toes rotated inward.
      Ventrogluteal—place child on side with the upper leg flexed and placed in front of the lower leg.
Avoid tracking any medication through superficial tissues:
   Replace needle after withdrawing medication or wipe medication from needle with sterile gauze.
   If withdrawing medication from an ampule, use a needle equipped with a filter that removes glass particles and use a second needle for injection.
   Use the Z-track and/or air bubble technique as indicated.
   Avoid any depression of the plunger during insertion of needle.
Inject the medication slowly over period of 20 seconds.
Remove the needle quickly; hold a gauze sponge firmly against the skin near the needle when removing it to avoid the needle's pulling on the tissue.
Apply firm pressure with dry sterile gauze to the site after injection; massage the site to hasten absorption unless contraindicated.
Place a small Band-Aid on the puncture site; with young children decorate Band-Aid by drawing a smiling face or other symbol of acceptance.
Hold and cuddle young child and encourage parents to offer comforting; praise older child.
Allow expression of feelings.
5. Discard syringe and uncapped, uncut needle in puncture-resistant container located near site of use.
6. Record time of injection, drug, dose, and injection site.

Intravenous administration*

1. Prepare correct medication according to manufacturer's recommendations. Compute fractional dose, if indicated, and withdraw dosage needed.
2. Assess the status of the intravenous infusion to determine that it is functioning properly.
3. Inspect injection site to make certain the needle is secure.
4. Check adequacy of restraint to maintain infusion site.
5. Dilute the drug in an amount of solution in a graduate chamber of buret (such as a Volutrol) appropriate to the following:

---

*Directions for care of heparin lock and central venous catheter are in Home Care Instructions on p 549.

Size of the child
Size of the vein being used for infusion
Length of time over which the drug is to be administered (e.g., 30 minutes, 1 hour, 2 hours)
Rate at which the drug is to be infused
Strength of the drug or the degree to which it is toxic to subcutaneous tissues
6. Monitor infusion until medication has been infused. Medication is not completely administered until solution in tubing between buret chamber and needle site has infused also (amount of solution depends on tubing length).
7. Apply and maintain adequate restraining devices as needed.

Rectal administration
*Suppository**

Medications may need to be administered rectally if the oral route is not available.

Retention enema

1. Dilute drug in smallest amount of solution possible.
2. Insert well into rectum.
3. Hold or tape buttocks together for 5 to 10 minutes.

*See Home Care Instructions, pp 565 and 566.

Eye, ear, and nose administration
*Eye medication**

Eye drops are administered in the same manner as to adults. Children, however, require additional preparation.

Ear medication†

Depending on the child's age, the pinna is pulled differently. Such variations are discussed in the Home Care Instructions.

Nose drops‡

Nose drops are administered in the same manner as to adults. Depending on the child's age difference positions may be used.

*See Home Care Instructions, p. 554
†See Home Care Instructions, p. 556
‡See Home Care instructions, p. 557

Nasogastric, orogastric, or gastrostomy administration

1. Use elixir or suspension (rather than syrup) preparations of medication whenever possible.
   If administering tablets, crush the tablet to a very fine powder and dissolve the drug in a small amount of warm water.
   Never crush enteric-coated or sustained-release tablets or capsules.
   Avoid oily medications as they tend to cling to side of tube.
   Dilute viscous medication if possible.
   Do not mix medication with enteral formula unless fluid is restricted. If adding a drug:
   Check with pharmacist for compatibility.
   Shake formula well and observe for any physical reaction, such as separation or precipitation.
   Label formula container with name of medication, dosage, date, and time infusion started.
2. Have the medication at room temperature.
3. Measure medication in calibrated cup.
4. Check for correct placement of nasogastric or orogastric tube (see p. 230).
5. Attach syringe (with adaptable tip but without plunger) to tube.
6. Pour medication into syringe.
7. Unclamp tube and allow medication to flow by gravity.
   Adjust height of container to achieve desired flow rate, e.g., increase height for faster flow.
8. As soon as syringe is empty, pour in water to flush tubing.
   Amount of water depends on length and gauge of tubing.
   Determine amount before administering any medication by using a syringe to completely fill an unused nasogastric or orogastric tube with water. The amount of flush solution is usually 1½ times this volume.
   With certain drug preparations, such as suspensions, more fluid may be needed.
9. If administering more than one drug at the same time, flush the tube between each medication with clear water.
10. Clamp tube after flushing, unless tube is left open.

Intramuscular injection sites in children

Site

Discussion

VASTUS LATERALIS

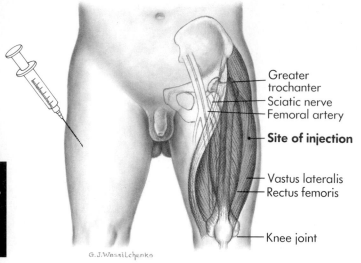

Greater trochanter
Sciatic nerve
Femoral artery
Site of injection
Vastus lateralis
Rectus femoris
Knee joint

G.J.Wassilchenko

Fig. 3-4

LOCATION

Palpate to find greater trochanter and knee joints; divide vertical distance between these two landmarks into quadrants; inject into middle of upper quadrant.

NEEDLE INSERTION AND SIZE

Insert needle at 45° angle toward knee in infants and in young children or needle perpendicular to thigh or slightly angled toward anterior thigh.

22 to 25 gauge, ⅝ to 1 inch*

ADVANTAGES

Large, well-developed muscle that can tolerate larger quantities of fluid (0.5 ml [infant] to 2.0 ml [child])

No important nerves or blood vessels in this location

Easily accessible if child is supine, side-lying, or sitting

A tourniquet can be applied above injection site to delay drug hypersensitivity reaction if necessary

DISADVANTAGES

Thrombosis of femoral artery from injection in midthigh area

Sciatic nerve damage from long needle injected posteriorly and medially into small extremity

VENTROGLUTEAL

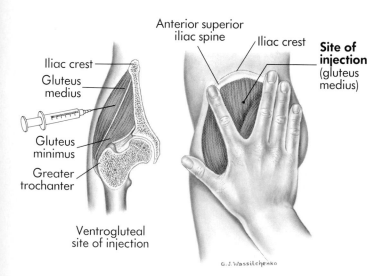

Anterior superior iliac spine
Iliac crest
Site of injection (gluteus medius)
Iliac crest
Gluteus medius
Gluteus minimus
Greater trochanter
Ventrogluteal site of injection

G.J.Wassilchenko

Fig. 3-5

LOCATION

Palpate to locate greater trochanter, anterior superior iliac tubercle (found by flexing thigh at hip and measuring up to 1 to 2 cm above crease formed in groin), and posterior iliac crest; place palm of hand over greater trochanter, index finger over anterior superior iliac tubercle, and middle finger along crest of ilium posteriorly as far as possible; inject into center of V formed by fingers.

NEEDLE INSERTION AND SIZE

Insert needle perpendicular to site but angled slightly toward iliac crest.

22 to 25 gauge, ½ to 1 inch

ADVANTAGES

Free of important nerves and vascular structures

Easily identified by prominent bony landmarks

Thinner layer of subcutaneous tissue than in dorsogluteal site, thus less chance of depositing drug subcutaneously rather than intramuscularly

Can accommodate larger quantities of fluid (0.5 ml [infant] to 2.0 ml [child])

Easily accessible if child is supine, prone, or side-lying

Less painful than vastus lateralis

DISADVANTAGES

Health professionals' unfamiliarity with site

Not suitable for use of a tourniquet

*Research has shown that a 1-inch needle is needed for adequate muscle penetration in infants 4 months old and possibly in infants as young as 2 months (Hick J and others: Optimum needle length for diphtheria-tetanus-pertussis inoculation of infants, Pediatrics 84(1):136-137, 1989). Other recommendations for needle size and volume of fluid are based on traditional practice and have not been verified by research.

Site

Discussion

DORSOGLUTEAL

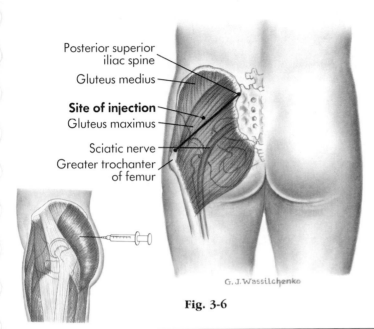

Posterior superior iliac spine
Gluteus medius
Site of injection
Gluteus maximus
Sciatic nerve
Greater trochanter of femur

G. J. Wassilchenko

Fig. 3-6

LOCATION

Locate greater trochanter and posterior superior iliac spine; draw imaginary line between these two points and inject lateral and superior to line into gluteus muscle.

NEEDLE INSERTION AND SIZE

Insert needle perpendicular to surface on which child is lying when prone.
20 to 25 gauge, ½ to 1½ inches

ADVANTAGES

In older child large muscle mass; well-developed muscle can tolerate greater volume of fluid (0.5 ml [infant] to 2.0 ml [child])
Child does not see needle and syringe
Easily accessible if child is prone or side-lying

DISADVANTAGES

Contraindicated in children who have not been walking for at least 1 year
Danger of injury to sciatic nerve
Thick, subcutaneous fat, predisposing to deposition of drug subcutaneously rather than intramuscularly
Not suitable for use of a tourniquet
Inaccessible if child is supine
Exposure of site may cause embarrassment in older child

DELTOID

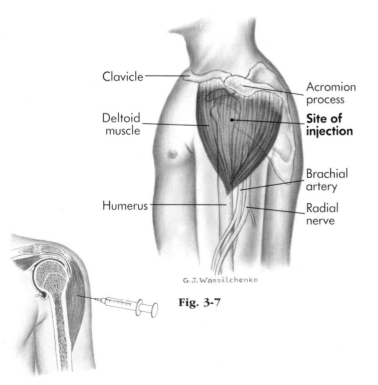

Clavicle
Deltoid muscle
Humerus

Acromion process
Site of injection
Brachial artery
Radial nerve

G. J. Wassilchenko

Fig. 3-7

LOCATION

Locate acromion process; inject only into upper third of muscle that begins about 2 finger-breadths below acromion.

NEEDLE INSERTION AND SIZE

Insert needle perpendicular to site but angled slightly toward shoulder.
22 to 25 gauge, ½ to 1 inch

ADVANTAGES

Faster absorption rates than gluteal sites
Tourniquet can be applied above injection site
Easily accessible with minimal removal of clothing

DISADVANTAGES

Small muscle mass; only limited amounts of drug can be injected (0.5 to 1.0 ml)
Small margins of safety with possible damage to radial nerve
Pain with repeated injections

Unit 3

PROCEDURES RELATED TO MAINTAINING FLUID BALANCE OR NUTRITION
Intravenous fluid administration

Intravenous therapy is employed for infants and children for the following reasons:
Fluid replacement
Fluid maintenance
A route for administration of medications or other therapeutic substances (e.g., blood, blood products, immunoglobulin)
Characteristics of pediatric administration sets:
Calibrated volume and control chamber with a limited capacity and an automatic cutoff mechanism
Drip chamber with microdropper delivering 60 drops/minute or 60 cc/hour
Small-gauge (23-25) butterfly needle, flexible plastic catheter (long-term therapy), or polyethylene tube via surgical cutdown procedure
For long-term administration, a heparin lock, central venous catheter,* or implanted port (see below)
Injection sites are as follows:
Scalp veins
Superficial veins of hand, foot, or arm
Maintain integrity of intravenous site.
Small, padded armboard
Sandbags
Restraints for infants and small children as needed (p. 219)

---

*See Home Care Instructions, pp 549 and 550-553.

Electronic infusion devices may be used:
Types
Pumps—have mechanisms to propel the solution at the desired rate under pressure; more accurate than controllers, especially for small infusion rates, but increase the risk of infiltration because of pressure used to infuse fluid; may employ a syringe pump (prefilled syringe is placed in a chamber) or volumetric pump (fluid is pulled from a container by a special disposable cassette)
Controllers—regulate gravity flow by counting drops with a sensor; are less accurate than pumps, are affected by patient movement, but are less likely to cause an infiltration than pumps
Precautions
Excess buildup of pressure
Drip rate faster than vein can accommodate
Needle out of vein lumen
Apparatus infusing an incorrect amount of fluid
Assess drip rate by assessing amount infused in a given length of time
Time drip rate if a discrepancy between amount infused and rate set on machine (applies primarily to controllers)

Long-term venous access devices

Device	Description	Advantages	Disadvantages
Hickman/Broviac catheter*	Silicone, radiopaque, flexible catheter with open ends One or two Dacron cuffs on catheter(s) enhances tissue ingrowth	Reduced risk of bacterial migration after tissue adheres to Dacron cuff Easy to use for self-administered infusions	Requires daily heparin flushes Must be clamped or have clamp nearby at all times Must keep exit site dry Heavy activity restricted until tissue adheres to cuff Risk of infection still present Protrudes outside body; susceptible to damage from sharp instruments and may be pulled out; may affect body image More difficult to repair Patient/family must learn catheter care
Groshong catheter	Clear, flexible, silicone, radiopaque catheter with closed tip and two-way valve at proximal end Dacron cuff on catheter enhances tissue ingrowth	Reduced time and cost for maintenance care; no heparin flushes needed Reduced catheter damage—no clamping needed because of two-way valve Increased patient safety due to minimum potential for blood backflow or air embolism Reduced risk of bacterial migration after tissue adheres to Dacron cuff Easily repaired Easy to use for self-administered IV infusions	Requires weekly irrigation with normal saline Must keep exit site dry Heavy activity restricted until tissue adheres to cuff Risk of infection still present Protrudes outside body; susceptible to damage from sharp instruments and may be pulled out; can affect body image Patient/family must learn catheter care
Implanted ports (Port-a-Cath, Infus-A-Port, MediPort*)	Totally implantable metal or plastic device that consists of self-sealing injection port with preconnected or attachable silicon catheter that is placed in large blood vessel Port-a-Cath has greater surface and thicker septum that increase ease of cannulation and provide more secure placement of needle in port	Reduced risk of infection Placed completely under the skin; therefore, cannot be pulled out or damaged No maintenance care and reduced cost for family Heparinized monthly and after each infusion to maintain patency No limitations on regular physical activity, including swimming No dressing needed No or only slight change in body appearance (slight bulge on chest)	Must pierce skin for access; pain with insertion of needle; can use local anesthetic before accessing port Special needle (Huber) with angled tip must be used to inject into port Skin preparation needed before injection Hard to manipulate for self-administered infusions Catheter may dislodge from port, especially if child "plays" with port site (twiddler syndrome) Vigorous contact sorts (football, soccer, hockey) generally not allowed

*Several other names exist for these devices.

Unit 3

Tube feeding

The purpose of tube feeding is to supply gastrointestinal feeding for the child who is unable to take nourishment by mouth because of anomalies of the throat or esophagus, impaired swallowing capacity, severe debilitation, respiratory distress, or unconsciousness.

*Gavage (nasogastric or orogastric tube) feeding**

Materials needed

A suitable tube selected according to the size of the child and the viscosity of the solution being fed. Feeding tubes are available in silicone rubber, polyurethane, polyethylene, or polyvinylchloride. Polyurethane and silicone rubber tubes are smaller in diameter and more flexible than the others and are often referred to as small bore tubes.

A receptacle for the fluid; for small amounts a 10 to 30 ml syringe barrel or Asepto syringe is satisfactory; for larger amounts a 50 ml syringe with a catheter tip is more convenient.

A syringe to aspirate stomach contents and/or to inject air after the tube has been placed.

Water or water-soluble lubricant to lubricate the tube; sterile water is used for infants.

Paper or nonallergenic tape to mark the tube and to attach the tube to the infant's or child's cheek.

A stethoscope to aid in determining the correct placement in the stomach.

The solution for feeding.

*See Home Care Instructions, p 558.

Procedure: placement of the tube

1. Place the child supine with the head slightly hyperflexed or in a sniffing position (nose pointed toward ceiling).
2. Measure the tube for approximate length of insertion and mark the point with a small piece of tape. Two standard methods of measuring length are:*

   Measuring from the nose to the earlobe and then to the end of the xiphoid process, or

   Measuring from the nose to the earlobe and then to a point midway between the xiphoid process and umbilicus.
3. Insert the tube that has been lubricated with sterile water or water-soluble lubricant through either the mouth or one of the nares to the predetermined mark. Since most young infants are obligatory nose breathers, insertion through the mouth causes less distress and helps to stimulate sucking. In older infants and children the tube is passed through the nose and alternated between nostrils. An indwelling tube is almost always placed through the nose.

   When using the nose, slip the tube along the base of the nose and direct it straight back toward the occiput.

   When entering through the mouth direct the tube toward the back of the throat.

   If the child is able to swallow on command, synchronize passing the tube with swallowing. To encourage an infant to swallow, blow a puff of air into the face. The stimulation elicits a reflexive swallow in infants under 11 months and in children with severe neurologic disorders.

4. Check the position of the tube by using *both* of the following:

   Attach the syringe to the feeding tube and apply negative pressure. Aspiration of stomach contents indicates proper placement, but aspiration of respiratory secretions may be mistaken for stomach contents. However, absence of fluid is not necessarily evidence of improper placement. The stomach may be empty or the tube may not be in contact with stomach contents. Note the amount and character of any fluid aspirated and return the fluid to the stomach.

   With the syringe, inject a small amount of air (0.5 to 1 ml in premature or very small infants to 5 ml in larger children) into the tube while simultaneously listening with a stethoscope over the stomach area. Sounds of gurgling or growling will be heard if the tube is properly situated in the stomach, although it is possible to hear the air entering the stomach even when the tube is positioned above the gastroesophageal sphincter.

5. Stabilize the tube by holding or taping it to the cheek, not to the forehead because of possible damage to the nostril. To maintain correct placement, measure and record the amount of tubing extending from the nose or mouth to the distal port when the tube is first positioned. Recheck this measurement before each feeding.

*NOTE: However, research on using these methods in premature infants has found both placements to be too high (in the esophagus), although the latter method provided better placement. (Weibley TT, and others, Gavage tube insertion in the premature infant, MCN 12:24-27, 1987.)

Procedure: feeding through the tube

1. Whenever possible hold the infant or young child during the feeding to associate the comfort of physical contact with the procedure. When this is not possible, place the infant or child supine or slightly toward the right side with head and chest slightly elevated.

   Use a folded blanket under the head and shoulders for infants and a pillow for small children.

   Raise the head of the bed for larger children.

2. Warm the formula to room temperature. Pour formula into the barrel of the syringe attached to the feeding tube. To start the flow, give a gentle push with the plunger, but then remove the plunger and allow the fluid to flow into the stomach by gravity. The rate of flow should not exceed 5 ml every 5 to 10 minutes in premature and very small infants and 10 ml/minute in older infants and children to prevent nausea and regurgitation. The rate is determined by the diameter of the tubing and the height of the reservoir containing the feeding and is regulated by adjusting the height of the syringe. A usual feeding may take from 15 to 30 minutes to complete.

3. Flush the tube with sterile water (1 or 2 ml for small tubes to 5 ml or more for large ones or see discussion of flushing for administering medication through nasogastric tubes on p. 225) to clear it of formula.

4. Cap or clamp indwelling catheters to prevent loss of feeding

   If the tube is to be removed, first pinch it firmly to prevent escape of fluid as the tube is withdrawn. Withdraw the tube quickly.

5. Position the child on the right side or abdomen for at least 1 hour in the same manner as following any infant feeding to minimize the possibility of regurgitation and aspiration. If the child's condition permits, bubble the youngster after the feeding.

6. Record the feeding, including the type and amount of residual, the type and amount of formula, and the manner in which it was tolerated. For most infant feedings any amount of residual fluid aspirated from the stomach is refed to prevent electrolyte imbalance and the amount subtracted from the prescribed amount of feeding. For example, if the infant is to receive 30 ml and 10 ml is aspirated from the stomach before the feeding, the 10 ml of aspirated stomach contents is refed plus 20 ml of feeding.

7. Between feedings give infants a pacifier to satisfy oral needs.

Gastrostomy feeding*

The gastrostomy tube is placed under general anesthesia or percutaneously using an endoscope under local anesthesia. The tube used can be a Foley, wing-tip, or mushroom catheter. For children on long-term gastrostomy feeding, a feeding button may be substituted for the initial tube. The button is a small, flexible silicone device that protrudes slightly from the abdomen, is cosmetically pleasing in appearance, affords increased comfort and mobility to the child, is easy to care for, is fully immersible in water, and has a one-way valve at the proximal end that minimizes reflux and eliminates the need for clamping.

Positioning and feeding of water, formula, or pureed foods are carried out in the same manner and rate as gavage feeding. With the feeding button, the child must remain fairly still, since the tubing easily disconnects from the button if the child moves. After gastrostomy feeding, residual may not be aspirated and is measured as the amount of feeding left in the tube and syringe.

After feedings the infant or child is positioned on the right side or in Fowler position, and the tube may be left open and suspended or clamped between feedings, depending on the child's condition. If the feeding button is used, the child needs frequent bubbling because the one-way valve prevents air from escaping.

If a Foley catheter is used as the gastrostomy tube, very slight tension is applied and the tube securely taped to maintain the balloon at the gastrostomy opening and prevent its progression toward the pyloric sphincter where it may occlude the stomach outlet. As a precaution the length of the tube should be measured postoperatively and then remeasured each shift to be sure it has not slipped.

---

*See Home Care Instructions, p 560.

Unit 3

PROCEDURES RELATED TO MAINTAINING CARDIORESPIRATORY FUNCTION
Respiratory therapy

Inhalation therapy involves changing the composition, volume, or pressure of inspired gases.

Oxygen therapy

Methods include use of a mask, hood, huts, nasal cannula, face tent, oxygen tent, or Isolette.

Method is selected on the basis of the following:
Concentration of inspired air needed
Ability of the child to cooperate in its use

Concentration is regulated according to the needs of the child (usually 40% to 50%).

Oxygen is dry; therefore, it must be humidified.

Use the following precautions with an oxygen hood.
Do not allow oxygen to blow directly on the infant's face.
Position hood to avoid rubbing against the infant's neck, chin, or shoulder.

Use the following precautions with an oxygen tent.
Plan nursing activities so tent is opened as little as possible.
Tuck open edges of tent carefully to reduce oxygen loss (oxygen is heavier than air).

Check temperature inside tent frequently.

Make certain cooling mechanism is functioning.

Keep child warm and dry.

Examine bedding and clothing periodically and change as needed

Inspect any toys placed in the tent for safety and suitability. Any source of sparks (e.g., some mechanical toys) is a potential fire hazard.

Monitor child's color, respirations, and O_2 saturation.

Periodically analyze oxygen concentration at a point near the child's head and adjust oxygen flow rate to maintain desired concentration.

Provide comfort and reassurance to the child. Make sure the child is able to see someone nearby.

Invasive and noninvasive oxygen monitoring

An essential goal in managing sick or injured children is to ensure the continuous delivery of adequate oxygen to vital organs. Although life-saving, oxygen therapy can cause a number of serious sequelae. In order to monitor oxygen therapy, blood oxygen levels are routinely measured.

Arterial blood gas

Direct sampling of the blood's oxygen content (measured as partial pressure of oxygen [Po_2] can be done on blood obtained from an indwelling arterial catheter or arterial puncture. Capillary punctures from the heel are also often performed but are less reliable for blood gas measurement.

Arterial punctures may be performed using the radial, brachial, or femoral arteries.
Arterial blood samples from punctures are painful, causing crying and breathholding, which affects the accuracy of blood gas values (decreases Po_2).
Use of intradermal lidocaine at the puncture site can reduce the pain and increase the validity of the analysis.

Usual site for heel puncture is outer aspects of heel.
Boundaries can be marked by an imaginary line extending posteriorly from a point between the fourth and fifth toes and running and parallel to the lateral aspect of the heel and another line extending posteriorly from the middle of the great toe and running parallel to the medial aspect of the heel.
Puncture should be no deeper than 2.4 mm.
Before puncture, warm heel by placing towel soaked in warm (39°-44° C) water on puncture site for 10 to 15 minutes.

Arterial blood is collected in heparinized tubes, with care taken to avoid any air bubbles in the collection tube, packed in ice to reduce blood cell metabolism, and analyzed as soon as possible.

After puncture, apply pressure with a dry sterile gauze on site for 5 to 10 minutes or until bleeding stops.

Pulse oximetry

Measures arterial hemoglobin oxygen saturation (Sao_2) by passage of two different wavelengths of light through blood-perfused tissues to a photodetector. Sao_2 and heart rate are displayed on digital readout.

Attach sensor to earlobe, finger, or toe; make certain light source and photodetector are in opposition

Avoid sites with restricted bloodflow, e.g., distal to a blood pressure cuff or indwelling arterial catheter

Secure sensor with tape to avoid interference created by patient movement

Advantages:
  Noninvasive technique
  No complicated preparation or calibration of sensor
  No special skin care needed
  Convenient sites can be used

Disadvantages:
  Requires peripheral arterial pulsation
  Limited use in hypotension or with vasoconstricting drugs
  Sensor affected by movement

Sao_2 is related to Po_2 but the values are not the same. As a rule of thumb, an Sao_2 of:
  98% = Po_2 of 100 mm Hg or greater
  90% = Po_2 of 60 mm Hg
  80% = Po_2 of 45 mm Hg
  60% = Po_2 of 30 mm Hg

In general, an Sao_2 of 90% signifies developing hypoxia.

Transcutaneous oxygen monitoring

Measures transcutaneous partial pressure of oxygen ($tcPo_2$) (amount of oxygen dissolved in blood). An electrode attached to the skin causes local hyperemia and arterial arterialization of blood within the capillaries beneath the electrode. A current, created as oxygen diffuses from the capillaries through the skin and a semipermeable membrane, is measured and converted to partial pressure of oxygen (Po_2). Displayed on digital readout.

NOTE: Anytime arterial blood gas measurements and $tcPo_2$ are compared in neonates, the two sampling sites must be both above or both below the ductus arteriosus (shunting of blood through the ductus will cause different blood oxygen contents above or below this point). If significant shunting is present, the sampling from both methods should be made above the shunt to measure the actual oxygen level in blood going to the lungs, brain, and eyes.

Place electrode on an area with good blood flow but thin subcutaneous skin
  Children—Place on chest
  Newborns and young infants—Chest, abdomen, back
  Thin infants—Place center of sensor over an intercostal space on chest

Avoid any pressure on electrode, e.g., infant lying on sensor

Keep temperature of electrode at 44° C or 45° C for term infants

Change placement of electrode every 12 hours; change more frequently if needed to prevent superficial burns

Recalibrate electrode each time it is moved

Aerosol therapy

The function is the inhalation of a solution in droplet (particle) form for direct deposition in the tracheobronchial tree.

Aerosols are liquid medications (bronchodilators, steroids, mucolytics, decongestants, antibiotics, and antiviral agent) suspended in a particulate form in air.

Aerosol generators propelled by air or air-oxygen mixtures generally fall into three categories:
  Small-volume jet nebulizers or hand-held nebulizers
  Ultrasonic nebulizers for sterile water or saline aerosol only
  Metered-dose inhalers (sometimes with a "spacer" device that acts as a reservoir and simplifies use of the inhaler)

Deposition of aerosol therapy is maximized by instructing the child to breathe through the mouth with slow, deep inhalations, followed by holding the breath for 5 to 10 seconds, and then slow exhalations while in an upright position.

Using an incentive spirometer can help a cooperative child learn this ventilatory pattern.

For infants and young children, maneuvers to produce deep breathing and coughing include feet tapping, tactile stimulation, and crying, while holding the infant upright.

Unit 3

Bronchial (postural) drainage*

The purpose is to facilitate drainage and expectoration of lung and bronchial secretions from specific areas by correct positioning of the patient, using gravity as an aid.

Aids to facilitate drainage

Consistency of lung secretions changed from viscid to more
    liquid by use of the following:
    Maintenance of adequate fluid balance (oral or intravenous)
    Medication (mucolytics)
Percussion and vibration
Cough stimulation
Breathing exercises

Indications

Pulmonary conditions: bronchitis, cystic fibrosis, pneumonia,
    asthma, lung abscess, obstructive lung disease
Postoperative prophylaxis: thoracotomy, stasis pneumonia
Prophylaxis
    In prolonged artificial ventilation
    In paralytic conditions
    In unconscious patient

*See Home Care Instructions, p 567.

Cardiopulmonary resuscitation (CPR)*

For signs of impending respiratory failure, see p. 335.

One-rescuer CPR

	Objectives	Actions		
		Adult (over 8 yr)	Child (1 to 8 yr)	Infant (under 1 yr)
A. AIRWAY	**1.** Assessment: Determine unresponsiveness.	Tap or gently shake shoulder.		
		Say, "Are you okay?"		Observe
	2. Get help.	Call out "Help!"		
	3. Position the victim.	Turn on back as a unit, supporting head and neck if necessary. (4-10 seconds)		
	4. Open the airway.	Head-tilt/chin-lift		

Reproduced with permission. Copyright, Healthcare Provider's Manual for Basic Life Support, American Heart Association, 1988, p 107.
*For a more detailed discussion of CPR in infants, children 1 to 8 years, and children over 8 years, see Home Care Instructions on pp 578 and 580.

	Objectives	Actions		
		Adult (over 8 yr)	**Child (1 to 8 yr)**	**Infant (under 1 yr)**
B. BREATHING	**5.** Assessment: Determine breathlessness.	Maintain open airway. Place ear over mouth, observing chest. Look, listen, feel for breathing. (3-5 seconds)		
	6. Give 2 rescue breaths.	Maintain open airway.		
		Seal mouth to mouth		Mouth to nose/mouth
		Give 2 rescue breaths, 1 to 1½ seconds each. Observe chest rise. Allow lung deflation between breaths.		
	7. Option for obstructed airway	**a.** Reposition victim's head. Try again to give rescue breaths.		
		b. Activate the EMS system.		
		c. Give 6-10 subdiaphragmatic abdominal thrusts (the Heimlich maneuver).		Give 4 back blows.
				Give 4 chest thrusts.
		d. Tongue-jaw lift and finger sweep	Tongue-jaw lift, but finger sweep only if you see a foreign object.	
		If unsuccessful, repeat a, c, and d until successful.		
C. CIRCULATION	**8.** Assessment: Determine pulselessness.	Feel for carotid pulse with one hand; maintain head-tilt with the other. (5-10 seconds)		Feel for brachial pulse; keep head-tilt.
	9. Activate EMS system.	If someone responded to call for help, send them to activate the EMS system.		
	Begin chest compressions: **10.** Landmark check	Run middle finger along bottom edge of rib cage to notch at center (tip of sternum).		Imagine a line drawn between the nipples.
	11. Hand position	Place index finger next to finger on notch:		Place 2-3 fingers on sternum, 1 finger's width below line. Depress ½-1 in.
		Two hands next to index finger. Depress 1½-2 in.	Heel of one hand next to index finger. Depress 1-1½ in.	
	12. Compression rate	80-100 per minute		At least 100 per minute
CPR CYCLES	**13.** Compressions to breaths.	2 breaths to every 15 compressions.	1 breath to every 5 compressions.	
	14. Number of cycles.	4 (52-73 seconds)	10 (60-87 seconds)	10 (45 seconds or less)
	15. Reassessment.	Feel for carotid pulse. (5 seconds)		Feel for brachial pulse.
		If no pulse, resume CPR, starting with 2 breaths.	If no pulse, resume CPR, starting with 1 breath.	
OPTION FOR ENTRANCE OF 2ND RESCUER: "I KNOW CPR. CAN I HELP?"	1st rescuer ends CPR.	End cycle with 2 rescue breaths.	End cycle with 1 rescue breath.	
	2nd rescuer checks pulse (5 seconds).	Feel for carotid pulse.		Feel for brachial pulse.
	If no pulse, 2nd rescuer begins CPR.	Begin one-rescuer CPR, starting with 2 breaths.	Begin one-rescuer CPR, starting with 1 breath.	
	1st rescuer monitors 2nd rescuer.	Watch for chest rise and fall during rescue breathing; check pulse during chest compressions.		
OPTION FOR PULSE RETURN	If no breathing, give rescue breaths.	1 breath every 5 seconds	1 breath every 4 seconds	1 breath every 3 seconds

Unit 3

*Two-rescuer CPR**

Step	Objective	Critical performance
1. AIRWAY	**One rescuer (ventilator):** Assessment: Determine unresponsiveness.	Tap or gently shake shoulder.
		Shout "Are you OK?"
	Position the victim.	Turn on back if necessary (4-10 sec).
	Open the airway.	Use a proper technique to open airway.
2. BREATHING	Assessment: Determine breathlessness.	Look, listen, and feel (3-5 sec).
	Ventilate twice.	Observe chest rise: 1-1.5 sec/inspiration.
3. CIRCULATION	Assessment: Determine pulselessness.	Feel for carotid pulse (5-10 sec).
	State assessment results.	Say "No pulse."
	Other rescuer (compressor): Get into position for compressions.	Hand, shoulders in correct position.
	Locate landmark notch.	Landmark check.
4. COMPRESSION/ VENTILATION CYCLES	**Compressor:** Begin chest compressions.	Correct ratio compressions/ventilations: 5/1
		Compression rate: 80-100/min (5 compressions/3-4 sec).
		Say any helpful mnemonic.
		Stop compressing for each ventilation.
	Ventilator: Ventilate after every 5th compression and check compression effectiveness.	Ventilate 1 time (1-1.5 sec/inspiration).
		Check pulse occasionally to assess compressions.
	(Minimum of 10 cycles.)	Time for 10 cycles: 40-53 sec.

Reproduced with permission. Copyright, Healthcare Provider's Manual for Basic Life Support, American Heart Association, 1988, p 106.
*(a) If CPR is in progress with one rescuer (layperson), the entrance of the two rescuers occurs after the completion of one rescuer's cycle of 5 compressions and 1 ventilation. The EMS should be activated first. The two new rescuers start with Step 6. (b) If CPR is in progress with one healthcare provider, the entrance of a second healthcare provider is at the end of a cycle after check for pulse by first rescuer. The new cycle starts with one ventilation by the first rescuer, and the second rescuer becomes the compressor. Applies to children 1 year and older.

Step	Objective	Critical performance
5. CALL FOR SWITCH	**Compressor:** Call for switch when fatigued.	Give clear signal to change.
		Compressor completes 5th compression.
		Ventilator completes ventilation after 5th compression.
6. SWITCH	Simultaneously switch:	
	Ventilator: Move to chest.	Move to chest.
		Become compressor.
		Get into position for compressions.
		Locate landmark notch.
	Compressor: Move to head.	Move to head.
		Become ventilator.
		Check carotid pulse (5 sec).
		Say "No pulse."
		Ventilate once (1-1.5 sec/inspiration)
7. CONTINUE CPR	Resume compression/ventilation cycles.	Resume Step 4.

Unit 3

Unit 3

Foreign body airway obstruction management*
Signs of life-threatening obstruction

The truly choking child *cannot speak, becomes cyanotic,* and *collapses.*

	Objectives	Actions		
		Adult (over 8 yr)	Child (1 to 8 yr)	Infant (under 1 yr)
CONSCIOUS VICTIM	1. Assessment: Determine airway obstruction.	Ask, "Are you choking?" Determine if victim can cough or speak.		Observe breathing difficulty.
	2. Act to relieve obstruction.	Perform subdiaphragmatic abdominal thrusts (Heimlich maneuver).		Give 4 back blows.
				Give 4 chest thrusts.
	Be persistent.	Repeat Step 2 until obstruction is relieved or victim becomes unconscious.		
VICTIM WHO BECOMES UNCONSCIOUS	3. Position the victim; call for help.	Turn on back as a unit, supporting head and neck, face up, arms by sides. Call out, "Help!" If others come, activate EMS.		
	4. Check for foreign body.	Perform tongue-jaw lift and finger sweep.	Perform tongue-jaw lift. Remove foreign object only if you actually see it.	
	5. Give rescue breaths.	Open the airway with head-tilt/chin-lift. Try to give rescue breaths.		
	6. Act to relieve obstruction.	Perform subdiaphragmatic abdominal thrusts (Heimlich maneuver).		Give 4 back blows.
				Give 4 chest thrusts.
	7. Check for foreign body.	Perform tongue-jaw lift and finger sweep.	Perform tongue-jaw lift. Remove foreign object only if you actually see it.	
	8. Try again to give rescue breaths.	Open the airway with head-tilt/chin-lift. Try to give rescue breaths.		
	9. Be persistent.	Repeat Steps 6-8 until obstruction is relieved.		
UNCONSCIOUS VICTIM	1. Assessment: Determine unresponsiveness.	Tap or gently shake shoulder. Shout, "Are you okay?"		Tap or gently shake shoulder.
	2. Call for help; position the victim.	Turn on back as a unit, supporting head and neck, face up, arms by sides. Call out, "Help!" If others come, activate EMS.		
	3. Open the airway.	Head-tilt/chin-lift		Head-tilt/chin-lift, but do not tilt too far.
	4. Assessment: Determine breathlessness	Maintain an open airway. Ear over mouth; observe chest. Look, listen, feel for breathing. (3-5 seconds)		
	5. Give rescue breaths.	Make mouth-to-mouth seal.		Make mouth-to-nose-and-mouth seal.
		Try to give rescue breaths.		
	6. Try again to give rescue breaths.	Reposition head. Try rescue breaths again.		
	7. Activate the EMS system.	If someone responded to the call for help, that person should activate the EMS system.		
	8. Act to relieve obstruction.	Perform subdiaphragmatic abdominal thrusts (Heimlich maneuver).		Give 4 back blows.
				Give 4 chest thrusts.
	9. Check for foreign body.	Perform tongue-jaw lift and finger sweep.	Perform tongue-jaw lift. Remove foreign object only if you actually see it.	
	10. Rescue breaths.	Open the airway with head-tilt/chin-lift. Try again to give rescue breaths.		
	11. Be persistent.	Repeat Steps 8-10 until obstruction is relieved.		

Reproduced with permission. Copyright, Healthcare Provider's Manual for Basic Life Support, American Heart Association, 1988, p 108.
*For a more detailed discussion of managing obstructed airway (choking) in infants and children see Home Care Instructions on pp 583 and 585.

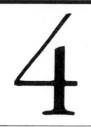

Nursing Care Plans

Unit 4

Unit 4

Unit 4

THE PROCESS OF NURSING INFANTS AND CHILDREN

The care of hospitalized children and their families requires the same systematic decision-making approach that is applied to nursing care for all patients. This problem-solving process involves both cognitive and operational skills and consists of five phases:

1. *Assessment*—the analysis and synthesis of collected data
2. *Problem identification*—the determination of the actual or potential problem or need stated as a *nursing diagnosis*
3. *Plan formulation*—a design of action sometimes stated as nursing orders, nursing interventions, or nursing functions
4. *Implementation*—the performance or execution of the plan
5. *Evaluation*—a measure of the outcome of nursing action(s) that either completes the nursing process or serves as a basis for reassessment

Nursing diagnoses

A nursing diagnosis, which places a patient in a diagnostic category for purposes of determining therapy, has been defined by several authorities. Two of these definitions follow:

Nursing diagnosis made by professional nurses describes actual or potential health problems that nurses, by virtue of their education and experience, are capable and licensed to treat.

Gordon, 1976

A nursing diagnosis is a clinical judgment about an individual, family, or community which is derived through a deliberate, systematic process of data collection and analysis. It provides the basis for prescriptions for definitive therapy for which the nurse is accountable. It is expressed concisely and it includes the etiology of the condition when known.

Shoemaker, 1984

The nursing diagnoses used in this segment are those compiled and approved at the National Conference on Classification of Nursing Diagnosis (Kim, McFarland, and McLane, 1988) and organized according to priority. Those selected for inclusion in this unit represent only one interpretation. Some diagnoses are closely related and it is often difficult to determine which diagnostic category best represents any given goal. A number of diagnoses do not appear. The diagnoses selected for inclusion and nursing interventions serve as a general guide for nursing care of children with health problems; therefore, others must be added by the user to individualize care for a specific child or family.

*Nursing diagnoses according to functional health patterns**

Health perception—health management pattern

Altered health maintenance	Potential for injury
Health-seeking behaviors (specify)	Potential for poisoning
Noncompliance (specify)	Potential for suffocation
Potential for infection	Potential for trauma

Nutritional-metabolic pattern

Altered nutrition: less than body requirements	Impaired skin integrity
Altered nutrition: more than body requirements	Impaired swallowing
Altered nutrition: potential for more than body requirements	Impaired tissue integrity
Altered oral mucous membrane	Ineffective breastfeeding
Fluid volume deficit (1)	Ineffective thermoregulation
Fluid volume deficit (2)	Potential altered body temperature
Fluid volume excess	Potential fluid volume deficit
Hyperthermia	Potential for aspiration
Hypothermia	Potential impaired skin integrity

Elimination pattern

Altered patterns of urinary elimination	Perceived constipation
Bowel incontinence	Reflex incontinence
Colonic constipation	Stress incontinence
Constipation	Total incontinence
Diarrhea	Urge incontinence
Functional incontinence	Urinary retention

*Nursing diagnoses include those approved by the North American Diagnosis Association in 1988. Functional Health Patterns from Gordon (1987) and personal communication, 1988.

Activity-exercise pattern

Activity intolerance
Altered growth and development
Altered (specify type) tissue perfusion (renal, cerebral, cardio-
  pulmonary, gastrointestinal, peripheral)
Bathing/hygiene self-care deficit
Decreased cardiac output
Diversional activity deficit
Dressing/grooming self-care deficit
Dysreflexia
Fatigue

Feeding self-care deficit
Impaired gas exchange
Impaired home maintenance management
Impaired physical mobility (level 0 to 4)*
Ineffective airway clearance
Ineffective breathing pattern
Potential activity intolerance
Potential for disuse syndrome
Toileting self-care deficit

Sleep-rest pattern

Sleep pattern disturbance

Cognitive-perceptual pattern

Altered thought processes
Chronic pain
Decisional conflict (specify)
Knowledge deficit (specify)

Pain
Sensory/perceptual alterations (specify) (visual, auditory, kin-
  esthetic, gustatory, tactile, olfactory)
Unilateral neglect

Self-perception—self-concept pattern

Anxiety
Body image disturbance
Fear
Hopelessness
Personal identity disturbance

Powerlessness
Self-esteem disturbance
  Chronic low self-esteem
  Situational low self-esteem

Role-relationship pattern

Altered family processes
Altered parenting
Altered role performance
Anticipatory grieving
Dysfunctional grieving

Impaired social interaction
Impaired verbal communication
Parental role conflict
Potential altered parenting
Potential for violence: self-directed or directed at others
Social isolation

Sexuality-reproductive pattern

Altered sexuality patterns
Rape-trauma syndrome
Rape-trauma syndrome: compound reaction

Rape-trauma syndrome: silent reaction
Sexual dysfunction

Coping—stress tolerance pattern

Defensive coping
Family coping: potential for growth
Impaired adjustment
Ineffective denial

Ineffective family coping: compromised
Ineffective family coping: disabling
Ineffective individual coping
Post-trauma response

Value-belief pattern

Spiritual distress (distress of the human spirit)

*Suggested code for functional level classification: 0 Completely independent; 1 Requires use of equipment or device; 2 Requires help from another person for assistance, supervision, or teaching; 3 Requires help from another person and equipment or device; 4 Is dependent, does not participate in activity.

Unit 4

*Nursing diagnoses according to NANDA taxonomy**

Human response pattern: Choosing

Family coping: potential for growth
Ineffective family coping: compromised
Ineffective family coping: disabling
Health-seeking behaviors (specify)
Decisional conflict

Impaired adjustment
Defensive coping
Ineffective denial
Noncompliance
Ineffective individual coping

Human response pattern: Communicating

Impaired verbal communication

Human response pattern: Exchanging

Altered (specify type) tissue perfusion (renal, cerebral, cardio-
   pulmonary, gastrointestinal, peripheral)
Bowel incontinence
Colonic constipation
Constipation
Perceived constipation
Decreased cardiac output
Diarrhea
Fluid volume deficit (1)
Fluid volume deficit (2)
Fluid volume excess
Potential fluid volume deficit
Altered nutrition: less than body requirements
Altered nutrition: more than body requirements
Altered nutrition: potential for more than body requirements
Potential for aspiration
Potential for disuse syndrome
Potential for injury
Potential for poisoning
Potential for suffocation
Potential for trauma

Dysreflexia
Hyperthermia
Hypothermia
Potential altered body temperature
Potential for infection
Ineffective thermoregulation
Impaired gas exchange
Ineffective airway clearance
Ineffective breathing pattern
Altered mucous membranes
Impaired skin integrity
Impaired tissue integrity
Potential impaired skin integrity
Functional incontinence
Reflex incontinence
Stress incontinence
Total incontinence
Urge incontinence
Urinary retention
Altered patterns of urinary elimination

Human response pattern: Feeling

Anxiety
Chronic pain
Pain
Fear
Anticipatory grieving
Dysfunctional grieving

Post-trauma response
Potential for violence; self-directed or directed at others
Rape-trauma syndrome
Rape-trauma syndrome: compromised
Rape-trauma syndrome: silent reaction

Human response pattern: Knowing

Altered thought processes
Knowledge deficit (specify)

---

*Modified from McFarland GK and McFarlane EA: Nursing diagnosis and intervention, St. Louis, 1989, The C.V. Mosby Co.

Human response pattern: Moving

Activity intolerance
Potential activity intolerance
Diversional activity deficit
Fatigue
Impaired physical mobility
Sleep-pattern disturbance
Altered growth and development
Altered health maintenance

Bathing/hygiene self-care deficit
Dressing/grooming self-care deficit
Feeding self-care deficit
Impaired home maintenance management
Impaired swallowing
Ineffective breastfeeding
Toileting self-care deficit

Human response pattern: Perceiving

Hopelessness
Powerlessness
Body-image disturbance
Personal identity disturbance
Self-esteem disturbance
Chronic low self-esteem

Situational low self-esteem
Sensory/perceptual alterations (specify) (visual, auditory, kinesthetic, gustatory, tactile, olfactory)
Unilateral neglect

Human response pattern: Relating

Altered family processes
Altered sexuality patterns
Altered parenting
Altered role performance
Parental role conflict

Potential altered parenting
Sexual dysfunction
Impaired social interaction
Social isolation

Human response pattern: Valuing

Spiritual distress (distress of the human spirit)

NURSING CARE OF THE CHILD AND FAMILY DURING STRESS AND ILLNESS

Illness and hospitalization constitute crises in the life of the child. In the hospital children must deal with a strange environment, a number of unfamiliar caregivers, and a general disruption of their usual life-style. Often, they must submit to painful procedures, loss of independence, and an endless series of unknowns. Their interpretation of events, their responses to the experience, and the significance they place on these experiences are directly related to the developmental level. Therefore, in order to meet the needs of hospitalized children, it is essential that the pediatric nurse has a knowledge of normal growth and development, including some understanding of children's cognitive process and the meaning that hospitalization has for children at any age.

NURSING CARE PLAN
THE CHILD IN THE HOSPITAL

MEANING OF ILLNESS AND HOSPITALIZATION TO THE CHILD

Infant

Change in familiar routine and surroundings; responds with global reaction

Separation from love-object

Toddler

Fear of separation, desertion; separation anxiety highest in this age-group

Relates illness to a concrete condition, circumstances, or behavior

Preschool

Fear of bodily harm or mutilation, castration, intrusive procedures

Separation anxiety less intense than toddler but strong

Causation same as toddler; often considers own role in causation, i.e., illness as a punishment for wrongdoing

School-age

Fears physical nature of illness

Concern regarding separation from age-mates and ability to maintain position in peer group

Perceives an external cause for illness, although located in body

Adolescent

Anxious regarding loss of independence, control, identity

Concern about privacy

Perceives malfunctioning organ or process as cause of illness

Able to explain illness

CHILD'S CONCEPT OF ILLNESS RELATED TO COGNITIVE DEVELOPMENT (BIBACE AND WALSH, 1980)

Age 2 to 7 years (preoperational thought)

Phenomenism:

Perceives an external, unrelated, concrete phenomenon as the cause of illness; e.g., "being sick because you don't feel well"

Contagion:

Perceives cause of illness as proximity between two events that occurs by "magic"; e.g., "getting a cold because you are near someone who has a cold"

Age 7 to 10+ years (concrete operational thought)

Contamination:

Perceives cause as a person, object, or action external to the child that is "bad" or "harmful" to the body; i.e., "getting a cold because you didn't wear a hat"

Internalization:

Perceives illness as having an external cause but as being located inside the body; i.e., "getting a cold by breathing in air and bacteria"

Age 13 years and older (formal operational thought)

Physiologic:

Perceives cause as malfunctioning or nonfunctioning organ or process; can explain illness in sequence of events

Psychophysiologic:

Realizes that psychologic actions and attitudes affect health and illness

ASSESSMENT

Take health history, especially regarding clues to child's past experience with hospitalization, illness, and factors related to reason for hospitalization (e.g., emergency treatment, diagnosis, etc.); determine type of preparation, if any (see box).

Perform physical assessment; see Unit 1.

Observe for manifestations of specific disorder for which child is admitted

Observe for evidence of psychologic reactions to the illness and/or hospitalization (see box)

Assist with diagnostic procedures and tests—Routine admission tests (e.g., urinalysis) and special tests and procedures. (See guidelines for preparing children for procedures, p. 211.)

GUIDELINES FOR ADMISSION

Preadmission

Assign a room based on developmental age, seriousness of diagnosis, communicability of illness, and projected length of stay

Prepare roommate(s) for the arrival of a new patient; when children are too young to benefit from this consideration, prepare parents

Prepare room for child and family, with admission forms and equipment nearby to eliminate need to leave child

Admission

Introduce primary nurse to child and family

Orient child and family to inpatient facilities, especially to assigned room and unit; emphasize positive areas of pediatric unit

Room: explain call light, bed controls, television, etc.; direct to bathroom, telephone, etc.

Unit: Direct to playroom, desk, dining area, or other areas

Introduce family to roommate and his or her parents

Apply identification band to child's wrist, ankle, or both (if not done)

Explain hospital regulations and schedules (e.g., visiting hours, mealtimes, bedtime, limitations [give written information if available])

Perform nursing admission history (see box)

Take vital signs, blood pressure, height, and weight

Obtain specimens as needed and order needed laboratory work

Support child and perform or assist health professional with physical examination (for purposes of nursing assessment)

Guidelines for emergency admission

Lengthy preparatory admission procedures often impossible and inappropriate for emergency situations

Unless an emergency is life threatening, children need to participate in their care to maintain a sense of control

Focus on essential components of admission counseling including:

Appropriate introduction to the family

Use of child's name, not terms such as "honey" or "dear"

Determination of child's age and some judgment about developmental age (if the child is of school age, asking about the grade level will offer some evidence for concurrent intellectual ability)

Information about child's general state of health, any problems that may interfere with medical treatment, such as sensitivity to medication, and previous experience with hospital facilities

Information about the chief complaint from both the parents and the child

Guidelines for admission to intensive care unit

Prepare child and parents for elective ICU admission, such as for postoperative care after cardiac surgery

Prepare child and parents for unanticipated ICU admission by focusing primarily on the sensory aspects of the experience and on usual family concerns, e.g., persons in charge of child's care, schedule for visiting, area where family can wait

Prepare parents regarding child's appearance and behavior when they first visit child in ICU

Accompany family to bedside to provide emotional support and answer questions

Prepare siblings for their visit; plan length of time for sibling visitation; monitor siblings' reactions during visit to prevent them from becoming overwhelmed

MANIFESTATIONS OF SEPARATION ANXIETY IN YOUNG CHILDREN

Phase of protest

Observed behaviors during later infancy

Cries

Screams

Searches for parent with eyes

Clings to parent

Avoids and rejects contact with strangers

Additional behaviors observed during toddlerhood

Verbally attacks strangers, i.e., "go away"

Physically attacks strangers, i.e., kicks, bites, hits, pinches

Attempts to escape to find parent

Attempts to physically force parent to stay

Behaviors may last from hours to days

Protest, such as crying, may be continuous, ceasing only with physical exhaustion

Approach of stranger may precipitate increased protest

Phase of despair

Observed behaviors

Inactive

Withdraws from others

Depressed, sad

Uninterested in environment

Uncommunicative

Regresses to earlier behavior, i.e., thumb sucking, bedwetting, use of pacifier, use of bottle

Behaviors may last for variable length of time

Child's physical condition may deteriorate from refusal to eat, drink, or move

Phase of detachment

Observed behaviors

Shows increased interest in surroundings

Interacts with strangers or familiar caregivers

Forms new but superficial relationships

Appears happy

Detachment usually occurs after prolonged separation from parent; rarely seen in hospitalized children

Behaviors represent a superficial adjustment to loss

NURSING ADMISSION HISTORY ACCORDING TO FUNCTIONAL HEALTH PATTERNS*

Health-perception—health-management pattern

Why has your child been admitted?

How has your child's general health been?

What does your child know about this hospitalization?

Ask the child why he or she came to the hospital.

If answer is "For an operation or for tests," ask the child to tell you about what will happen before, during, and after the operation or tests.

Has your child ever been in the hospital before?

How was that hospital experience?

What things were important to you and your child during that hospitalization? How can we be most helpful now?

What medications does your child take at home?

Why are they given?

When are they given?

How are they given (if a liquid, with a spoon; if a tablet, swallowed with water, or other)?

Does your child have any trouble taking medication? If so, what helps?

Is your child allergic to any medications?

Nutrition-metabolic pattern

What are the family's usual mealtimes?

Do family members eat together or at separate times?

What are your child's favorite foods, beverages, and snacks?

Average amounts consumed or usual size portions

Special cultural practices, such as family eats only ethnic food

What foods and beverages does your child dislike?

What are your child's feeding habits (bottle, cup, spoon, eats by self, needs assistance, any special devices)?

How does your child like the food served (warmed, cold, one item at a time)?

How would you describe your child's usual appetite (hearty eater, picky eater)?

Has being sick affected your child's appetite?

Are there any known or suspected food allergies; is your child on a special diet?

Are there any feeding problems (excessive fussiness, spitting up, colic); any dental or gum problems that affect feeding?

What do you do for these problems?

Elimination pattern

What are your child's toilet habits (diaper, toilet trained—day only or day and night, use of word to communicate urination or defecation, potty chair, regular toilet, other routines)?

What is your child's usual pattern of elimination (bowel movements)?

Do you have any concerns about elimination (bed-wetting, constipation, diarrhea)?

What do you do for these problems?

Have you ever noticed that your child sweats a lot?

Sleep-rest pattern

What is your child's usual hour of sleep and awakening?

What is your child's schedule for naps; length of naps?

Is there a special routine before sleeping (bottle, drink of water, bedtime story, nightlight, favorite blanket or toy, prayers)?

Is there a special routine during sleep time, such as waking to go to the bathroom?

What type of bed does your child sleep in?

Does your child have a separate room or share a room; if shares, with whom?

What are the home sleeping arrangements (alone or with others, such as a sibling, parent, or other person)?

What is your child's favorite sleeping position?

Are there any sleeping problems (falling asleep, waking during night, nightmares, sleep walking)?

Are there any problems awakening and getting ready in the morning?

What do you do for these problems?

Activity-exercise pattern

What is your child's schedule during the day (nursery school, daycare center, regular school, extracurricular activities)?

What are your child's favorite activities or toys (both active and quiet interests)?

What is your child's usual television viewing schedule at home?

What are your child's favorite programs?

Are there any TV restrictions?

Does your child have any illness or disabilities that limit activity? If so, how?

What are your child's usual habits and schedule for bathing (bath in tub or shower, sponge bath, shampoo)?

What are your child's dental habits (brushing, flossing, fluoride supplements or rinses, favorite toothpaste); schedule of daily dental care?

Does your child need help with dressing or grooming, such as hair combing?

Are there any problems with the above (dislike of or refusal to bathe, shampoo hair, or brush teeth)?

What do you do for these problems?

Are there special devices that your child requires help in managing (eyeglasses, contact lenses, hearing aid, orthodontic appliances, artificial elimination appliances, orthopedic devices)?

NOTE: Use the following code to assess functional self-care level for feeding, bathing/hygiene, dressing/grooming, toileting:

O: Full self-care

I: Requires use of equipment or device

II: Requires assistance or supervision from another person

III: Requires assistance or supervision from another person and equipment or device

IV: Is dependent and does not participate

---

*The focus of the admission history is the child's psychosocial environment. Most of the questions are worded in terms of parental responses. Depending on the child's age, they should be addressed directly to the child when appropriate.

Cognitive-perceptual pattern

Does your child have any hearing difficulty?

Does the child use a hearing aid?

Have "tubes" been placed in your child's ears?

Does your child have any vision problems?

Does the child wear glasses or contact lenses?

Does your child have any learning difficulties?

What is the child's grade in school?

For information on pain, see p. 279.

Self-perception— self-concept pattern

How would you describe your child (e.g., takes time to adjust, settles in easily, shy, friendly, quiet, talkative, serious, playful, stubborn, easygoing)?

What kinds of things make your child angry, annoyed, anxious, or sad? What helps?

How does your child act when annoyed or upset?

What have been your child's experiences with and reactions to temporary separation from you (parent)?

Does your child have any fears (places, objects, animals, people, situations)? How do you handle them?

Do you think your child's illness has changed the way he or she thinks about self (e.g., more shy, embarrassed about appearance, less competitive with friends, stays at home more)?

Role-relationship pattern

Does your child have a favorite nickname?

What are the names of other family members or others who live in the home (relatives, friends, pets)?

Who usually takes care of your child during the day/night (especially if other than parent, such as babysitter, relative)?

What are the parents' occupation and work schedules?

Are there any special family considerations (adoption, foster child, stepparent, divorce, single parent)?

Have any major changes in the family occurred lately (death, divorce, separation, birth of a sibling, loss of a job, financial strain, mother beginning a career, other)? Describe child's reaction.

Who are your child's play companions or social groups (peers, younger or older children, adults, prefers to be alone)?

Do things generally go well for your child in school or with friends?

Does your child have "security" objects at home (pacifier, thumb, bottle, blanket, stuffed animal or doll)? Did you bring any of these to the hospital?

How do you handle discipline problems at home? Are these methods always effective?

Does your child have any speech or hearing problems? If so, what are your suggestions for communicating with him?

Will your child's hospitalization affect the family's financial support or care of other family members, such as other children?

What concerns do you have about your child's illness and hospitalization?

Who will be staying with your child while hospitalized?

How can we contact you or another close family member outside of the hospital?

Sexuality-reproductive pattern

(Answer questions that apply to your child's age-group.)

Has your child begun puberty (developing physical sexual characteristics, menstruation)? Have you or your child had any concerns?

Does your daughter know how to do breast self-examination?

Does your son know how to do testicular self-examination?

How have you approached topics of sexuality with your child?

Do you feel you might need some help with some topics?

Has your child's illness affected the way he or she feels about being a boy or a girl? If so, how?

Do you have any concerns with behaviors in your child, such as masturbation, asking many questions or talking about sex, not respecting others' privacy or wanting too much privacy?

Initiate a conversation about adolescent's sexual concerns with open-ended to more direct questions and using the terms "friends" or "partners" rather than "girlfriend" or "boyfriend":

Tell me about your social life.

Who are your closest friends? (If one friend is identified, could ask more about that relationship, such as how much time they spend together, how serious they are about each other, if the relationship is going the way the teenager hoped it would.)

Might ask about dating and sexual issues, such as the teenager's views on sex education, "going steady," "living together," or premarital sex.

Which friends would you like to have visit in the hospital?

Coping-stress tolerance pattern

(Answer questions that apply to your child's age-group.)

What does your child do when tired or upset?

If upset, does your child want a special person or object? If so, explain.

If your child has temper tantrums, what causes them and how do you handle them?

Whom does your child talk to when worried about something?

How does your child usually handle problems or disappointments?

Have there been any big changes or problems in your family recently? How did you handle them?

Has your child ever had a problem with drugs or alcohol or tried suicide?

Do you think your child is "accident prone"? If so, explain.

Value-belief pattern

What is your religion?

How is religion or faith important in your child's life?

What religious practices would you like continued in the hospital, such as prayers before meals/bedtime; visit by minister, priest, or rabbi, prayer group?

NURSING DIAGNOSIS: Anxiety/fear related to separation from accustomed routine and support system; unfamiliar surroundings

GOAL

Prevent or minimize separation

INTERVENTIONS

Provide consistency of nursing personnel as much as possible; assign a primary nurse

Arrange workload and schedule to allow personal contact with the child

Encourage parents to room-in whenever possible

Provide an atmosphere of warmth and acceptance for both child and parents

Encourage parents and others to cuddle, fondle, and otherwise demonstrate affection for the child

Recognize the child's separation behaviors as normal
Allow the child to cry
Provide support through physical presence

Maintain the child's contact with parents and siblings
Talk about the child's parents frequently
Encourage the child to talk about and remember parents
Stress the significance of the parents' visits, telephone calls, or letters

Help the parents understand the behaviors of separation anxiety and suggest ways of supporting the child
Explain to the child when they leave and when they will return
Tell the hospitalized child the reason for leaving
Convey the expected time of return in terms of anticipated events. For example, if the parents will return in the morning, they can say they will see the child, "After the sun comes up," or, "When (a favorite program) is on television"
Use a clock or calendar for an older child
Visit for short but frequent times rather than one long time; encourage parents and relatives to take turns visiting
Allow siblings to visit
Leave favorite home articles, such as a blanket, toy, bottle, feeding utensil, or article of clothing, with the child
Respect treasured objects or older objects of older children, such as a stuffed animal
Encourage the family to provide photographs of family members and tape recordings of the parents' voices, such as reading a story, singing a song, saying prayers before bedtime, or relating events at home

Play family tape recordings at lonely times, such as before sleep

Encourage the child to talk about family members
Suggest that the family leave small gifts for the child to open each day; if the parents know when their next visit will be, have them leave the number of packages that correspond to the days between visits

Assign a "foster grandparent" or consistent volunteer to be with the child if available

EXPECTED OUTCOMES

Child has consistent caregivers

Parents visit as much as possible

Parents cooperate in care (specify)

Child accepts and responds positively to comforting measures

Child discusses the family, including pets

Parents demonstrate an understanding of separation behaviors

Siblings visit as much as possible

Family provides the child with familiar and/or cherished articles from home

Assigned person spends time with the child (specify amount of time)

GOAL

Allow expression of feelings

INTERVENTIONS

Accept expression of feelings

Provide an atmosphere that encourages free expression of feelings

Provide opportunities for the child to verbalize, "play out," or otherwise express feelings without fear of punishment

EXPECTED OUTCOME

Child verbalizes or plays out feelings or concerns

GOAL

Keep child calm

INTERVENTIONS

Do nothing to make child more anxious than he already is

Maintain calm, relaxed, and reassuring manner

Establish rapport with child and parents

Instill confidence in both parents and child

Try to avoid intrusive procedures

EXPECTED OUTCOMES

Child exhibits no signs of apprehension

Parents relate readily with personnel and calmly with child

Child rests quietly and calmly

GOAL

Establish a trusting relationship with the child

INTERVENTIONS

Be positive in approach to the child

Be honest with the child

Convey to the child the behaviors expected

Be consistent in expectations and in relationships with the child

Treat the child fairly and help him feel that he is being treated fairly

Encourage parents to maintain a truthful relationship with the child

Make certain the child has call light or other signal device within reach

EXPECTED OUTCOMES

Child develops rapport with primary nurse

Child maintains trust of family

GOAL

Help the child to feel cared for as a person

INTERVENTIONS

Maintain the child's identity
  Address the child by name or usual nickname
  Avoid assigning a nickname to the child or converting a given
    name to its counterpart in another language, such as using
    Joe instead of José
Avoid communicating any signals of rejection, distaste, or other
  negative feelings to the child
Criticize or communicate disapproval of unacceptable *behavior*
  not disapproval of the *child*
Communicate (verbally and nonverbally) that the child is a
  valued person

EXPECTED OUTCOMES

Child interacts with staff
*Staff demonstrates respect for the child

GOAL

Reduce or alleviate fear of the unknown

INTERVENTIONS

Explain routines, items, procedures, and events in a language
  appropriate to the child's developmental level; use simple
  language
Reassure the child and repeat reassurance as necessary
Absolve the child from any guilt about being hospitalized
Allow the parent(s) to participate in the child's care
Allow the child to handle items that may seem strange or threat-
  ening
Give encouragement and positive feedback for cooperation in
  care

EXPECTED OUTCOMES

Child exhibits understanding of information presented (specify
  information and means of demonstration)
Child discusses procedures and activities without evidence of
  anxiety

GOAL

Allow for regression during periods of illness

INTERVENTIONS

Recognize that regressive behavior is a feature of illness
Accept regressive behavior and help the child with dependency
Assist the child in reconquering the negative counterpart of the
  psychosocial stage to which regressed (e.g., overcome mis-
  trust; facilitate development of trust)

EXPECTED OUTCOME

*Staff and parents exhibit an attitude of acceptance of regressive
  behaviors

GOAL

Provide comfort measures

---

*Nursing outcome.

INTERVENTIONS

Provide pacifier to meet oral needs, if appropriate
Hold infant or young child when this does not interfere with
  therapy
Touch, talk, and otherwise comfort child who cannot be held
Provide sensory stimulation and diversion appropriate to child's
  level of development
Encourage family members to visit and allow them to comfort
  and care for child to the extent possible

EXPECTED OUTCOMES

Child engages in nonnutritive sucking
Child exhibits no signs of distress
Family is involved in care

NURSING DIAGNOSIS: Anxiety/fear related to distressing procedures, events

GOAL

Prepare for hospitalization

INTERVENTIONS

Prepare the child as needed
Select appropriate preparatory materials
Involve the parents
Modify preparation in special situations, e.g. day hospital, emer-
  gency admission, or ICU (see box, p. 247)

EXPECTED OUTCOME

Child is prepared for hospital experience

GOAL

Decrease fear of bodily injury

INTERVENTIONS

Recognize developmental fears associated with illness and pro-
  cedures
Provide age-appropriate explanations for procedures, especially
  those that are intrusive or involve the genitals
Reassure the child that certain body parts can be removed with-
  out producing harm (such as blood, tonsils, or appendix)
Provide privacy for any procedure that exposes the body
Protect the child from seeing unclothed patients
Use interventions that preserve the child's concept of body
  integrity (such as bandages over puncture sites)

EXPECTED OUTCOME

Child displays minimal fear of bodily injury

GOAL

Support child during tests and procedures

INTERVENTIONS

Prepare child for procedures according to age and level of
  understanding (see p. 211)

Unit 4

Remain with child
Prepare child and family for surgery if prescribed
Answer questions and explain purposes of activities
Keep informed of progress

EXPECTED OUTCOME

Child remains calm and cooperative during procedures

NURSING DIAGNOSIS: Powerlessness related to the health care environment

GOAL

Modify the hospital environment to resemble home

INTERVENTIONS

Determine from the parents or other caregiver the child's customary routine and manner of handling (see nursing admission history, p. 248)
Maintain a routine similar to the one the child is accustomed to at home
Minimize a hospital-like environment as much as possible; allow the child to sit at table to eat meals, wear own pajamas or street clothes
Use terms familiar to the child, such as those for body functions

EXPECTED OUTCOME

Child's routines and environment are similar to those at home (specify)

GOAL

Provide opportunities for acceptable control

INTERVENTIONS

Allow the child choices whenever possible, such as food selection, clothing, options for time of basic care (bath, play, bedtime), selection of television channels
Use time structuring with an older child, a jointly planned and written schedule of daily activities
Permit freedom on the unit within defined and enforced limitations
Limit use of restraints
Encourage self-care according to the child's abilities
Assign tasks to an older child, especially in extended hospitalization—such as making the bed, supervising younger children, distributing menus, collating charts
Respect the child's need for privacy

EXPECTED OUTCOMES

Child participates in planning care (specify)
Child moves about the unit but respects limits
Child participates in care activities (specify activities)
Child assumes responsibility for tasks (specify)
*Child's need for privacy is maintained

NURSING DIAGNOSIS: Diversional activity deficit related to impaired mobility musculoskeletal impairment, confinement to hospital or home, effects of illness

GOAL

Provide opportunity for activities

INTERVENTIONS

Schedule therapies and periods of rest to allow for activities
Involve the child in planning care to the extent of capabilities
Arrange for and encourage interaction with others as feasible
Encourage visits from family and friends
Provide opportunity to socialize with noninfectious children

EXPECTED OUTCOMES

Child helps plan care and schedule
Child interacts with family and other children

GOAL

Provide diversion

INTERVENTIONS

Spend time with child
Change position of bed in room periodically to alter sensory stimuli, if child is confined to bed
Provide activities appropriate to the child's condition, physical limitations, and developmental level
Encourage family to fondle and hold infant or child
Maintain accustomed routine at home and, when possible, if hospitalized
Provide diversional activities or consult with a child-life specialist
Encourage interaction with other children
Choose a roommate compatible in age, sex, and physical abilities
Monitor time spent watching television versus interactive or creative activities
Allow ample time for play
Make play materials available to the child
Encourage play activities and diversions appropriate to the child's age, condition, and capabilities
Use play as a teaching stratgy and an anxiety-reducing technique

EXPECTED OUTCOMES

Child engages in activities appropriate for age, interests, and physical limitations (specify activities)
Child receives attention and comfort
Child engages in age-appropriate play (specify)

NURSING DIAGNOSIS: Activity intolerance related to generalized weakness, fatigue, imbalance between oxygen supply and demand

GOAL

Conserve energy

---

*Nursing outcome

INTERVENTIONS

Assess child's level of physical tolerance

Anticipate child's need, as evidenced by irritability, short attention span, and fretfulness and assist child in those activities of daily living that may be beyond tolerance

Provide entertainment and quiet diversional activities appropriate to age and interest of the child

Provide diversional play activities that promote rest and quiet but prevent boredom and withdrawal

Choose an appropriate roommate of similar age and interests and one who requires restricted activity

Instruct child to rest when feeling tired

Balance rest and activity when ambulatory

EXPECTED OUTCOMES

Child plays and rests quietly and engages in activities appropriate to age and capabilities (specify)

Child exhibits no evidence of intolerance

Child tolerates increasingly more activity

GOAL

Promote rest

INTERVENTIONS

Provide quiet environment

Organize activities for maximum sleep time

Schedule visiting to allow for sufficient rest

Keep visiting periods with friends and family short

Encourage parents to remain with child

*Administer sedatives and analgesics as indicated if ordered for restlessness and pain

Encourage frequent rest periods

Enforce regular sleep times

Implement measures to ensure sleep, such as quiet, darkened room

EXPECTED OUTCOMES

Child remains calm, quiet, and relaxed

Child gets a sufficient amount of rest (specify)

NURSING DIAGNOSIS: Potential for injury/trauma related to unfamiliar environment, therapies, hazardous equipment

GOAL

Promote safety

INTERVENTIONS

Employ environmental safety measures

Report any potential hazards (e.g., slippery floors, poor illumination, electrical hazards, damaged or malfunctioning furniture or equipment, unprotected windows, stairwells)

Dispose of small breakable items appropriately (thermometers, bottles)

Keep potentially hazardous articles out of child's reach

Check bathwater for temperature before bathing infant or child

---

*Dependent nursing activity.

Maintain surveillance of children in bathtubs

Keep crib sides up and securely fastened, siderails on children who may fall out of bed; use safety restraints when applicable

Maintain hand contact while caring for a child in a crib with siderails down

Transport infants and children appropriately
    Held with proper support
    Fasten safety belt on gurney, wheelchair

Alert ancillary hospital personnel regarding child's physical tolerance and need for assistance during activity

EXPECTED OUTCOME

Child remains free of injury

GOAL

Prevent complications from restraining devices, if used

INTERVENTIONS

Remove restraints from extremities as often as possible

Change position at least every 2 hours

Frequently observe circulation, position, and pressure points

EXPECTED OUTCOME

Extremities remain free of constriction and pressure

NURSING DIAGNOSIS: Bathing/hygiene self-care deficit related to physical or cognitive disability, mechanical restrictions

GOAL

Promote self-help

INTERVENTIONS

Assist with bathing

Allow child to help plan own daily routine and choose from alternatives when appropriate

Encourage participation in self-care activities according to developmental level and capabilities

Provide devices, equipment, and methods to assist the child in self-care

Assist with dressing, grooming

EXPECTED OUTCOME

Child engages in self-help activities to maximum capabilities

---

NURSING DIAGNOSIS: Dressing/grooming self-care deficit related to physical or cognitive disability, mechanical restrictions

NURSING DIAGNOSIS: Toileting self-care deficit related to physical or cognitive disability, mechanical restrictions

GOAL

Facilitate elimination

INTERVENTIONS

Sit in upright position when possible

Employ special devices where appropriate (e.g., fracture pan, commode, elevated toilet seat); modify utensils when indicated

Carry out bowel training program with hydration, high fiber diet, stool softeners, and mild laxatives if needed

Provide privacy

EXPECTED OUTCOME

Child has daily bowel movement

NURSING DIAGNOSIS: Altered patterns of urinary elimination related to discomfort, positioning

GOAL

Stimulate voiding

INTERVENTIONS

Position as upright as possible to void

Hydrate to adequate urinary output for age

Stimulate bladder emptying with warm water, running water, stroking suprapubic area

Catheterize as indicated

EXPECTED OUTCOME

Child voids without difficulty

See also:

Nursing care plan: The child with a chronic illness or disability, p. 259

Nursing care plan: The child undergoing surgery, p. 267

Nursing care plan: The child in pain, p. 279

Nursing care plan: The child with special nutritional needs, p. 277

Nursing care plan: The child with elevated body temperature, p. 271

Nursing care plan: The child with fluid and electrolyte disturbance, p. 272

Nursing care plan: The child at risk for infection, p. 288

Nursing care plan: The child who is terminally ill or dying, p. 292

Nursing care plan for specific health problem(s)

NURSING CARE PLAN:
THE FAMILY OF THE ILL OR HOSPITALIZED CHILD

A family is the coexistence of more than one human being involving continuous, presumably permanent, sharing of living facilities, a perception of reciprocal obligations, a sense of commonness, and sharing of certain obligations toward each other and toward others (Mauksch, 1974).

Factors that influence parental responses to illness of a child:

The seriousness of the threat to their child

Previous experience with illness or hospitalization

Medical procedures involved in diagnosis and treatment

Available support systems

Personal ego strengths

Previous coping abilities

Additional stresses on the family system

Cultural and religious beliefs

Communication patterns among family members

Factors that influence sibling's responses to illness/ hospitalization of the child:

Fear of contracting the illness

Younger age

Close relationship to sick sibling

Out-of-home residence during period of hospitalization

Minimal explanation of the sick child's illness

Perceived changes in parenting, such as increased parental anger

ASSESSMENT

See Family assessment, p. 58.

Observe behavior of family members.

NURSING DIAGNOSIS: Anxiety/fear related to situational crisis, threat to role functioning, change in environment

GOAL

Help family adjust to the hospital

INTERVENTIONS

Introduce family to significant staff members
Describe hospital routine that affects the child
Acclimate family to the new and strange surroundings
  Physical layout of unit including playroom, unit kitchen, toilet, telephone, where they can stay
Direct family to areas they may need to use outside the unit (e.g., dining room, chapel)
Provide an atmosphere that promotes questioning, expression of doubts and feelings
Be available to family
Be alert to signs of tension in family members
Provide for privacy

EXPECTED OUTCOMES

Family demonstrates familiarity with hospital environment
Family members ask questions

GOAL

Make family feel important as members of the health team

INTERVENTIONS

Employ a polite approach and demeanor
Greet family by name when they arrive on the unit
Encourage frequent visiting
Include family in planning patient care
Encourage family to select and assume specific roles in the child's care
Offer encouragement for their efforts
Ask family to share with the staff what they know about the child's care and needs
Convey an attitude of collegiality with family—not competition

EXPECTED OUTCOME

Family becomes involved in planning and carrying out care for the child

GOAL

Reduce apprehension

INTERVENTIONS

Allow for expression of feelings about the child's hospitalization and illness
Provide needed information
Prepare family for what to expect (e.g., procedures, behaviors)
Explore family's concerns and feelings of irritation, guilt, anger, disappointment, inadequacy
Explore family's fears and anxieties regarding the child's status and expectations of results of procedures or therapy
Introduce parents to other families who have a child in the hospital—especially a child who is similarly affected

Provide something constructive for family to focus on (e.g., keeping record of intake and output, pain relief record, ensuring a specified amount of fluid intake, collecting a specimen)

EXPECTED OUTCOMES

Family members verbalize feelings and concerns
Family demonstrates an understanding of procedures and behaviors (specify manner of demonstration and learning)
Family interacts with other families
Family complies with directions (specify)

GOAL

Prepare family for special procedures (x-ray, diagnostic tests, surgery)

INTERVENTIONS

Assess family's understanding of the procedure and its purpose
Provide needed information, clarify misconceptions
Explain special preparation needed (e.g., NPO, shaving, preprocedure medication or equipment)
Describe
  Where the child will be during the procedure
  Whether the family can be with the child
  Where the family can wait
  Approximate length of time procedure requires
Reassure family that they will be notified regarding progress of the procedure

EXPECTED OUTCOME

Family demonstrates an understanding of procedures and tests (specify)

GOAL

Support the family during child's absence

INTERVENTIONS

Provide a comfortable place for the family to wait
Suggest activities to help reduce anxiety (e.g., go to the coffee shop or dining room, take a short walk [specify activity])
Be available to family
Make contact with family at frequent intervals to relay information, provide comforts

EXPECTED OUTCOME

Family takes advantage of suggestions (specify)

GOAL

Help family adjust to the child's appearance and behavior following procedure(s) or in special care unit

INTERVENTIONS

Remain calm
Describe the environment, if appropriate (e.g., ICU)
Apply principles of learning to explanations
  Begin with small amounts of information
  Begin with very general information
  Allow ample time for family to absorb information and to ask questions

Explain how the child will look and the reasons for his appearance and equipment
Explain what the child is experiencing
Prepare the child and surroundings to lessen the impact of first impression
  Tidy the bed
  Personalize the bed and bedside with a toy or other item(s)
  Provide chairs for the family
  Be prepared for possible adverse reaction (e.g., fainting)
Convey an attitude of caring *about* as well as *for* the child
Accompany the family to the child's bedside

EXPECTED OUTCOME

Family comes to child's bedside without evidence of distress

GOAL

Alleviate fears

INTERVENTIONS

Help family distinguish between realistic and unfounded fears
Help eliminate unfounded fears
Discuss with family their fears regarding
  Child's signs and symptoms
  Child's anxiety
  Dire consequences of disease or therapy
  Deterioration of child's condition
  Tests and procedures
  Death
Answer questions honestly and compassionately

EXPECTED OUTCOME

Family members verbalize fears and explore nature and ramifications of these fears

NURSING DIAGNOSIS: Powerlessness related to health care environment

GOAL

Provide a sense of control

INTERVENTIONS

Encourage family visiting at times convenient for them (there will be cultural variations in the amount and type of visiting)
Allow expression of concerns regarding the child's care and progress
Explore the family's feelings regarding prescribed therapies
Permit the family as much control as possible in the child's management
  Encourage participation in the child's care
  Include family in setting goals for care
  Involve family in scheduling and other aspects of care
  Explain what family can do for the child and how to handle the child to maintain therapy (e.g., how to pick up the child with an IV)
  Employ family's suggestions regarding the child's care whenever possible

EXPECTED OUTCOMES

Family schedules visiting times
Family readily discusses feelings and concerns
Family contributes to care and management of the child
*Family's suggestions are incorporated into plan of care

NURSING DIAGNOSIS: Altered family processes related to situational crisis (threat to role functioning, hospitalization of a child)

GOAL

Help family understand the child's illness

INTERVENTIONS

Recognize family concern and need for information and support
Assess family's understanding of the diagnosis and the plan of care
Reinforce and clarify health professional's explanation of the child's condition, suggested procedures and therapies, and the prognosis
Use every opportunity to increase the family's understanding of the disease and its therapies
Repeat information as often as necessary
Interpret technical information
Help family interpret the infant's or child's behaviors and responses
Do not appear rushed—if time is inappropriate, set a date for discussion as soon as feasible
  Keep appointment meticulously

EXPECTED OUTCOME

Family demonstrates an understanding of the disease and its therapies (specify knowledge)

GOAL

Help alleviate guilt feelings

INTERVENTIONS

Provide accurate and specific information regarding the causes of the illness
Clarify misconceptions and false assumptions

EXPECTED OUTCOME

Family verbalizes their understanding of the cause of the illness (specify)

GOAL

Support family

INTERVENTIONS

Respect parental rights
Convey an attitude of respectful caring for both the child and the family
Support and emphasize the strengths and abilities of the family
Provide feedback and praise for compliance

*Nursing outcome.

Refer to other professionals for additional interpersonal and concrete support (e.g., social service, clergy)

EXPECTED OUTCOMES

Family exhibits behaviors that indicate a feeling of self-respect
Family avails itself of supportive services

GOAL

Help family cope with the child's behavior

INTERVENTIONS

Determine family's understanding of the normal childhood responses to stress of illness and hospitalization
Explain child's regression, magical thinking, egocentricity, separation anxiety, fears
Explain behavioral reactions generally expected of the child (specify according to age and developmental level)
Explain what the child is (family are) permitted to do in coping with the child's behavior
Reinforce family's endeavors

EXPECTED OUTCOME

Family demonstrates an understanding of the child's unfamiliar behaviors (specify manner of demonstration—verbalization, physical attitude, behaviors with child)

GOAL

Help family assist the child to cope with hospitalization

INTERVENTIONS

Help parents determine the best way to prepare the child for hospitalization, procedures
Provide family with precise information about what will take place so they know what the child is likely to experience
Encourage family to trust the child's capacity to cope
Impress upon family the need for honesty in relating to the child
Encourage family to use play as a coping strategy
Suggest appropriate items to bring to the child (e.g., pajamas, favorite toys)
See also The child in the hospital, p. 246

EXPECTED OUTCOMES

Family helps in planning strategies
Family is honest with the child and staff
Family uses play as a tool for relating with the child

GOAL

Promote and foster positive family relationships

INTERVENTIONS

Recognize that family members know the child best and are "cued in" to the child's needs
Allow unlimited visiting times
Encourage family to bring other significant family members to visit (e.g., siblings, grandparents, and [where permitted] pets)
Encourage family to provide the child with significant, but manageable, items from home

EXPECTED OUTCOMES

Child and family exhibit behaviors that indicate positive coping
Family visits child at appropriate times and in appropriate numbers
Child demonstrates an attitude of security with familiar persons and things

GOAL

Promote family health

INTERVENTIONS

Stress the importance of maintaining family members' health during the child's illness and hospitalization
Encourage adequate rest
    Provide sleeping facilities where possible
    Encourage members to alternate visiting with the child to allow some time at home
    Explore means for respite care of dependent family members
Convey to family the assurance that the child will receive optimum care in their absence
Provide relief for family from direct care of child as needed
Promote adequate nutrition
    Provide meals for parents if possible
    Direct family to nutritious resources for meals
    Encourage regular mealtimes away from unit

EXPECTED OUTCOMES

Family shows no evidence of illness
Family members appear well rested
Family members eat regularly

GOAL

Promote a smooth transition from hospital to home

INTERVENTIONS

Assess the learning needs of the family
Outline and carry out a teaching plan
Determine services needed and make necessary referrals
Include family in planning and problem solving
Maintain open communication between family and health care providers

EXPECTED OUTCOME

Child and family demonstrate the ability to provide needed care in the home

GOAL

Prepare for discharge

INTERVENTIONS

Assess the family's knowledge
Teach family the skills needed to carry out the therapeutic program (specify)
    Allow ample time for preparation
    Teach necessary techniques and observations
    Help family by demonstration
        Distribute appropriate Home Care Instructions or other educational materials or both
    Encourage questions and expression of feelings and concerns

Unit 4

Allow sufficient time for family to perform procedures under supervision

Inform parents of

Signs of progress to observe for

Any unfavorable signs to be alert for

Problems that can be anticipated (e.g., care of equipment or devices)

Behaviors that indicate special needs (e.g., pain medication, imminent seizures)

A course of action to follow (e.g., seizure care, CPR)

Make certain family knows how to contact appropriate persons if or when needed

Prepare family for possible posthospital behaviors of the child

Ensure family's comprehension of the child's needs before discharge

EXPECTED OUTCOMES

Family demonstrates the procedures needed to care for the child in the home (specify learning and method of demonstration)

Family is aware of how to seek help

GOAL

Maintain continuity of care

INTERVENTIONS

Inform family of community resources available

Refer to agencies as appropriate (specify)

Help identify support group(s) for family

Be available to family by telephone or other means

Schedule follow-up appointments as needed

Prepare family for possible unexpected posthospital behaviors (see box)

EXPECTED OUTCOMES

Family seeks appropriate assistance

Family keeps appointments

See also:

Nursing care plan: The child in the hospital, p. 246

Nursing care plan: The child with a chronic illness or disability, p. 259

Nursing care plan: The child who is terminally ill or dying, p. 292

POSTHOSPITAL BEHAVIORS IN CHILDREN

Young children

Some initial aloofness toward parents; may last from a few minutes (most common) to a few days

Frequently followed by dependency behaviors:

Tendency to cling to parents

Demand parents' attention

Vigorously oppose any separation, e.g., staying at nursery school or with a baby-sitter

Other negative behaviors include:

New fears, e.g., nightmares

Resistance to going to bed, night waking

Withdrawal and shyness

Hyperactivity

Temper tantrums

Food finickiness

Attachment to blanket or toy

Regression in newly learned skills, e.g., self-toileting

Older children

Negative behaviors include:

Emotional coldness, followed by intense, demanding dependence on parents

Anger toward parents

Jealousy toward others, i.e., siblings

NURSING CARE PLAN:
THE CHILD WITH A CHRONIC ILLNESS OR DISABILITY

Chronic illness—A condition that interferes with daily functioning for more than 3 months in a year, causes hospitalization of more than 1 month in a year, or (at time of diagnosis) is likely to do either of these (Hobbs and Perrin, 1985).

Disability—Broadly, refers to a loss of function (Reynolds, 1984).

Developmental disability—Any severe, chronic disability that is attributable to a mental (cognitive) and/or physical impairment, is manifested before age 22 years, is likely to continue indefinitely, results in substantial limitation of function, and requires special services (Golden, 1984).

ASSESSMENT

Perform physical assessment with special emphasis on specific condition

Take careful history of possible causative factors (initial assessment), progress and management of condition, child and family coping

Observe for manifestations of specific condition

Assist with diagnostic procedures and tests appropriate to specific condition

---

NURSING DIAGNOSIS: Altered growth and development related to chronic illness or disability, parental reactions (overbenevolence), repeated hospitalization

Infant

See Summary of growth and development during infancy, p. 134

GOAL

Promote development of a sense of trust

INTERVENTIONS

Encourage consistent caregivers in hospital or other care settings

Meet infant's needs promptly as they arise

EXPECTED OUTCOMES

Infant has consistent caregivers

Infant's needs are met promptly

GOAL

Promote parent-child attachment/bonding

INTERVENTIONS

Encourage parents to visit frequently or "room in" during hospitalization and to participate in care

Emphasize healthy, perfect qualities of infant

Help parents learn special care needs of infant for them to feel competent

EXPECTED OUTCOMES

Parents and infant demonstrate attachment behaviors

Parents learn to care for infant

GOAL

Facilitate sensorimotor development

INTERVENTIONS

Expose infant to pleasurable experiences via all intact senses (touch, hearing, sight, taste, movement)

Encourage age-appropriate developmental skills (i.e., sitting unsupported, holding bottle, finger feeding, crawling)

Encourage all family members to participate in stimulation

Enroll in infant stimulation program, if appropriate

EXPECTED OUTCOMES

Infant engages in appropriate sensorimotor experiences

Infant learns age-appropriate skills (specify)

GOAL

Facilitate development of a sense of separateness from parent (older infant)

INTERVENTION

Encourage parents to take periodic respites from burdens of care responsibilities

EXPECTED OUTCOME

Infant has opportunities to separate from parent

Unit 4

Toddler

See Summary of growth and development during toddlerhood, p. 140

GOAL

Promote development of a sense of autonomy

INTERVENTIONS

Encourage independence in as many areas as possible within child's capabilities (i.e., toileting, dressing, feeding)
Offer simple choices to allow opportunities for control
Reinforce the concept that negative and ritualistic behavior are normal and expected
Institute age-appropriate discipline and limit-setting, keeping in mind the limitations of child's condition

EXPECTED OUTCOMES

Child engages in independent activities appropriate for age and limitations
Parents demonstrate an understanding of typical toddler behavior
Family carries out appropriate discipline strategies

GOAL

Promote locomotion

INTERVENTIONS

Provide opportunities for gross motor skill activity
Help family modify toys or locomotion equipment to facilitate movement

EXPECTED OUTCOME

Child achieves appropriate motor skills and independent locomotion

GOAL

Promote development of language

INTERVENTIONS

Provide opportunities for child to use language
Encourage nonverbal communication wherever appropriate
Provide alternative means of communication when speech is severely impaired, e.g., symbols

EXPECTED OUTCOME

Child communicates needs and wants appropriately (specify)

GOAL

Facilitate learning through sensorimotor experience, beginning preoperational thought

INTERVENTION

Provide a variety of play experiences, especially sensory play, e.g., water play, sandbox, finger paint, swing

EXPECTED OUTCOME

Child engages in appropriate sensorimotor experiences

Preschool

See Summary of growth and development during preschool years, p. 142

GOAL

Promote development of a sense of initiative and purpose

INTERVENTIONS

Encourage mastery of self-help skills
Provide devices that make task easier (i.e., self-dressing or feeding)

EXPECTED OUTCOME

Child achieves independence as expected for age and capabilities

GOAL

Develop social relationships with peers

INTERVENTIONS

Encourage socialization, such as inviting friends to play, daycare experience
Provide age-appropriate play, especially cooperative play opportunities
Help child deal with criticisms
Help family realize that too much protection prevents child from realities of world and may foster social isolation
Encourage relationships with same-sex and opposite-sex peers and adults

EXPECTED OUTCOMES

Child forms relationships with peers and adults
Child demonstrates beginning ability to deal with criticism

GOAL

Facilitate learning through preoperational thought (magical thinking)

INTERVENTIONS

Use simple means to explain aspects of child's condition
Clarify that cause of illness or disability is not child's fault or a punishment

EXPECTED OUTCOME

Child has beginning understanding of condition without self-blame

GOAL

Facilitate control of body wastes

INTERVENTIONS

Encourage bowel and bladder control
Help child and family learn any special skills needed, e.g., bowel training techniques, ostomy care

EXPECTED OUTCOME

Child achieves bowel and bladder control

School-age

See Summary of growth and development during school-age years, p. 146

GOAL

Promote development of sense of industry and accomplishment

INTERVENTIONS

Educate teachers and classmates about child's condition, abilities, and special needs
Encourage school attendance
    Schedule medical visits at times other than school
    Provide opportunity to make up missed work
Provide opportunities for informal education, learning, and accomplishment
    Encourage sports activities (i.e., Special Olympics)
    Encourage socialization (i.e., Girl Scouts, Campfire Girls, having a best friend or joining a club)

EXPECTED OUTCOME

Child attends school and has opportunities to achieve according to own interests and capabilities

GOAL

Promote learning through concrete operations

INTERVENTIONS

Provide child with knowledge about condition

EXPECTED OUTCOME

Child demonstrates an understanding of condition

GOAL

Promote development of appropriate masculine or feminine social role

INTERVENTIONS

Encourage involvement in culturally and socially defined sex role activities
Provide appropriate sex role models
Encourage interaction with same sex and opposite sex peers

EXPECTED OUTCOME

Child develops the appropriate sex role

Adolescent

See Summary of growth and development during adolescence, p. 148

GOAL

Promote development of personal and sexual identity

INTERVENTIONS

Discuss with teenager the difficulties he/she is experiencing as a part of normal adolescence (i.e., rebelliousness, risk-taking, lack of cooperation)
Encourage activities appropriate for age, such as attending mixed-sex parties, sports activities, driving a car (when possible)
Help parents understand that adolescent has same sexual needs and concerns as any other teenager

EXPECTED OUTCOMES

Adolescent forms relationships with same sex and opposite sex peers
Adolescent demonstrates the appearance and manner of his/her gender
Parents demonstrate an understanding of adolescent sexual needs and concerns

GOAL

Achieve independence from family

INTERVENTIONS

Involve adolescent and family in discussion regarding teenager's potential for independence outside the home
Explore appropriate educational/vocational pursuits
Encourage socialization with peers, including peers with special needs and those without special needs

EXPECTED OUTCOMES

Adolescent achieves independence according to child's potential
Adolescent develops a realistic concept of his/her capabilities and engages in suitable educational/vocational activities

GOAL

Promote learning through abstract reasoning

INTERVENTIONS

Explore with adolescent future issues (e.g., employment, marriage, financial support)
Discuss planning for future and how condition can affect choices (i.e., inheritance of disease and child-bearing)

EXPECTED OUTCOME

Adolescent demonstrates an understanding of the condition and how it affects future choices

---

NURSING DIAGNOSIS: Altered family processes related to situational crisis (child with a chronic disease or disability)

GOAL

Help family adjust to the diagnosis

INTERVENTIONS

Provide opportunity for family to adjust to discovery of diagnosis
Anticipate the usual grief reaction to loss of "perfect" child
Explore family's feelings regarding the child and their ability to cope with the disorder
Encourage family to express their concerns
Repeat information as often as necessary
Serve as a role model regarding attitudes and behavior toward the child

EXPECTED OUTCOMES

Parents verbalize feelings and concerns regarding implications of the disease
Family demonstrates an attitude of acceptance and adjustment

GOAL

Increase family's understanding of the disorder

INTERVENTIONS

Assist family to understand the disorder, its therapies, and implications
Reinforce information given by others
Clarify misconceptions
Provide accurate information at a rate family can absorb
Discuss advantages and limitations of therapeutic plan
Encourage family to ask questions and express concerns

EXPECTED OUTCOME

Family demonstrates an understanding of the disease (specify)

GOAL

Reduce family's fears and anxieties

INTERVENTIONS

Explore family's concerns and feelings of irritation, guilt, anger, disappointment, inadequacy
Help family distinguish between realistic fears and eliminate unfounded fears
Discuss with parents their fears regarding
    Dealing with the child's anxiety about his condition
    Fear of dreadful developments
    Fear of death
    Fear of tests and procedures
    Child's ability to compete with peers
Explore their feelings regarding prescribed therapies

EXPECTED OUTCOME

Family members discuss their fears and concerns

GOAL

Promote positive adaptation to the child

INTERVENTIONS

Explore family's reaction to the child and the disorder
Assess family's coping skills, abilities, and resources
Help family to achieve a realistic view of the child and capabilities and limitations
Foster positive family relationships
Assess interpersonal relationships within the family, especially behaviors that reflect family attitudes toward the affected child
Intervene appropriately if there is evidence of maladaptation
Encourage parents in their attempts to promote child's development
Emphasize positive aspects of the child's abilities or attributes
Help family gain confidence in their ability to cope with the child, the disorder, and its impact on other family members

EXPECTED OUTCOMES

Family verbalizes feelings and concerns regarding the special needs of the child and their effect on the family process

Family members demonstrate an attitude of confidence in their ability to cope

GOAL

Promote family's ability to provide child's care

INTERVENTIONS

Help family develop a thorough plan of care
Teach skills needed to provide optimum care
Interpret child's behavior to parents (e.g., anger, depression, regression, physical modifications as a result of disorder)
Help family plan for the future

EXPECTED OUTCOME

Family sets realistic goals for selves, child, and others

GOAL

Foster growth-promoting family relationships

INTERVENTIONS

Identify family support systems (immediate family, extended family, friends, health service providers)
Assess systematically the number, affiliation, and interrelationships (if any) of persons the family sees as important
Assist family to assign specific tasks to specific people
Reinforce positive coping mechanisms
Encourage family members to discuss their feelings about each other
Impress upon parents the importance of providing as normal a life as possible for the affected child
Help family feel adequate in their maternal-paternal roles by emphasizing growth and developmental progress of their child
Help family foster child's development by stimulating child to age-appropriate goals consistent with his activity tolerance

EXPECTED OUTCOMES

Family demonstrates positive, growth-promoting behaviors
Family avails itself of support

GOAL

Provide support

INTERVENTIONS

Be available to the family
Listen to family members—singly or collectively
Allow for expression of feelings including feelings of guilt, helplessness, and their perception of the impact that the condition may have (or does have) on the family
Refer to community agencies or special organizations providing assistance—financial, social, and support
Refer for genetic counseling if appropriate
Help family learn to expect feelings of frustration and anger toward the child; reassure that it is not a reflection on their parenting
Assist family in problem solving
Encourage interaction with other families who have a similarly affected child
    Introduce to families
    Provide information regarding support groups
Help families learn when to accept and when to "fight"

EXPECTED OUTCOMES

Family maintains contact with health providers
Family demonstrates an understanding of the needs of the child
and the impact the condition will have on them
Problems are dealt with early
Family becomes involved with local agencies and support
groups

GOAL

Prepare family for hospitalized child's discharge

INTERVENTIONS

Teach skills needed for home care
Assess home situation, including family's strengths, weaknesses,
and support systems
Help devise an individualized plan of care based on assessment
of family's needs and resources
Encourage family involvement in care while still in the hospital
Encourage family to ask questions regarding posthospital care
Explore family's attitudes toward the child's entry (or reentry)
into the home
Help family acquire needed drugs, supplies, and equipment
Refer to special agencies based on need assessment
Arrange for regular follow-up care to reassess effectiveness of
home management

EXPECTED OUTCOMES

Family demonstrates an understanding of needed skills (specify
skills and method of demonstration)
Family members avail themselves of resources within their community (specify)
Family complies with home care program

GOAL

Continue ongoing evaluation

INTERVENTIONS

Participate in follow-up care
Coordinate team management of child and family
Be alert to comments by child or family members that indicate
possible problems
Assess interpersonal relationships within the family, especially
behaviors that reflect family attitudes toward the child
Be alert for cues that signal undue anxiety and guilt; preoccupation with causative factors, constant analysis of effects of
therapies, experimentation with diets and folk remedies,
seeking magical cures
Be alert for overprotective behaviors such as assuming self-care
activities for child, restricting child's activities of interaction
with peers
Allow family to express discouragement at interference with
activities and what appears to be slow progress

EXPECTED OUTCOMES

Family participates in follow-up care
Family expresses both positive and negative reactions to child's
progress
*Signs that may indicate family's difficulty in adjusting to the
child's condition are identified early.

---

*Nursing outcome

GOAL

Support siblings of affected child

INTERVENTIONS

Assess siblings to identify areas of concern
Communicate honestly with siblings about the child's disease
or disability
Provide opportunity for siblings to ask questions and express
feelings but avoid lengthy explanations before they ask
Help parents talk to siblings about the child's condition and
interpret the siblings' needs and questions
Encourage parents to spend special time with their child (or
children) who are not ill or disabled
Help siblings and family understand that it is normal for them
to have negative feelings about the child
Prepare siblings in advance for any household changes
Allow sibling(s) to participate in the child's care and therapy as
appropriate
Help siblings learn how to explain the child's condition to their
peers and others
Acknowledge siblings' strengths and abilities to cope
Refer to sibling groups and networks composed of siblings of
children with the same or similar conditions
Assess siblings periodically to determine their adjustment to the
family situation

EXPECTED OUTCOMES

Siblings verbalize or otherwise demonstrate their feelings and
concerns
Parents include siblings in discussions of the disabled child
Parents make an effort to spend time with other children
Siblings exhibit an understanding of household changes
Siblings assist with affected child's care (specify)
Siblings become involved in support groups (specify)

**NURSING DIAGNOSIS: Anxiety/fear related to tests,
procedures, hospitalization, etc. (specify)**

GOAL

Prepare for tests and procedures, hospitalization, etc. (specify)

INTERVENTIONS

See Preparation for procedures, p. 211
See Nursing care plan: The child in the hospital, p. 246

EXPECTED OUTCOME

Child copes with stresses of procedures, tests, etc. (specify)

NURSING DIAGNOSIS: Potential for injury (specify)

GOAL

Decrease risk of injury

INTERVENTIONS

Assess environment for hazards if indicated
Teach safety precautions
Encourage activities that are compatible with the disease or
disability

EXPECTED OUTCOME

Child remains free of injury and complications

GOAL

Help child adjust to restricted activities

INTERVENTIONS

Help devise alternatives for restricted activities and help child cope with physical limitations

EXPECTED OUTCOME

Child demonstrates appropriate adaptation to limitations (specify)

GOAL

Prevent complications

INTERVENTIONS

Stress importance of sound health practices and frequent health supervision

Make certain child and family understand the therapeutic measures prescribed

Encourage older child to choose activities but take responsibility for own safety

Plan with allied personnel (e.g., teachers, coaches, counselors) appropriate activities

Confer with school nurse (or other person) regarding any special needs of the child

Discuss with parents any indicated limit-setting

EXPECTED OUTCOME

Child maintains optimum health

NURSING DIAGNOSIS: Diversional activity deficit related to environmental lack of diversion, physical limitations (specify), hospitalization

GOAL

Provide diversion

INTERVENTIONS

Provide appropriate stimulation

Encourage activities appropriate to age, interests, and capabilities of child

Encourage physical exercise that does not overtax the child (if indicated)

Incorporate therapeutic needs in play activities as appropriate

Supervise and encourage activities of daily living

Encourage child's natural tendency to be active

Encourage interaction with family and peers

Include child in planning and scheduling care

EXPECTED OUTCOMES

Child engages in age-appropriate activities within the limits of capabilities

Child accepts efforts of family and caregivers

GOAL

Discourage sedentary habits

INTERVENTIONS

Encourage child to participate in normal childhood activities commensurate with interests and capabilities

Encourage and reinforce age-appropriate behaviors, experiences, and socialization with peers

Discourage physical inactivity

EXPECTED OUTCOME

Child engages in nonsedentary activities within the limits of disability

---

NURSING DIAGNOSIS: Impaired social interaction related to hospitalization, confinement to home, frequent illness, activity intolerance, fatigue (specify)

GOAL

Promote interpersonal relationships

INTERVENTIONS

Encourage to maintain usual activities

Arrange for continued interpersonal contacts while hospitalized or otherwise confined

Provide opportunities for interaction with others, especially peers

Encourage regular school attendance (including daycare, beginning school, return to school)

Arrange for rest periods at school if needed

Promote peer contact wherever possible

Encourage recreational outlets and after-school activities appropriate to the child's interests and capabilities

Discourage activities that increase isolation from others

EXPECTED OUTCOMES

Child engages in appropriate activities

Child associates with peers and family

Child attends school with reasonable regularity

NURSING DIAGNOSIS: Self-care deficit (specify) related to specific impairment (specify)

GOAL

Promote self-help (self-care)

INTERVENTIONS

Teach child about the disease and therapies

Encourage child to assist in own care as age and capabilities permit

Provide and/or help devise methods to facilitate maximum functioning

Incorporate play that encourages desired behavior

Select toys and activities that allow maximum participation by the child

Modify environment if needed (specify)

Assist with self-care activities where needed (specify)
Avoid undue persistence to accomplish a goal
Provide incentives to achieve desired behavior
Instruct when to seek assistance from family or health care providers

EXPECTED OUTCOME

Child engages in self-help activities commensurate with capabilities (specify activities and extent of involvement)

GOAL

Enhance child's sense of competence and mastery

INTERVENTIONS

Capitalize on child's assets; help child compensate for liabilities
Praise child for accomplishments and "near" accomplishments, such as partial completion of a task
Ensure adequate rest before attempting energy-expending activities
Emphasize the child's abilities and focus on realistic endeavors
Emphasize positive coping behaviors
Discourage activities that are beyond the child's capabilities; promote and reinforce successful endeavors
Encourage participation in own care to the extent that child is able
Teach and encourage responsibility for use of equipment, appliances, testing, medication (specify)
Help child become adept at self-management to maximum capabilities

EXPECTED OUTCOMES

Child takes responsibility for self-care according to age and capabilities (specify)
Child engages in appropriate activities without undue fatigue

---

NURSING DIAGNOSIS: Body image disturbance related to perception of disability (self and others), feeling of differentness, inability to participate in specific activities (specify)

GOAL

Meet child's emotional needs

INTERVENTIONS

Convey an attitude of understanding, caring, and acceptance
Avoid conveying an attitude of intrusion
Maintain open communications with child
Relate to the child on appropriate cognitive level
Serve as a role model for others

EXPECTED OUTCOME

Child maintains a positive attitude (specify behaviors)

GOAL

Determine extent of disturbance

INTERVENTIONS

Encourage verbalization of feelings and perceptions, especially feelings of "differentness"
Explore feelings concerning disease or disability and its implications: stress of being "different," physical limitations, difficulty competing, relationships with peers, self-image
Encourage child to discuss feelings about how he/she thinks others feel about the disorder

EXPECTED OUTCOME

Child openly discusses feelings and concerns about the condition, therapies, and perceived reactions of others

GOAL

Help child cope with actual and perceived differentness

INTERVENTIONS

Acknowledge feelings and facilitate sharing feelings with family and other health professionals
Clarify misconceptions child may have acquired
Assist child to identify positive aspects of situation

EXPECTED OUTCOME

Child discusses the disorder and feelings regarding limitations imposed by it

GOAL

Assist child in adjusting to the disorder and its effects

INTERVENTIONS

Help child assess own strengths and assets; emphasize strengths
Identify coping behaviors
Support positive coping mechanisms and extinguish negative ones
Help child set realistic goals
Encourage as much independence as condition allows
Introduce child to other children who have adjusted well to this or a similar disorder
Suggest involvement with special groups and facilities for children with similar problems

EXPECTED OUTCOMES

Child identifies own assets and strengths realistically
Child verbalizes positive suggestions for adjusting to the disability
Child becomes involved with special group activities

GOAL

Help child build self-esteem and a positive self-concept

INTERVENTIONS

Encourage an appealing physical appearance: good body hygiene, clean straight teeth, good grooming, stylish clothing, makeup for teenage girls
Assist with improving appearance and grooming
Point out positive aspects of own coping, appearance, and other capabilities

Unit 4

Promote constructive thinking in child; encourage to maximize strengths
Reinforce positive behaviors
Assist child to determine and engage in activities that foster self-esteem
Promote independence

EXPECTED OUTCOMES

Child demonstrates a positive appearance and attitude (specify)
Child appears clean, well groomed, and attractively dressed
Child exhibits behaviors that indicate elevated self-esteem (specify)

GOAL

Provide child with appropriate feeling of control

INTERVENTIONS

Channel need for control and feeling of effectiveness in appropriate directions
Encourage child to monitor own care as appropriate
Provide opportunities for child to make choices and participate in care when appropriate
Assist the child with vocational planning when appropriate

EXPECTED OUTCOME

Child becomes actively involved in own care and management

GOAL

Help prepare hospitalized child for discharge

INTERVENTIONS

Begin early in hospitalization to discuss "going home"
Help child develop independence and self-help capabilities
Encourage visits from friends to help child assess the impact of any change in appearance or behavior that might interfere with returning to previous environments

EXPECTED OUTCOME

Child verbalizes and otherwise demonstrates interest in going home

See also:
Nursing care plan: The child in the hospital, p. 246
Nursing care plan: The family of the ill or hospitalized child, p. 254
Nursing care plan: The child who is terminally ill or dying, p. 292
Nursing care plan: Child and family compliance, p. 296

NURSING CARE OF COMMON PROBLEMS OF ILL AND HOSPITALIZED CHILDREN

Children are admitted to the hospital for a variety of health problems. Some experiences are the same for all children (e.g., admission); others are shared by a number of children in their unique circumstances. The following are some of the problems that are experienced frequently but not universally by children in the hospital.

NURSING CARE PLAN:
THE CHILD UNDERGOING SURGERY

I. Preoperative care

ASSESSMENT

Perform physical assessment (see p. 10)
Assess the child's understanding of the impending surgery and postoperative expectations

Assess child for any evidence of infection
Review results of laboratory tests for abnormal findings

NURSING DIAGNOSIS: Potential for injury related to surgical procedure, anesthesia

GOAL

Ensure legal authorization

INTERVENTIONS

Check chart for signed informed consent form or obtain informed consent
  Contact physician to determine if parents have been informed of procedure (informed consent is physician's responsibility)
Obtain and/or witness signature if not obtained earlier

EXPECTED OUTCOME

*Appropriate permissions are obtained

GOAL

Provide hygienic preparation

INTERVENTIONS

Bathe child, groom hair
Provide mouth care
Check for loose teeth
  Inform anesthesiologist if detected

---

*Nursing outcome

Cleanse operative site according to prescribed method, if ordered

EXPECTED OUTCOME

Child is cleansed and prepared appropriately (specify)

GOAL

Provide physical preparation

INTERVENTIONS

Carry out special procedures as prescribed, e.g., colonic enemas
Administer antibiotics as ordered, observing for known side effects
Order and/or assist with special tests such as radiographs
Consult with physician for appropriate change in schedule or route of administration of any medication child ordinarily receives
Attire child appropriately (e.g., special operating room gown)
  Allow child to wear underwear or pajama bottoms, if possible
  Label personal articles and clothing
Remove any makeup and/or nail polish (to observe for cyanosis)
Remove jewelry and/or prosthetic devices (e.g., mouth retainers)

EXPECTED OUTCOME

Child is prepared appropriately (specify)

GOAL

Prevent complications

INTERVENTIONS

Maintain child NPO (nothing by mouth) usually 12 hours before surgery (prevents aspiration from vomiting during anesthesia [gag reflex is depressed]; last feeding indicated by physician)

Maintain infant NPO 2-4 hours

Be sure child is well hydrated before NPO begins, especially infants

Take and record vital signs

Report any deviations from admission readings, especially elevated temperature, which may indicate infection

Have child void before preoperative medication is administered to prevent bladder distention or incontinence during anesthesia

Record time of last voiding if unable to void

Be certain allergies are clearly indicated on chart

Check laboratory values for any sign of systemic abnormality, such as infection (increased white blood cells), anemia (decreased hemoglobin and/or hematocrit), or bleeding tendencies (reduced platelets or prolonged bleeding or clotting time

EXPECTED OUTCOMES

Child is NPO for designated time preoperatively

Child voids

Pertinent information about child is visible

GOAL

Ensure safety

INTERVENTIONS

Ascertain that identification band is securely fastened

Check identification band with surgical personnel

Fasten siderails of bed or crib

Use restraints during transport by use of stretcher (or other conveyance)

Do not leave child unattended

Explain what is happening, unless child is asleep

EXPECTED OUTCOME

Child is safe from immediate harm

GOAL

Prepare to receive child on return from surgery

INTERVENTIONS

Collect needed equipment for assessment and recording (e.g., record sheets, IV pole, restraints, thermometer, BP apparatus)

Turn down covers or prepare surgical bed as appropriate

EXPECTED OUTCOME

*Room is prepared for child's return from surgery

---

*Nursing outcome.

NURSING DIAGNOSIS: Anxiety/fear related to separation from support system, unfamiliar environment, knowledge deficit

GOAL

Increase child's sense of security

INTERVENTIONS

Institute preoperative teaching

Orient child to strange surroundings

Explain where parents will be while child is in operating room

EXPECTED OUTCOME

Child demonstrates minimum insecurity or anxiety

GOAL

Prepare child and family for expected surgical procedure and postoperative care

INTERVENTIONS

Prepare for postoperative procedures, as indicated, such as nasogastric tube, intravenous fluids, nothing by mouth, dressing changes, and wound drains if necessary

Explain reason for surgery: if special operative procedure is to be performed, explain basic principles and brief outline of care needed

Explain all preoperative procedures, such as blood work and any other laboratory test

In emergency situation, explain most essential components of surgery, such as where child will be before and after surgery, anesthesia, and dressing on abdomen

Accept behavioral reactions of parents and child

EXPECTED OUTCOMES

Child and family demonstrate an understanding of forthcoming events (specify methods of learning and evaluation)

*Family's behavioral reactions are accepted and supported

GOAL

Achieve optimum relaxation and sedation before child arrives in operating room

INTERVENTIONS

Administer preoperative sedation (preferably oral), as ordered

Place unfamiliar equipment out of child's view

Place child in quiet room with minimal distraction

Do not leave child unattended

Explain what is happening, unless child is asleep

Encourage parents to stay with child as long as permitted

Permit parent to hold child until falls asleep, if desired

Encourage parents to accompany child as far as possible, preferably through induction of anesthesia

Allow for significant objects to accompany child (e.g., a favorite toy)

EXPECTED OUTCOMES

Child falls asleep or lies quietly

Child is not left alone

---

*Nursing outcome.

NURSING DIAGNOSIS: Altered family processes related to a surgical procedure

GOAL

Support and reassure family

INTERVENTIONS

Reinforce and clarify information given by the physician
Explain associated diagnostic tests and procedures such as x-ray examinations, ECG
Explain child's schedule
    When the child will receive premedication
    Time the child will leave for surgery
    Where parents can wait for the child to return
    Room to which the child will return
    Postprocedural care and routines
Explore family's feelings regarding the procedure and its implications
Include parents in the preparation of the child
Be available to family
See also The family of the ill or hospitalized child, p. 254

EXPECTED OUTCOMES

Family demonstrates an understanding of procedure (specify demonstration) and related information (specify)
Family complies with directives (specify)

Postoperative care

ASSESSMENT

Ensure that preparations are made to receive child
Obtain baseline information:
    Take vital signs, including BP; keep BP cuff in place, deflated in order to lessen amount of disturbance to child
    Take and record more frequently if any value fluctuates
    Inspect operative area
        Check dressing if present
        Outline any bleeding area on dressing or cast with pen
        Reinforce, but do not remove, loose dressing
        Observe areas below surgical site for blood that may have drained toward bed
        Assess for bleeding and other symptoms in areas not covered with a dressing, such as throat following tonsillectomy
    Assess skin color and characteristics

Assess level of consciousness, activity
Notify physician of any irregularities
Assess for evidence of pain (see The child in pain, p. 279)
Review surgeon's orders after completing initial assessment
Monitor vital signs as ordered
Check dressings for bleeding or other abnormalities
Check bowel sounds
Observe for signs of shock, abdominal distention, bleeding
Assess for bladder distention
Observe for signs of dehydration
Detect presence of infection
    Take vital signs every 2-4 hours, as ordered
    Collect or request needed specimens
    Inspect wound for signs of infection—redness, swelling, heat, pain, purulent drainage

NURSING DIAGNOSIS: Potential for injury related to surgical procedure, anesthesia

GOAL

Receive child on return from surgery

INTERVENTIONS

Place child in bed (unless transported in own bed or crib) using techniques appropriate to type of surgery
Hang IV and connect any needed equipment (e.g., suction apparatus, traction)
Place in position of comfort in accordance with surgeon's orders
Perform stat (immediate) activities

EXPECTED OUTCOME

Child is transferred to bed without injury and with minimum stress

GOAL

Promote wound healing and prevent wound infection

INTERVENTIONS

Use proper hand washing techniques, especially if wound drainage is present
Employ careful wound care
    Keep wound clean and dry
    Change dressings if indicated, whenever soiled; carefully dispose of soiled dressings
    Carry out special wound care as prescribed: irrigation, drain care, etc.
    Cleanse with prescribed preparation (if ordered)
    Apply antibacterial solutions and/or ointments as ordered
    Report any unusual appearance or drainage
Pin diapers below abdominal dressing to prevent contamination
When child begins oral feedings, provide nutritious diet as ordered
See Potential for infection, p. 288

EXPECTED OUTCOME

Child exhibits no evidence of wound infection

GOAL

Prevent other complications

INTERVENTIONS

Ambulate as prescribed
Maintain child NPO until fully awake
Encourage to void when awake
    Offer bedpan
    Boys may be allowed to stand at bedside
Notify physician if unable to void
Maintain abdominal decompression, chest tubes, or other equipment, if prescribed
Provide diet as prescribed; advance as appropriate

EXPECTED OUTCOME

Child exhibits no evidence of complications

NURSING DIAGNOSIS: Anxiety/fear related to surgery, unfamiliar environment, separation from support systems, discomfort

GOAL

Relieve anxiety

INTERVENTIONS

Maintain calm, reassuring manner
Encourage expression of feelings
Explain procedures and other activities before initiating
Answer questions and explain purposes of activities
Keep informed of progress
Remain with child as much as possible
Give encouragement and positive feedback for cooperation in care
See also The child in the hospital, p. 246
Encourage parental visiting as soon as child is awake
If emergency procedure, review child's memory of previous events

EXPECTED OUTCOMES

Child rests quietly and calmly
Discusses procedures and activities without evidence of anxiety

---

NURSING DIAGNOSIS: Pain related to surgical incision

GOAL

Relieve pain

INTERVENTIONS

See The child in pain, p. 279
Do not wait until child experiences severe pain to intervene
Avoid palpating the operative area unless necessary
Insert rectal tube, if indicated
Encourage to void, if appropriate
Administer mouth care
Lubricate nostril to decrease irritation from nasogastric tube, if present
Allow the child position of comfort if not contraindicated
Perform nursing activities and procedures (e.g., dressing change, deep breathing) after analgesia

* Administer analgesics prescribed
* Administer antiemetics as ordered
Monitor effectiveness of analgesics

EXPECTED OUTCOME

Child rests quietly and exhibits minimum or no evidence of pain (specify)

NURSING DIAGNOSIS: Potential fluid volume deficit related to NPO prior to and/or after surgery, loss of appetite, vomiting

GOAL

Promote adequate hydration

INTERVENTIONS

Monitor intravenous infusion at prescribed rate
    Attach pediatric intravenous apparatus if not done in operating room
Offer fluids as soon as ordered or child tolerates
    Start with small sips of water and advance as tolerated
    Avoid giving brown- or red-colored fluids (to distinguish old and fresh blood from oral fluids) in oral or abdominal surgery
Encourage to drink
    Tempt with favorite fluids
See also The child with fluid and electrolyte disturbance, p. 272

EXPECTED OUTCOMES

Child exhibits no evidence of dehydration
Child takes and retains fluid when allowed (specify)

NURSING DIAGNOSIS: Potential for infection related to weakened condition, presence of infective organisms

GOAL

Prevent respiratory complications

INTERVENTIONS

Assess need for pain medication before respiratory hygiene
Assist to turn, deep breathe
    Splint operative site with hand or pillow if possible before coughing (if coughing prescribed)
    Stimulate infant to cry
Assist with use of spirometer or blow bottle
Perform percussion and vibration, if indicated
Suction secretions if needed

EXPECTED OUTCOME

Lungs remain clear

---

*Dependent nursing action

NURSING DIAGNOSIS: Altered family processes related to situational crisis (emergency hospitalization of child), knowledge deficit

GOAL

Support and reassure child and family

INTERVENTIONS

Explain all procedures
Prepare child and family for surgery
Keep family informed of child's progress
Encourage expression of feelings
Review child's memory of events, if an emergency procedure
Refer to public health nurse if indicated
Refer to appropriate agency or persons for specific help (e.g., social service, clergy)
See also The child in the hospital, p. 246
See also The family of the hospitalized child, p. 254

EXPECTED OUTCOMES

Family discusses child's condition and therapies comfortably
Family demonstrates an awareness of child's progress (specify method of evaluation)
Family members avail themselves of appropriate assistance

GOAL

Instruct family regarding needed knowledge for home care

INTERVENTIONS

If dressing changes are required at home, teach parents sterile or aseptic procedures; provide written list of necessary equipment and instructions
Instruct parents regarding administration of medications (if ordered) including possible side effects and untoward reactions
Instruct parents in care and management of special procedures such as ostomy care, irrigations

EXPECTED OUTCOME

Family demonstrates an understanding of instructions (specify methods of learning and evaluation)

NURSING CARE PLAN
THE CHILD WITH ELEVATED BODY TEMPERATURE

Set point—The temperature around which body temperature is regulated
Hyperthermia—A situation in which body temperature exceeds the set point, which usually results from the body creating more heat than it can eliminate (such as in heat stroke, aspirin toxicity, or hyperthyroidism)

Fever—An elevation in set point such that body temperature is regulated at a higher level—Rectal temperature above 38° C (100.4° F); oral temperature above 37.8° C (100° F); axillary temperature above 37.2° C (99° F)
High fever   temperature above 40.4° C (105° F)
Harmful fever—Temperature above 41.7° C (107° F)

ASSESSMENT

Observe for clinical manifestations of fever

NURSING DIAGNOSIS: Ineffective thermoregulation related to inflammatory process, elevated environmental temperature (fever)

GOAL

Reduce body temperature

INTERVENTIONS

Reduce environmental temperature
Place in lightweight clothing
Expose skin to air
Increase air circulation
Avoid chilling; if child shivers, apply more clothing or blankets
*Administer antipyretic drug (acetaminophen in prescribed dosage, see p. 285)
Apply cool compresses to areas of skin such as the forehead
Monitor temperature to determine effectiveness of treatment

EXPECTED OUTCOME

Body temperature remains within the acceptable limits—see inside front cover

---

*Dependent nursing action.

NURSING DIAGNOSIS: Hyperthermia related to increased heat production

GOAL

Reduce body temperature

INTERVENTIONS

Apply cooling blanket or mattress
Give cool bath—20 to 30 minutes' duration

Wrap child in cool, moist towels—Change as needed; continue approximately 30 minutes
Avoid chilling
Monitor temperature to prevent excessive body cooling

EXPECTED OUTCOME

Temperature is reduced to acceptable limits—see inside front cover

NURSING CARE PLAN
THE CHILD WITH FLUID AND ELECTROLYTE DISTURBANCE

Dehydration
Isotonic (isosmotic, isonatremic)—Electrolyte and water deficits are present in approximately balanced proportion
Hypotonic (hyposmotic, hyponatremic)—Electrolyte deficit exceeds the water deficit

Hypertonic (hyperosmotic, hypernatremic)—water loss in excess of electrolyte loss
Fluid excess—Increased fluid retention
Edema—Abnormally large amounts of fluid in the interstitial spaces

ASSESSMENT

Take careful health history, especially regarding current health problem, e.g., length of illness, events that may have precipitated symptoms
Perform physical assessment
Observe for manifestations of fluid and electrolyte disturbances (Table 4-1)
Perform specific assessments:
　Intake and output—Accurate measurements of fluid intake and output are vital to the assessment of dehydration. This includes oral and parenteral intake and losses from urine, stools, vomiting, fistulas, nasogastric suction, sweat, and wound drainage.

Urine—Assess frequency, volume, and consistency of urine
Stools—Assess frequency, volume, and consistency of stools
Vomitus—Assess for volume, frequency, and type of vomiting
Sweating—Can be only estimated from frequency of clothing and linen changes
Vital signs—Temperature (normal, elevated, or lowered depending on degree of dehydration), pulse, and blood pressure
Skin—Assess for color, temperature, feel, turgor, and presence or absence of edema
Mucous membranes—Assess for moisture, color, and presence of and consistency of secretions; condition of tongue
Fontanel (infants)—Sunken, soft, normal
Sensory alterations—Presence of thirst
Assist with diagnostic procedures and tests—Urinalysis, blood chemistry, CBC, blood gases

Table 4-1. MANIFESTATIONS OF FLUID AND ELECTROLYTE DISTURBANCES

Observation	Significant variation	Probable imbalance	Comments
Take temperature	Elevated	Early water depletion Sodium excess	Elevated temperature will increase rate of water loss
	Lowered	Fluid volume deficit	Caused by reduced energy output Shock is outcome of severe fluid deficit
Take pulse	Rapid, weak, thready, easily obliterated	Circulatory collapse may result from fluid deficit, hemorrhage, plasma-to-interstitial fluid shift	Pulse rate should include assessment of volume and quality as well as rate
	Bounding, easily obliterated	Impending circulatory collapse Sodium deficit	Pulse may be influenced by activity or emotions
	Bounding, not easily obliterated	Fluid volume excess Interstitial fluid-to-plasma shift	
	Weak, irregular, rapid	Severe potassium deficit	
	Weak, irregular, slowing	Severe potassium excess	
	Increased	Sodium excess Magnesium deficit	
	Decreased	Magnesium excess	
Take respiration	Slow, shallow	Respiratory alkalosis	Rapid respirations increase water loss
	Rapid, deep	Metabolic acidosis	Not a reliable sign of respiratory alkalosis in infants
	Dyspnea	Fluid volume excess either general or pulmonary	
	Moist rales	Fluid volume excess Pulmonary edema	
	Shallow	Potassium excess or deficit	
	Stridor	Severe calcium deficit	
Take blood pressure	Increased	Fluid volume excess	Blood pressure not a reliable sign in young children
	Decreased	Sodium deficit Diminished vascular volume (loss or plasma-to-interstitial fluid shift) Severe potassium excess or deficit	Elasticity of blood vessels may keep blood pressure stable
Inspect skin for: Color	Pallor	Protein deficit	
	Flushed	Fluid deficit Fluid compartment shifts Sodium excess	
Temperature	Cold extremities	Severe fluid volume deficit, even with fever Severe sodium depletion	Caused by decreased peripheral blood flow
Feel	Dry	Fluid depletion	
	Clammy, cold	Sodium excess Sodium deficit Plasma-to-interstitial fluid shift Hypotonic dehydration	
	Poor capillary filling	Fluid volume deficit	
Turgor	Poor to very poor	Fluid depletion	Pinch of skin from abdomen or inner thigh is lifted and remains raised for several seconds

Continued.

Unit 4

Table 4-1. MANIFESTATIONS OF FLUID AND ELECTROLYTE DISTURBANCES—cont'd

Observation	Significant variation	Probable imbalance	Comments
Pitting edema	Slight to severe	Fluid volume excess Plasma-to-interstitial fluid shift	Obese infants may appear normal
Inspect mucous membranes	Dry Longitudinal wrinkles on tongue Sticky; rough, red, dry tongue	Fluid volume depletion Sodium excess Hypertonic dehydration	
Observe salivation and tearing	Absent	Fluid volume deficit	
Palpate fontanel	Sunken	Fluid volume deficit	
Palpate eyeballs	Sunken Soft	Fluid volume deficit	
Observe for sensory alterations	Tingling in fingers and toes	Calcium deficit Alkalosis	Sensory alterations unreliable in infants and young children who are unable to communicate symptoms
	Abdominal cramps	Sodium deficit Potassium excess	
	Muscle cramps	Calcium deficit Potassium deficit	
	Lightheadedness Nausea	Respiratory alkalosis Calcium excess Potassium excess Potassium deficit	
	Thirst	Fluid deficit Sodium excess Calcium excess	May be difficult to assess in infants May be masked by nausea Any condition that reduces intravascular volume will stimulate thirst receptors
Observe for neurologic signs	Hypotonia	Potassium deficit Calcium excess	
	Flaccid paralysis	Severe potassium deficit Severe potassium excess	
	Weakness Hypertonia	Metabolic acidosis	
	Positive Chvostek sign Tremors, cramps, tetany	Calcium deficit Alkalosis with diminished calcium ionization Calcium deficit	Children may suffer calcium deficit easily, since growing bones do not readily relinquish calcium to circulation
	Twitching	Magnesium deficit	

Continued.

Table 4-1. MANIFESTATIONS OF FLUID AND ELECTROLYTE DISTURBANCES—cont'd

Observation	Significant variation	Probable imbalance	Comments
Observe behavior	Lethargy	Fluid volume deficit	Behavioral changes among the first indications of dehydration as reported by parents
	Irritability	Fluid volume deficit	
	Comatose condition	Hypotonic fluid deficit	
		Profound acidosis or alkalosis	
	Lethargy with hyperirritability on stimulation	Hypertonic fluid deficit	
	Extreme restlessness	Potassium excess	
Weigh child	Loss	Fluid deficit	
	Up to 5%	Mild	
	5% to 9%	Moderate	
	10% or higher	Severe	
		Protein or calorie deficiency	
	Gain	Edema—general or pulmonary	
		Ascites	
Collect urine specimen			
Volume	Increased (polyuria)	Interstitial fluid-to-plasma shift	Normal range*
		Increased renal solute load	Newborn: 50-300 ml/d
	Diminished	Mild fluid deficit	Infant: 350-550 ml/d
	Oliguria	Moderate to severe fluid deficit	Child: 500-1000 ml/d
		Plasma-to-interstitial fluid shift	Adolescent: 700-1400 ml/d (varies with intake and other factors)
		Sodium deficit	
		Potassium excess	
		Severe sodium excess	
		Renal insufficiency	
Specific gravity	Low (1.010 or less)	Adequate hydration	Used to monitor hydration status in infants
		Fluid excess	Fixed low reading occurs in renal disease
		Renal disease	
		Sodium deficit	
	High (1.030 or more)	Fluid deficit	
		Sodium excess	
		Glycosuria	
		Proteinuria	
pH	Acid	Acidosis—metabolic or respiratory	
		Alkalosis accompanied by severe potassium deficit	
	Alkaline	Alkalosis—metabolic or respiratory	
		Hyperaldosteronism	
		Acidosis accompanied by chronic renal infection and renal tubular dysfunction	
		Diuretic therapy with carbonic anhydrase inhibitors	

*Data from Behrman RE and Vaughan, VC, III, editors: Nelson textbook of pediatrics, ed 3, Philadelphia, 1987, WB Saunders Co.

Unit 4

NURSING DIAGNOSIS: Fluid volume deficit (1) related to failure of regulatory mechanisms, such as renal, hypothalamic

NURSING DIAGNOSIS: Fluid volume deficit (2) related to active loss from renal, gastrointestinal (vomiting, diarrhea, nasogastric tube), or respiratory (hyperventilation) tracts; from skin (diaphoresis, wounds)

GOAL

Replace fluid losses

INTERVENTIONS

Administer fluids as ordered
  Intravenous
    *Administer fluid as prescribed
    Maintain desired drip rate
    *Add appropriate electrolytes as prescribed
    Maintain integrity of infusion site
  Oral
    *Feed electrolyte-containing solutions as prescribed

EXPECTED OUTCOMES

Child receives sufficient fluids to replace losses
Child exhibits signs of adequate hydration (specify)

GOAL

Prevent interference with therapeutic regimen

INTERVENTIONS

Apply appropriate restraining methods where indicated
Provide pacifier for infants who are receiving nothing by mouth

EXPECTED OUTCOMES

Child does not interfere with fluid therapy
Infant engages in nonnutritive sucking

NURSING DIAGNOSIS: Potential fluid volume deficit related to loss of appetite, NPO therapy, self-care deficit, immobility, altered sensorium

GOAL

Maintain hydration

INTERVENTIONS

See above

EXPECTED OUTCOME

See above

GOAL

Prevent dehydration

────────
*Dependent nursing action.

INTERVENTIONS

See above
Employ play for promoting fluid intake
  Make freezer pops using child's favorite juice
  Cut Jell-O into fun shapes
  Make game of taking sip when turning page of book or in games like "Simon Says"
  Use small medicine cups; decorate the cups
  Color water with food coloring or Kool-Aid
  Have tea party; pour at small table
  Let child fill a syringe and squirt it into child's mouth or use it to fill small decorated cups
  Cut straws in half and place in small container (much easier for child to suck liquid)
  Decorate straw—cut out small design with two holes and pass straw through; place small sticker on straw
  Use a "crazy" straw
  Make a "progress poster"; give rewards for drinking a predetermined quantity

EXPECTED OUTCOMES

Child drinks a sufficient amount of fluid (specify type and amount)
Child exhibits evidence of adequate hydration, e.g., moist mucous membranes, good skin turgor, adequate urinary output for age

NURSING DIAGNOSIS: Fluid volume excess related to overhydration; failure of regulatory mechanisms

GOAL

Prevent increased fluid intake

INTERVENTIONS

Regulate fluid intake carefully
Monitor intravenous infusion to maintain prescribed intake
Employ strategies to prevent undesired intake
  Use small containers for fluid intake
  Divide allowed intake into small volumes spread over entire day
  Spray mouth with atomizer (mist) to prevent feeling of dryness
  Keep lips lubricated

EXPECTED OUTCOME

Child receives no more fluid than allowed

GOAL

Promote fluid loss

INTERVENTION

*Administer diuretic as prescribed, preferably early in day to minimize night voiding

EXPECTED OUTCOME

Child eliminates excess fluid

────────
*Dependent nursing action.

NURSING CARE PLAN
THE CHILD WITH SPECIAL NUTRITIONAL NEEDS

The child who has an imbalance between nutrient intake and nutrient expenditure or need. See specific nursing care plan for the child with disease-related nutritional alterations.

ASSESSMENT

Take a dietary history (see p. 85)
Assess nutritional status (see Clinical assessment of nutritional status, p. 85)

Review laboratory analyses of hemoglobin, hematocrit, albumin, creatinine, nitrogen, or any other specific nutrient measurement (see p. 589)
Observe child's eating behaviors

NURSING DIAGNOSIS: Altered nutrition: less than body requirements related to fatigue, neuromuscular impairment, unconsciousness

GOAL

Provide nourishment

INTERVENTIONS

Provide feedings appropriate to age and capabilities
Feed when child is well rested
*Administer appropriate diet by gavage, gastrostomy, or nasogastric tubes
*Administer supplementary vitamins and iron as ordered

EXPECTED OUTCOME

Child consumes an adequate amount with minimum effort (specify amount)

NURSING DIAGNOSIS: Altered nutrition: less than body requirements related to receiving nothing by mouth

GOAL

Provide nourishment

INTERVENTIONS

Administer intravenous fluids and/or hyperalimentation as prescribed
Provide nonnutritive sucking for infants
Provide mouth care for children
    Moist swabs, emollient for lips
    Spray mouth with mist

---

*Dependent nursing action.

EXPECTED OUTCOMES

Child receives sufficient nourishment
Infant engages in nonnutritive sucking
Child's mucous membranes remain moist

NURSING DIAGNOSIS: Altered nutrition: less than body requirements related to loss of appetite, refusal to eat

GOAL

Promote nutritional intake

INTERVENTIONS

Use information from dietary history to make eating time as much like home as possible.
Encourage parents or other family members to feed child or to be present at mealtimes.
Have children eat at tables in groups; bring nonambulatory children to eating area in wheelchairs, beds, strollers, gurneys, or wagons.
Use familiar eating utensils, such as a favorite plate, cup, or bottle for small children.
Make mealtimes pleasant; avoid any procedures immediately before or after eating; make sure child is rested and pain-free.
Have a nurse present at mealtimes to offer assistance, prevent disruptions, and praise children for their eating.
Serve small, frequent meals rather than three large meals or serve three meals and nutritious between-meal snacks.
Bring in foods from home, especially if food preparation is markedly different from hospital; consider cultural differences.
Provide finger foods for young children.
Involve children in food selection and preparation whenever possible.

Unit 4

Serve small portions, and serve each course separately, such as soup first, followed by meat, potatoes, and vegetables, and ending with dessert; with young children camouflage size of food by cutting meat thicker so less appears on plate or by folding a cheese slice in half; offer second helpings; ensure a variety of foods, textures, and colors.

Provide food selections that are favorites of most children, such as peanut butter/jelly sandwiches, hot dogs, hamburgers, macaroni and cheese, pizza, spaghetti, tacos, fried chicken, and corn on the cob.

Avoid foods that are highly seasoned, have strong odors, are served hot, or are all mixed together, unless typical of cultural practices.

Provide fluid selections that are favorites of most children, such as fruit punch, cola, ginger ale, sweetened tea, ice pops, sherbet, ice cream, milk and milk shakes, eggnog, pudding, gelatin, clear broth, or creamed soups.

Offer nutritious snacks, such as frozen yogurt or pudding, ice cream, oatmeal or peanut butter cookies, hot cocoa, cheese slices or "kisses," pieces of raw vegetable or fruit, and dried fruit or cereal.

Make food attractive and different, for example:

Serve a "picnic lunch" in a paper bag.

Pack food in a Chinese-food container; decorate container.

Put a "face" or a "flower" on a hamburger or sandwich with pieces of vegetable.

Use a cookie-cutter to shape a sandwich.

Serve pudding, yogurt, or juice frozen as a popsicle.

Make slurpies or snowcones by pouring flavored syrup on crushed ice.

Add vegetable coloring to water or milk.

Serve fluids through brightly colored or unusually shaped straws.

Make "bowtie" sandwiches by cutting them in triangles and placing two points together.

Slice sandwiches into "fingers."

Grate mounds of cheese.

Cut apples horizontally to make circles.

Put a banana on a hotdog bun and spread with peanut butter.

Break uncooked spaghetti into toothpick lengths and skewer cheese, cold meat, vegetables, or fruit chunks.

Praise child for what he does eat.

Do *not* punish children for not eating by removing their dessert or putting them to bed.

EXPECTED OUTCOME

Child consumes an adequate amount of appropriate foods (specify type and amount)

NURSING DIAGNOSIS: Feeding deficit related to physical disability, mechanical restrictions, cognitive impairment

GOAL

Promote self-feeding (specify amount and type of self-help)

INTERVENTIONS

Modify utensils to facilitate self-help

Place dishes and utensils within reach based on disability (specify)

Place plate on child's chest (if unable to sit or turn)

Employ a length of clean clear plastic tubing for drinking (if straw too short)

Serve easy-to-handle foods

Make meals as interesting and attractive as possible

Protect child and bed linens from possible spills etc. with bib, towels, etc.

EXPECTED OUTCOME

Child assists with feeding as much as possible within limitations (specify amount of self-help)

GOAL

Feed child

INTERVENTIONS

Allow child some autonomy in passive feeding

Include child in food selection and sequence of eating foods served (within limits of diet and sound nutrition)

Offer small bites, semisolid foods, and fluids through a straw for children lying in prone position

Provide diet appropriate for age

EXPECTED OUTCOMES

Child participates in feeding activity according to ability

Child consumes a sufficient amount (specify)

NURSING CARE PLAN
THE CHILD IN PAIN

"An unpleasant sensory and emotional experience associated with actual or potential tissue damage, or described in terms of such damage. Pain is always a subjective experience."
(International Association for the Study of Pain, 1986).

"Pain is whatever the experiencing person says it is, existing whenever he says it does"
(McCaffery and Beebe, 1989).

CHILD'S CONCEPT OF PAIN RELATED TO COGNITIVE DEVELOPMENT (HURLEY AND WHELAN, 1988):
Age 2 to 7 years (preoperational thought)

Relates to pain primarily as physical, concrete experience
Thinks in terms of magical disappearance of pain
May view pain as punishment for wrongdoing
Tends to hold someone accountable for own pain and may strike out at person

Age 7 to 10+ years (concrete operational thought)

Relate to pain physically; i.e., headache, stomachache
Able to perceive of psychologic pain, such as someone dying
Fears bodily harm and annihilation (body destruction and death)
May view pain as punishment for wrongdoing

Age 13 years and older (formal operational thought)

Able to give reason for pain; i.e., fell and hit nerve
Perceives several types of psychologic pain
Has limited life experiences to cope with pain as adult might cope despite mature understanding of pain
Fears losing control during painful experience

ASSESSMENT

Use a variety of pain assessment sources (see Table 4-2)
Obtain pain history before pain is expected, e.g., on admission to hospital, preoperatively
Obtain information from child and family regarding *previous* pain experiences, child's coping strategies, understanding of pain (see box, p. 280)
Consider pathology associated with underlying condition or expected pain associated with a procedure
Observe coping strategies the child uses during a painful procedure, such as talking, moaning, lying rigidly still, squeezing a hand, breath-holding
Obtain information regarding *current* pain—Duration, type, location
Have parent or child describe pain in terms of interruption of daily activities
Evaluate child's behavior(s) that indicate discomfort and pain (see box on p. 280)
Evaluate physiologic changes that may indicate pain—Increased heart rate, respirations, blood pressure; sweating, dilated pupils, flushing or pallor; muscle tension; nausea; decreased oxygen saturation
Observe for specific reactions that indicate local pain—Pulling ears, rolling head from side to side, lying on side with legs flexed on abdomen, limping, refusing to move a body part

Employ pain assessment tools and strategies
Have child indicate location of pain by marking body part on a human figure drawing (p. 211), point to area with one finger on self, doll, stuffed animal, or to "where mommy or daddy would put a Band-Aid"
Use pain rating scale (see examples in Table 4-3)
Select a scale suitable for the child's age, abilities, and preference
Use the same scale with child each time pain is assessed
Teach child to use scale before pain is expected (e.g., preoperatively)
Observe for improvement in behavior following administration of analgesic; use pain assessment record to monitor effectiveness of interventions (see box, p. 281)

Table 4-2. SOURCES OF ASSESSMENT DATA

Age	Self-report	Behavior	Physical signs
0-3	Not available	Primary	Secondary
3-6	Primary (limited) Often requires special scales	Primary if self-report available	Secondary
>6	Primary	Secondary	Secondary

Unit 4

PAIN EXPERIENCE INVENTORY

Questions for parents

Describe any pain your child has had before.

How does your child usually react to pain?

Does your child tell you or others when he is hurting?

How do you know when your child is in pain?

What do you do to ease discomfort for your child when your child is hurting?

What does your child do to get relief when hurting?

Which of these actions work best to decrease or take away your child's pain?

Is there anything special that you would like me to know about your child and pain? (If yes, have parent[s] describe.)

Questions for child

Tell me what pain is.

Tell me about the hurt you have had before.

What do you do when you hurt?

Do you tell others when you hurt?

What do you want others to do for you when you hurt?

What don't you want others to do for you when you hurt?

What helps the most to take away your hurt?

Is there anything special that you want me to know about you when you hurt? (If yes, have child describe.)

From Hester N and Barcus C: Assessment and management of pain in children. In Pediatrics: nursing update 1(14):3, Princeton, NJ, 1986, Continuing Professional Education Center, Inc.

DEVELOPMENTAL CHARACTERISTICS OF CHILDREN'S RESPONSES TO PAIN

Young infants

Generalized body response of rigidity or thrashing, possibly with local reflex withdrawal of stimulated area

Loud crying

Facial expression of pain (brows lowered and drawn together, eyes tightly closed, and mouth open and squarish)

Demonstrates no association between approaching stimulus and subsequent pain

Older infants

Localized body response with deliberate withdrawal of stimulated area

Loud crying

Facial expression of pain and/or anger (same facial characteristics as pain but eyes are open)

Physical resistance, especially pushing the stimulus away *after* it is applied

Young child

Loud crying, screaming

Verbal expressions of "Ow," "Ouch," "It hurts"

Thrashing of arms and legs

Attempts to push stimulus away *before* it is applied

Uncooperative; needs physical restraint

Requests termination of procedure

Clings to parent, nurse, or other significant person

Requests emotional support, such as hugs or other forms of physical comfort

May become restless and irritable with continuing pain

All of these behaviors may be seen in anticipation of actual painful procedure

School-age child

May see all behaviors of young child, especially *during* actual painful procedure but less in anticipatory period

Stalling behavior, such as "Wait a minute" or "I'm not ready"

Muscular rigidity, such as clenched fists, white knuckles, gritted teeth, contracted limbs, body stiffness, closed eyes, wrinkled forehead

Adolescent

Less vocal protest

Less motor activity

More verbal expressions, such as "It hurts" or "You're hurting me"

Increased muscle tension and body control

Sources: Craig et al, 1984; Katz, Kellerman, and Siegel, 1980.

PAIN ASSESSMENT RECORD

Directions:

1. Record time of administering drug and assess analgesic effect 30 minutes later and then hourly.
2. State "Reason for drug administration" in behavioral terms, e.g., "child says he hurts" or "child crying and irritable."
3. Use column "Reason for drug administration" to record behavior during reassessment, e.g., "child says he feels better" or "child playing."
4. Use pain rating scale if child understands its use and only when child is awake. Name of scale: _____ ;
   Rating: No pain = _____ and Worst pain = _____ .
5. Suggested guidelines for safe minimal respiratory rates for children receiving narcotics are 10 to 16 breaths/minute. Consider child's age (with age respiratory rate decreases) and physiologic status (shallow respiration, decreased oxygen saturation, decreased consciousness) when evaluating respirations.

Date	Time	Drug administered	Reason for drug administration	Pain rating	Respirations	Signature

Unit 4

Table 4-3. PAIN RATING SCALES FOR CHILDREN

Pain scale	Instructions	Comments
Faces Scale* (Wong and Baker, 1988)	Explain to child that each face is for a person who feels happy because there is no pain (hurt) or sad because there is some or a lot of pain. Face 0 is very happy because there is no hurt. Face 1 hurts just a little bit. Face 2 hurts a little more. Face 3 hurts even more. Face 4 hurts a whole lot, but Face 5 hurts as much as you can imagine, although you don't have to be crying to feel this bad. Ask child to choose face that best describes how the pain feels.	Can be used with children as young as 3 years.

      0   1   2   3   4   5

Pain scale	Instructions	Comments
Poker Chip (Hester, 1979, 1989)	Use four red plastic (poker) chips. Explain to child that these are "pieces of hurt." One piece is a "little bit of hurt," and four pieces is the "most hurt." Ask child to choose number of pieces that describes the pain. If child replies "no pain," record a 0.	Recommended for children as young as 4½ years.
Color Tool (Eland, 1985)	Ask child to identify things that have hurt in the past and what has hurt the worst. Give child 8 crayons or markers (yellow, orange, red, green, blue, purple, brown, and black) in a random order. Ask child which color is like the worst pain experienced. Place that crayon or marker aside and ask child to identify crayon that is like a hurt not quite as bad as the worst hurt. Place that crayon aside and ask which other crayon is like something that hurts just a little. Place that crayon with the others and ask child which crayon is like no hurt at all. Show four crayon choices to child in order from worst hurt color to no hurt color. Ask child to show on body outline where it hurts using crayon of color that most nearly is like the pain feeling. When colors are ranked, assign them a numeric value of 0 to 3.	Recommended for children as young as 4 years provided children know their colors and are not color blind.
Oucher† (Beyer, 1988)	Consists of six photographs of child's face representing "no hurt" to "biggest hurt you could ever have." Child chooses face that most nearly describes the pain. Also includes a vertical scale with numbers from 0 to 100. Child chooses number that best describes the pain.	Photographic scale may be appropriate for children as young as 3 years; use numeric scale for children who can count to 100 by ones.
Numeric Scale	Explain to child that at one end of the line is a 0, which means that a person feels no pain (hurt). At the other end is a 10, which means the person feels the worst pain imaginable. The numbers 1 to 9 are for a very little pain to a whole lot of pain. Ask child to choose the number that best describes how the pain feesl.	May be appropriate for children as young as 5 years, although children who cannot count may have difficulty with scale.

No pain   Worst pain

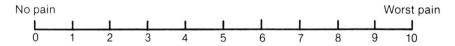

  0 1 2 3 4 5 6 7 8 9 10

Pain scale	Instructions	Comments
Simple Descriptive Scale	Explain to child that at one end of line is *no pain* because person feels no hurt. At the other end is *worst pain* because person feels the worst pain imaginable. The words in between are *mild* for just a little pain, *moderate* for a little more, *quite a lot* for even more, and *very bad* for a whole lot of pain. Ask child to choose word that best describes how the pain feels.	May be appropriate for children as young as 5 years, although words may need explanation.

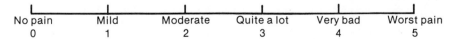

No pain   Mild   Moderate   Quite a lot   Very bad   Worst pain
    0   1   2   3   4   5

---

*Available from Purdue Frederick Company, 100 Connecticut Avenue, Norwalk, CT 06856 (1-800-243-5667, ext 4010).

†Available from Judith E. Beyer, PhD, RN, School of Nursing, University of Colorado Health Sciences Center, Campus Box C-288, 4200 E 9th Avenue, Denver, CO 80262 (303) 270-4317.

(Figures may be photocopied for clinical use.)

NURSING DIAGNOSIS: Pain related to (specify)

GOAL

Reduce perception of pain and promote coping strategies

INTERVENTIONS

Employ nonpharmacologic strategies to help child manage pain
Select appropriate strategy (see Guidelines for nonpharmacologic pain management)
Use strategy familiar to child or describe several strategies and let child select one
Involve parent in selection of strategy
Select appropriate person(s) to assist child with strategy
Develop individualized child and family goals for decreasing pain and increasing coping strategies
Teach child to use specific nonpharmacologic strategies before pain occurs or before it becomes severe
Assist or have parent assist child with using strategy during actual pain

EXPECTED OUTCOMES

Child exhibits reduced or tolerable pain level
Child learns and implements effective coping strategies
Parent learns coping skills and is effective in assisting child to cope

GOAL

Relieve pain

INTERVENTIONS

Plan to administer prescribed analgesic before procedure so that its peak effect coincides with inducement of pain (see Table 4-B)
Plan preventive schedule of medication around the clock, not as needed, when pain is continuous and predictable, e.g., postoperatively
Administer analgesia by mouth or into intravenous line whenever possible (avoid injection)
Prepare child for administration of analgesia
Use supportive statements
  Reinforce the effect of the analgesic by telling that the child he will begin to feel better in X amount of time (according to drug use); use a clock or timer to measure onset of relief with the child; reinforce the cause and effect of pain—analgesic, so the child becomes conditioned to *expecting* relief.
  Avoid saying "I am going to give you an injection for pain," since this is another pain in addition to the existing pain; if the child refuses an injection, explain that the little hurt from the needle will take away the bigger hurt for a long time.
  Avoid statements such as, "This is enough medicine to take away anyone's pain," or "By now you shouldn't need so much pain medicine."
  Give the child control whenever possible (e.g., choosing which leg for an injection, taking bandages off, holding the tape or other equipment).
*Administer prescribed analgesic
  Titrate dosage for maximum pain relief

---

*Dependent nursing action.

Begin with recommended dosage for age and weight (see Tables 4-A and B)
Increase dosage and/or decrease dose interval between dosages if pain relief is inadequate
If using parenteral route, change to oral route as soon as possible using equianalgesic dosages (Table 4-B)
  Convert directly by giving next dose of analgesic orally in equivalent dosage without any parenteral form of the same drug
OR

  Convert gradually to oral form using the following steps:
    Convert half the parenteral dose to a po dose
    Administer half the parenteral dose and the po dose
    Assess pain relief
    If pain relief is inadequate, increase the po dose as needed
    If sedation occurs, decrease the po dose as needed
    When the parenteral and po doses are effective, discontinue the parenteral dose and give twice the po dose
Avoid combining narcotics with so-called "potentiators"
Avoid using placebos to verify if pain is real

EXPECTED OUTCOMES

Child exhibits absence of or minimal evidence of pain
Child accepts administration of analgesia with minimal distress

NURSING DIAGNOSIS: Potential for poisoning or injury related to sensitivity, overuse, decreased gastrointestinal motility

GOAL

Prevent respiratory distress

INTERVENTIONS

Have emergency drugs and equipment in case of respiratory depression from narcotics
Decrease drug dosage if excessive sedation or decreased respiratory rate occurs
Have emergency drugs and equipment available
*Administer naloxone (Narcan) for respiratory depression

EXPECTED OUTCOME

Child's respirations remain within acceptable limits (see inside front cover for normal variations)

GOAL

Prevent minor side effects from becoming serious

INTERVENTIONS

*Administer stool softener or laxative to prevent constipation
Stop or decrease medication if evidence of rash

EXPECTED OUTCOMES

Child has regular bowel movements
Child exhibits no evidence of rash

GOAL

Manage tolerance and physical dependency

---

*Dependent nursing action.

Table 4-A. NONSTEROIDAL ANTI-INFLAMMATORY DRUGS (NSAIDs) APPROVED FOR CHILDREN*

Drug (trade name)	Dose	Comments
Acetaminophen (Tylenol and other brands)	10 to 15 mg/kg/dose every 4 to 6 hours not to exceed 5 doses in 24 hr.	Available in drops (80 mg/0.8 ml), elixir (160 mg/5 ml), tablets (80 mg), and swallowable caplets (160 mg) (see also p. 535) Non-prescription
Choline magnesium trisalicylate (Trilisate)	Children 37 kg or less: 50 mg/kg/day divided into 2 doses Children >37 kg: 2250 mg/day divided into 2 doses	Available in elixir 500 mg/5 ml Prescription
Ibuprofen PediaProfen	Children 6 months to 12 years: 5 to 10 mg/kg/dose every 6 to 8 hours not to exceed 40 mg/kg/day for fever Children over 12 years: 200 to 400 mg/dose every 6 to 8 hours	Available in suspension 100 mg/5 ml Prescription Recommended for fever reduction in children 6 months to 12 years, but is also indicated for use in juvenile rheumatoid arthritis and mild to moderate pain in children over 12 years
(Children's Advil)	Children 12 months and older: 30 to 40 mg/kg/day divided in 3 or 4 doses	Available in suspension 100 mg/5 ml Prescription Dosage is recommendation for juvenile rheumatoid arthritis; dosage for fever is same as for PediaProfen but for children 12 months and over
Naproxen (Naprosyn)	Children >2 years: 10 mg/kg/day divided in 2 doses	Available in elixir 125 mg/5 ml Prescription
Tolmetin (Tolectin)	Children >2 years: 20 mg/kg/day divided in 3 or 4 doses	Available in scored 200 mg tablets Prescription

*All NSAIDs in the table except acetaminophen have significant anti-inflammatory, antipyretic, and analgesic actions. Acetaminophen has a weak anti-inflammatory action and its classification as an NSAID is controversial. As analgesics, NSAIDs are effective for mild to moderate pain. Patients respond differently to various NSAIDs; therefore, changing from one drug to another may be necessary for maximum benefit.

Acetylsalicylic acid (aspirin) is also an NSAID but is not recommended for children because of its possible association with Reye syndrome. The NSAIDs in the table have no known association with Reye syndrome. However, caution should be exercised in prescribing any salicylate-containing drug (e.g., Trilisate) for children with known or suspected viral infection.

Side effects of ibuprofen, naproxen, and tolmetin include nausea, vomiting, diarrhea, constipation, gastric ulceration, bleeding nephritis, and fluid retention.

Acetaminophen and choline magnesium trisalicylate are well tolerated in the gastrointestinal tract and do not interfere with platelet function. NSAIDs except acetaminophen should not be given to patients with allergic reactions to salicylates. All the NSAIDs should be used cautiously in patients with renal impairment.

References: FDA-approved product information as of November 1989.

Table 4-B. DOSAGE AND THERAPEUTIC ACTIVITY OF SELECTED OPIOIDS FOR CHILDREN

Drug (route)	Initial dose (a)	Conversion factor IM to PO (b)	Equivalent IM dose (mg) (c)	Therapeutic activity for IM route except as noted (d)
Morphine (IV, IM, SC, PO)	0.1-0.2 mg/kg IM	3-6	10	O = 15-60 min. P = 0.5-1 hr. D = 3-7 hr.
Fentanyl (Sublimaze) (IV)	2-3 μg/kg IV	—	0.1	IV route: O = 7-8 min. P = No data D = 1-2 hr.
Codeine (IM, PO)	0.5-1 mg/kg PO	1.5	130	O = 15-30 min. P = 0.5-1 hr. D = 4-6 hr.
Methadone (Dolophine) (IM, PO)	0.1-0.2 mg/kg PO	2	10	O = 30-60 min. P = 0.5-1 hr. D = 4-6 hr. (d)
Hydromorphone (Dilaudid) (IV, SC, PO)	0.015-0.03 mg/kg IM	5	1.5	O = 15-30 min. P = 0.5-1 hr. D = 4-5 hr.
Levorphanol (Levo-Dromoran) (SC, IV, PO)	0.02-0.04 mg/kg IM	2	2	O = 30-90 min. P = 0.5 1 hr. D = 4-8 hr.
Meperidine (e) (Demerol) (IV, IM, PO)	1 to 2 mg/kg IV or IM	4	75	O = 10-45 min. P = 0.5-1 hr. D = 2-4 hr.

(a) These dosages are considered initial starting doses for moderate to severe pain in children who have not developed tolerance to the drug. The optimal dose is determined by titration: increasing or decreasing the dose according to the child's response. Dosages for hydromorphone and levorphanol are based on the equianalgesic dose of parenteral morphine.

(b) To convert an IM dose to a PO dose, multiply the IM dose by the conversion factor. Based on clinical experience, IM and IV doses are considered equianalgesic. However, some clinicians suggest that ½ the IM dose equals the IV dose, especially for an initial IV bolus dose. For morphine a conversion factor of 3 is recommended for repetitive dosing.

(c) When converting from one drug to another drug, be certain that the dosages of the drugs are equivalent. For example, 5 mg of IV morphine is equal to 0.75 mg of IV or 4 mg of PO hydromorphone.

(d) O = onset; P = peak; D = duration. With IV administration, times may be shorter, and with PO administration, times may be longer. Times for all drugs are approximate and may be shorter in children due to their more rapid metabolism of the drug. With repeated dosing, duration of methadone and levorphanol increases. Sustained-release preparations of oral morphine are available (MS Contin, 8-12 hours: Roxanol-SR, 8 hours).

(e) Should not be used chronically, particularly in patients with compromised renal function or for treatment of sickle cell crisis pain, because of accumulation of the metabolite, normeperidine, which causes central nervous system irritability (anxiety, tremors, myoclonus, and generalized seizures).

Principal reference: American Pain Society: Principles of analgesic use in the treatment of acute pain and chronic cancer pain, ed. 2, Skokie, IL, 1989, American Pain Society.

Unit 4

INTERVENTIONS

Recognize signs of tolerance—Decreasing pain relief, decreasing duration of pain relief

Recognize signs of withdrawal following discontinuation of drug (physical dependence)—Lacrimation, rhinorrhea, yawning, sweating;

    Later signs—Restlessness, irritability, tremors, anorexia, dilated pupils, gooseflesh

*Help treat tolerance and physical dependence appropriately

Never refer to child who is tolerant or physically dependent as addicted

---

*Dependent nursing action.

EXPECTED OUTCOME

Child receives appropriate therapy for tolerance or dependency

See also Preparation for procedures, p. 211
See also Administration of medications, p. 222

GUIDELINES FOR NONPHARMACOLOGIC PAIN MANAGEMENT

General strategies

Form a trusting relationship with child and family

    Express concern regarding their reports of pain

    Take an active role in seeking effective pain management strategies

Use general strategies to prepare child for painful procedure (see p. 211)

Prepare the child before potentially painful procedures but avoid "planting" the idea of pain. For example, instead of saying

    "This is going to (or may) hurt," say "Sometimes this feels like pushing, sticking, or pinching and sometimes it doesn't bother people. You tell me what it feels like to you."

    Use "non-pain" descriptors when possible, e.g., "It feels like intense heat," rather than, "It's a burning pain."

    This allows for variation in sensory perception, avoids suggesting pain, and gives the child control in describing reactions.

Avoid evaluative statements or descriptions, such as "This is a terrible procedure" or "It really will hurt a lot."

Stay with the child during a painful procedure

    Encourage parents to stay with child if child and parent desire; encourage parent to talk softly to child and to remain near child's head

    Involve parents in learning specific nonpharmacologic strategies and assisting child in their use

Educate the child about the pain, especially when explanation may lessen anxiety (e.g., that the pain the child is experiencing is expected after surgery and does not indicate that something is wrong; reassure the child that he is not responsible for the pain).

For long-term pain control give the child a doll that becomes "the patient" and allow child to do everything to the doll that is done to the child; pain control can be emphasized through the doll by stating, "Dolly feels better after the medicine."

Specific strategies
Distraction

Involve parent and child in identifying strong distractors.

Involve child in play; use radio, tape recorder, record player; have child sing or use rhythmic breathing

Have the child concentrate on yelling or saying "ouch" by focusing on "yelling loud or soft as you feel it hurt; that way I know what's happening."

Use humor, such as watching cartoons, telling jokes or funny stories, or acting silly with the child

Relaxation

With an infant or young child:

    Hold in a comfortable, well-supported position, such as vertically against the chest and shoulder.

    Rock in a wide, rhythmic arc in a rocking chair or sway back and forth, rather than bouncing the child.

    Repeat one or two words softly, such as "Mommy's here."

With a slightly older child:

    Ask the child to take a deep breath and "go limp as a rag doll" while exhaling slowly, then ask the child to yawn (demonstrate if needed).

    Help the child assume a comfortable position (e.g., pillow under neck and knees).

    Begin progressive relaxation: starting with the toes, systematically instruct the child to let each body part "go limp" or "feel heavy"; if the child has difficulty with relaxing, instruct him to tense or tighten each body part and then relax it.

    Allow child to keep eyes open since children may respond better if eyes are open than closed during relaxation

Guided imagery

Have the child identify some highly pleasurable real or pretend experience

Have the child describe the details of the event, including as many senses as possible, e.g., "feel the cool breezes," "see the beautiful colors," "hear the pleasant music"

Have child write down or record script

Encourage the child to concentrate only on the pleasurable event during the painful time; enhance the image by recalling specific details, such as reading the script or playing the record.

Combine with relaxation

GUIDELINES FOR NONPHARMACOLOGIC PAIN MANAGEMENT—cont'd

Positive self-talk

Teach child positive statements to say when in pain, e.g., "I will be feeling better soon," "When I go home, I will feel better," "Relaxing will make me hurt less."

Thought-stopping

Identify positive facts about the painful event, such as "It does not last long."

Identify reassuring information, such as, "If I think about something else, it does not hurt as much."

Condense positive and reassuring facts into a set of brief statements and have the child memorize them, e.g.: "Short procedure, good veins, little hurt, nice nurse, go home."

Have the child repeat the memorized statements whenever thinking about or experiencing the painful event.

Cutaneous stimulation

Includes simple rhythmic rubbing; use of pressure, electric vibrator; massage with hand lotion, powder, or menthol cream; application of heat or cold, such as an ice cube on the site before giving injection or application of ice to the site opposite the painful area (e.g., if right knee hurts, place ice on left knee).

A more sophisticated method is transcutaneous electrical nerve stimulation (TENS) (use of controlled low voltage electricity to the body via electrodes placed on the skin).

Behavioral contracting

Informal—May be used with children as young as 4 or 5:

Use stars or tokens as rewards

Uncooperative or procrastinating children (during a procedure) can be given a limited amount of time (measured by a visible timer) to complete the procedure

Proceed as needed if child is unable to comply

Reinforce cooperation with a reward if the procedure is accomplished within specified time

Formal—Use written contract, which includes the following:

Realistic (seems possible) goal or desired behavior

Measurable behavior, e.g., agrees not to hit anyone during procedures

Contract written, dated, and signed by all persons involved in any of the agreements

Identified rewards or consequences are reinforcing

Goal can be evaluated

Unit 4

NURSING CARE PLAN:
THE CHILD AT RISK FOR INFECTION

Invasion of the body by pathogenic microorganisms that re-produce and multiply, causing disease by local cellular injury, secretion of a toxin, or antigen-antibody reaction to the host.

ASSESSMENT

Take careful health history especially regarding evidence of contact with infective organisms, conditions that predispose the child to infection, and medications (such as steroids, chemotherapeutic agents) that reduce the body's natural defenses

Observe for evidence of infection:
  Elevated temperature
  Swelling, tenderness, pain, and reddness at site of infection
  Lethargy
  Loss of appetite
  Evidence of leukocytosis—elevated WBC, appearance of pus
Monitor vital signs for early signs of infectious processes
  Report any temperature elevation to physician
Assist with diagnostic procedures and tests—collect specimens for culture, radiography, thoracentesis, venipuncture

NURSING DIAGNOSIS: Potential for infection related to impaired body defenses, presence of infective organisms

GOAL

Prevent infection

INTERVENTIONS

Promote good health practices
  Maintain adequate nutrition
  Maintain good hygienic habits
Protect child from contact with infected persons
Observe good hand washing
Place child in room with noninfectious children; restrict visitors with active illnesses
Advise visitors (and hospital personnel) to practice good hand washing
Restrict contact with persons who have infections, including family, other children, friends, and members of staff
Observe medical asepsis
Keep child dry and warm

EXPECTED OUTCOMES

Child and family apply good health practices
Child exhibits no evidence of infection

GOAL

Prevent spread of infection to others

INTERVENTIONS

Employ body substance isolation (BSI) (see pp. 289-291)
Implement category-specific isolation precautions according to hospital policy
Implement disease-specific isolation precautions according to hospital policy
Instruct others (parents, members of staff) in appropriate precautions
Teach affected children protective methods to prevent spread of infection for example hand washing, handling genital area, care after using bedpan or toilet
Endeavor to keep infants and small children from placing hand and objects in contaminated areas
Assess home situation and implement protective measures as feasible in individual circumstances
* Administer antimicrobial medications if prescribed
Support body's natural defenses, e.g., good nutrition

EXPECTED OUTCOME

Others remain free from infection

_____

*Dependent nursing action.

COMPARISON OF BODY SUBSTANCE ISOLATION AND UNIVERSAL PRECAUTIONS

	Body substance isolation (BSI)*	Centers for Disease Control (CDC) universal precautions (UP)†	Comments
Purpose	Reduces risk of cross-transmission of organisms, including human immunodeficiency virus (HIV), between patients Depends on the interaction between the caregiver and patient, regardless of diagnosis	Minimizes risk of bloodborne infection (HIV, hepatitis B virus) Must also use category- or disease-specific isolation precautions for diagnosed infections Depends on type of patient contact and diagnosis	Major difference between BSI and UP: BSI considers all patients potentially infectious for all pathogens (interaction-driven); UP considers all patients potentially infectious only for bloodborne infections and requires additional protections once diagnosis is made (diagnosis-driven) *Category-specific isolation precautions*—diseases for which similar isolation precautions are indicated. Instructions include all precautions necessary to prevent transmission of the most infectious disease in each category. Categories are: strict isolation, contact isolation, respiratory isolation, tuberculosis isolation, enteric precautions, drainage/secretion precautions, and blood/body fluid precautions *Disease-specific isolation precautions*—each disease is listed with only precautions needed to prevent transmission of that disease
Body substances considered potentially infectious	All, including: Blood Feces Urine Vomitus Wound and other drainage Oral secretions	Blood Semen Vaginal secretions Cerebrospinal fluid Synovial fluid Pleural fluid Peritoneal fluid Pericardial fluid Amniotic fluid Fluids NOT included unless they contain visible blood: Feces Nasal secretions Sputum Sweat Tears Urine and vomitus	UP do not apply to human breast milk or saliva except in special situations: Frequent exposure to breast milk; i.e., in breast milk banking During dental procedures where saliva may be contaminated with blood
Handwashing	Performed for 10 seconds with soap, running water, and friction anytime the hands are visibly soiled and between most patient contacts even if gloves are worn	Immediately and thoroughly wash hands and other skin surfaces that are contaminated with body fluids to which UP apply	Handwashing is the single most important strategy for preventing infection transmission

*Lynch P, and others: Rethinking the role of isolation practices in the prevention of nosocomial infections, Ann Intern Med 107:243-246, 1987.

†Update: Universal precautions for prevention of transmission of human immunodeficiency virus, hepatitis B virus, and other bloodborne pathogens in health-care settings, MMWR 37(24):377-387, 1988.

NOTE: The American Academy of Pediatrics has published guidelines on infection control, but because they are limited only to HIV infection and depend on the prevalence of HIV infection in an area, which is rarely known, they are not included. (Task Force on Pediatric AIDS: Pediatric guidelines for infection control of human immunodeficiency virus (acquired immunodeficiency virus) in hospitals, medical offices, schools, and other settings, Pediatrics 82(5):801-807, 1988.)

Unit 4

Continued

COMPARISON OF BODY SUBSTANCE ISOLATION AND UNIVERSAL PRECAUTIONS—cont'd

	Body substance isolation (BSI)	Centers for Disease Control (CDC) universal precautions (UP)	Comments
Handwashing— cont'd	Not necessary between sequential low-risk patient contacts involving intact skin, such as taking vital signs or administering medications		
Gloves	Must be used when contact with mucous membranes, nonintact skin, or moist body substances is likely to occur; changed between patient contacts	Must be worn when touching fluids to which universal precautions apply. Use during phlebotomy depends on risk of exposure to blood and prevalence of blood-borne pathogens. General guidelines include: If operator has breaks in skin. If operator is receiving training in phlebotomy. If hand contamination with blood is likely; i.e., performing phlebotomy on uncooperative patient. Finger and/or heel sticks on infants and children	Washing or disinfecting gloves for reuse is not recommended. Washing with surfactants may cause "wicking"; i.e., the enhanced penetration of liquids through undetected holes in the glove. Disinfecting agents can deteriorate the glove. General CDC control practices for saliva include use of gloves for digital examination of mucous membranes and endotracheal suctioning
Gowns or plastic aprons	Worn when it is likely that body substances will soil the clothing; changed between patient contacts	Same as BSI	With young children use of a gown or plastic apron with adequate shoulder and chest protection may be needed during feeding and bubbling
Masks and/or eye protection	Worn when likely that the eyes and/or nose and mouth will be splashed with body substances or when personnel are working directly over large open skin lesions; masks may be recommended for some airborne infections, if the health care worker is not immune	Same as BSI	Benefit of masks in preventing transmission of airborne infection is questionable. Eyeglasses generally provide adequate eye protection

COMPARISON OF BODY SUBSTANCE ISOLATION AND UNIVERSAL PRECAUTIONS—cont'd

	Body substance isolation (BSI)	Centers for Disease Control (CDC) universal precautions (UP)	Comments
Needle/syringe units and other sharps	Used needles not generally removed from disposable syringes, recapped or broken; all sharp instruments are disposed of in a rigid, puncture-resistant container located preferably near the site of use, such as patient's room and treatment rooms	Same as BSI	Needles punctures are a leading cause of nosocomial (hospital-acquired) transmission of blood-borne pathogens Gloves cannot prevent penetrating injuries caused by needles or other sharp instruments Adherence to proper handling of sharp instruments is essential
Trash and linen	Bagged securely in leak-proof containers and disposed of or cleaned according to institutional policy	Same as BSI	CDC recommendations include extensive discussions of environmental considerations for HIV transmission, although there is no evidence of casual or environmental transmission of HIV
Private rooms	Desirable for children who soil the environment with body substances; required for children with airborne, communicable diseases unless they can share a room with a roommate or roommates known to be immune to the disease	Not addressed other than to use disease- or category-specific isolation precautions	According to CDC, diseases affecting children which require use of a private room for strict or respiratory isolation precautions are varicella (chicken pox), diphtheria, mumps, pertussis, measles, erythema infectiosum, epiglottitis, meningitis (*H. influenzae,* meningococcal), pneumonia (*H. influenzae,* meningococcal), and meningococcemia

Unit 4

NURSING CARE PLAN:
THE CHILD WHO IS TERMINALLY ILL OR DYING

Terminal illness—A condition wherein a life is near or approaching its end

Grief—Physical and emotional responses to bereavement, separation, or loss

Grief reaction—Complex of somatic and psychologic symptoms associated with some extreme sorrow or loss

Anticipatory grief—Grieving before an actual loss

ASSESSMENT

Perform physical assessment

Obtain health history of the terminal illness and therapies

Assess child's conception of self in relation to the disease; identify stage of knowledge acquisition (Bluebond-Langner, 1978):

Stage 1 Disease is a serious illness.
　New identity of "sick" child.

Stage 2 Discovery of the relationship of medication and recovery.
　Learns the taboos of disease and death.

Stage 3 Marked by an understanding of the purposes and implications of special procedures.
　Sense of well-being begins to fade and perceives self as different from other children.

Stage 4 Illness is viewed as a permanent condition.
　Sense of always being sick and never getting better.

Stage 5 Realization that there is only a finite number of medications.
　Awareness (directly or indirectly) of the fatal prognosis.

Observe for signs of approaching death:

　Loss of sensation and movement in the lower extremities, progressing toward the upper body

　Sensation of heat, although body feels cool

　Loss of senses

　　Tactile sensation decreases

　　Sensitive to light

　　Hearing is last sense to fail

　Confusion, loss of consciousness, slurred speech

　Muscle weakness

　Loss of bowel and bladder control

　Decreased appetite/thirst

　Difficulty swallowing

　Change in respiratory pattern

　　Cheyne-Stokes respirations (waxing and waning of depth of breathing with regular periods of apnea)

　　"Death rattle" (noisy chest sounds from accumulation of pulmonary and pharyngeal secretions)

　Weak, slow pulse; decreased blood pressure

Assess family's response to impending death

Observe for manifestations of the normal grief reaction in family members (Modified from Lindemann, 1944) (see box)

Assess family's support systems, coping capacities, evidence of burnout

See also assessment of specific disorder

NORMAL GRIEF REACTION

Sensations of Somatic Distress

Feeling of tightness in the throat

Choking, with shortness of breath

Marked tendency toward sighing

Empty feeling in abdomen

Lack of muscular power

Intense subjective distress described as tension or mental pain

Preoccupation with Image of the Deceased

Hears, sees, or imagines that the dead person is present

Slight sense of unreality

Feeling of emotional distance from others

May believe that he is approaching insanity

Feelings of Guilt

Searches for evidence of failure in preventing the death

Accuses himself of negligence or exaggerates minor omissions

Feelings of Hostility

Loss of warmth toward others

Tendency toward irritability and anger

Wish not to be bothered by friends or relatives

Loss of Usual Pattern of Conduct

Restlessness, inability to sit still, aimless moving about

Continual searching for something to do or what he thinks he ought to do

Lack of capacity to initiate and maintain organized patterns of activity

NURSING DIAGNOSIS: Altered growth and development related to terminal illness and/or impending death

GOAL

Support child during terminal phase

INTERVENTIONS

Encourage children to talk about their feelings and provide safe, acceptable outlets for aggression

Answer questions as honestly as possible while maintaining a positive, hopeful approach

Explain all procedures and therapies, especially physical effect child will experience

Help child distinguish between consequences of therapies and manifestations of disease process

Structure hospital environment to allow for maximum self-control and independence within the limitations imposed by child's developmental level and physical condition

Respect the child's need for privacy without neglecting the child

Provide for presence of customary support systems

Encourage the parents to remain near the child as much as possible; if parents are unable to visit frequently, assign a primary nurse

EXPECTED OUTCOMES

Child expresses feelings freely

Child demonstrates an understanding of symptoms

GOAL

Provide physical comfort and nurturing at time of dying

INTERVENTIONS

Offer any foods child desires

Avoid excessive encouragement to eat or drink

Avoid foods with strong odors

Serve foods that require the least energy to eat (soups, shakes)

Feed slowly

Provide mouth care before and after eating; lubricate lips with petrolatum

Keep bedsheets untucked

Keep child uncovered if sheets are bothersome

Apply loose, cool clothing

Keep fresh air circulating in room (open window, use small fan)

Change child's position only as tolerated

Give cool sponge baths

Use pillows or other supports to prop child in comfortable position

Carry (if possible) to other areas for diversion if desired

Place absorbent pads under hips

Help child to toilet if he desires

Limit care to essentials

  May need to forego usual hygienic measures such as bath or clothing change but provide comfort measures (e.g., mouth care, wiping forehead, gentle back rub)

Avoid bright, direct light, but do not keep room too dim

Administer anticholinergic drugs (atropine or scopolamine) to reduce secretions (lessens "death rattle," which can be distressing to family)

Position with head slightly elevated or in well-supported sitting position if tolerated

Provide pain relief as needed (see Nursing care plan, The child in pain, p. 279)

EXPECTED OUTCOME

Child exhibits minimal or no evidence of physical discomfort

GOAL

Provide emotional support at time of dying

INTERVENTIONS

Talk to child even though may not appear awake

Sit at head of bed where child can easily see face

Talk to child in clear, distinct voice, not whispers

Avoid conversation about the child in his presence

Offer calm reassurance and orient child to surroundings when awake

Phrase questions for yes or no answers

Do not disturb child with repeated measurements of vital signs

Play favorite music (may soothe child)

Preserve physical closeness with family members (e.g., parent may want to rock child in chair or lie next to child in bed)

EXPECTED OUTCOME

Child appears calm and relaxed

NURSING DIAGNOSIS: Altered nutrition: less than body requirements related to loss of appetite, disinterest in food

GOAL

Provide nutriments

INTERVENTIONS

Offer any food and fluids child desires

Provide small meals and snacks several times a day

Avoid excess encouragement to eat or drink

Avoid foods with strong odors

Provide pleasant environment for eating

Serve foods that require the least energy to eat (soups, shakes)

Feed slowly

*Administer antiemetic as prescribed if nausea/vomiting is a problem

Provide mouth care before and after eating; lubricate lips with petrolatum

EXPECTED OUTCOME

Child consumes some nutriments

NURSING DIAGNOSIS: Fear/anxiety related to diagnosis, tests, and therapies and prognosis

GOAL

Reduce anxiety

---

*Dependent nursing action.

INTERVENTIONS

Limit interventions to palliation only; discuss need for nonpalliative treatment with family and physician
Explain all procedures and other aspects of care to child
Remain with child or provide for constant attendance
Determine what child has been told about prognosis
Determine what the family wishes the child to know about the prognosis
Answer child's questions as openly and honestly as possible
Involve parents in child's care
Remain nonjudgmental regarding child's behavior

EXPECTED OUTCOME

Child discusses fears without evidence of stress

NURSING DIAGNOSIS: Anticipatory grieving related to potential loss of a child

GOAL

Support family

INTERVENTIONS

Identify stage of grieving process the family is experiencing
Provide opportunities for family to express emotions
Help parents deal with their feelings, allowing them more emotional reserve to meet the needs of their children
Encourage the parents to remain as near to the child as possible, yet be sensitive to the parents' needs
Provide information regarding child's status, anticipated reactions
Help parents to understand behavioral reactions of their children, especially that concern for present crises, such as loss of hair, may be much greater than for future ones, including possible death
Facilitate family's assistance with child's care
Provide comfort measures for child and family
Encourage family to maintain own health care needs
Provide as much privacy as possible
Assess family's need for referral services, e.g., hospice services, specific organizations for grieving families
Encourage parents to honestly answer questions about dying rather than avoiding or fabricating euphemisms
Encourage parents to share their moments of sorrow with their children
Provide preparation for postdeath services
Discuss with family their preferences for care if death is imminent
Arrange for appropriate spiritual care in accordance with family's beliefs and/or affiliations
Maintain contact with family
Provide support for families who choose home care for their child
See Guidelines for supporting grieving families (boxed material)

EXPECTED OUTCOMES

Family expresses fear, concerns, and any special desires for terminal child
Family demonstrates an understanding of child and his needs (specify)

Family avail themselves of services
See also:
   Nursing care plan: The child in the hospital, p. 246
   Nursing care plan: The family of the hospitalized child, p. 254
   Nursing diagnosis: Anticipatory grieving (newborn), p. 306

GOAL

Provide interpersonal comfort

INTERVENTIONS

Offer calm reassurance to child
Reassure child of the love of others
Continue to set some limits for the child to provide a sense of security
Spend time with the child when not directly involved in care
Reinforce to the child that what is happening is not the child's fault
Involve child in routine activities as tolerated
Maintain a "normal" atmosphere
Talk to the child even though may not appear to be awake
   Situate self and others where easily visible to child
   Speak to child in clear, distinct voice; avoid whispering
   Avoid conversation about the child's condition in presence of child
Play favorite music and read stories to child
Orient child to surroundings when awake
Phrase questions for "yes" or "no" answers when possible to conserve child's energy

EXPECTED OUTCOME

Child exhibits no evidence of loneliness

NURSING DIAGNOSIS: Anticipatory grief related to imminent death of a child

GOAL

Support family

INTERVENTIONS

Be available to the family
Convey an attitude of caring for both child and family
Encourage at least one family member to stay with child
Help family to provide care of the child as they desire without forcing involvement
* Administer medications or other agents as prescribed to reduce unpleasant manifestations
   Oxygen for respiratory distress
   Anticonvulsants for seizures
   Anticholinergic drugs to reduce secretions ("death rattle")
   Analgesics for pain
   Stool softeners/laxatives for constipation
   Antiemetics for nausea/vomiting
Help and encourage family to express feelings appropriately
Encourage family to meet their own physical needs
Provide privacy
Provide for physical comfort of the family
Provide emotional support and comfort to the family
Encourage family to talk to child

---

*Dependent nursing action.

Involve family and other children in decision-making whenever possible, especially regarding alternatives for terminal care (hospital, home, hospice)

Support and assist family in giving explanations to other family members regarding child's status

Maintain a nonjudgmental attitude toward behavior of family members

EXPECTED OUTCOMES

Family members discuss their feelings
Family are actively involved in child's care

GOAL

Support family's decision to take child home to die, if they wish

INTERVENTIONS

Teach family physical care of the child

Provide family with means for contacting health professionals at any time, e.g., phone numbers

Maintain daily contact with family, e.g., telephone call, home visit

*Refer to community agencies as appropriate

Reassure family that they can readmit child to the hospital at any time

Help plan with family what to do when the child dies

EXPECTED OUTCOMES

Family demonstrates the ability to provide care for the child
Family contacts appropriate support groups

*__The Compassionate Friends,__ P.O. Box 3696, Oak Brook, IL 60522-3696, (708) 990-0010.

GUIDELINES FOR SUPPORTING GRIEVING FAMILIES*

General

Stay with the family; sit quietly if they prefer not to talk; cry with them if desired

Accept the family's grief reactions; avoid judgmental statements, e.g., "You should be feeling better by now"

Avoid offering rationalizations for the child's death, e.g., "You should be glad your child isn't suffering anymore"

Avoid artificial consolation, e.g., "I know how you feel" or "You are still young enough to have another baby"

Deal openly with feelings such as guilt, anger, and loss of self-esteem

Focus on feelings by using a feeling word in the statement, e.g., "You're still feeling all the pain of losing a child"

Refer the family to an appropriate self-help group or for professional help if needed

At the time of death

Reassure the family that everything possible is being done for the child, if they wish lifesaving interventions

Do everything possible to ensure the child's comfort, especially relieving pain

Provide the child and family the opportunity to review special experiences or memories in their lives

Express personal feelings of loss and/or frustrations, e.g., "We will miss him so much" or "We tried everything; we feel so sorry that we couldn't save him"

Provide information that the family requests and be honest

Respect the emotional needs of family members, such as siblings, who may need brief respites from the dying child

Make every effort to arrange for family members, especially parents, to be with the child at the moment of death, if they wish to be present

Allow the family to stay with the dead child for as long as they wish and to rock, hold, or bathe the child

Provide practical help when possible, such as collecting the child's belongings

Arrange for spiritual support, such as clergy; pray with the family if no one else can stay with them

After the death

Attend the funeral or visitation if there was a special closeness with the family

Initiate and maintain contact, e.g., sending cards, telephoning, inviting them back to the unit, or making a home visit

Refer to the dead child by name; discuss shared memories with the family

Discourage the use of drugs or alcohol as a method of escaping grief

Encourage all family members to communicate their feelings rather than to remain silent to avoid upsetting another member

Emphasize that grieving is a painful process that often takes *years* to resolve

---

*The *family* refers to all significant persons involved in the child's life, such as the parents, siblings, grandparents, or other close relatives or friends.

NURSING CARE PLAN:
CHILD AND FAMILY COMPLIANCE (ADHERENCE)

The extent to which the patient's or family's behavior coincides with the prescribed regimen, in terms of taking medications, following diets, or executing other life-style changes.

Factors that enhance compliance

Child/family factors
High self-esteem
Positive body image
High degree of autonomy
Supportive and well-adjusted family
Effective family communication
Family expectation for successful completion of therapy

Care setting factors
Perceived satisfaction with care
Positive interactions with practitioners
Continuity of care
Individualized care
Minimal waiting time for appointments
Convenient care setting

Treatment factors
Simple regimen
Minimal disruption in usual life-style
Short duration
Inexpensive
Visible benefits
Tolerable side effects

ASSESSMENT

Assessment of compliance should include a combination of at least two of the following methods:

Clinical judgment—Make a subjective inference about the family compliance. This is a very poor method that is subject to bias and inaccuracy unless the criteria used in evaluating compliance are carefully validated.

Self reporting—Question the family about their adherence to the prescribed treatments. Although simple to execute, most people, even when they admit to lapses in treatment, overestimate their compliance by about 20%.

Direct observation—Observe the child or family performing the treatment. Although this approach is very effective in identifying errors related to the correct procedure, it is difficult to employ outside the health care setting, and the family's awareness of being observed frequently affects their performance.

Monitoring appointments—Record the family's attendance at scheduled appointments. Keeping appointments indicates general levels of compliance, but only indirectly implies compliance with the prescribed care.

Monitoring therapeutic response—Monitor the child's responses in terms of benefit from treatment, preferably recorded on a graph or chart. Unfortunately, few treatments yield directly measurable results, such as decreased blood pressure or weight loss, making this a less satisfactory method for most types of therapies.

Pill counts—Count the number of pills remaining in the original container and compare to the amount missing and the number of days the medication should have been taken. Although a simple method, families may forget to bring the container or deliberately alter the number of pills to avoid detection. This method is also poorly suited to liquid medication that is so commonly prescribed for children.

Chemical assay—Measurement of plasma drug levels for certain drugs (e.g., digoxin and phenytoin) provides information about the amount of drug recently ingested. This method is expensive, reflects only short-term compliance, and requires precise timing of the assay for accurate results.

NURSING DIAGNOSIS: Noncompliance related to (specify)

GOAL

Promote compliance

INTERVENTIONS

Encourage child and family to adhere to the prescribed treatment plan
Implement strategies to improve compliance (see box)

EXPECTED OUTCOMES

Child and family provide evidence of compliance (specify)
Child exhibits evidence of benefits from therapy (specify)

STRATEGIES TO IMPROVE COMPLIANCE

The best results occur when at least two strategies are employed

Organizational strategies—Those interventions that are concerned with the care setting and the therapeutic plan

Give specific appointments and names of specific health care professionals to be seen

Increase the frequency of appointments

Designate a primary practitioner

Use mail and telephone reminders

Reduce waiting time for appointments of treatments

Reduce the cost of treatment, e.g., suggest generic brands of medications or supplement with free samples

Reduce the disruption of the treatment on the family's lifestyle

Use "cues" to minimize forgetfulness, e.g., pill dispensers, watches with alarms, charts to record completed therapy; reminders such as messages on the refrigerator or morning coffee pot; and treatment schedules that incorporate the treatment plan into the daily routine, e.g., physical therapy after the evening bath

Educational strategies—Those interventions that are concerned with instructing the family about the treatment plan

Establish rapport; reduce anxiety and fear

Assess what the family knows and expects to learn, and address any concerns the family express before beginning teaching

Assess the family's learning style; determine if they are people who like to have everything explained in detail or if they prefer knowing only the major facts

Identify factors that may impede learning, e.g., language, illiteracy, cognitive impairments, sensory impairments (hard of hearing, poor vision), physical impairments (lack of strength, poor coordination)

Use a variety of teaching materials (lecture, demonstration, video or slide presentation, written material)

Provide written materials, especially in any regimen requiring multiple or complex treatments, that are readable by the average individual (about a fourth grade reading level)

Speak the family's language, avoid jargon, and clarify all terms

Be specific when giving information; divide the information into small steps

Keep information short, simple, and concrete

Introduce most important information first

Use "verbal" headings to organize information, e.g., "There are two things you need to learn: how to give the medicine and what side effects to look for. First, how to give.... Second, what side effects...."

Stress importance of the instructions and the expected benefits; explain the detrimental effects of inadequate treatment but avoid fear tactics

Evaluate the teaching by eliciting feedback to ensure that the family understands the information

Repeat information as needed

Behavioral strategies—Those interventions designed to modify behavior directly

Involve significant others

Teach self-management skills, e.g., problem-solving

Provide positive reinforcement for accomplishment

Give verbal praise

Use concrete rewards, e.g., child's earning stars or tokens, a special privilege, or gift

Institute appropriate disciplinary techniques, e.g., time out for young children or withholding privileges for older children, for noncompliance

Implement behavioral contracting—A process in which the exact elements of desired behavior are explicitly outlined in the form of a written contract

Essential components of a contract:

Goal or desired behavior is realistic and seems attainable

Behavior is measurable, e.g., agreeing to take the drug before leaving for school without reminding

Contract is written and signed by all those involved in any of the agreements

Contract is dated, and if appropriate, a date is specified when a goal should be reached, e.g., number of pounds to be lost in 2 weeks

Reinforce with identified rewards or consequences

Goal can be evaluated, e.g., counting the number of pills or using a scale for weight determination

Use psychosocial services (e.g., counseling psychotherapy, group therapy) when indicated

Unit 4

NURSING CARE PLAN:
THE NORMAL NEWBORN AND FAMILY

A recently born infant, usually 38 to 42 weeks gestational age; includes the infant from birth to 4 weeks of age

ASSESSMENT

See Newborn assessment, p. 10
See Assessment of gestational age, p. 18
Observe states of sleep and activity:

Regular Sleep: 4-5 hr/day, 10-20 min/sleep cycle
Closed eyes
Regular breathing
No movement except for sudden bodily jerks

Irregular Sleep: 12-15 hr/day, 20-45 min/sleep cycle
Closed eyes
Irregular breathing
Slight muscular twitching of body

Drowsiness: Variable
Eyes may be open
Irregular breathing
Active body movement

Alert Inactivity: 2-3 hr/day
Responds to environment by active body movement and staring at close-range objects

Waking and Crying: 1-4 hr/day
May begin with whimpering and slight body movement
Progresses to strong, angry crying and uncoordinated thrashing of extremities

Observe parental attachment behaviors:
When the infant is brought to the parents, do they reach out for the child and call the child by name?
Do the parents speak about the child in terms of identification—whom the infant looks like; what appears special about their child over other infants?
When parents are holding the infant, what kind of body contact is there—do parents feel at ease in changing the infant's position; are fingertips or whole hands used; are there parts of the body they avoid touching or parts of the body they investigate and scrutinize?
When the infant is awake, what kinds of stimulation do the parents provide—do they talk to the infant, to each other, or to no one; how do they look at the infant—direct visual contact, avoidance of eye contact, or looking at other people or objects?
How comfortable do the parents appear in terms of caring for the infant? Do they express any concern regarding their ability or disgust for certain activities, such as changing diapers?
What type of affection do they demonstrate to the newborn, such as smiling, stroking, kissing, or rocking?
If the infant is fussy, what kinds of comforting techniques do the parents use, such as rocking, swaddling, talking, or stroking?

NURSING DIAGNOSIS: Ineffective airway clearance related to excess mucus, improper positioning

GOAL

Establish and maintain a patent airway

INTERVENTIONS

Suction mouth and nasopharynx with bulb syringe as needed
Lavage stomach of amniotic fluid and check for tracheoesophageal anomalies (not routinely done in all hospitals)
Position infant on side or abdomen with head slightly lower than chest (about 15 degrees) to facilitate drainage of secretions
Perform as few procedures as possible on infant during first hour and have oxygen ready for use if respiratory distress should develop

Take vital signs according to institutional policy and more frequently if necessary
Position infant on right side or abdomen after feeding to prevent aspiration
Keep diapers, clothing, and blankets loose enough to allow maximum lung (abdominal) expansion
Clean nares of any crusted secretions during bath or when necessary
Check for patent nares

EXPECTED OUTCOMES

Airway remains patent
Breathing is regular and unlabored
Respiratory rate is within normal limits (see inside front cover for normal variations)

Unit 4

NURSING DIAGNOSIS: Potential altered body temperature related to immature temperature control, change in environmental temperature

GOAL

Maintain stable body temperature

INTERVENTIONS

Wrap infant snugly in a warmed blanket

Place infant in a preheated environment (under radiant warmer or next to mother)

Place infant on a padded, covered surface

Take infant's temperature on arrival at nursery or mother's room; proceed according to hospital policy regarding method and frequency of monitoring

Maintain room temperature between 24° and 25.5° C (75° to 78° F) and humidity about 40% to 50%

Give initial bath according to hospital policy
    Prevent chilling of infant during daily bath
    Postpone bath if there is any question regarding stabilization of body temperature

Dress infant in a shirt and diaper and swaddle in a blanket or cover with blanket

Provide infant with a head covering if heat loss is a problem

Keep infant away from drafts, air conditioning vents, or fans

Place infant in a recessed cubicle with walls high enough to shield from cross ventilation

Warm all objects used to examine or cover infant, for example, place them under radiant warmer

Uncover only one area of body for examination or procedures

Postpone circumcision until after postnatal recovery period

Be alert to signs of hypothermia or hyperthermia

EXPECTED OUTCOME

Infant's temperature remains at optimum level (36.5° to 37.5° C [97.7° to 99.5° F])

NURSING DIAGNOSIS: Potential for infection related to deficient immunologic defenses, environmental factors

GOAL

Protect infant from infection

INTERVENTIONS

Wash hands before and after caring for each infant

Make certain appropriate eye prophylaxis has been carried out

Keep infant from potential sources of infection, e.g., persons with respiratory or skin infections, improperly prepared food sources, other unclean items

Clean vulva in posterior direction to prevent fecal contamination of vagina or urethra; stress this to parents

While cleaning penis, do not retract foreskin; gently wipe away smegma

Maintain asepsis during circumcision

*If infant has been circumcised, cover area with a petrolatum jelly gauze (if ordered)

Keep umbilical stump clean and dry
    Place diapers below umbilical stump
    Assess cord daily for odor, color, and drainage

Check eyes daily for evidence of inflammation or discharge

* Apply antibacterial agent or alcohol or both to cord as ordered

EXPECTED OUTCOMES

Infant exhibits no evidence of infection

Eyes remain clear with no evidence of irritation

Genital area is free of irritation

Cord appears dry, surrounding area free of infection

NURSING DIAGNOSIS: Potential for trauma related to physical helplessness

GOAL

Ensure infant's identity

INTERVENTIONS

Make certain infant is properly identified
    Ensure that identification bracelet(s) properly and securely placed
    Check often to ensure correct infant identity

EXPECTED OUTCOMES

Infant is identified

Identification bracelet remains in place

GOAL

Prevent physical injury

INTERVENTIONS

Never leave infant unsupervised on a raised surface without sides

Always close diaper pins and place them away from infant's body

Keep pointed or sharp objects out of infant's reach

Keep own fingernails short and trimmed; avoid jewelry that can scratch infant

Employ appropriate methods of handling and transporting infant

EXPECTED OUTCOME

Infant remains free of physical injury

GOAL

Prevent bleeding

INTERVENTIONS

* Administer vitamin K intramuscularly, using vastus lateralis muscle as site of injection

Check circumcision site; assess any oozing

---

*Dependent nursing action.

EXPECTED OUTCOME

Infant exhibits no evidence of bleeding

NURSING DIAGNOSIS: Altered nutrition: less than body requirements (potential) related to immaturity, parental knowledge deficit

GOAL

Prepare for feeding

INTERVENTIONS

Determine parental feeding preference (breast or bottle)
Offer initial intake according to hospital policy, practitioner's protocol, and individual preference
Assess strength of suck and coordination with swallowing

EXPECTED OUTCOMES

Family determines feeding method
Infant demonstrates strong suck

GOAL

Provide optimum nutrition

INTERVENTIONS

Prepare for demand feeding of breast-fed infants; night feedings determined by condition and preferences of the mother
Offer bottle-fed infants 2 to 3 ounces of formula every 3 to 4 hours or on demand
Support and assist breast-feeding mothers during initial feedings
Avoid routine water or supplemental feedings for breast-feeding infants
Encourage father or other supportive person to remain with mother to help her and infant with positioning, relaxation, and reinforcement
Encourage father to participate in bottle-feeding
Place infant on right side after feeding to prevent regurgitation
Observe stool pattern

EXPECTED OUTCOMES

Infant retains feedings
Infant receives an adequate amount of nutrients (specify amount and frequency of feedings)
Infant loses less than 10% of birth weight

NURSING DIAGNOSIS: Altered family processes related to maturational crisis, birth of term infant, change in family unit

GOAL

Facilitate parent-infant attachment process

INTERVENTIONS

As soon after delivery as possible, encourage parents to see and hold infant; place newborn close to face of parents so that visual contact can be established
Ideally, perform eye care after initial meeting of infant and parents, usually about 1 hour after birth
Identify for parents specific behaviors manifested by infant, for example, alertness, ability to see, vigorous suck, rooting behavior, and attention to human voice
Discuss with parents their expectations of fantasy child vs real child, if indicated
Encourage parents to "talk out" their labor and delivery experience; identify any events that signify loss of control to either parent, especially mother
Identify behavioral steps in attachment process and evaluate those aspects that could be considered positive and those that may represent inadequate or delayed parenting
Encourage family to call for infant frequently if not rooming-in
Observe and assess the reciprocity of cues between infant and parent
Assist parents in recognizing attention-nonattention cycles and in understanding their significance
Assess variables affecting development of attachment through observing infant and parent and interviewing each parent or other significant caregiver

EXPECTED OUTCOMES

Parents establish contact with infant immediately or soon after birth
Parents demonstrate attachment behaviors, such as touch, eye contact, naming and calling infant by name, talking to infant, participating in caregiving activities
Parents recognize attention-nonattention cycles

GOAL

Facilitate siblings' adjustment to newborn

INTERVENTIONS

Allow to visit and touch newborn when feasible
Explain physical differences in newborn, such as bald head, umbilical stump and clamp, circumcision
Explain to siblings realistic expectations regarding newborn abilities and needs
  Requires complete care
  Is not a playmate
Encourage siblings to participate in care at home
Encourage parents to spend individual time with other children at home

EXPECTED OUTCOME

Siblings express interest in newborn and realistic expectations for their age

GOAL

Prepare for discharge and home care

INTERVENTIONS

Instruct in newborn care
  Feeding (formula or breast)
  Bathing
  Umbilical and circumcision care
  Recognize states of activity for optimum interaction (see box below)
Encourage participation in parenting classes, if offered
Discuss importance and proper use of federally approved car restraints
  Refer to organizations that may rent car restraints

If parent-infant attachment is at risk, refer to appropriate agencies (social services, family and child services, at-risk programs)

EXPECTED OUTCOMES

Family demonstrates ability to provide care for infant
Family keeps appointments for follow-up care
Infant rides home in federally approved car restraint
Family members avail themselves of needed services

IMPLICATIONS FOR PARENTING RELATIVE TO INFANT'S STATES OF SLEEP AND ACTIVITY

Regular sleep

External stimuli do not arouse infant
Continue usual house noises
Leave infant alone, if sudden loud noise awakens infant and he cries

Irregular sleep

External stimuli that did not arouse infant during regular sleep may minimally arouse him
Periodic groaning or crying is usual; do not interpret as an indication of pain or discomfort

Drowsiness

Most stimuli arouse infant
Pick infant up during this time rather than leave in crib

Alert inactivity

Satisfy infant's needs such as hunger
Place infant in area of home where activity is continuous
Place toys in crib or playpen
Place objects within 17.5-20 cm (7-8 inches) of infant's view

Waking and crying

Remove intense internal or external stimuli
Stimuli that were effective during alert inactivity are usually ineffective
Rock, swaddle, bring finger to mouth for self-quieting, or give pacifier to decrease crying

Unit 4

NURSING CARE PLAN:
THE HIGH-RISK INFANT AND FAMILY

High-risk infants are newborns, regardless of gestational age or birth weight, who have a greater than average chance of morbidity or mortality because of conditions or circumstances that are superimposed on the normal course of events associated with birth and the adjustment to extrauterine existence.

Classification According to Size

Low-birth-weight (LBW) infant—An infant whose birth weight is less than 2500 g regardless of gestational age

Very-low-birth-weight (VLBW) infant—An infant whose weight is less than 1500 g

Appropriate-for-gestational-age (AGA) infant—An infant whose weight falls between the 10th and 90th percentiles on intrauterine growth curves

Small-for-date (SFD) or small-for-gestational-age (SGA) infant—An infant whose rate of intrauterine growth was slowed and who was delivered at or later than term; the infant's birth weight falls below the 10th percentile on intrauterine growth curves

Intrauterine growth retardation (IUGR)—Found in infants whose intrauterine growth is retarded (sometimes used as a more descriptive term for the SGA infant)

Large-for-gestational-age (LGA) infant—An infant whose birth weight falls above the 90th percentile on intrauterine growth curves

Classification According to Gestational Age

Premature (preterm) infant—An infant born before completion of 37 weeks of gestation, regardless of birth weight

Term infant—An infant born between the beginning of the 38 weeks and the completion of the 42 weeks of gestation, regardless of birth weight

Postmature (postterm) infant—An infant born after 42 weeks of gestational age, regardless of birth weight

NOTE: See also nursing care plan for specific health problem(s).

ASSESSMENT

See Assessment of gestational age, p. 18
See Newborn assessment, p. 10
Observe for clinical manifestations of prematurity:
  Very small, scrawny appearance
  Skin—Red to pink with visible veins
  Fine, feathery hair; lanugo on back and face
  Little or no evidence of subcutaneous fat
  Head larger in relation to body
  Sucking pads prominent
  Lies in "relaxed attitude"
  Limbs extended
  Lax, easily manipulated joints
  Ear cartilages poorly developed
  Few fine wrinkles on palms and soles
  Clitoris prominent in female
  Scrotum underdeveloped, nonpendulous, with minimal rugae and undescended testes
  Weak grasping, sucking, and swallowing reflexes
  Other neurologic signs are absent or diminished
  Unable to maintain body temperature
  Dilute urine
  Pliable thorax
  Periodic breathing, hypoventilation
  Frequent episodes of apnea

Observe for clinical manifestations of postmaturity:
  Absence of lanugo
  Little if any vernix caseosa, deep yellow or green in color
  Abundant scalp hair
  Long fingernails
  Whiter skin than term newborns
  Skin frequently cracked, parchmentlike, and desquamating
  Wasted physical appearance
  Long, thin appearance

General assessment

Weigh as ordered.
Described general body shape and size, presence and location of edema, amount of body fat.
Describe any apparent deformities.

Respiratory assessment

Describe shape of chest (barrel, concave), symmetry, presence of incisions, chest tubes, or other deviations.
Describe use of accessory muscles substernal, intercostal, or subclavicular retractions; nasal flaring.
Determine respiratory rate and regularity.
Describe breath sounds: rales, rhonchi, wheezing, wet diminished sounds, areas of absence of sound, grunting.

ASSESSMENT—cont'd

Describe secretions.

Determine whether suctioning is needed.

Describe cry.

Describe ambient oxygen and method of delivery; if intubated, describe size of tube, type of ventilator, and settings.

Cardiovascular assessment

Determine heart rate and rhythm.

Describe heart sounds, including any suspected murmurs.

Determine the point of maximum intensity, the point where the heartbeat sounds loudest (a change in the point of maximum intensity may indicate a mediastinal shift).

Describe infant's color (alterations may be of cardiac, respiratory, or hematopoietic origin): cyanosis, pallor, plethora, jaundice.

Determine blood pressure; indicate extremity used.

Describe peripheral pulses; palpate bilaterally.

Determine central venous pressure (if central venous pressure line is part of infant's apparatus).

Describe monitors and their parameters.

Gastrointestinal assessment

Determine presence of any indication of abdominal distention: increase in circumference, shiny skin, erythema or discoloration.

Observe feeding behavior (strength of suck, coordination of sucking and swallowing).

Determine any signs of regurgitation, especially following feeding; character and amount of residual if gavage fed; if nasogastric tube in place, describe type of suction, drainage (color, consistency, pH, guaiac).

Describe amount, color, consistency, and odor of any emesis.

Describe amount, color, and consistency of stools; check for occult blood or appearance in stool, reducing substances.

Describe bowel sounds: presence or absence.

Genitourinary assessment

Describe any abnormalities of genitalia.

Describe amount (as determined by weight), color, pH, labstick findings, and specific gravity of urine (to screen for adequacy of hydration).

Check weight (the most accurate measure for assessment of hydration).

Neurologic-musculoskeletal assessment

Describe infant's movements: random, purposeful, jittery, twitching, spontaneous, elicited.

Describe infant's position or attitude: flexed, extended.

Describe reflexes observed: Moro, sucking, Babinski, and other expected reflexes.

Determine level of response.

Determine changes in head circumference (if indicated).

Determine pupillary responses.

Temperature assessment

Determine axillary temperature.

Determine relationship to environmental temperature.

Skin assessment

Describe any discoloration, reddened area, or signs of irritation, especially where monitoring equipment, infusion lines, or other apparatus comes in contact with skin; also check and note any skin preparation used (e.g., povidone-iodine).

Determine texture and turgor of skin: dry, smooth, flaky, peeling, etc.

Describe any rash or skin lesion.

Determine whether intravenous infusion catheter or needle is in place and observe for signs of infiltration.

Describe parenteral infusion lines: location, type (arterial, venous, hyperalimentation, central venous pressure); type of infusion and relevant information; type of infusion pump and rate of flow; type of needle (butterfly, Quik Cath), appearance of insertion site.

NURSING DIAGNOSIS: Ineffective breathing pattern related to neuromuscular impairment (immature respiratory center), decreased energy, and fatigue

GOAL

Support respiratory efforts

INTERVENTIONS

Position for optimum air exchange (head supported when on side)

Observe for deviations from desired functioning; recognize signs of distress

Suction as necessary to remove accumulated mucus from nasopharynx, trachea, and (where necessary) endotracheal tube

Carry out percussion, vibration, and postural drainage to loosen secretions in respiratory tree

Position prone or on side; turn head to side to prevent aspiration

Observe for signs of respiratory distress—nasal flaring, retractions, tachypnea

Maintain ambient oxygen at level to ensure satisfactory skin color with minimum respiratory effort and energy expenditure

Carry out regimen prescribed for supplemental oxygen therapy (maintain ambient oxygen concentration at minimum FIO_2 level to maintain good color and energy expenditure)

Apply and manage monitoring equipment correctly

Understand functioning of respiratory support apparatus
  Assisted ventilation apparatus
  Controlled ventilation apparatus
  Insufflation bags with masks and/or endotracheal adaptor
  Oxygen hoods
  Humidifier warmers

EXPECTED OUTCOMES

Breathing is regular and unlabored
Respiratory rate is within normal limits (specify)

NURSING DIAGNOSIS: Ineffective thermoregulation related to immature temperature control

GOAL

Provide neutral thermal environment

INTERVENTIONS

Place infant in humidified Isolette, radiant warmer, or warmly clothed in open crib
Monitor temperature hourly in unstable infants (take axillary temperature; check function of servocontrolled mechanism when used)
Check temperature of infant in relation to temperature of heating unit
Avoid situations that might predispose infant to chilling, such as exposure to cool air

EXPECTED OUTCOME

Infant's temperature remains at optimum level

NURSING DIAGNOSIS: Potential for infection related to deficient immunologic defenses

GOAL

Protect infant from infection

INTERVENTIONS

Carry out meticulous handwashing before handling infant
Ensure that all equipment in contact with infant is scrupulously clean or sterile
Prevent personnel with infections from coming into direct contact with infant
Isolate other infants who have infections according to agency policy
*Administer prophylactic antibiotics as ordered

EXPECTED OUTCOME

Infant exhibits no evidence of infection

NURSING DIAGNOSIS: Altered nutrition: less than body requirements (potential) related to inability to ingest nutrients because of weakness, helplessness

GOAL

Provide nutrition

INTERVENTIONS

*Maintain parenteral fluid or hyperalimentation therapy as ordered
Bottle-feed infant if strong sucking and swallowing reflexes are present (usually at gestational age of 33 to 35 weeks)
Follow unit protocol for advancing volume and concentration of formula
Gavage feed if infant tires easily or has weak sucking, gag, or swallowing reflexes
Assist mothers with breast-feeding if feasible and desirable

EXPECTED OUTCOMES

Infant receives an adequate amount of nutrients
Infant demonstrates a steady weight gain

NURSING DIAGNOSIS: Potential fluid volume deficit related to physiologic characteristics of preterm infant, helplessness

GOAL

Maintain hydration

INTERVENTIONS

Monitor therapies that increase insensible water loss, e.g., phototherapy
Ensure adequate intake
Assess state of hydration, e.g., skin tugor, temperature, weight, urine specific gravity
Regulate parenteral fluids
Avoid administering hypertonic fluids, e.g., undiluted medications

EXPECTED OUTCOME

Infant exhibits no evidence of dehydration

NURSING DIAGNOSIS: Activity intolerance related to imbalance between oxygen supply and demand, physical weakness

GOAL

Conserve energy

INTERVENTIONS

Maintain neutral thermal environment
Concentrate activities to allow for longer periods of rest
Administer gavage feeding when infant tires easily
Ensure minimum handling of infant

EXPECTED OUTCOME

Infant rests 1 hour (uninterrupted) at regularly scheduled intervals (specify)

NURSING DIAGNOSIS: Potential impaired skin integrity related to immature skin structure, immobility

GOAL

Prevent skin breakdown

INTERVENTIONS

Cleanse skin with clear water or approved cleanser
Avoid use of alkaline-based or hexachlorophene cleansing products or lotions
Use only transpore tape to secure items to the skin
Apply protective preparation to skin on which tape or adhesive-backed items, e.g., electrodes, may be attached
Exert extreme care when performing activities involving skin, e.g., removing dressings, electrodes, tape
Place infant on water pillow or fleece
Turn at least every 2 hours

EXPECTED OUTCOME

Skin remains clean and intact with no evidence of irritation or injury

NURSING DIAGNOSIS: Altered growth and development related to preterm birth, unnatural environment, separation from parents

GOAL

Facilitate growth and development

INTERVENTIONS

Provide optimum nutrition
Provide developmental intervention as appropriate (see box, p. 307)
Recognize signs of overstimulation (flaccidity, yawning, staring, eye floating, active averting, irritability, crying)
Promote parent-infant bonding

EXPECTED OUTCOMES

Infant exhibits a steady weight gain
Infant responds to appropriate stimuli

NURSING DIAGNOSIS: Altered family processes related to situational/maturational crisis, knowledge deficit (birth of a preterm and/or ill infant), interruption of bonding process

GOAL

Keep parents informed of infant's progress

INTERVENTIONS

Answer questions, allow expression of concern regarding care and prognosis
Encourage mother and father to visit and/or call unit
Emphasize positive aspects of infant status
Be honest but not overly candid, overly optimistic, or pessimistic

EXPECTED OUTCOME

Parents express feelings and concerns regarding the infant and his prognosis

GOAL

Facilitate parent-infant attachment process

INTERVENTIONS

Initiate parents' visit as soon as possible
Encourage parents to
    Visit infant frequently
    Touch, fondle, and caress infant
    Become actively involved in infant's care
    Bring clothing to dress up infant as soon as condition permits
Reinforce parents' endeavors
Be alert to signs of tension in parents
Allow parents to spend time alone with infant
Help parents interpret infant responses; comment regarding any positive infant response
Help parents by demonstrating techniques and offer support

EXPECTED OUTCOMES

Parents visit infant soon after birth and at frequent intervals
Parents relate positively with infant
Parents provide care for the infant and demonstrate an attitude of comfort in relationships with the infant

GOAL

Facilitate sibling-infant attachment

INTERVENTIONS

Allow siblings to visit infant when feasible
Explain environment, events, and strange appearance of infant, e.g., why infant cannot come home, "special" bed
Provide photos of infant or other items if siblings unable to visit

EXPECTED OUTCOMES

Siblings visit infant in nursery
Siblings exhibit an understanding of explanations (specify)
Siblings receive infant-related items (specify)

GOAL

Prepare for infant's discharge

INTERVENTIONS

Assess readiness of family (especially mother) to care for infant
Teach necessary techniques and observations
Arrange for public health referral if indicated
Reinforce follow-up care
Refer to appropriate agencies or services for needed assistance
Encourage and facilitate involvement with parent group
Teach family infant cardiopulmonary resuscitation technique and response to choking incident (see Home care instructions, p. 234)
*Refer to appropriate support group(s)

*Parent Care, 1½ South Union Street, Alexandria, VA 22314-3323, (703) 836-4678; The Compassionate Friends, P.O. Box 3696, Oak Brook, IL 60522-3696, (708) 990-0010.
See also appropriate disorder (if applicable) for specific support groups and agencies.

Unit 4

EXPECTED OUTCOMES

Family demonstrates the ability to provide care for the infant
Family members take advantage of available services
Family members keep appointments for follow-up care

NURSING DIAGNOSIS: Anticipatory grieving related to grave prognosis and/or death of infant

GOAL

Help parents understand reality of death

INTERVENTIONS

Provide family with the opportunity to hold their infant before death and, if possible, be present at the time of death
Arrange for or perform appropriate baptism rite for infant
Provide family with the opportunity to see, touch, hold, caress, examine, and talk to their infant privately after death
Allow family to bathe infant after death if they desire
Comply with family's wish regarding nurse's attendance
Keep baby's body available for a few hours to allow time for family who are hesitant an opportunity to see dead infant if they change their minds
Provide a photograph taken before or after infant's death to allow family to refer to at a later time to make infant seem more real
    Take photograph of infant being held or touched by an adult; avoid morgue type photograph

Provide other tangible remembrances of child's death, e.g., name tags, armband, lock of hair (removed for intravenous insertion)
Encourage family to name the infant if they have failed to do so

EXPECTED OUTCOME

Family discuss the reality of the death and convey an attitude of acceptance

GOAL

Support family

INTERVENTIONS

Be available to family
Provide appropriate religious support, e.g., clergyman
Discuss the death with family
Talk with family openly and honestly about funeral arrangements
    Have information available regarding inexpensive services in the community
    Inform family of all options available
Provide opportunity for the family to call the unit if they have any questions
Contact family after the death to assess coping and status of grieving process
Refer family to appropriate support group(s)*

EXPECTED OUTCOME

Family copes with infant's death appropriately

---

*Parent Care, 1½ South Union Street, Alexandria, VA 22314-3323, (703) 836-4678; The Compassionate Friends, P.O. Box 3696, Oak Brook, IL 60522-3696; see also appropriate disorder (if applicable) for specific groups and agencies.

Unit 4

SUGGESTIONS FOR DEVELOPMENTAL INTERVENTION

General guidelines

Individualize interventions for each infant

Offer only during periods of alertness

Limit to one or two types of stimulus per session

Provide intervention for short periods

Space periods according to infant's tolerance

Titrate interventions according to infant cues

Terminate stimulation if infant displays evidence of overstimulation:*

Color changes—Mottled, gray, flushed

Gagging, gasping, spitting up

Straining as if or actually producing a bowel movement

Yawning, sighing

Flaccidity—Truncal, extremity, facial

Hyperextensions—Leg, arm, trunk, finger

Facial grimacing, tongue extension

Hyperflexion—Trunk, extremity

Frantic, diffuse activity

Visual

Place magazine photographs (black and white schematic faces) in visual range (19 to 22 cm) in "en face" position.

Cover mattress with black and white patterned material for length of intervention (may be too stimulating for some infants).

Provide black and white mobiles with varied hanging shapes.

Initiate eye-to-eye contact; repeat as tolerated.

Alternate holding black and white pattern still and moving it across the infant's visual field.

Tactile

Press skin appropriately

Stroke skin slowly and gently in head-to-toe direction; begin with trunk and move to more sensitive areas such as face.

Provide alternate textures, e.g., sheepskin, satin, velvet.

Provide boundaries, foot bracing, blankets.

Auditory

Play tape of parents' voices.

Play classical music recording or music box (jazz or rock is less effective).

Speak with a variety of voice inflections; alternate adult and baby talk.

Call infant by name at each interaction.

Vestibular

Place on waterbed with oscillations and waves per minute determined on an individual basis; alternate oscillation with rest periods (may not be acceptable intervention in some units).

Rock in chair.

Place in sling (hammock) and rock.

Provide passive range-of-motion exercises to knee and hip joints.

Close infant's fist around cloth toy.

Lift head to upright position, tip to right and then to left, stopping at midline.

Slowly change position during handling.

Olfactory

Pass open breast milk or formula container under nose.

Pass various sweet smelling items under nose, e.g., cherry syrup, cinnamon, nutmeg, strawberry extract.

Gustatory

Place infant's hand or a pacifier in mouth when sucking movements are observed or during gavage feeding.

Place 2 drops of milk in infant's mouth with each tube feeding

Modified from Chaze BA and Ludington Hoe SM: Sensory stimulation in the NICU, Am J Nurs 84:68-71, 1984.
*Als H: Toward a synactive theory of development: promise for the assessment and support of infant and individuality, Infant Mental Health J, 3:229-243 1982.

Unit 4

Neonatal complications

Metabolic abnormalities in the newborn

	Hypoglycemia	Hypocalcemia
Definition	Blood glucose concentration significantly lower than that in the majority of infants of the same age and weight	Abnormally low levels of calcium in circulating blood
Types	Early transitional neonatal: large or normal-size infants who appear to suffer from hyperinsulinism	Early onset: appears in first 48 hours, appears in preterm infants who experienced perinatal hypoxia
	Classic transient neonatal: infants who suffered intrauterine malnutrition that depleted glycogen and fat stores	Late onset, cow's milk–induced hypocalcemia (neonatal tetany): apparent after first 3 to 4 days (high phosphorus-to-calcium ratio of cow's milk depresses parathyroid activity, reducing serum calcium levels)
	Secondary: a response to perinatal stresses that increase infant's metabolic needs relative to glycogen stores	
	Recurrent, severe: caused by an enzymatic or metabolic-endocrine defect	
Clinical manifestations	Vague, often indistinguishable from other conditions	Early onset: jitteriness, apnea, cyanotic episodes, edema, high-pitched cry, abdominal distention
	Cerebral signs: jitteriness, tremors, twitching, weak or high-pitched cry, lethargy, limpness, apathy, convulsions, and coma	Late onset: twitching, tremors, seizures
	Other: cyanosis, apnea, rapid irregular respirations, sweating, eye rolling, refusal to eat	
	Signs often transient but recurrent	
Laboratory diagnosis	Plasma glucose concentrations less than 35 mg/100 ml in first 72 hours: 45 mg/100 ml thereafter (LBW infants: less than 25 mg/dl)	Serum calcium less than 7 mg/100 ml
		Ionized calcium less than 3 to 3.5 mg/100 ml
Treatment	Intravenous glucose administration	Early onset: increased milk feedings, administration of calcium supplements (sometimes)
	Preventive: early feeding in normoglycemic infants	Late onset: administration of calcium gluconate orally or intravenously (slowly); vitamin D
Nursing	See Nursing care plan: The high-risk infant and family, p. 302	See Nursing care plan: The high-risk infant and family, p. 302
	Identify infants with hypoglycemia	Identify infants with hypocalcemia
	Reduce environmental factors that predispose to hypoglycemia, e.g., cold stress, respiratory	Administer calcium as prescribed
	Employ proper feeding techniques	Observe for signs of acute hypercalcemia, e.g., vomiting, bradycardia
	Administer glucose as prescribed	Manipulate environment to reduce stimuli that might precipitate a seizure or tremors, e.g., picking up infant suddenly, sudden jarring of crib

See also Nursing care plan: The child with hyperbilirubinemia, p. 373.

Respiratory complications in the newborn

Description	Specific manifestations	Treatment	Nursing considerations
Respiratory distress syndrome (RDS)			
See p. 326			
Meconium aspiration syndrome (MAS)			
Aspiration of amniotic fluid containing meconium into fetal or newborn trachea in utero or at first breath	Meconium stained at birth	Vigorous suction of hypopharynx at birth	See Nursing care of infant with respiratory distress syndrome, p. 326
	Tachypnea	Treat for respiratory distress	
	Hypoxia		
	Depressed		
	Hyperventilation (early)		
	Hypoventilation (later)		

Description	Specific manifestations	Treatment	Nursing considerations
Apnea of prematurity			
Lapse of spontaneous breathing for 20 or more seconds, followed by bradycardia and color change	Persistent apneic spells	Observe for apnea Administer theophylline	Monitor respiratory and heart rates Observe for presence of respirations Observe color Apply gentle tactile stimulation Suction nose and oropharynx if still apneic Apply artificial ventilation with mask and resuscitation (AMBU) with sufficient pressure to lift rib cage Assess for and manage any precipitating factors, e.g., temperature, humidity, distention, ambient oxygen
Pneumothorax			
Presence of extraneous air in the pleural space as a result of alveolar rupture	Tachypnea Grunting, flaring nares Retractions Absent or diminished breath sounds Shift in point of maximum intensity of heart sounds	Evacuate trapped air from pleural space through chest tubes and waterseal drainage	Maintain close vigilance of infants with respiratory distress or those on assisted ventilation Provide appropriate care of chest drainage apparatus
Bronchopulmonary dysplasia (BPD)			
A pathologic process related to alveolar damage from lung disease, prolonged exposure to high oxygen concentrations, use of positive-pressure ventilation, and endotracheal intubation	Nonspecific Susceptibility to upper respiratory infections Frequent hospitalization for respiratory dysfunction	Nonspecific Support respiratory efforts Prevent and/or control respiratory infections	Provide opportunities for additional rest, fluids, and calories Provide small, frequent feedings to avoid overextending stomach, which interferes with respiration Observe for signs of over- or under-hydration

Cardiovascular complications in the newborn

Description	Clinical manifestations	Therapeutic management	Nursing considerations
Patent ductus arteriosus (PDA)			
	Increased P_{CO_2} Recurrent apnea Bounding peripheral pulses Typical systolic or continuous murmur	Regulate fluids Provide respiratory support Administer indomethacin	See nursing care plan: The high-risk infant and family, p. 302 Collect specimens as needed Assess renal function Observe for bleeding tendencies
Persistent pulmonary hypertension (PPH)			
Severe pulmonary hypertension and large right-to-left shunt through foramen ovale and ductus arteriosus	Hypoxia when agitated Marked cyanosis Tachypnea with grunting and retractions Decreased peripheral pulses	Regulate fluids Give supplemental oxygen Give assisted ventilation Administer vasodilators (sometimes)	See Nursing care plan: The high-risk infant and family, p. 302; Nursing care plan: The infant with respiratory distress syndrome p. 326 Reduce stress to infant, especially noxious stimuli that cause crying and struggling Decrease physical manipulation and disturbance
Anemia			
Loss of blood from hemorrhage in organs (during delivery), blood diseases Contributing: decreased fetal hemoglobin and shortened red blood cell survival time in preterm infant	Pallor Dyspnea Tachycardia Tachypnea Diminished activity	Administer iron-fortified formula and/or supplemental iron Transfuse with packed red blood cells for severe anemia	Monitor blood drawn for tests Administer iron as prescribed

Unit 4

Cardiovascular complications in the newborn—cont'd

Description	Clinical manifestations	Therapeutic management	Nursing considerations
Polycythemia/hyperviscosity syndrome			
Venous hematocrit 65% or greater owing to twin-to-twin or mother-to-fetus transfusion or increased red blood cell production	High incidence of: Cardiovascular symptoms (PPH, cyanosis, apnea) Seizures Hyperbilirubinemia Gastrointestinal abnormalities	Correct metabolic imbalances Implement partial exchange transfusion Provide appropriate therapy for associated problems	See Nursing care plans: The high-risk infant and family, p. 302; The infant with hyperbilirubinemia, p. 373
Hemorrhagic disease of the newborn			
Bleeding disorder resulting from transient deficiency of vitamin K–dependent blood factors	Oozing blood from umbilicus or circumcision Bloody or black stools Hematuria Ecchymosis Epistaxis	Administer prophylactic vitamin K	Administer vitamin K into vastus lateralis muscle
Retinopathy of prematurity (ROP)			
Replacement of retina by fibrous tissue and blood vessels	Progressive vascular growth of retina Eventual blindness	Arrest proliferation process—cryotherapy Administer prophylactic vitamin E (sometimes) Use supplemental oxygen judiciously, and monitor carefully	See Nursing care plan: The high-risk infant and family, p. 302 Monitor oxygen concentration

Cerebral complications in the newborn

Description	Clinical manifestations	Therapeutic management	Nursing considerations
Hypoxic-ischemic brain injury			
Nonprogressive neurologic (brain) impairment caused by intrauterine or postnatal asphyxia resulting in hypoxemia and/or cerebral ischemia	Appears in first 24 hours after hypoxic episode Seizures Abnormal muscle tone (usually hypotonia) Disturbance of sucking and swallowing Apneic episodes Stupor or coma	Provide vigorous supportive care Provide adequate ventilation Maintain cerebral perfusion Prevent cerebral edema Treat seizures	See Nursing care plan: The high-risk infant and family, p. 302 Observe for signs that indicate cerebral hypoxia Monitor ventilatory and intravenous therapy and nutrition Observe for and manage seizures Support family Provide guidelines for family management of permanent neurologic damage
Periventricular/intraventricular hemorrhage (PVH/IVH)			
Hemorrhage into and around ventricles caused by ruptured vessels as result of an event that increases cerebral blood flow to area	Tense, bulging anterior fontanel Separated sutures Neurologic signs Twitching Stupor Apnea Seizures Evident on ultrasonography and/or tomography	Supportive care: Provide ventilatory support Maintain oxygenation Regulate fluid and electrolytes, acid-base balance Suppress or prevent seizures	See Nursing care plan: The high-risk infant and family, p. 302 Prevent increased cerebral blood pressure Elevate head Avoid pressure-producing procedures Support family

Description	Clinical manifestations	Therapeutic management	Nursing considerations
Intracranial hemorrhage			
Hemorrhage into the subdural or subarachnoid spaces; intracerebellar	Same as above	Same as above	Same as for PVH/IVH
Neonatal seizures			

Sudden, violent involuntary contractions of a group of muscles	Subtle seizures:
	  Clonic horizontal eye deviation
	  Repetitive blinking or fluttering of eyelids
	  Drooling
	  Sucking or other oral-buccal-lingual movements
	  Arm movements resembling rowing or swimming
	  Leg movements described as pedaling or bicycling
	  Apnea
	Generalized tonic seizures:
	  Usually manifest as extensions of all four limbs, similar to decerebrate rigidity
	  Occasionally upper limbs are maintained in stiffly flexed position resembling decorticate rigidity
	  Appear more frequently in premature infants
	Multifocal clonic seizures:
	  Rhythmic jerking movements, about 1 to 3 per second
	  May migrate randomly from one part of the body to another
	  Simultaneous involvement of separate areas often occurs
	  Convulsive movements may start at different times and at different rates
		Correct metabolic derangements
		Supportive care:
		  Respiratory
		  Cardiovascular
		Suppress seizure activity with anticonvulsants
		Treat underlying cause
			Recognize that a seizure is occurring
			Observe and record seizure accurately (see p. 403)
			Administer oxygen, anticonvulsants, and other therapies as prescribed
			See Nursing care plan: The high-risk infant and family, p. 302

Neonatal tremors			

Involuntary trembling, quivering, or jitteriness	Repetitive shaking of an extremity or extremities
	Observed with crying, may occur with changes in sleeping state, or may be elicited with stimulation
	Relatively common in newborn
	Mild jitteriness may be considered normal during first 4 days of life
	Can be distinguished from seizures by several characteristics:
	  Not accompanied by ocular movement
	  Dominant movement in jitteriness is tremor
	  Seizure movement is clonic jerking that cannot be stopped by flexion of affected limb
	  Jitteriness is highly sensitive to stimulation; seizures are not
		No therapy required
		Evaluate if persist beyond the fourth day of life
			Distinguish between tremors and seizures

Unit 4

Infections of the newborn

Description	Clinical manifestations	Therapeutic management	Nursing considerations
Sepsis, septicemia			
Generalized bacterial infection in the bloodstream	Fever frequently absent; body temperature commonly normal or suboptimum Indication of local inflammatory response rare Subtle, vague, and nonspecific signs: "Failure to do well" "Does not look right" Nonspecific respiratory distress Respiratory distress: Apnea Irregular, grunting respirations Retractions Gastric distress: Vomiting (vomitus may be bile stained) Diarrhea Abdominal distention Absent stools as a result of paralytic ileus Poor sucking and feeding Skin manifestations may include: Cyanosis Pallor Mottling Jaundice Lesions associated with specific organisms Central nervous system involvement: Irritability Apathy Tremors Convulsions Coma Signs of increased intracranial pressure related to meningitis, a frequent sequela of sepsis	Aggressive administration of antibiotics Transfusion with polymorphonuclear leukocytes Supportive therapy: Oxygen Fluid and electrolyte management Blood transfusions, if indicated Electronic monitoring of vital signs Neutral thermal environment	See Nursing care plan: The high-risk infant and family, p. 302 Elevate head of bed Administer antibiotics and other medications as prescribed Collect needed specimens for laboratory examination Be alert for evidence of extensions of infection (e.g., meningitis) and superimposed infections (e.g., candidiasis) Prevent spread of infection to other infants (see p. 288) Observe for signs of septic shock (see p. 371)
Necrotizing enterocolitis (NEC)			
Acute inflammation of the bowel characterized by ischemic necrosis of the GI mucosa that may lead to perforation and peritonitis	Nonspecific clinical signs: Lethargy Poor feeding Hypotension Vomiting Apnea Decreased urine output Unstable temperature Specific signs: Distended (often shiny) abdomen Blood in the stools or gastric contents Gastric retention	Discontinuation of all oral feedings for 24 to 48 hours Abdominal decompression via nasogastric suction Intravenous antibiotics Correction of fluid and electrolyte derangements Parenteral feedings	See Nursing care plan: The high-risk infant and family, p. 302 Administer antibiotics as prescribed Monitor intravenous fluids and feedings Check abdomen for distention frequently Listen for presence of bowel sounds Assist with diagnostic procedures Prevent pressure on abdomen—loose or no diapering, position on side or back Advance to normal diet as prescribed Prevent spread of infection
Bullous impetigo (impetigo neonatorum)			
Superficial skin infection most often caused by *Staphylococcus aureus*	Eruption of bullous vesicular lesions on previously untraumatized skin	Warm compresses followed by gentle cleansing and application of topical antibiotic several times daily	Prevent spread of infection See Nursing care plan: The normal newborn and family, p. 298

Neonatal complications associated with maternal conditions

Description	Clinical manifestations	Therapeutic management	Nursing considerations
Infant of the diabetic mother (IDM)			
Characterized by hypoglycemia associated with increased insulin activity in the blood	Large for their gestational age Very plump and full-faced Liberal coat of vernix caseosa Plethora Listlessness and lethargy Hypoglycemia that appears shortly after birth Clinical signs appear in mothers with poor control of their diabetes	Careful observation of mother and fetus during gestation Blood glucose determination Feedings of 5% to 10% glucose begun 1 hour after birth followed by formula, if tolerated IV infusion for critically ill infants	See Nursing care plan: The normal newborn and family, p. 298 Observe for signs of hypoglycemia (p. 308), hyperbilirubinemia (p. 373), and respiratory distress (p. 326)
Drug-addicted infant (narcotic)			
Passively addicted to drug to which the mother is addicted	Tremors Restlessness and irritability Hypertonicity of muscles Hyperactive reflexes Frequent sneezing Frequent yawning Low-grade fever Tachypnea High-pitched, shrill cry Uncoordinated, ineffectual sucking and swallowing reflexes Regurgitation and vomiting after feedings Diarrhea—a later manifestation Minimum sleeping Sweating Seizures	Intramuscular administration of chlorpromazine or phenobarbital followed by oral administration Diazepam for selected infants Paregoric administration for GI symptoms	See Nursing care plan: The normal newborn and family, p. 298 Reduce external stimuli that might trigger hyperactivity and irritability Reduce infant's ability to self-stimulate by wrapping snugly and holding infant tightly Carefully monitor intake and output—both fluid and food Protect hyperactive infants from skin abrasions Monitor activity level and its relationship to other activities

Congenital disorders acquired from maternal infections

Fetal or newborn effect	Comments and nursing considerations*
Acquired Immune Deficiency Syndrome (AIDS) (human immunodeficiency virus [HIV])	
Growth failure Prominent boxlike forehead Short nose with flattened columella Well-formed, triangular philtrum Microcephaly Flat nasal bridge Mild upward or downward obliquity of eyes Long palpebral fissures with blue sclerae Patulous lips Ocular hypertelorism	Transmitted transplacentally; during delivery; in breast milk No treatment currently available other than supportive care
Coxsackie Virus (group B)	
Poor feeding, vomiting, diarrhea, fever: cardiac enlargement, arrhythmias, congestive heart failure: lethary, seizures, meningeal involvement	Transmitted: first trimester or late in pregnancy
***Chlamydia* Infection (*Chlamydia trachomatis*)**	
Conjunctivitis, pneumonia	Transmitted: last trimester or intrapartum Apply prophylactic medication to eyes at time of birth Treatment: antibiotics

*Isolation precautions depend on institutional policy (see p. 289).

Unit 4

Congenital disorders acquired from maternal infections—cont'd

Fetal or newborn effect	Comments and nursing considerations
Cytomegalic Inclusion Disease—CID (cytomegalovirus [CMV])	
Microcephaly, cerebral calcifications, chorioretinitis	Transmitted: throughout pregnancy
Jaundice, hepatosplenomegaly	Affected individuals excrete virus
Petechial or purpuric rash	Virus detected in urine by electron microscopy
Neurologic sequelae: seizure disorders, sensorimotor deafness, mental retardation	Avoid kissing affected child
	Pregnant women should avoid close contact with known cases
	Treatment: antimetabolites, antiviral agent
Gonococcal Disease *(Neisseria gonorrhoeae)*	
Ophthalmitis	Transmitted: last trimester or intrapartum
Neonatal gonococcal arthritis, septicemia, meningitis	Apply prophylactic medication to eyes at time of birth
	Obtain smears for culture
	Treatment: penicillin
Hepatitis B (virus)	
May be asymptomatic	Transmitted: transplacentally, contaminated maternal secretions during delivery; possibly through breast-feeding, especially if mother has cracked nipples
Acute hepatits, changes in liver function	Treatment: hepatitis B immune globulin to all infants of HBsAg-positive mothers
Herpes, Neonatal (herpes simplex virus)	
Cutaneous lesions: vesicles at 6 to 10 days of age, may be no lesions	History of genital infection in mother/partner in 50% of cases
Disseminated disease resembles sepsis	Transmitted: intrapartum either ascending and/or direct contact; incubation period 6 to 10 days
Visceral involvement: granulomas	Rarely acquired as intrauterine infection during first trimester and intrapartum
Early nonspecific signs: fever, lethargy, poor feeding, irritability, vomiting	Cesarean section a preventive measure for mothers with active lesions
May include hyperbilirubinemia, seizures, flaccid or spastic paralysis, apneic episodes, respiratory distress, lethargy, or coma	
Listeriosis *(Listeria)*	
Acquired in late pregnancy: stillborn or acutely ill; may die within an hour after birth	Transmitted: transplacentally or by aspiration of secretions at birth
Late onset: septicemia; meningitis	Segregate infants until cultures are negative
Rubella, Congenital (rubella virus)	
Eye defects: cataracts (unilateral or bilateral), microphthalmia, retinitis, glaucoma	Transmitted: first trimester; early second trimester
Central nervous system signs: microcephaly, seizures, severe mental retardation	Pregnant women should avoid contact with all affected persons, including infants with rubella syndrome
Congenital heart defects: patent ductus arteriosus	Emphasize vaccination of all unimmunized prepubertal children, susceptible adolescents, and adult females of childbearing age
Auditory: high incidence of delayed hearing loss	Caution women against pregnancy for at least 3 months after vaccination
Intrauterine growth retardation	
Hyperbilirubinema, spinal fluid abnormalities, thrombocytopenia, hepatomegaly	
Syphilis, Congenital *(Treponema pallidum)*	
Copper-colored maculopapular cutaneous lesions (after 7th day), mucous membrane patches, hair loss, nail exfoliation, sniffles (syphilitic rhinitis), profound anemia, poor feeding, pseudo-paralysis of one or more limbs	Transmitted: transplacentally, usually after 18th week of pregnancy
	Most severe form of syphilis
	Strict isolation of infant
	Treatment: penicillin
Toxoplasmosis *(Toxoplasma gondii)*	
Hydrocephaly, cerebral calcifications, chorioretinitis (classic triad)	Transmitted: throughout pregnancy
Microcephaly	Predominant host for organism is cats
Encephalitis, myocarditis, hepatosplenomegaly, anemia, jaundice, diarrhea, vomiting, seizures, purpura	May be transmitted through cat feces, poorly cooked or raw infected meat
	Caution pregnant women to avoid contact with cat feces, e.g., emptying cat litter boxes
	Treatment: sulfonamides, pyrimethamine

Fetal or newborn effect	Comments and nursing considerations
Varicella (Chickenpox) (varicella virus)	
Skin lesions, microcephaly, limb deformities, encephalomyocarditis, visceral involvement	Transmitted: first trimester or intrapartum Strict isolation of infant

Congenital disorders acquired from maternal use of selected chemicals

Fetal or newborn effect	Comments and nursing considerations
Alcohol (fetal alcohol syndrome [FAS])	
Facial features: hypoplastic maxilla, micrognathia, hypoplastic philtrum, short palpebral fissures Neurologic: mental retardation, motor retardation, microcephaly, hypotonia Growth: prenatal growth retardation, persistent postnatal growth lag	Exact quantity of alcohol needed to produce teratogenic effects in fetus is not known All women, especially those with histories of heavy drinking, should be counseled regarding risks to fetus Provide mother with resources for treatment to decrease or eliminate alcoholic intake
Cocaine	
Neurologic: seizures, tremors, irritability, intolerant of cuddling efforts, abnormal sleep patterns Respiratory: increased periodic breathing. Low-birth weight Incessant crying, poor suck	Counsel and educate mothers regarding risks of cocaine use Refer mother for treatment
Tobacco smoking	
Fetal growth retardation Increased perinatal deaths Increased spontaneous abortions Postnatal: growth and intellectual and emotional developmental deficits; increased risk of SIDS Increased risk of cancer in childhood	Women should be counseled regarding the risk to fetus Provide with resources to help eliminate smoking

Neonatal abnormalities

Common autosomal aberrations

Syndrome	Chromosomal abnormality and nomenclature	Average incidence (live births)*	Major clinical manifestations
Cri du chat	Deletion of short arm of B (No. 5) chromosome—46,XY,5p−	1:50,000	Distinctive weak, high-pitched, mewlike cry resembling the cry of a cat; small head; hypertelorism; failure to thrive; severe mental retardation—profound with age
Trisomy 13 (Patau)	Trisomy of group D (No. 13) chromosome—47,XY,13+	1:4000-15000	Multiple anomalies, including cleft lip and palate (frequently bilateral); ear malformations; microphthalmia; polydactyly; eye defects; mental retardation; early death
Trisomy 18 (Edwards)	Trisomy of group E (No. 18) chromosome—47,XY,18+	1:3500-8000	Deformed and low-set ears; micrognathia; rocker-bottom feet; overlapping (index over third) fingers; prominent occiput; hypertelorism; failure to thrive and early death; mental retardation
Trisomy 21 (Down)	Trisomy of group G (No. 21) chromosome—47,XY,21+ (trisomy); 46,XY,D−,G−(DqGq)+ (translocation); 46,XY/47,XY,21+ (mosaic)	1:700*	Brachycephaly with flat occiput; inner epicanthal folds; small ears, nose, and mouth with protruding tongue; muscular hypotonia; broad, short hands with stubby fingers and transverse palmar crease; broad, stubby feet with wide space between big and second toes; mental retardation; variable life expectancy

From Nora JJ and Fraser FC: Medical genetics, ed 3 Philadelphia, 1989, Lea & Febiger.
*Risk related to maternal age—age < 30 yrs = 1:1500; age 35 yrs = 1:300, age 40 = 1:100; age > 45 yrs = 1:25

Unit 4

NURSING CARE OF THE CHILD WITH RESPIRATORY DYSFUNCTION

Interference with the ability of the pulmonary system to exchange oxygen and carbon dioxide adequately

NURSING CARE PLAN
THE CHILD WITH RESPIRATORY DYSFUNCTION

ASSESSMENT

History:

Family history of allergies, genetic disorders

Patient history of previous respiratory dysfunction; recent evidence of exposure to infection, allergens or other irritants, trauma

See physical assessment of the chest and lungs, p. 40.

See physical assessment of respirations, p. 26.

Observe respirations for:

Rate—Rapid (tachypnea), normal, or slow for the particular child

Depth—Normal depth, too shallow (hypopnea), too deep (hyperpnea); usually estimated from the amplitude of thoracic and abdominal excursion

Ease—Effortless, labored (dyspnea), orthopnea, associated with intercostal and/or substernal retractions (inspiratory "sinking in" of soft tissues in relation to the cartilaginous and bony thorax), pulsus paradoxus (blood pressure falls with inspiration and rises with expiration), flaring nares, head bobbing (head of sleeping child with suboccipital area supported on mother's forearm bobs forward in synchrony with each inspiration), grunting, or wheezing

Labored breathing—Continuous, intermittent, becoming steadily worsening, sudden onset, at rest or on exertion, associated with wheezing, grunting, associated with pain

Rhythm—Variation in rate and depth of respirations

Observe for:

Evidence of infection—Check for elevated temperature, enlarged cervical lymph nodes, inflamed mucous membranes, and purulent discharges from the nose, ears, or lungs (sputum)

Cough—Observe the characteristics of the cough (if present); for example, under what circumstances the cough is heard (e.g., night only, on arising), the nature of the cough (paroxysmal, with or without wheeze, "croupy" or "brassy"), frequency of cough, associated with swallowing or other activity

Wheeze—Expiratory or inspiratory, high-pitched or musical, prolonged, slowly progressive or sudden, associated with labored breathing

Cyanosis—Note distribution (peripheral, perioral, facial, trunk as well as face), degree, duration, associated with activity

Chest pain—May be a complaint of older children. Note location and circumstances: localized or generalized, referred to base of neck or abdomen, dull or sharp, deep or superficial, associated with rapid, shallow respirations or grunting

Sputum—Supervised older children may provide sputum sample. Note volume, color, viscosity, and odor

Bad breath—May be associated with some lung infections

NURSING DIAGNOSIS: Ineffective airway clearance related to mechanical obstruction, inflammation, increased secretions, discomfort, perceptual and cognitive impairment, pain

GOAL

Maintain patent airway

INTERVENTIONS

Aspirate (suction) secretions from airway as needed

Insert oral airway if indicated

Avoid neck hyperextension

Position to prevent aspiration of secretions

Semiprone position

Side-lying position

Assist child to expectorate sputum

Provide nebulization with appropriate solution and equipment as prescribed

*Administer expectorants, if prescribed

Perform percussion, vibrations, and drainage if prescribed

Give nothing by mouth to prevent aspiration of fluids (severe tachypnea)

---

*Dependent nursing action

EXPECTED OUTCOMES

Airways remain clear
Child breathes easily; respirations are within normal limits (see inside front cover)

NURSING DIAGNOSIS: Potential for suffocation related to airway obstruction (internal, external), inadequate environmental oxygen

GOAL

Prevent suffocation

INTERVENTIONS

Remove impediment to air exchange where possible, e.g., pillow over face, secretions
Avoid situations that predispose to airway obstruction or oxygen depletion

EXPECTED OUTCOME

Infant or child breathes without difficulty

NURSING DIAGNOSIS: Ineffective breathing pattern related to inflammatory process, pain, neurologic or musculoskeletal impairment

GOAL

Ease respiratory efforts

INTERVENTIONS

Allow position of comfort
Promote rest
Maintain patent airway
Provide high-humidity atmosphere
Position for comfort and maximum lung expansion
Implement measures to reduce anxiety and apprehension
Organize activities to allow for minimal expenditure of energy

EXPECTED OUTCOMES

Child rests and sleeps quietly
Respirations are unlabored
Respirations remain within normal limits (see inside front cover for normal variations)

GOAL

Increase oxygen supply to lungs

INTERVENTIONS

Position for maximum ventilatory efficiency such as high-Fowler position or sitting, leaning forward
Avoid constricting clothing, linens, restraints
Place in Croupette with cool vapor, if prescribed
*Provide oxygen as prescribed and/or needed
*Provide nebulization, if prescribed

---

*Dependent nursing action.

EXPECTED OUTCOMES

Child breathes easily
Respirations remain within normal limits (see inside front cover for normal variations)

GOAL

Promote expectoration of mucous secretions

INTERVENTIONS

Ensure adequate fluid intake
Provide humidified atmosphere
Assist child to cough effectively
Remove accumulated mucus; suction, if needed

EXPECTED OUTCOME

Older child expectorates secretions appropriately and without undue stress and fatigue

GOAL

Reduce anxiety and apprehension

INTERVENTIONS

Provide constant attendance during acute phase of illness
Encourage presence of parents
Provide comfort and cuddling when possible
Remove restraining devices when and as often as possible
Provide quiet diversion appropriate to child's age and condition
*Administer medications that promote breathing (bronchodilators, expectorants)

EXPECTED OUTCOMES

Child exhibits no signs of distress
Parents remain with child and provide comfort
Child engages in quiet activities appropriate for age, interest, and condition

---

NURSING DIAGNOSIS: Activity intolerance related to imbalance between oxygen supply and demand

GOAL

Conserve energy

INTERVENTIONS

Promote effective breathing
Promote rest
Implement measures to reduce apprehension
Disturb as little as possible

EXPECTED OUTCOME

Child rests quietly and engages in activities suitable to energy level
See Nursing diagnosis: Activity intolerance, p. 252

---

*Dependent nursing action

NURSING DIAGNOSIS: Pain related to inflammatory process, surgical incision

GOAL

Relieve pain

INTERVENTIONS AND EXPECTED OUTCOMES

See Nursing care plan: The child in pain, p. 279

NURSING DIAGNOSIS: Fear/anxiety related to hospitalization, difficulty breathing

GOAL

Keep child calm

INTERVENTIONS

Explain unfamiliar procedures and equipment to the child
Remain with child during procedures
Employ calm, reassuring manner
Provide constant attendance
Hold and cuddle child whenever possible—preferably by parent or other familiar person
Provide security devices such as familiar toy, blanket
Encourage parental attendance and, when possible, involvement in child's care
Do nothing to make the child more anxious than already is
Maintain a relaxed manner
Establish rapport with the child and parents
Instill confidence in both parents and child

Try to avoid any intrusive procedures
*Administer sedatives as indicated if ordered for restlessness and pain

EXPECTED OUTCOMES

Child responds positively to comforting measures
Parents relate readily with personnel and calmly with child
Child remains calm and cooperative

NURSING DIAGNOSIS: Altered family processes related to illness and/or hospitalization of a child

GOAL

Reduce parental anxiety

INTERVENTIONS

Recognize parental concern and need for information and support
Explain therapy and child's behavior
Provide support as needed
Encourage to become involved in child's care

EXPECTED OUTCOME

Parents ask appropriate questions, discuss the child's condition and care calmly, and become involved positively in child's care
See Nursing care plan: The family of the hospitalized child, p. 254
See Nursing care plan: The child in the hospital, p. 246

---

*Dependent nursing action.

NURSING CARE PLAN
THE CHILD WITH ACUTE RESPIRATORY INFECTION

Inflammatory process involving any or all parts of the respiratory tract caused by viral, bacterial, or mycoplasma
Upper respiratory tract—Consists of the nose, pharynx, and larynx
Croup syndromes—Involves structurally stable, nonreactive portion of the airway, the epiglottis and larynx

Lower respiratory tract—Consists of the rigid trachea; bronchi and bronchioles, with smooth muscle that has ability to constrict
Lungs—The primary respiratory unit

ASSESSMENT

See Nursing care plan: The child with respiratory dysfunction, p. 316

Assist with diagnositc procedures and test—radiography, throat culture, thoracentesis, venipuncture for blood analysis

Observe for general manifestations of acute respiratory tract infection:

Altered breathing—Respirations may be altered to a greater or lesser degree depending on the location and extent of the infective process

Cough—Coughing is a common manifestation. A cough may be described as dry, moist, hacking, barking, brassy, croupy, productive, or nonproductive

Nasal blockage—The small nasal passages of the infant are easily blocked by mucosal swelling and exudation. Infants have difficulty breathing through their mouths; therefore, this occlusion can interfere with respiration and feeding

Fever—Most children manifest an elevated temperature with respiratory infections. In children 6 months to 3 years, the temperature may reach 39.5° to 40.5° C (103° to 105° F), even with mild infections

Febrile seizures—In some small children, a sudden temperature rise to 40° C (104° F) or higher will precipitate febrile convulsions

Anorexia—Loss of appetite is a symptom common to most childhood illnesses, and it almost invariably accompanies acute infections in small children

Vomiting—Small children vomit readily with illness, and vomiting occurs so frequently at the onset of infection that its appearance for no obvious reason is a clue to the advent of infection

Meningism—Signs associated with meningitis but without actual inflammation of the meninges include headache, stiffness in the back and neck, and positive Kernig and Brudzinski signs

Diarrhea—Mild, transient diarrhea often accompanies respiratory infections in small children, particularly viral infections

Abdominal pain—Abdominal pain, sometimes indistinguishable from the pain of appendicitis, is a common complaint in small children with acute respiratory infections

Assess respiratory status:

Monitor respirations for rate, depth, pattern, presence of retractions, and flaring nares

Auscultate lungs

Evaluate breath sounds (type and location)

Detect presence of rales or rhonchi

Detect areas of consolidation

Evaluate effectiveness of chest therapy

Observe for presence or absence of retractions, nasal flaring

Observe color of skin and mucous membranes for pallor and cyanosis

Observe for presence of hoarseness, stridor, and cough

Monitor heart rate and regularity

Observe behavior

Restlessness

Irritability

Apprehension

Observe for signs of

Chest pain

Abdominal pain

Dyspnea

Observe for manifestations of respiratory infection (specific)

I. Upper respiratory tract infection

Nasopharyngitis—Viral infection, *acute rhinitis* or *coryza*, equivalent of the "common cold" in adults

Edema and vasodilation of mucosa

Younger child

Fever

Irritability, restlessness

Sneezing

Vomiting and/or diarrhea, sometimes

Older child

Dryness and irritation of nose and throat

Sneezing, chilly sensation

Muscular aches

Cough, sometimes

Pharyngitis—Throat (including the tonsils) is principal anatomic site

Younger child

Fever

General malaise

Anorexia

Moderate sore throat

Headache

Mild to moderate hyperemia

Older child

Fever (may reach 40° C)

Headache

Anorexia

Dysphagia

Abdominal pain

Vomiting

Mild to fiery red, edematous pharynx

Hyperemia of tonsils and pharynx; may extend to soft palate and uvula

Often abundant follicular exudate that spreads and coalesces to form pseudomembrane on tonsils

Cervical glands enlarged and tender

Influenza—("Flu") caused by three antigenically distinct orthomyxoviruses: types A and B, which cause epidemic disease, and type C

May be subclinical, mild, moderate, or severe

Overt illness:

Dry throat and nasal mucosa

Dry cough

Tendency toward hoarseness

Sudden onset of fever

Flushed face

Photophobia

Myalgia

Hyperesthesia

Prostration (sometimes)

Subglottal croup common (especially in infants)

Unit 4

ASSESSMENT—cont'd

II. Croup syndromes

Acute laryngitis, laryngotracheitis, laryngotracheobronchitis—Most common form of croup; may be localized or one manifestation of a variety of conditions; most common at ages 3 months to 3 years; mean age—21 months

Wide range of manifestations from few symptoms to severe obstructive laryngitis

Infection rapidly descends, with first laryngeal symptoms—hoarseness, brassy cough, stridor, respiratory distress

Fever and prostration increase

Respiratory distress, especially inspiratory dyspnea with substernal and suprasternal retractions

Bronchi involvement becomes evident with increased dyspnea

Expiratory difficulty with labored and prolonged expirations

Scattered rales of various types; rhonchi

Diminished breath sounds bilaterally

Pallor or cyanosis

Irritability and restlessness

Acute spasmodic laryngitis (spasmodic croup)—Distinct clinical entity characterized by sudden paroxysmal attacks of laryngeal obstruction that occur chiefly at night; usually affects small children ages 1 to 3 years

Appears primarily at night

Child suddenly wakens with characteristic barking, metallic cough, hoarseness, noisy inspirations, and restlessness; child appears anxious, frightened, and prostrated

Accessory muscles of respiration used and inspiratory retractions sometimes evident

Dyspnea aggravated by excitement

May be some cyanosis

Attack wears off in a few hours and child appears well the following day except for some hoarseness and cough

May be repeated 1 or 2 nights in succession

No fever

Usually self-limited

Acute epiglottitis—Severe, rapidly progressive infection of the epiglottis and surrounding area; chiefly ages 3-7 years*

Abrupt onset; rapidly progressive

High fever; appears ill

Sore throat

Difficulty or inability to swallow

Drooling of saliva; retching

Difficulty in breathing progressing to severe respiratory distress in minutes or hours

Child will sit upright, leaning forward, with chin thrust out and mouth open—tripod position

Thick, muffled voice

Croaking, "froglike" sound on inspiration

Anxious and frightened expression

Suprasternal and substernal retractions may be visible

Seldom struggle to breathe (breathing slowly and quietly provides better air exchange)

Sallow color of mild hypoxia to frank cyanosis

Throat red, inflamed

Distinctive large, cherry-red, edematous epiglottis

III. Lower respiratory tract infections

Tracheitis—Infection of trachea

Follows previous URI

Begins with signs and symptoms similar to croup

Croupy cough, stridor, unaffected by position

Copious purulent secretions—may be severe enough to cause respiratory arrest

High fever, toxicity

No response to laryngotracheobronchitis

Asthmatic bronchitis—Exaggerated response of bronchi to infection. Occurs in late infancy and early childhood; spasm and exudation similar to asthma in older children

Sudden onset at night

Previous URI

Wheezing

Productive cough

Moderate signs of emphysema

Bronchitis—Usually occurs in association with URI; affects children in first 4 years of life URI; seldom occurs as an isolated entity in childhood

Abrupt onset

Persistent dry, hacking cough (worse at night) becoming productive in 2-3 days

Tachypnea

Low-grade fever

May have chest pain aggravated by coughing

Bronchiolitis—Maximum obstruction at bronchiolar level consists of hypersecretion, edema, and inflammatory reaction and confined to smaller bronchioles; usually affects children 2-12 months; rare after age 2 years

Begins as simple URI with serous nasal discharge

May be accompanied by moderate temperature elevation

Gradually develops increasing respiratory distress, paroxysmal cough, dyspnea, and irritability

Tachypnea with flaring nares and intercostal and subcostal retractions

Emphysema with barrel chest and palpable liver and spleen from depressed diaphragm

Shallow respiratory excursion

Fine rales and prolonged expiratory phase; diminished breath sounds, hyperresonance, and scattered consolidation

May be wheezing

*Avoid throat examination in suspected epiglottitis

ASSESSMENT—cont'd

IV. Pneumonias

Viral pneumonia—Occurs more frequently than bacterial pneumonia; seen in children of all age-groups

May be acute or insidious

Symptoms variable

   Mild: low-grade fever, slight cough, malaise

   Severe: high fever, severe cough, prostration

Cough usually unproductive early in disease

A few rhonchi or fine crepitant rales heard on auscultation

Atypical pneumonia—More prevalent where there are crowded living conditions

May be sudden or insidious

General systemic symptoms:

   Fever

   Chills (older children)

   Headache

   Malaise

   Anorexia

   Myalgia

Followed by:

   Rhinitis

   Sore throat

   Dry, hacking cough

      Nonproductive early, then seromucoid sputum, to muco-purulent or blood streaked

   Fine crepitant rales over various lung areas

Pneumococcal pneumonia—Usually lobar but may be lobular; areas of consolidation (usually patchy) in one or more lobes; most common in first 4 years and declines with increasing age; uncommon in infants less than 1 year of age

Infants

   Fretfulness and diminished appetite followed by abrupt onset of fever

   May be accompanied by convulsions

   Restlessness, apprehension, respiratory distress, appears acutely ill, flushed cheeks, circumoral cyanosis

   Decreased breath sounds and crackling rales; exaggerated breath sounds on opposite side; pleural friction rub may be heard

Older children

   Usually follows a URI

   Shaking chill followed by high fever, chest pain, tachypnea

   Drowsiness with intermittent periods of restlessness, anxiety

   Occasionally, delirium

   Circumoral cyanosis

   Hacking, unproductive cough (initially)

   Splinting of side caused by pleurisy pain

   Chest—dullness; diminished breath sounds, tactile and vocal fremitus; consolidation on second or third day evidenced by dullness, increased fremitus, tubular breath sounds, and disappearance of rales

   With resolution—moist rales; productive cough with large amounts of blood-tinged mucus

   Resolution begins about 24 hours after initiation of therapy

Staphylococcal pneumonia—Localized abscesses in older children; more diffuse in infants; greatest incidence in first 2 years of life, usually less than 1 month of age

Abrupt onset of fever

Listlessness and lethargy when undisturbed

Irritability on arousal

Anorexia

Nasal discharge, cough

Grunting respirations

Progressively severe dyspnea that may include subcostal and sternal retractions and cyanosis

Shocklike state may be present

Symptoms of complications: for example, pneumothorax, empyema, septicemia

Some infants have gastrointestinal disturbances: for example, vomiting, diarrhea, and sometimes abdominal distention

Rapid progression of symptoms characteristic

Chest—early, diminished breath sounds

   Rales, and rhonchi with effusion or pneumothorax

   Dullness on percussion

   Respiratory lag on affected side; exaggerated excursion on opposite side

Streptococcal pneumonia—Interstitial bronchopneumonia; less common than other bacterial pneumonias

May appear without evidence of illness

Symptoms similar to those of pneumococcal pneumonia

Onset sudden

High temperature

Chills

Signs of respiratory distress

At times, extreme prostration

Occasionally, only mild symptoms

Tachypnea, usually mild

Rales generally unilateral and exaggerated by deep inspiration

NURSING DIAGNOSIS: Potential for suffocation (airway obstruction) related to inflammatory process in airway(s)

GOAL

Prevent respiratory arrest

INTERVENTIONS

Avoid throat examination (epiglottitis)

Have emergency equipment available

Be prepared to assist with tracheostomy

   Have tracheostomy equipment at bedside

   Obtain parental permission for procedure

EXPECTED OUTCOME

Child breathes normally

NURSING DIAGNOSIS: Ineffective breathing pattern related to inflammatory process

Unit 4

GOAL

Facilitate breathing

INTERVENTIONS

Promote rest
Position for optimum chest expansion
*Administer oxygen as prescribed
*Administer antiinflammatory medications as prescribed
*Administer antibiotics as prescribed

EXPECTED OUTCOME

Child breathes normally

NURSING DIAGNOSIS: Potential for injury related to presence of infective organisms

GOAL

Help eradicate infective organisms

INTERVENTIONS

*Administer antibiotics as prescribed
Provide nutritious diet according to child's preferences and ability to consume nourishment

EXPECTED OUTCOME

Child exhibits evidence of diminishing symptoms

GOAL

Prevent spread of infection to others

INTERVENTIONS AND EXPECTED OUTCOMES

See Nursing care plan: The child at risk for infection, p. 288

NURSING DIAGNOSIS: Activity intolerance related to generalized weakness, imbalance between oxygen supply and demand

---

*Dependent nursing action.

GOAL

Promote rest

INTERVENTIONS AND EXPECTED OUTCOMES

See Nursing diagnosis: Activity intolerance, p. 252

NURSING DIAGNOSIS: Fear/anxiety related to hospitalization, discomfort, difficulty breathing

GOAL

Relieve anxiety

INTERVENTIONS AND EXPECTED OUTCOMES

See Nursing diagnosis: Fear/anxiety, p. 250 and p. 251

GOAL

Facilitate nonverbal communication

INTERVENTIONS

Observe child's behavior closely to detect nonverbal messages
Teach signing, use pictures or other means to communicate needs and concerns

EXPECTED OUTCOME

Child communicates needs and concerns

NURSING DIAGNOSIS: Altered family processes related to a child with an acute illness

GOAL

Support family

INTERVENTIONS AND EXPECTED OUTCOMES

See Nursing care plan: The family of the ill or hospitalized child, p. 254

See also Nursing care plan: The child in the hospital, p. 246
Nursing care plan: The child with elevated temperature, p. 271
Nursing diagnosis: Fluid volume deficit, p. 276

NURSING CARE PLAN
THE CHILD WITH A TONSILLECTOMY

Surgical removal of tonsils (and adenoids, usually)

ASSESSMENT

Preoperative

See Nursing care plan: The child undergoing surgery, p. 267.
Perform routine physical assessment
Note any evidence of bleeding tendencies
Note any evidence of infection
Examine laboratory results for bleeding and clotting times; report any abnormalities

Postoperative

See Nursing care plan: The child undergoing surgery, p. 269
Assess for evidence of hemorrhage
  Take pulse and respiration frequently
  Assess skin color
  Restlessness
  More than usual frequency of swallowing
  Frequent clearing of throat
  Nausea and vomiting
Inspect throat for signs of oozing
  Insert tongue depressor carefully
  Use good light source
Inspect any vomitus for evidence of fresh bleeding (blood-tinged mucus expected; may be small amounts of old blood)

Unit 4

NURSING DIAGNOSIS: Altered oral mucous membranes related to raw, denuded surfaces of tonsil sockets

GOAL

Prevent bleeding

INTERVENTIONS

Discourage child from coughing frequently or clearing the throat
Avoid use of gargles or hard objects (such as toothbrush) in the mouth
Avoid foods that are irritating (e.g., high acid fruit juices, raw vegetables) or highly seasoned
Encourage cool liquid or semi-soft foods

EXPECTED OUTCOMES

Child does not aggravate the operative site
There is no evidence of bleeding

NURSING DIAGNOSIS: Impaired swallowing related to inflammation and pain

GOAL

Prevent dehydration

INTERVENTIONS

Offer cool, bland liquids; soft, bland foods
Provide pain relief (see p. 279)
Position for optimal swallowing

EXPECTED OUTCOME

Child consumes an adequate amount of nourishment

GOAL

Prevent aspiration of secretions

INTERVENTIONS

Assist child to expectorate
Position on side or stomach while sleeping

EXPECTED OUTCOME

Child disposes of mucus and drainage appropriately

NURSING DIAGNOSIS: Pain related to surgical site

GOAL

Relieve pain

INTERVENTIONS

Avoid offering irritating liquid and solid foods
Employ nonpharmacologic pain reduction techniques (see p. 284)
*Administer analgesics as prescribed

EXPECTED OUTCOMES

Child rests quietly and exhibits no evidence of pain
See also Nursing care plan: The child in pain, p. 279

GOAL

Prevent irritation to operative site

INTERVENTIONS

Offer diet as tolerated
  Cool liquid diet for 12-24 hours
  Soft diet thereafter
  Advance to regular diet as recommended
Avoid substances that irritate denuded areas, e.g.,
  Acid juices
  Rough foods
  Highly seasoned foods
Avoid placing hard objects in mouth

EXPECTED OUTCOME

Child exhibits no evidence of discomfort

NURSING DIAGNOSIS: Anxiety/fear related to unfamiliar event, discomfort

GOAL

Reduce anxiety

---
*Dependent nursing intervention.

INTERVENTIONS

Explain source of discomfort
See Nursing care plan: The child in the hospital, p. 246
See Nursing care plan: The child undergoing surgery, p. 267
Anticipate needs
Keep child and bed free from any blood-tinged excretions
Reassure child regarding any blood-tinged drainage
Keep emesis basin within easy reach

EXPECTED OUTCOME

Child rests quietly and readily attends to verbal and nonverbal communication
Child communicates needs and wants in a calm manner

NURSING DIAGNOSIS: Potential fluid volume deficit related to nothing by mouth, prior to surgery, reluctance to swallow

GOAL

Promote adequate hydration

INTERVENTIONS

See Nursing diagnosis: Potential for fluid volume deficit, p. 276

EXPECTED OUTCOME

Child remains well hydrated

NURSING DIAGNOSIS: Altered family processes related to a child hospitalized for surgery

GOAL

Support family

INTERVENTIONS AND EXPECTED OUTCOMES

See Nursing care plan: The family of the ill or hospitalized child, p. 254

See also Nursing care plan: The child in the hospital, p. 246

NURSING CARE PLAN
THE CHILD WITH ACUTE OTITIS MEDIA

Otitis media—An inflammation of the middle ear without reference to etiology or pathogenesis

Acute otitis media (AOM)—A rapid and short onset of signs and symptoms lasting approximately 3 weeks

Otitis media with effusion (OME)—An inflammation of the middle ear in which a collection of fluid is present in the middle ear space

Subacute otitis media—Middle ear effusion lasting from 3 weeks to 3 months

Chronic otitis media with effusion—Middle ear effusion that persists beyond 3 months

ASSESSMENT

Observe for evidence of acute ear infection:
  Follows an upper respiratory infection
  Otalgia (earache)
  Purulent otorrhea may be present
  Fever
  Muted cerumen in external auditory canal
  Purulent discharge may or may not be present
Infant or very young child
  Crying
  Fussy, restless, irritable
  Tendency to rub, hold, or pull affected ear
  Rolls head side to side
  Difficulty comforting child
  Loss of appetite
Older child
  Crying and/or verbalizes feelings of discomfort
  Irritability
  Lethargy
  Loss of appetite
Otoscopic examination reveals bright red, bulging tympanic membrane; obscured bony landmarks; absent light reflex
May be visible fluid level behind eardrum

NURSING DIAGNOSIS: Pain related to pressure caused by inflammatory process

GOAL

Relieve pain

INTERVENTIONS

Position for comfort according to needs of individual child
Apply external heat (with heating pad on low setting) or cool compresses
Avoid chewing by offering liquid or soft foods
Position with affected ear in dependent position; have child lie on affected side
*Administer analgesics

EXPECTED OUTCOME

Child sleeps and rests quietly and exhibits no signs of discomfort

---

*Dependent or independent nursing function.

NURSING DIAGNOSIS: Potential for infection/injury related to inadequate treatment, presence of infective organisms

GOAL

Prevent reinfection

INTERVENTIONS

Emphasize the importance of following instructions, especially regarding administration of antibiotics
  Maintain regularity of administration
  Complete the course of therapy
  See Home Care Instructions, p. 272
Employ simple preventive practices such as
  Sit or hold child upright for feedings
  Promote aeration of middle ear
    Encourage gentle nose blowing
    Employ the modified Valsalva maneuver, i.e., pinch the nose, close the lips, and force air up the eustachian tube
    Use blowing games
    Chew gum
  Eliminate tobacco smoke and known allergens from child's environment

EXPECTED OUTCOMES

Child remains free of infection
Family complies with directives (specify)

GOAL

Prevent complications (especially hearing loss)

INTERVENTIONS

See above
Stress importance of follow-up care
Stress importance of regular hearing tests to assess early signs of impairment
Teach parents to recognize signs of hearing impairment in the infant or child (p. 463)
Avoid excessive water in ear if polyethylene tubes or myringotomy was part of the therapy

EXPECTED OUTCOME

Child remains free of complications

NURSING DIAGNOSIS: Altered family processes related to a child with an infection

GOAL

Support family

INTERVENTION

Prepare family for surgical procedure, if appropriate (insertion of pressure equilizer tubes)

EXPECTED OUTCOME

Family demonstrates an understanding of procedure

GOAL

Prepare family for discharge and home care

INTERVENTIONS

Cleanse external meatus of draining ear with sterile cotton swabs or pledgets soaked in sterile normal saline
Avoid water from baths or shampoo from dampening wicks, if inserted to facilitate drainage after surgery
Avoid contaminated water (from baths, swimming pools, freshwater lakes) entering the external ear
    Suggest use of a good earplug
Notify health professional if grommet (tiny, white, plastic spool-shaped tube) falls out of the ear canal
    No immediate intervention needed

EXPECTED OUTCOME

Child recovers from infection and/or surgery without complications

See also:
Nursing care plan: The child in the hospital, p. 246
Nursing care plan: The family of the ill or hospitalized child, p. 254

NURSING CARE PLAN
THE INFANT WITH RESPIRATORY DISTRESS SYNDROME

An acute lung disease of the newborn, which occurs at birth or soon afterward; it occurs almost exclusively in preterm infants

Also known as hyaline membrane disease or idiopathic respiratory distress syndrome

ASSESSMENT

Perform newborn assessment (see p. 10)
Perform systematic assessment, with special emphasis on respiratory assessment, (see p. 26 and p. 40)
Observe for manifestations of respiratory distress syndrome:
    Dyspnea
    Tachypnea (up to 80 to 120 breaths/min)
    Pronounced substernal retractions
    Fine inspiratory rales heard over both lungs
    Audible expiratory grunt
    Flaring of the external nares
    Cyanosis

As the disease progresses:
    Flaccidity
    Inertness
    Unresponsiveness
    Frequent apneic episodes
    Diminished breath sounds
Severe disease associated with:
    Shocklike state
    Diminished cardiac return
    Low arterial blood pressure
Assist with diagnostic procedures and tests—Radiography, pulse oximetry, blood gas analysis and pH

NURSING DIAGNOSIS: Ineffective airway clearance related to flexible rib cage, fatigue, weak or absent cough reflex

GOAL

Remove secretions from airway

INTERVENTIONS

Suction airway as needed
  Insert catheter quickly and gently to a predetermined depth
    0.5 cm beyond end of ET tube
  Apply intermittent suction during withdrawal
  Obstruct airway with catheter for no longer than 5 seconds
Apply percussion and vibration to thoracic wall modified for infant, e.g., use infant face mask with opening occluded (see also p. 234)

EXPECTED OUTCOME

Infant exhibits no evidence of secretions in airway

GOAL

Facilitate drainage of secretions

INTERVENTIONS

Position on side with head supported in alignment with small folded blanket or towel
Position on back, with small shoulder roll to keep neck slightly extended in "sniffing" position
Position on abdomen with head turned to side

EXPECTED OUTCOME

Infant does not aspirate secretions

NURSING DIAGNOSIS: Ineffective breathing pattern related to pliant chest wall, deficient secretion of surfactant, fatigue

GOAL

Facilitate respiratory efforts

INTERVENTIONS

Position for optimum lung expansion
  Elevate head of crib slightly
  Maintain head and neck in neutral position and in good alignment
Monitor controlled ventilation apparatus
* Administer oxygen as prescribed
* Administer surfactant as prescribed

----
*Dependent nursing action

EXPECTED OUTCOME

Infant breathes with minimal effort

NURSING DIAGNOSIS: Impaired gas exchange related to inability to maintain lung expansion, presence of hyaline membrane

GOAL

Facilitate gas exchange

INTERVENTIONS

Facilitate respiratory efforts (see above)
* Assist with extracorporeal membrane oxygenation (ECMO) if implemented

EXPECTED OUTCOME

Infant breathes with minimal effort

NURSING DIAGNOSIS: Potential for infection related to accumulation of pulmonary secretions, ineffective immune response, presence of infective organisms

GOAL

Prevent infection

INTERVENTIONS

Prevent contact with contaminated articles and infected persons
Carry out conscientious handwashing
* Administer prophylactic antibiotics as prescribed

EXPECTED OUTCOME

Infant exhibits no evidence of infection

NURSING DIAGNOSIS: Altered family processes related to an infant with a serious illness

GOAL

Support family

INTERVENTIONS AND EXPECTED OUTCOMES

See Nursing diagnosis: Altered family processes, p. 256
See also: Nursing care plan: The high-risk infant and family, p. 302

----
*Dependent nursing action.

Unit 4

NURSING CARE PLAN
THE CHILD WITH BRONCHIAL ASTHMA

A reversible obstructive process of a hyperactive tracheobronchial tree caused by musosal edema, increased viscid secretions, and smooth muscle constriction—usually in response to an allergen

ASSESSMENT

Perform physical assessment

Obtain family history, especially regarding presence of atopy in members

Obtain health history, including any evidence of atopy (e.g., eczema, rhinitis), evidence of possible precipitating factor(s), previous episodes of shortness of breath, wheezing, and coughing; any complaints of itching at the front of neck or upper part of back

Observe for manifestations of bronchial asthma:

Cough:
Hacking, paroxysmal, irritative, and nonproductive
Becomes rattling and productive of frothy, clear, gelatinous sputum

Shortness of breath
Prolonged expiratory phase
Audible wheeze
Often appears pale
May have a malar flush and red ears
Lips deep, dark-red color
May progress to cyanosis of nail beds, circumoral
Restlessness
Apprehension
Anxious facial expression

Sweating may be prominent as the attack progresses
Older children may sit upright with shoulders in a hunched-over position, hands on the bed or chair, and arms braced
Speaks with short, panting, broken phrases

Chest:
Hyperresonance on percussion
Coarse, loud breath sounds
Sonorous rales throughout the lung fields
Prolonged expiration
Coarse rhonchi
Generalized inspiratory and expiratory wheezing; increasingly high pitched

With repeated episodes:
Barrel chest
Elevated shoulders
Use of accessory muscles of respiration
Facial appearance—flattened malar bones, circles beneath the eyes, narrow nose, prominent upper teeth

Assist with diagnostic procedures and tests—Radiography, pulmonary function tests, collect specimens for blood and sputum analysis for eosinophilia, assist with sensitivity testing, supervise elimination diet

Assess environment for presence of possible allergenic factors

Assess parent-child relationships

NURSING DIAGNOSIS: Potential for suffocation related to interaction between individual and allergen(s)

GOAL

Prevent asthmatic attack

INTERVENTIONS

Use prophylactic medication(s) according to instructions

Teach child and family correct use of bronchodilators, corticosteroids

Teach child and family how to avoid conditions or circumstances that precipitate asthmatic attack

Avoid contact with offending allergens

Assist parents in eliminating allergens that trigger attack
Meal planning to eliminate allergenic foods
Removal of pets
Modification of environment; "allergy proof" home (see box on p. 330)

Assist parents in obtaining and/or installing device to control environment (humidifier, air conditioner, electronic air filter)

Avoid extremes of environmental temperature

Avoid undue excitement and/or physical exertion

Teach child and family to recognize early signs and symptoms so that an impending attack can be controlled before it becomes distressful

Teach child to understand how equipment works

Teach child correct use of inhalers and peak flow meters

EXPECTED OUTCOMES

Family makes every effort to remove or avoid possible allergens or precipitating events

Family is able to detect signs of an impending attack early and implement appropriate actions

GOAL

Maintain optimum health

INTERVENTIONS

Encourage sound health practices
  Balanced, nutritious diet
  Adequate rest
  Hygiene
  Appropriate exercise
  Avoid exposure to infection
Prevent infection
  Avoid exposure to infection
  Employ meticulous care of equipment to avoid bacterial and/or fungal growth
  Employ good handwashing

EXPECTED OUTCOMES

Child and parents conform to sound health practices
Child exhibits no evidence of infection

NURSING DIAGNOSIS: Ineffective breathing pattern related to allergenic response in bronchial tree

GOAL

Improve ventilatory capacity

INTERVENTIONS

Instruct and/or supervise
  Breathing exercises
  Controlled breathing
Assist child and family in selecting appropriate to the child's capabilities and preferences
Encourage regular exercise
Encourage good posture
Encourage physical exercise involving stop-and-start activity that does not overtax the respiratory mechanism
Discourage physical inactivity

EXPECTED OUTCOMES

Child breathes easily and without dyspnea
Child engages in activities according to abilities and interest (specify)

NURSING DIAGNOSIS: Activity intolerance related to imbalance between oxygen supply and demand

GOAL

Promote rest

INTERVENTIONS

Encourage activities appropriate to the child's capabilities (specify)
Provide ample opportunities for rest and quiet activities

EXPECTED OUTCOMES

Child engages in appropriate activities (specify)
Child appears rested

NURSING DIAGNOSIS: Body image disturbance related to inability to compete with agemates, perception of the disorder

GOAL

Promote positive self-image

INTERVENTIONS AND EXPECTED OUTCOMES

See Nursing diagnosis: Altered body image, p. 265

NURSING DIAGNOSIS: Altered family processes related to having a child with a chronic illness

GOAL

Promote positive adaptation to the disorder

INTERVENTIONS

Foster positive family relationships
Be alert to signs of parental rejection or overprotection
Intervene appropriately if there is evidence of maladaptation
Use every opportunity to increase the parents' and child's understanding of the disease and its therapies
Be alert to signs that the child may be using symptoms to manipulate interpersonal relationships
*Refer family to appropriate support groups and community agencies

EXPECTED OUTCOME

Family cope with symptoms and effects of the disease and provide a normal environment for the child
See also Nursing care plan: The child with a chronic illness or disability, p. 259

*Asthma and Allergy Foundation of America (AAFA), 1717 Massachusetts Avenue NW, Suite 305, Washington, DC 20036; (202) 265-0265 American Lung Association, 1740 Broadway, New York, NY 10019, (212) 315-8700. In Canada: Canadian Lung Association, 75 Albert St., Suite 908, Ottawa, Ontario KIP 5E7; The Lung Association, 573 King St. East, Suite 201, Toronto, Ontario M5A 1M5.

Unit 4

SUGGESTIONS FOR "ALLERGY PROOFING" THE HOME

House dust—most common cause of respiratory allergy in children

Use bedroom for sleeping, not playing.

Avoid feather pillows, which collect dust; if used, encase in an impermeable plastic casing. Dacron pillows are preferred.

Encase mattresses and box springs in an impermeable covering.

Dust room daily and thoroughly clean weekly, when the child is not present.

Use sheets, bedspreads, and curtains made of washable, smooth cotton or synthetic fabric and clean frequently. Window shades are preferable to curtains or venetian mini-blinds, which collect dust.

Keep floors bare, with only a cotton or synthetic (not wool) "scatter rug."

Remove the following from the room:

Stuffed animals

Upholstered and stuffed furniture, except those stuffed exclusively with foam rubber; in general, the less furniture, the better

Plants and aquariums, which can harbor molds

All pets (if one is already there, keep outdoors at all times)

Keep closet free of stored articles, especially woolen clothing.

Keep windows and doors closed.

Cover walls with washable paint or wallpaper.

Heating system—forced air circulates dust.

Minimum treatment—cover vent or duct with cheesecloth, which is washed frequently.

Preferable treatment—close heating ducts off in room and use an electric heater (which is placed so as to prevent severe burns to the child).

If possible use an air-cleaning machine, such as an electronic air purifier. Small units can be used in the child's room.

Mildew exposure

Avoid cellars as play areas.

Clean showers and tile areas well and spray with an antimold agent such as Lysol.

Keep vaporizers clean and free of mold.

Keep plants and aquariums out of child's room.

NURSING CARE PLAN
THE CHILD IN STATUS ASTHMATICUS

An acute, severe, and prolonged asthma attack in which bronchospasm does not respond to oral medications. Hypoxia, cyanosis, and unconsciousness may follow.

ASSESSMENT

Perform physical assessment

See Nursing care plan: The child with respiratory dysfunction, Assessment, p. 316

Observe for labored breathing, bilateral wheezing, prolonged expiration, irritative tight cough, excessive respiratory secretions

Assist with diagnostic procedures and tests—blood gases and pH, oximetry; assess urine for concentration and specific gravity

NURSING DIAGNOSIS: Potential for suffocation related to bronchospasm, mucous secretions, edema

GOAL

Increase ventilatory capacity

INTERVENTION

Position for optimum lung expansion
    High Fowler position
    Provide overbed table with pillows on which to lean if more comfortable for child
*Initiate oxygen therapy with appropriate equipment—tent, cannula, mask
*Administer or arrange for positive-pressure breathing if ordered

EXPECTED OUTCOME

Child breathes more easily

GOAL

Relieve bronchospasm

INTERVENTIONS

*Administer prescribed bronchodilator (usually aminophylline)
Carefully regulate flow rate of aminophylline infusion; monitor pulse, respiration, and blood pressure before, during, and after administration

EXPECTED OUTCOME

Child breathes more easily

GOAL

Reduce mucosal inflammation and edema

INTERVENTIONS

*Administer corticosteroids as prescribed
Provide cool, moist environment

EXPECTED OUTCOME

Child breathes more easily

GOAL

Liquify and remove bronchial secretions

INTERVENTIONS

Promote hydration—Oral or intravenous fluids
Provide humidified atmosphere
Provide adequate hydration
Assist child to cough effectively
Suction secretions
*Administer expectorants

---

*Dependent nursing action.

EXPECTED OUTCOME

Child is able to manage secretions without undue stress and fatigue

NURSING DIAGNOSIS: Fluid volume deficit related to difficulty taking fluid and nourishment, insensible fluid loss from lungs

GOAL

Promote adequate hydration

INTERVENTIONS

Maintain intravenous infusion
Offer cool liquids as tolerated

EXPECTED OUTCOME

Child exhibits no evidence of dehydration

NURSING DIAGNOSIS: Fear/anxiety related to hospitalization, difficulty breathing

GOAL

Reduce anxiety and apprehension

INTERVENTIONS

Explain procedures and equipment before use
Provide continuous attendance
Provide reassurance with calm words and manner
Encourage parents to remain near child
See Nursing diagnosis: Fear/anxiety, p. 250

EXPECTED OUTCOME

Child rests quietly and facial expression does not appear tense or anxious

NURSING DIAGNOSIS: Potential for infection related to mucous secretions as media for growth, presence of infectious organisms

GOAL

Prevent infection

INTERVENTIONS

Keep child from contact with sources of infection
*Administer prophylactic antibiotics if ordered

EXPECTED OUTCOME

Child remains free of infection

---

*Dependent nursing action.

Unit 4

NURSING DIAGNOSIS: Fatigue related to difficulty breathing

GOAL

Promote rest and reduce fatigue

INTERVENTIONS

Carry out measures to improve ventilation and facilitate breathing
Organize care to allow for maximum rest
Disturb as little as possible when resting or asleep

EXPECTED OUTCOME

Child rests quietly

NURSING DIAGNOSIS: Potential for injury (hypoxemia) related to imbalance between oxygen supply and demand

GOAL

Prevent or help correct acidosis

INTERVENTIONS

*Administer sodium bicarbonate or tromethamine as ordered
*Administer oxygen to reduce anaerobic metabolism (and subsequent increase in acid metabolites)

EXPECTED OUTCOME

Child exhibits no evidence of respiratory acidosis

---

*Dependent nursing action.

GOAL

Prevent drug (theophylline) toxicity

INTERVENTIONS

Interview parents to determine medications given before admission to avoid possible overdose
Monitor condition frequently during and after administration of drugs, including oxygen
Monitor serum blood levels

EXPECTED OUTCOME

Child demonstrates no evidence of theophylline toxicity

NURSING DIAGNOSIS: Altered family processes related to emergency hospitalization of child

GOAL

Reduce parental anxiety

INTERVENTIONS

Keep parents informed of child's condition
Encourage expression of feelings
Allow parents to be with the child as much as possible
Point out any evidence of improvement

EXPECTED OUTCOME

Family verbalize concerns and spend time with the child

See also:
Nursing care plan: The family of the ill or hospitalized child, p. 254
Nursing care plan: The child in the hospital, p. 246
Nursing care plan: The child with respiratory failure, p. 335

Unit 4

NURSING CARE PLAN
THE CHILD WITH CYSTIC FIBROSIS

A genetic multisystem disorder characterized by chronic obstruction and infection of airways and by maldigestion and its consequences

Unit 4

ASSESSMENT

Perform a physical assessment (see p. 10)

Take a health and a family history

Observe for any of the following clinical manifestations of cystic fibrosis:

Meconium ileus:
Abdominal distention
Vomiting
Failure to pass stools
Rapid development of dehydration

Gastrointestinal:
Large, bulky, loose, frothy, extremely foul-smelling stools
Voracious appetitie (early in disease)
Loss of appetite (later disease)
Weight loss
Marked tissue wasting
Failure to grow
Distended abdomen
Thin extremities
Sallow skin
Evidence of deficiency of fat-soluble vitamins A, D, E, K
Anemia

Pulmonary:
Initial manifestations:
Wheezy respirations
Dry, nonproductive cough
Eventually:
Increased dyspnea
Paroxysmal cough
Evidence of obstructive emphysema and patchy areas of atelectasis
Progressive involvement:
Overinflated, barrel-shaped chest
Cyanosis
Clubbing of fingers and toes
Repeated episodes of bronchitis and bronchopneumonia

Assist with diagnostic procedures that include:
Chest radiography for evidence of generalized obstructive emphysema, atelectasis, bronchopneumonia
Sweat chloride concentrations (greater than 60 mEq/L is diagnostic)
Pancreatic enzyme measurements from stool specimens
Fat-absorption tests of stool specimens
Screening newborns (not in general use)

NURSING DIAGNOSIS: Ineffective airway clearance related to secretion of thick, tenacious mucus

See Nursing diagnosis, p. 316

NURSING DIAGNOSIS: Ineffective breathing pattern related to mechanical airway obstruction caused by thick mucus

See Nursing diagnosis, p. 317

NURSING DIAGNOSIS: Altered nutrition: less than body requirements related to inability to digest nutrients, loss of appetite (advanced disease)

See Nursing care plan: The child with special nutritional needs, p. 277

GOAL

Promote digestion

INTERVENTIONS

*Administer pancreatic enzymes, with meals and snacks as prescribed

EXPECTED OUTCOME

Child takes medication

GOAL

Prevent malnutrition

INTERVENTIONS

Provide healthful diet with any modifications that may be prescribed

---

*Dependent nursing function.

Provide adequate salt, especially when sweating (e.g., fever, hot weather)

*Administer water-miscible vitamins, iron as prescribed

EXPECTED OUTCOME

Child eats a balanced diet and exhibits a satisfactory weight gain

---

NURSING DIAGNOSIS: Altered growth and development related to inadequate digestion of nutrients, chronic illness

GOAL

Promote nutrition

INTERVENTIONS

See Altered nutrition above

EXPECTED OUTCOME

Child exhibits normal growth

GOAL

Promote normal development
See Nursing care plan: The child with a chronic illness or disability, p. 259

NURSING DIAGNOSIS: Potential for infection related to impaired body defenses, presence of mucus as medium for growth of organisms

GOAL

Prevent infection

INTERVENTIONS

See Nursing diagnosis: Potential for infection, p. 288
Instruct family, and child if old enough, in administration of prophylactic antibiotics
Instruct family to have child immunized yearly against influenza

EXPECTED OUTCOME

Child is free of infection

---

*Dependent nursing function.

NURSING DIAGNOSIS: Altered family processes related to a child with a chronic and potentially fatal illness

GOAL

Support family

INTERVENTION

*Refer to appropriate support groups and agencies

EXPECTED OUTCOMES

Family demonstrates the ability to cope with child's illness (specify behaviors)
Family contact and become involved with appropriate agencies

NURSING DIAGNOSIS: Impaired social interaction related to frequent hospitalizations, confinement to home, fatigue

GOAL

Encourage social interaction

INTERVENTIONS AND EXPECTED OUTCOMES

See Nursing diagnosis: Impaired social interaction, p. 264

NURSING DIAGNOSIS: Anticipatory grief related to perceived potential loss of child

GOAL

Support family

INTERVENTIONS AND EXPECTED OUTCOMES:

See Nursing diagnosis: Anticipatory grief, p. 306

See also:
Nursing care plan: The child with a chronic illness or disability, p. 259
Nursing care plan: The child in the hospital, p. 246
Nursing care plan: The family of the ill or hospitalized child, p. 254

---

*Cystic Fibrosis Foundation,** 6931 Arlington Rd., Bethesda, Md 20814-3205, (800) FIGHT CF or (301) 951-4422. In Canada: **Canadian Cystic Fibrosis Foundation,** 586 Eglinton Ave. East, Suite 204, Toronto, Ontario M4P 1P2.

Unit 4

NURSING CARE PLAN
THE CHILD WITH RESPIRATORY FAILURE

Inability of the cardiac and pulmonary systems to maintain an adequate exchange of oxygen and carbon dioxide in the lungs

Respiratory insufficiency:
1. Increased work of breathing with preservation of gas exchange function near normal (ventilatory insufficiency)
2. Inability to maintain normal blood gas tensions and development of hypoxemia and acidosis secondary to carbon dioxide retention

Respiratory failure—Inability of the respiratory apparatus to maintain adequate oxygenation of the blood, with or without carbon dioxide retention

Respiratory arrest—Cessation of respiration

Apnea—Absence of airflow (breathing)
Central—respiratory efforts are absent
Obstructive—respiratory efforts are present
Mixed—both central and obstructive components are present

ASSESSMENT

See Nursing care plan: The child with respiratory dysfunction, assessment, p. 316

Be alert to the possiblity of respiratory failure in children with conditions that predispose to failure:

Obstructive lung disease—Increased resistance to airflow in either the upper or the lower respiratory tract

Restrictive lung disease—Impaired lung cxpansion resulting from loss of lung volume, decreased distensibility, or chest wall disturbance

Primary inefficient gas transfer—Insufficient alveolar ventilation for carbon dioxide removal or impaired oxygenation of pulmonary capillary blood as a result of dysfunction of the respiratory control mechanism or a diffusion defect

Observe for manifestations of respiratory failure:

Cardinal Signs
Restlessness
Tachypnea
Tachycardia
Diaphoresis

Early but Less Obvious Signs
Mood changes, such as euphoria or depression
Headache
Altered depth and pattern of respirations

Hypertension
Exertional dyspnea
Anorexia
Increased cardiac output and renal output
Central nervous system symptoms (decreased efficiency, impaired judgment, anxiety, confusion, restlessness, and irritability)
Flaring nares
Chest wall retractions
Expiratory grunt
Wheezing and/or prolonged expiration

Signs of More Severe Hypoxia
Hypotension or hypertension
Dimness of vision
Somnolence
Stupor
Coma
Dyspnea
Depressed respirations
Bradycardia
Cyanosis, peripheral or central

Assist with diagnostic procedures and tests—Blood gases and pH, oximetry, radiography, pulmonary function tests

---

NURSING DIAGNOSIS: Impaired gas exchange related to altered oxygen supply, altered pulmonary blood flow, alveolar-capillary membrane changes

GOAL

Improve ventilatory capacity

INTERVENTIONS

Position for optimum lung expansion—Head elevated, in neutral position

Administer supplemental oxygen (nasal prongs, mist tent, Isolette, hood, mechanical ventilator)
Monitor mechanical ventilation
Administer bronchodilators, corticosteroids, as prescribed
Have emergency tracheostomy or intubation equipment available
Assist with application of artificial airway

EXPECTED OUTCOME

Child's ventilatory capacity and gas exchange improve

Unit 4

NURSING DIAGNOSIS: Potential for suffocation related to mechanical or functional obstruction to air flow

GOAL

Restore ventilation

INTERVENTIONS

Implement appropriate emergency management of airway obstruction, p. 238 and/or cardiopulmonary resuscitation, p. 234

EXPECTED OUTCOME

Child resumes breathing

NURSING DIAGNOSIS: Altered family processes related to situational crisis (seriously ill child)

GOAL

Support family

INTERVENTIONS

Keep family informed of child's progress
Explain procedures and therapies
Reinforce information regarding child's condition
Arrange for presence of family support systems, if possible

EXPECTED OUTCOME

Family exhibit evidence of understanding and coping (specify)
See also:
Nursing care plan: The family of the ill or hospitalized child, p. 254
Nursing care plan: The child in the hospital, p. 246

NURSING CARE OF THE CHILD WITH GASTROINTESTINAL DYSFUNCTION

The gastrointestinal tract consists of the alimentary canal (mouth, esophagus, stomach, intestines, colon, and rectum), liver, pancreas, and gallbladder.

NURSING CARE PLAN
THE CHILD WITH GASTROINTESTINAL DYSFUNCTION

ASSESSMENT

Take careful health history, including history of present illness
Observe for manifestations of gastrointestinal dysfunction:

Spitting up and/or regurgitation, characteristic of infants:
Regurgitation—return of undigested food from the stomach, usually accompanied by burping
Spitting up—dribbling of unswallowed formula from the infant's mouth immediately after a feeding
Vomiting—Forceful ejection of stomach contents, involves a complex reflex that is associated with widespread autonomic discharge that causes salivation, pallor, sweating, and tachycardia. Vomiting is ordinarily accompanied by nausea
Projectile vomiting—Vomitus is forcefully ejected as far as 2 to 4 feet (0.6 to 1.2 m) from the child and is not associated with nausea
Hematemesis—Vomiting of blood that may result from swallowing blood from the oropharynx or from bleeding in the upper GI tract
Nausea—Unpleasant sensation vaguely referred to the epigastrium, with an inclination to vomit
Stools—Number, type, consistency, presence or absence of blood, and associated signs and symptoms provide clues to the etiology of gastrointestinal dysfunction
Constipation—Regular passage of firm or hard stools or of small, hard masses with associated symptoms such as difficulty expelling the stools, blood-streaked bowel movements, and abdominal discomfort. Suggested lower limit of frequency is six movements per week in children less than 3 years and 4 per week in older children. The apparent difficulty in passing stools is not a reliable sign, especially in infancy
Diarrhea—Increase in the number of stools or a decrease in their consistency as a result of alterations of water and electrolyte transport by the alimentary tract. Diarrhea may be acute or chronic
Mild diarrhea—Few loose stools each day without other evidence of illness
Moderate diarrhea—Several loose or watery stools daily
Elevated temperature, often
Vomiting
Fretfulness and irritability

Signs of dehydration usually absent, although may not gain weight or may even show weight loss
Severe diarrhea—Numerous to continuous stools
Signs of moderate to severe dehydration evident (see p. 343)
Drawn, flaccid expressions
Eyes lack luster
Cry lacks vigor, is often whining and higher pitched than usual
Irritable
Seeks comfort and attention of parent
Displays purposeless movements and inappropriate responses to people and familiar things
May become lethargic, moribund, or comatose
Abdominal pain, specific or nonspecific—Associated with a number of GI disorders
Abdominal enlargement or distention—A common observation in a child with GI dysfunction
Dysphagia—Difficulty in swallowing, can be the result of structural abnormalities or neurologic or neuromuscular impairment
Bowel sounds, or their absence—Provide information about some GI disorders
Jaundice—Yellow discoloration of the skin associated with liver dysfunction
Disability in sucking and swallowing—Are manifestations often observed in infants
Failure to thrive—Deceleration from established growth pattern or consistently below the fifth percentile for height and weight on standard growth charts

Manifestations of possible bowel obstruction include:
Colicky abdominal pain—From peristalsis attempting to overcome the obstruction
Abdominal distention—As a result of accumulation of gas and fluid above the level of the obstruction
Vomiting—Often the earliest sign of a high obstruction; a later sign of lower obstruction
Constipation and obstipation—Early signs of low obstructions; later signs of higher obstructions
Dehydration—From losses of large quantities of fluid and electrolytes

ASSESSMENT—cont'd

Rigid and boardlike abdomen—From increased distention

Bowel sounds—Gradually diminish and cease

Respiratory distress—Occurs as the diaphragm is pushed up into the pleural cavity

Shock—Plasma volume diminishes as proteins are lost from the bloodstream into the intestinal lumen

Assist with diagnostic procedures—Upper GI series, lower GI series, fiberoptic endoscopy, esophagoscopy, sigmoidoscopy, colonoscopy, manometry, radiography, mucosal biopsy

Collect specimens for stool examination, blood analyses (RBC, WBC, enzyme studies)

NURSING DIAGNOSIS: Impaired swallowing related to pain, neuromuscular impairment, presence of mechanical devices (e.g., ET tube)

GOAL

Facilitate swallowing

INTERVENTIONS

Position to prevent aspiration
  Elevate head of bed
Check neurologic function before attempting feeding
Stroke anterior aspect of throat (external) in distal to proximal direction to encourage swallowing

EXPECTED OUTCOME

Child swallows without aspiration

GOAL

Provide fluids and nourishment by alternative means

INTERVENTIONS

Feed child by enternal means
  Nasogastric tube (continuous or intermittent) (see p. 231)
  Gastrostomy (p. 231)
*Feed child by parenteral means
  Total parenteral nutrition

EXPECTED OUTCOMES

Child consumes sufficient calories and nutrients
Child demonstrates satisfactory weight gain

NURSING DIAGNOSIS: Diarrhea related to dietary indiscretions, food sensitivity, helminths, microorganisms

See Nursing care plan: The child with fluid and electrolyte disturbance, p. 272
See Nursing care plan for specific condition

GOAL

Reduce excessive intestinal losses

INTERVENTIONS

Modify diet as appropriate
  High-fiber diet (see box that follows)
  Increase fluid intake
*Administer stool softeners as prescribed
*Administer enemas and/or suppositories as prescribed

EXPECTED OUTCOME

Child exhibits normal bowel elimination
See also specific gastrointestinal disorder for appropriate application

See also:
Nursing care plan: The child in the hospital, p. 246
Nursing care plan: The family of the ill or hospitalized child, p. 254

NURSING DIAGNOSIS: Constipation related to immobility, neuromuscular impairment, medications

GOAL

Facilitate bowel elimination

INTERVENTIONS

Modify diet as appropriate
  High-fiber diet (see box that follows)
  Increase fluid intake
*Administer stool softeners as prescribed
*Administer enemas and/or suppositories as prescribed

EXPECTED OUTCOME

Child exhibits normal bowel elimination
See also specific gastrointestinal disorder for appropriate application

See also:
Nursing care plan: The child in the hospital, p. 246
Nursing care plan: The family of the ill or hospitalized child, p. 254

---

*Dependent nursing action.

*Dependent nursing action.

HIGH-FIBER FOODS

Food group	Selections	Food group	Selections
Bread, grains	Whole-grain bread or rolls Whole-grain cereals Bran Pancakes, waffles and muffins with fruit or bran Unrefined (brown) rice	Vegetables—cont'd	Cooked vegetables, such as those listed above and asparagus, beans, brussels sprouts, corn, potatoes, rhubarb, squash, string beans, turnips
Vegetables	Raw vegetables, especially broccoli, cabbage, carrots, cauliflower, celery, lettuce, and spinach	Fruits	Raw fruits, especially those with skins or seeds, other than ripe banana or avocado Raisins, prunes, or other dried fruits
		Miscellaneous	Nuts, seeds, legumes, popcorn

NURSING CARE PLAN
THE CHILD WITH APPENDICITIS

Inflammation of the fusiform appendix

ASSESSMENT

Take careful history of illness
Observe for clinical manifestations of appendicitis
  Colicky abdominal pain
  Rebound tenderness
  Fever
  Rigid abdomen
  Decreased or absent bowel sounds
  Vomiting (commonly follows onset of pain)
  Constipation or diarrhea may be present

Anorexia
Tachycardia, rapid shallow breathing
Pallor
Restlessness
Irritability
Ruptured appendix: sudden relief of pain followed by increased diffuse pain, abdominal rigidity, distention, and toxic manifestations (chills, fever, restlessness)
Assist with diagnostic procedures—White blood count, abdominal radiography

Preoperative care

NURSING DIAGNOSIS: Pain related to inflamed appendix

GOAL

Relieve discomfort

INTERVENTIONS

See Nursing care plan, The child in pain, p. 279
Allow position of comfort
*Administer analgesia, if prescribed

EXPECTED OUTCOME

Child rests quietly

*Dependent nursing action.

NURSING DIAGNOSIS: Potential for injury related to possibility of rupture

GOAL

Prevent rupture

INTERVENTIONS

Avoid application of heat or cold to abdomen
Apply ice pack to abdomen if it provides relief
Avoid palpating the abdomen unless necessary

EXPECTED OUTCOME

Status remains unchanged

NURSING DIAGNOSIS: Potential fluid volume deficit related to decreased intake secondary to loss of appetite, vomiting

See Potential for fluid volume deficit, p. 276

Postoperative care

See Postoperative care: The child undergoing surgery

Ruptured appendix

ASSESSMENT

Assess for evidence of infection
Assess status of bowel activity
  Gently palpate abdomen to determine the degree of distention (if present)

Auscultate abdomen for sounds of peristaltic activity
Observe and record type and amount of any bowel movement

NURSING DIAGNOSIS: Potential for infection related to presence of infective organisms in abdomen

GOAL

Prevent spread of infection

INTERVENTIONS

Position in low Fowler position to localize and prevent upward spread of infection
Implement appropriate isolation precautions
  Careful wound care and disposal of wound dressings
*Administer antibiotics as prescribed

EXPECTED OUTCOME

Infection remains confined to lower right quadrant of abdomen

NURSING DIAGNOSIS: Potential for injury related to absence of bowel activity

GOAL

Prevent abdominal distention

INTERVENTIONS

Allow nothing by mouth
Insert rectal tube if indicated

EXPECTED OUTCOME

Child does not exhibit signs of discomfort; abdomen remains soft

NURSING DIAGNOSIS: Altered family processes related to a child with a serious illness

GOAL

Support family

INTERVENTIONS AND EXPECTED OUTCOME

See Nursing care plan: The family of the ill or hospitalized child, p. 254
See also Nursing care plan: The child in the hospital, p. 246

---

*Dependent nursing action.

NURSING CARE PLAN
THE CHILD WITH ACUTE INFECTIOUS GASTROENTERITIS

Inflammation of the stomach and intestines caused by various bacteria and viruses (bacterial gastroenteritis, infectious gastroenteritis)

See Table 4-4—Enteropathic causes of infectious gastroenteritis

ASSESSMENT

Obtain careful history of illness including:
  Possible food poisoning from contamination (especially milk or egg products)
  Possible infection elsewhere (skin or lungs)
Perform routine physical assessment
Observe for manifestations of acute gastroenteritis (see Table 4-7)
Assess diarrhea (see p. 337)
Assess state of dehydration (Table 4-8)
Record fecal output—number, volume, characteristics
Observe and record presence of associated signs—tenesmus, cramping, vomiting

Assist with diagnostic procedures and tests
  Collect specimens as needed
  Make appropriate diagnostic tests and record
    Stools—pH, blood, sugar, frequency
    Urine—pH, specific gravity, frequency
Detect source of infection
  Examine other members of household and refer for treatment where indicated
  Collect stool specimens from household members where indicated

Table 4-7. ENTEROPATHOLOGIC CAUSES OF INFECTIOUS GASTROENTERITIS

Organism	Characteristics/manifestations	Comments
Viral agents		
Rotavirus Incubation period: 2-3 days	Abrupt onset Fever (38° C or above) lasting approximately 48 hours Associated upper respiratory tract infection Diarrhea may persist for more than a week	Incidence higher in cool weather (80% in winter) Affects all age groups; 6- to 24-month-old infants more vulnerable Usually mild and self-limited
Norwalk-like organisms Incubation period: 1-2 days	Fever Loss of appetite Nausea/vomiting Abdominal pain Diarrhea Malaise	Source of infection: drinking water, recreation water, food (including shellfish) Affects all ages Benign; seldom lasts more than 3 days Self-limited

Bacterial agents
Pathogenic
  Escherichia coli
    Incubation period: highly variable
	Onset gradual or abrupt
	Variable clinical manifestations
	Moist—green, watery diarrhea with mucus; becomes explosive
	Vomiting may be present from onset
	Abdominal distention
	Diarrhea
	Fever; appears toxic
		Incidence higher in summer
		Usually interpersonal transmission but may transmit via inanimate objects
		A cause of nursery epidemics
		With symptomatic treatment only, may continue for weeks
		Full breast-feeding has a protective effect
		Symptoms generally subside in 3-7 days
		Relapse rate approximately 20%

Continued.

Table 4-7. ENTEROPATHOLOGIC CAUSES OF INFECTIOUS GASTROENTERITIS—cont'd

Organism	Characteristics/manifestations	Comments
Bacterial agents—cont'd		
Salmonella groups (nontyphoidae)—gram-negative, nonencapsulated, nonsporulating Incubation period: 6-72 hours for intraluminal 7-21 days for extraluminal	Rapid onset Variable symptoms—mild to severe Nausea, vomiting, and colicky abdominal pain followed by diarrhea, occasionally with blood and mucus Chills not uncommon Hyperactive peristalsis and mild abdominal tenderness Symptoms usually subside within 5 days May have fever, headache, and cerebral manifestations, e.g., drowsiness, confusion, meningismus, or seizures Infants may be afebrile and nontoxic May result in life-threatening septicemia and meningitis	Two thirds of patients are younger than 20 years of age Highest incidence in children younger than 9 years of age, especially infants More prevalent July through October, lowest from January through April Transmission primarily via contaminated food and drink Most common sources are poultry and eggs In children—pets, e.g., dogs, cats, hamsters, and especially pet turtles Communicable as long as organisms are excreted
S. typhi	Variable in infants Older children—irregular fever, headache, malaise, lethargy Diarrhea occurs in 50% at early stage Cough is common In a few days, fever rises and is consistent; fatigue, cough, abdominal pain, anorexia, and weight loss develop; diarrhea begins	Rapid invasion of bloodstream from minor sites of inflammation Decreased incidence in last decade Acute symptoms may persist for a week or more
Shigella groups—gram-negative, nonmotile, anaerobic bacilli Incubation period: 1-7 days	Onset variable but usually abrupt Fever and cramping abdominal pain initially Fever—may reach 40.5° C Convulsions in about 10%—usually associated with fever Patient appears sick Headache, nuchal rigidity, delirium	Approximately 60% of cases in children younger than age 9 years with more than one third between ages 1 and 4 years Peak incidence late summer Transmitted directly or indirectly from infected persons Communicable for 1-4 weeks
Vibrio cholerae (cholera) groups Incubation period: usually 1-3 days; range from few hours to 5 days	Sudden onset of profuse, watery diarrhea without cramping, tenesmus, or anal irritation, although children may complain of cramping Stools are intermittent at first, then almost continuous Stools are whitish, almost clear, with flecks of mucus—"rice water stools"	Rare in infants younger than 1 year old Mortality high in both treated and untreated infants and small children Transmitted via contaminated food and water Attack confers immunity
Food poisoning		
Staphylococcus Incubation period: 4-6 hours	Nausea, vomiting Severe abdominal cramps Profuse diarrhea Shock may occur in severe cases May be a mild fever	Transferred via contaminated food—inadequately cooked or refrigerated, e.g., custards, mayonnaise, cream-filled or -topped desserts Self-limited; improvement apparent within 24 hours Excellent prognosis
Clostridium perfringens Incubation period: 8-24 hours	Moderate to severe crampy, midepigastric pain	Self-limited illness Transmission by commercial food products—most often meat and poultry
Botulism		
Clostridium botulinum Incubation period: 12 hr–3 days	Nausea, vomiting Diarrhea CNS symptoms with curare-like effect Dry mouth, dysphagia	Transmitted by contaminated food products Variable severity—mild symptoms to rapidly fatal within a few hours Antitoxin administration

Table 4-8. CLINICAL MANIFESTATIONS OF DEHYDRATION

	Isotonic (loss of water and salt)	Hypotonic (loss of salt in excess of water)	Hypertonic (loss of water in excess of salt)
Skin			
Color	Gray	Gray	Gray
Temperature	Cold	Cold	Cold or hot
Turgor	Poor	Very poor	Fair
Feel	Dry	Clammy	Thickened, doughy
Mucous membranes	Dry	Slightly moist	Parched
Tearing and salivation	Absent	Absent	Absent
Eyeball	Sunken and soft	Sunken and soft	Sunken
Fontanel	Sunken	Sunken	Sunken
Body temperature	Subnormal or elevated	Abnormal	Subnormal or elevated
Pulse	Rapid	Very rapid	Moderately rapid
Respirations	Rapid	Rapid	Rapid
Behavior	Irritable to lethargic	Lethargic to comatose; convulsions	Marked lethargy with extreme hyper-irritability on stimulation

---

NURSING DIAGNOSIS: Fluid volume deficit related to active losses in stools

See Nursing care plan: The child with fluid and electrolyte disturbance, p. 272

GOAL

Reestablish diet appropriate for age

INTERVENTIONS

Gradually reintroduce foods as indicated (specify)
Observe response to feedings
Describe feeding behavior

EXPECTED OUTCOME

Child takes prescribed nourishment

NURSING DIAGNOSIS: Potential impaired skin integrity related to frequent loose stools

GOAL

Prevent skin breakdown

INTERVENTIONS

Change diaper and wash and dry area thoroughly after each soiling (a hair dryer on low or cool setting can be helpful)
Cleanse buttocks and genital area well
Apply protective lotion or ointment
Expose reddened area to heat and air where feasible (risk of contamination great in explosive diarrhea)

EXPECTED OUTCOME

Skin exhibits no evidence of discoloration or irritation

NURSING DIAGNOSIS: Potential for infection related to presence of infectious organisms

GOAL

Prevent spread of infection

INTERVENTIONS

Isolate affected child from contact with others
Implement protective techniques as dictated by hospital policy, including
  Disposal of excreta and laundry
  Appropriate handling of specimens
Maintain careful handwashing

EXPECTED OUTCOMES

Others remain free of infection
See also Nursing diagnosis: Potential for infection, p. 288

GOAL

Prevent future infection

INTERVENTIONS

Instruct in preparation and storage of food, based on assessment of individual family needs and facilities
Instruct in care and disposal of waste materials
Teach and emphasize importance of good hygiene and sanitation

EXPECTED OUTCOME

Child and family remain free of infection

NURSING DIAGNOSIS: Altered family processes related to a child with a serious illness

GOAL

Support family

INTERVENTIONS AND EXPECTED OUTCOMES

See Nursing care plan: The family of the ill or hospitalized child, p. 254
See also Nursing care plan: The child in the hospital, p. 246

NURSING CARE PLAN
THE CHILD WITH INFLAMMATORY BOWEL DISEASE

Chronic inflammatory reaction involving the mucosa and submucosa of the lower alimentary tract

Ulcerative colitis—Involves primarily the colon and rectum. Recurrent ulceration in the colon, chiefly of the mucosa and submucosa.

Crohn disease—Involves chiefly the terminal ileum, colon, and rectum. Patchy, deep ulcers that may cause fistulas. Also known as *regional enteritis*.

ASSESSMENT

See Assessment of gastrointestinal dysfunction

Observe for manifestations of inflammatory bowel disease (IBD) (see box)

Assist with diagnostic procedures and tests—Rectosigmoidoscopy, barium enema, stool examination, biopsy, blood studies

Assess parent-child relationships
  Explore the child's attitudes and feelings
  Explore the parent's attitudes and feelings
  Elicit clues to possible parent-child disharmony, school problems, and other sources of stress

COMPARISON OF ULCERATIVE COLITIS AND CROHN DISEASE

Characteristics	Ulcerative Colitis	Crohn Disease
Rectal bleeding	Common	Uncommon
Diarrhea	Often severe	Moderate to absent
Pain	Less frequent	Common
Anorexia	Mild or moderate	Can be severe
Weight loss	Moderate	Severe
Growth retardation	Usually mild	Often marked
Anal and perianal lesions	Rare	Common
Fistulas and strictures	Rare	Common

NURSING DIAGNOSIS: Anxiety related to persistent diarrhea

GOAL

Reduce distress of diarrhea

INTERVENTIONS

Provide ready access to bedpan or bathroom

Keep hand-cleansing materials readily available

Empty and clean bedpan as soon as possible after use

Provide room deodorizer

EXPECTED OUTCOMES

Child uses bedpan or bathroom facilities before soiling occurs

Room is free of bowel odors

GOAL

Relieve inflammation

INTERVENTIONS

*Administer sulfasalazine as prescribed

*Administer corticosteroids if prescribed

*Administer antibiotics if ordered

EXPECTED OUTCOME

Child exhibits abatement of symptoms

NURSING DIAGNOSIS: Altered nutrition: less than body requirements related to loss of appetite and poor assimilation of nutrients

GOAL

Promote nourishment

INTERVENTIONS

See Nursing care plan: The child with special nutritional needs, p. 277

Serve meals and snacks around medication schedule when symptoms are controlled

Avoid high fiber foods and foods that are known to aggravate condition

EXPECTED OUTCOME

Child consumes sufficient nourishment (specify)

—————
*Dependent nursing action.

NURSING DIAGNOSIS: Altered family processes related to child's illness

GOAL

Prepare child and family for temporary or permanent colostomy or ileostomy

INTERVENTIONS

Explain procedure and relationship to disease process
Consult with enterostomal therapist for joint teaching sessions
Teach ostomy care (see p. 564)
*Refer to appropriate agency and/or support group

*****Colitis and Ileitis Foundation,** 444 Park Ave. South, New York, NY 10016, (212) 679-1570; **United Ostomy Association,** 36 Executive Park, Suite 120, Irvine, CA 92714-6744, (714) 660-8624; **International Association for Enterostomal Therapy.** 2081 Business Center Drive, Suite 290, Irvine, CA 92715, (714) 476-0268. In Canada: **Canadian Foundation for Ileitis and Colitis,** 21 St. Clair Ave. E., Suite 301, Toronto, Ontario M4T 1L9, (416) 920-5035; **United Ostomy Association, Canada,** 5 Hamilton Ave., Hamilton, Ontario L8V 2S3, (416) 389-8822.

EXPECTED OUTCOME

Child and family demonstrate an understanding of procedures, surgery, enterostomy care

See also:
Nursing care plan: The family of the ill or hospitalized child, p. 254
Nursing care plan: The child in the hospital, p. 246
Nursing care plan: The child with a chronic illness or disability, p. 259

NURSING CARE PLAN
THE CHILD WITH PEPTIC ULCER DISEASE

An erosion of the mucosal wall of the stomach, pylorus, or duodenum caused by the action of the acid gastric juice

Unit 4

ASSESSMENT

Perform routine physical assessment
Observe for manifestations of peptic ulcer disease (PUD):

Neonates (usually gastric)
Usually perforation
Often massive hemorrhage
Almost the same as seen in stress ulcers

Infants to 2-year-old children (gastric or duodenal, primary or secondary)
Poor eating, vomiting, crying spells after feeding, abdominal distention, tarry stools, melena
Vague discomfort
Irritability
Usually bleed rather than perforate

2- to 6-year-old children (gastric or duodenal)
No really positive physical findings
May have vomiting related to eating, generalized or periumbilical pain, melena, hematemesis
Wake at night crying with pain
Perforation more likely in secondary ulcers

6- to 9-year-old children (usually duodenal and primary)
Pain—burning or gnawing sensation in epigastrium related to fasting state, melena, hematemesis, vomiting
Often with obstruction

Over 9 years (usually duodenal)
Same as above
More typical of adult type
Take a careful health history, especially regarding pattern of pain
Assist with diagnostic procedures and tests—Radiography, barium swallow, endoscopy, blood studies, stool examination for occult blood, gastric acid measurement (occasionally)
Observe for signs of hemorrhage

NURSING DIAGNOSIS: Pain related to ulceration

GOAL

Relieve pain

INTERVENTIONS

Implement nonpharmacologic pain management (see p. 286)
*Implement measures to reduce gastric secretions

EXPECTED OUTCOME

Child exhibits no evidence of pain
See also Nursing care plan: The child in pain, p. 279

NURSING DIAGNOSIS: Potential for injury related to increased gastric secretion

GOAL

Help reduce gastric acidity

INTERVENTIONS

Avoid foods that increase gastric secretions
*Administer antacids every 1 to 2 hours as ordered to absorb or neutralize acids
*Administer anticholinergic drugs to decrease gastric motility and acid secretion
*Administer histamine$_2$ (H$_2$) receptor antagonist if ordered
Encourage compliance with drug regimen

EXPECTED OUTCOME

Child and family comply with medication regimen

GOAL

Reduce stress

*Dependent nursing action.

INTERVENTIONS

Place in quiet environment
Employ measures to reduce anxiety
    Spend as much time as possible with child
    Schedule activities around rest periods
    Explain procedures and therapies
Explore feelings and attitudes for clues to stress-provoking situations
Help child and family to recognize and avoid stress-producing situations

EXPECTED OUTCOMES

Child discusses feelings and concerns
Child exhibits an attitude of relaxation

GOAL

Regulate eating practices

INTERVENTIONS

Provide and encourage well-balanced nutritious diet
Maintain regular meal schedule
Encourage small, frequent meals evenly spaced throughout day
Avoid overeating
Discourage drinking large amounts of fluids with meals

EXPECTED OUTCOME

Child demonstrates an understanding of the relationship of food to symptoms and the elements of sound nutrition

NURSING DIAGNOSIS: Altered family processes related to a child with a potentially life-threatening condition

GOAL

Support family

INTERVENTIONS AND EXPECTED OUTCOMES

See Nursing care plan: The family of the ill or hospitalized child, p. 254
See also Nursing care plan: The child in the hospital, p. 246

*Dependent nursing action.

NURSING CARE PLAN
THE CHILD WITH ACUTE HEPATITIS

Inflammation of the liver
Hepatitis of viral etiology is caused by at least four types of virus. These are:

Hepatitis virus A (HAV)
Hepatitis virus B (HBV)

Hepatitis D (HDV)
Non-A, non-B virus (NANBV)

ASSESSMENT

Perform routine physical assessment
Take careful health history especially regarding:
  Contact with a person known to have hepatitis
  Questionable sanitation practices (e.g., drinking impure water)
  Eating certain foods (e.g., clams or oysters, especially from polluted water)
  Recent blood transfusions

Ingestion of hepatotoxic drugs (e.g., salicylates, sulfonamides, several antineoplastic agents)
Parenteral administration of illicit drugs or sexual contact with persons who use these drugs (include careful examination for signs of needle marks)
Observe for manifestations of hepatitis (see box)
Assist with diagnostic procedures and tests—blood examination for presence of antibodies, liver function tests

COMPARISON OF HEPATITIS TYPES A AND B

Characteristics	Type A	Type B
Onset	Usually rapid, acute	More insidious
Fever	Common and early	Less frequent
Anorexia	Extreme	Mild to moderate
Nausea and vomiting	Common	Less common
Rash	Rare	Common
Arthralgia	Rare	Common
Pruritus	Rare	Sometimes present
Jaundice	Present	Present

NURSING DIAGNOSIS: Potential for infection related to presence of hepatitis virus

GOAL

Prevent spread of infection

INTERVENTIONS

Carry out universal precautions for handling body secretions (see p. 289)
Clean items contaminated with body secretions in disinfectant after use on affected child
Discourage affected child from sharing toys with other children
*Administer hyperimmune gamma globulin prophylactically, if prescribed

___
*Dependent nursing action.

Use special care in use and disposal of blood or invasive instruments

EXPECTED OUTCOME

Others do not contract the disease

NURSING DIAGNOSIS: Altered family processes related to an ill child

GOAL

Support and educate family
Prepare family for home care
  Teach importance of handwashing
  Teach importance of handling and disposing of feces
Caution family against administering any medication (e.g., acetaminophen, ferrous sulfate) since liver may be unable to detoxify the drug sufficiently

EXPECTED OUTCOME

Family demonstrates the ability to provide home care for the child (specify learning and method of demonstration)

See also:
Nursing care plan: The child in the hospital, p. 246
Nursing care plan: The family of the ill or hospitalized child, p. 254

Unit 4

NURSING CARE PLAN
THE CHILD WITH CELIAC DISEASE

A malabsorption disease characterized by hypersensitivity to gluten

ASSESSMENT

Perform routine physical assessment

Take careful health history especially regarding bowel habits related to intake

Observe for manifestations of celiac disease (CD):

Impaired fat absorption:

Steatorrhea (excessively large, pale, oily, frothy stools)

Exceedingly foul-smelling stools

Impaired absorption of nutrients:

Malnutrition

Muscle wasting (especially prominent in legs and buttocks)

Anemia

General wasting

Abdominal distention

Behavioral changes common:

Irritabilty

Fretfulness

Uncooperativeness

Apathy

Celiac crisis (in very young children)

Acute, severe episodes of profuse watery diarrhea and vomiting

May be precipitated by

Infections (especially gastrointestinal)

Prolonged fluid and electrolyte depletion

Emotional disturbance

Assist with diagnostic procedures and tests—Stool collection, intestinal biopsy, gluten challenge

---

NURSING DIAGNOSIS: Altered nutrition: less than body requirements related to malabsorption

GOAL

Reduce irritation of intestinal mucosa

INTERVENTIONS

Provide gluten-free diet tailored to child's appetite and capacity to absorb

*Administer corticosteroids if prescribed

EXPECTED OUTCOME

Child consumes specified diet and displays no evidence of malabsorption

GOAL

Provide nourishment

INTERVENTIONS

Provide for prescribed diet

Arrange conference with dietitian to help select foods compatible with diet and child's preferences

---

*Dependent nursing action.

Administer supplemental water-miscible vitamins and minerals as ordered

Monitor parenteral nutrition line when employed

EXPECTED OUTCOMES

Child consumes prescribed diet

Child exhibits appropriate growth

GOAL

Prepare family for lifelong dietary control

INTERVENTIONS

Explain reason for eliminating gluten from diet

Give written list of common food sources of wheat, rye, barley, and oats

Emphasize suitable substitutes, especially rice and corn

Stress importance of reading labels of prepared food for hidden sources of gluten

In addition to gluten-restricted diet, emphasize other dietary principles, such as high calories, high protein, low fat, low residue, and vitamin supplements

Make referral to public health nurse for continued dietary counseling after hospital discharge

EXPECTED OUTCOMES

Family demonstrates an understanding of dietary restrictions (specify learning and method of demonstration)

Child and family comply with prescribed diet

NURSING DIAGNOSIS: Potential for injury related to celiac crisis

GOAL

Prevent complications from celiac crisis

INTERVENTIONS

Monitor intravenous fluids closely

Give mouth care during period when nothing is given by mouth

Observe child closely for signs of metabolic acidosis (weakness, irritability, decreasing level of consciousness, irregular heartbeat, poor muscular control)

Observe child closely for signs of dehydration

Monitor nasogastric suctioning and record drainage

Observe for signs of shock

Administer steroids as ordered; when discontinued by decreasing doses, observe for return of signs suggestive of celiac disease

If hyperalimentation is required, observe all precautions to prevent infection

EXPECTED OUTCOME

Child recovers from crisis uneventfully

NURSING DIAGNOSIS: Altered family processes related to a child with a chronic illness

GOAL

Support family

INTERVENTIONS AND EXPECTED OUTCOMES

*Refer to appropriate support group(s) and agencies

See also Nursing care plan: The child with a chronic illness or disability, p. 259

---

*__American Celiac Society,__ Dept. N83, 45 Gifford Ave., Jersey City, NJ 07304, (201) 432-1207; **Celiac Sprue Association/United States of America,** 3213 Rocklyn Dr., Des Moines, IA 50322, (515) 270-9689. In Canada: **The Canadian Celiac Association, Inc.,** 1087 Meyerside Dr., Suite 5, Mississauga, Ontario L5T 1M5, (416) 673-8200.

NURSING CARE PLAN
THE CHILD WITH HIRSCHSPRUNG DISEASE (MEGACOLON)

Mechanical obstruction caused by inadequate motility in part of the large intestine.

(Unit 4)

ASSESSMENT

Perform routine physical assessment

Take careful health history especially relative to bowel pattern

Assess general hydration and nutritional status

Observe for manifestations of Hirschsprung disease:

Newborn period

Failure to pass meconium within 24 to 48 hours after birth

Reluctance to ingest fluids

Bile-stained vomitus

Abdominal distention

Infancy

Failure to thrive

Constipation

Abdominal distention

Episodes of diarrhea and vomiting

Ominous signs (often signify the presence of enterocolitis)

Explosive, watery diarrhea

Fever

Severe prostration *extreme exhaustion*

Childhood (symptoms more chronic)

Constipation

Ribbonlike, foul-smelling stools

Abdominal distention

Visible peristalsis

Fecal masses easily palpable

Child usually poorly nourished and anemic

Monitor bowel elimination pattern

Measure abdominal circumference *while supine*

Assist with diagnostic procedures and tests—Radiography, colon biopsy, anorectal manometry

[handwritten margin note: inflammation of both small & large intestine]

NURSING DIAGNOSIS: Constipation related to defective bowel motility

GOAL

Promote elimination

INTERVENTIONS

*Administer enemas as prescribed—Avoid tap water, concentrated saline, soap, or phosphate preparations

EXPECTED OUTCOME

Child eliminates bowel contents

GOAL

Prepare bowel for surgical correction

INTERVENTIONS

*Administer saline enemas as prescribed
*Administer systemic antibiotics as prescribed to sterilize bowel
*Administer antibiotic colon irrigations as prescribed

EXPECTED OUTCOME

Bowel is prepared for surgical procedure

GOAL

Prepare child and family for surgical procedure (colostomy)

INTERVENTIONS

See preparation for procedures, p. 211
See Nursing care plan: The child undergoing surgery, preoperative care, p. 267
Stress to child and family that the colostomy is temporary

---

*Dependent nursing action.

EXPECTED OUTCOME

Child and family demonstrate an understanding of the surgery and its implications

NURSING DIAGNOSIS: Altered family processes related to situational crisis (hospitalized child)

GOAL

Support family

INTERVENTIONS AND EXPECTED OUTCOMES

See Nursing care plan: The family of the ill or hospitalized child, p. 254

GOAL

Prepare the child and family for home care

INTERVENTIONS

Teach colostomy care (See Home care instructions on caring for a child with a colostomy, p. 564)
Enlist the aid of enterostomal therapist if available

EXPECTED OUTCOME

Child and family demonstrate the ability to provide ostomy care at home

See also Nursing care plan: The child in the hospital, p. 254

NURSING CARE PLAN
THE CHILD WITH INTUSSUSCEPTION

An invaginating, or telescoping, of a portion of the intestine into an adjacent portion.

ASSESSMENT

Perform routine physical assessment
Take careful health history, especially family's description of symptoms
Observe stooling pattern and behavior preoperatively and post-operatively
Observe child's behavior
Observe for manifestations of intussusception:
  Sudden acute abdominal pain
    Child screams and draws the knees onto the chest
    Child appears normal and comfortable during intervals between episodes of pain
Vomiting
Apathy
Passage of red currant jelly–like stools (stool mixed with blood and mucus)
Tender, distended abdomen
Palpable sausage-shaped mass in upper right quadrant
Empty lower right quadrant (Dance sign)
Eventual fever, prostration, and other signs of peritonitis

NURSING DIAGNOSIS: Pain related to invaginating bowel

GOAL

Relieve pain

INTERVENTIONS

See Nursing care plan: The child in pain, p. 279

EXPECTED OUTCOME

Child exhibits minimal discomfort

NURSING DIAGNOSIS: Potential for injury related to invaginating bowel

GOAL

Prepare child and family for surgical or nonsurgical correction

INTERVENTIONS

See Preparation for procedures, p. 211
See Nursing care plan: The child undergoing surgery, p. 267

EXPECTED OUTCOME

Child and family demonstrate an understanding of the prescribed therapy

NURSING DIAGNOSIS: Altered family processes related to a child with a life-threatening disorder

GOAL

Support family

INTERVENTIONS AND EXPECTED OUTCOMES

See Nursing care plan: The family of the ill or hospitalized child, p. 254
See also Nursing care plan: The child in the hospital, p. 246

NURSING CARE PLAN
THE CHILD WITH ENTEROBIASIS (PINWORMS)

Intestinal infestation with the nematode *Enterobius vermicularis,* the common pinworm

ASSESSMENT

Perform routine physical assessment
Observe for manifestations of pinworms:
  Intense perianal itching (principal symptom)
    Evidence of itching in young children includes:
      General irritability
      Restlessness
      Poor sleep
      Bed-wetting
      Distractibility
      Short attention span

Perianal dermatitis and excoriation secondary to itching
If worms migrate, possible vaginal and urethral infection
Assist with diagnostic procedures and tests—Collect stool for laboratory testing for ova and parasites; tape test (a loop of transparent tape, sticky side out, is placed around the end of a tongue depressor, which is then pressed firmly against the child's perianal area) collected on awakening

---

NURSING DIAGNOSIS: Potential for injury related to presence of organisms

GOAL

Help eradicate organisms

INTERVENTIONS

*Teach family to administer antihelminthics as prescribed

EXPECTED OUTCOME

Child exhibits no evidence of pinworms

NURSING DIAGNOSIS: Potential for infection related to presence of organisms

GOAL

Prevent spread of infestation

INTERVENTIONS

Teach family preventive measures
  Handwashing after toileting and before eating
  Keep child's fingernails short
  Daily bathing or showering

Discourage child from biting nails, placing fingers in mouth, and scratching anal area
Dress in one-piece outfit to prevent access to anal area

EXPECTED OUTCOME

Child and others remain free of infestation

NURSING DIAGNOSIS: Altered family processes related to a child with an infestation

GOAL

Support family

INTERVENTIONS

Help family comply with therapy
Help family cope and community cope with repeated infestations
Refer to appropriate support groups and agencies, especially regarding repeated infestations

EXPECTED OUTCOME

Family complies with therapy
Family becomes involved with support group(s)

---

*Dependent nursing action.

NURSING CARE PLAN
THE CHILD WITH GIARDIASIS

Inflammatory, intestinal infestation with the protozoan *Giardia lamblia*

ASSESSMENT

Perform routine physical assessment

Take careful health history, especially relative to contact with water (e.g., mountain lakes, streams, and pools), possible contaminated food, and animals

Observe for manifestations of giardiasis:

Infants and young children
 Diarrhea
 Vomiting
 Anorexia
 Failure to thrive

Children over 5 years of age
 Abdominal cramps
 Intermittent loose stools
 Constipation
 Stools may be:
 Malodorous
 Watery
 Pale
 Greasy

Most infections resolve spontaneously in 4 to 6 weeks

Rarely, chronic form occurs
 Intermittent loose, foul-smelling stools
 Possibility of:
 Abdominal bloating
 Flatulence
 Sulfur-tasting belches
 Epigastric pain
 Vomiting
 Headache
 Weight loss

Assist with diagnostic procedures and tests—Multiple stool specimens for identification of organisms and/or cysts, and CIE and ELISA tests

NURSING DIAGNOSIS: Potential for injury related to presence of organisms

GOAL

Help eradicate organism

INTERVENTIONS

*Administer, or teach family to administer, antiprotozoal agents

EXPECTED OUTCOME

Child exhibits no evidence of infestation

NURSING DIAGNOSIS: Potential for infection related to presence of organisms

GOAL

Prevent spread of infestation

INTERVENTIONS

Always wash hands and fingernails with soap and water before eating and handling food and after toileting.

Avoid placing fingers in mouth and biting nails.

Discourage children from scratching bare anal area.

Change diapers as soon as soiled and dispose of in plastic bags in closed receptacle out of children's reach.

Disinfect toilet seats and diaper changing areas; use dilute household bleach (10% solution) or Lysol and wipe clean with paper towels.

Drink water that is specially treated, especially if camping.

Wash all raw fruits and vegetables or food that has fallen on the floor.

Avoid growing foods in soil fertilized with human excreta.

Teach children to defecate only in a toilet, not on the ground.

Keep dogs and cats away from playgrounds or sandboxes.

Avoid swimming in pools frequented by diapered children.

Wear shoes outside.

EXPECTED OUTCOME

Child and others do not become infected with organism

*Dependent nursing action.

Unit 4

NURSING DIAGNOSIS: Altered family processes related to a child with an infestation

GOAL

Support family

INTERVENTIONS

Help family comply with therapy
Offer suggestions to decrease side effects of quinacrine

*Administer drug with meals
Crush tablets and mix with a strong flavoring (e.g., jam or syrup)
See Home care instructions, p. 542

EXPECTED OUTCOMES

Family complies with therapy
Child takes prescribed medication with minimum or no distress.

---

*Dependent nursing action.

Other common intestinal parasites

Parasites/clinical manifestations	Comments
ASCARIASIS—*ASCARIS LUMBRICOIDES* (COMMON ROUNDWORM)	
Light infections: asymptomatic Heavy infections: anorexia, irritability, nervousness, enlarged abdomen, weight loss, fever, intestinal colic Severe infections: intestinal obstruction, appendicitis, perforation of intestine with peritonitis, obstructive jaundice, lung involvement—pneumonitis	Transferred to mouth by way of contaminated food, fingers, or toys Largest of the intestinal helminths Affects principally young children 1-4 years of age Prevalent in warm climates
HOOKWORM DISEASE—*NECATOR AMERICANUS*	
Light infections in well-nourished individuals: no problems Heavier infections: mild to severe anemia malnutrition May be itching and burning ("ground itch") followed by erythema and a papular eruption in areas to which the organism migrates	Transmitted by discharging eggs on the soil and in turn picked up infection from direct skin contact with contaminated soil Wearing shoes is recommended, although children playing in contaminated soil expose many skin surfaces
STRONGYLOIDIASIS—*STRONGYLOIDES STERCORALIS* (THREADWORM)	
Light infection: asymptomatic Heavy infection: respiratory signs and symptoms, abdominal pain, distention, nausea and vomiting, diarrhea—large, pale stools, often with mucus Threat to life in children with weakened immunologic defenses	Transmission is same as for hookworm except autoinfection common Older children and adults affected more often than young children Severe infections may lead to severe nutritional deficiency
VISCERAL LARVA MIGRANS—*TOXOCARA CANIS* (DOGS) **INTESTINAL TOXOCARIASIS—*TOXOCARA CATI* (CATS)**	
Depends on reactivity of infected individual May be asymptomatic except for eosinophilia Specific diagnosis difficult	Transmitted by direct contamination of hands from contact with dog, cat, or objects or ingestion of soil Dogs and cats should be kept away from areas where children play; sandboxes especially important transmission areas Periodic deworming of diagnosed dogs and cats Control of dog population Continued education and laws to prevent indiscriminate canine defecation
TRICHURIASIS—*TRICHURIS TRICHURA* (WHIPWORM)	
Light infections: asymptomatic Heavy infections: abdominal pain and distention, diarrhea	Transmitted from contaminated soil, vegetables, toys, and other objects Most frequent in warm, moist climates Occurs most often in undernourished children living in unsanitary conditions

NURSING CARE PLAN
THE CHILD WITH CLEFT LIP AND/OR CLEFT PALATE

Cleft lip (CL)—A malformation resulting from failure of the maxillary and median nasal processes to fuse during embryonic development

Cleft palate (CP)—A midline fissure of the palate resulting from failure of the two sides to fuse during embryonic development

ASSESSMENT

Perform routine physical assessment
Inspect palate, both visually and by placing fingers directly on palate

Observe feeding behaviors

1. Preoperative care (cleft lip)

NURSING DIAGNOSIS: Altered nutrition: less than body requirements related to difficulty eating

GOAL

Provide adequate nutritional intake

INTERVENTIONS

Administer diet appropriate for age
Modify feeding techniques to adjust to defect
    Feed in sitting position
    Use special appliances
    Encourage frequent bubbling
    Assist with breast-feeding if method of choice

EXPECTED OUTCOME

Infant consumes an adequate amount of nutrients (specify amounts)

NURSING DIAGNOSIS: Potential altered parenting related to infant with a highly visible physical defect

GOAL

Facilitate family's acceptance of infant

INTERVENTIONS

Allow expression of feelings
Convey attitude of acceptance of infant and family
Indicate by behavior that child is a valuable human being
Describe results of surgical correction of defect
    Use photographs of satisfactory results

EXPECTED OUTCOMES

Family discusses feelings and concerns regarding the child's defect, its repair, and future prospects
amily exhibits an attitude of acceptance of infant

See also Nursing care plan: The child undergoing surgery, preoperative care, p. 267

2. Postoperative care (cleft lip)

NURSING DIAGNOSIS: Potential for trauma related to surgical procedure, immature reasoning

GOAL

Prevent trauma to suture line

INTERVENTIONS

Position on back or side
Maintain lip protective device
Use nontraumatic feeding techniques
Restrain arms to prevent access to operative site
    Use jacket restraints on older infant
Avoid placing objects in the mouth following cleft palate repair (suction catheter, tongue depressor, straw, pacifier, small spoon)
Prevent vigorous and sustained crying
Cleanse suture line gently after feeding and as necessary in manner ordered by surgeon
Teach cleansing and restraining procedures, especially when infant will be discharged before suture removal

EXPECTED OUTCOME

Operative site remains undamaged

GOAL

Prevent aspiration of secretions

INTERVENTIONS

Position to allow for mucus drainage (partial side-lying position, semi-Fowler position)

EXPECTED OUTCOME

Child manages secretions without aspiration

NURSING DIAGNOSIS: Altered nutrition: less than body requirements related to physical defect, surgical procedure

GOAL

Provide adequate nutritional intake

INTERVENTIONS

Administer diet appropriate for age
Involve family in determining best feeding methods
Modify feeding techniques to adjust to defect
    Feed in sitting position
    Use special appliances
    Encourage frequent bubbling
    Assist with breast-feeding if method of choice
Teach feeding and suctioning techniques to family
Monitor IV fluids (if prescribed)

EXPECTED OUTCOMES

Infant consumes an adequate amount of nutrients (specify amounts)
Family demonstrates ability to carry out postoperative care

NURSING DIAGNOSIS: Sensory-perceptual alterations (gustatory, tactile) related to feeding methods (some types), arm restraints

GOAL

Provide comfort measures

INTERVENTIONS

Remove restraints periodically while supervised
Provide cuddling and tactile stimulation
Involve parents in infant's care
Apply infant stimulation activities appropriate for infant's developmental level and tolerance (see p. 307)
*Administer analgesics and/or sedatives as ordered

EXPECTED OUTCOME

Child rests quietly, is not irritable, and responds appropriately

---

NURSING DIAGNOSIS: Altered family processes related to child with a physical defect

GOAL

Support family

INTERVENTIONS AND EXPECTED OUTCOMES

See Nursing care plan: The family of the hospitalized child, p. 254
†Refer family to appropriate agencies and support groups

See also Nursing care plan: The child with a chronic illness or disability, p. 259

---

*Dependent nursing action.
†**The Cleft Palate Foundation,** 1218 Grandview Avenue, Pittsburgh, PA 15211, (412) 481-1376; Hotline or Cleftline 1-800-24-CLEFT, for information and referral to associated agencies: **The American Cleft Palate Association** and **The National Cleft Palate Association. The National Association for the Craniofacially Handicapped,** Chattanooga, TN. In Canada: **Canadian Cleft Lip and Palate Family Association,** 180 Dungas Street West, Toronto, M501X8, (416) 593-1448; **About Face, the Craniofacial Family Society,** 123 Edward Street, Suite 1405, Toronto, M5G1E2, (416) 593-1448.

NURSING CARE PLAN
THE CHILD WITH HYPERTROPHIC PYLORIC STENOSIS

Hypertrophy of the pyloric musculature, which causes narrowing and variable degrees of obstruction to the outflow of gastric contents at the pyloric sphincter

ASSESSMENT

Perform routine physical assessment

Take health history, especially regarding eating behavior and vomiting pattern

Observe for manifestations of hypertrophic pyloric stenosis (HPS):
  Projectile vomiting
    May be ejected 3 to 4 feet from the child when side-lying, 1 foot or more when back-lying
    Occurs shortly after a feeding (may not occur for several hours)
    May follow each feeding or appear intermittently
    Nonbilious vomitus; may be blood-tinged

Infant hungry, avid nurser, eagerly accepts a second feeding after vomiting episode
No evidence of pain or discomfort except that of chronic hunger
Weight loss
Signs of dehydration
Distended upper abdomen
Readily palpable olive-shaped tumor in the epigastrium just to the right of the umbilicus
Visible gastric peristaltic waves that move from left to right across the epigastrium
Assist with diagnostic procedures and tests—Upper GI series, ultrasound, laboratory assessment of electrolyte status

---

NURSING DIAGNOSIS: Fluid volume deficit related to vomiting

GOAL

Prevent dehydration

INTERVENTIONS

*Maintain intravenous fluids as prescribed
Provide fluids as tolerated

EXPECTED OUTCOME

Child exhibits no evidence of dehydration

NURSING DIAGNOSIS: Altered nutrition: less than body requirements related to persistent vomiting

GOAL

Prevent vomiting (preoperative)

INTERVENTIONS

Give small, frequent feedings; feed slowly
Bubble before and frequently during feedings

---

*Dependent Nursing Action

Position in high Fowler position and slightly on right side after feeding
Handle minimally and gently after feeding

EXPECTED OUTCOME

Child does not vomit

GOAL

Provide nutrition

INTERVENTIONS

Feed diet for age
Begin with small feeding at frequent intervals to prevent overdistention

EXPECTED OUTCOME

Child consumes a sufficient amount of nourishment

NURSING DIAGNOSIS: Altered family processes related to a child with a life-threatening condition

GOAL

Support family

INTERVENTIONS AND EXPECTED OUTCOMES

See Nursing care plan: The family of the ill or hospitalized child, p. 254

NURSING CARE PLAN
THE CHILD WITH ESOPHAGEAL ATRESIA AND TRACHEOESOPHAGEAL FISTULA

A malformation caused by failure of the esophagus to develop a continuous passage; the esophagus may or may not form a connection with the trachea

Type A (5% - 8%)—Blind pouch at each end of esophagus, widely separated and with no communication to the trachea

Type B (rare)—Blind pouch at each end of esophagus with fistula to form trachea to upper esophageal segment

Type C (80% - 90%)—Proximal esophageal segment terminates in a blind pouch and the distal segment is connected to the trachea or primary bronchus by a short fistula at or near the bifurcation

Type D (rare)—Both upper and lower esophageal segments connected to trachea

Type E (less frequent than A or C)—Otherwise normal trachea and esophagus connected by a common fistula

ASSESSMENT

Perform routine newborn assessment (p. 10)

Observe for manifestations of esophageal atresia and tracheoesophageal fistula (TEF):

Excessive salivation and drooling

Three Cs of TEF:

Coughing

Choking

Cyanosis

May stop breathing

Assist with diagnostic procedures—Chest radiography, catheter gently passed into the esophagus meets with resistance if the lumen is blocked

Monitor frequently for signs of respiratory distress

NURSING DIAGNOSIS: Ineffective airway clearance related to abnormal opening between esophagus and trachea or obstruction to swallowing secretions

GOAL

Maintain patent airway and prevent aspiration

INTERVENTIONS

Remove accumulated secretions from oropharynx

Position for patent airway, lung expansion, and prevention of aspiration of saliva or stomach contents (depends on type of defect)

Supine with head elevated on an inclined plane (at least 30°)

Administer nothing by mouth

EXPECTED OUTCOMES

Airway remains patent

Infant does not aspirate secretions

Respiration remains within normal limits (see inside front cover)

NURSING DIAGNOSIS: Impaired swallowing related to mechanical obstruction

GOAL

Provide nutrition

INTERVENTIONS

Administer gastrostomy feedings when tolerated

Progress to oral feedings as prescribed according to child's condition

Provide for non-nutritive sucking

EXPECTED OUTCOME

Child receives sufficient nourishment and exhibits a satisfactory weight gain

GOAL

Teach child to take oral feedings (following late repair)

INTERVENTIONS

Introduce foods one at a time

Provide foods with various textures and flavors

Teach to chew foods well

Begin with slightly liquid feedings and progress to more solid food

Cut food in small non-cylindric pieces

Avoid foods like whole hot dogs or large pieces of meat

EXPECTED OUTCOME

The child takes an adequate amount of nourishment and displays no evidence of malnourishment

---

NURSING DIAGNOSIS: Potential for injury related to surgical procedure

GOAL

Prevent trauma to surgical site

INTERVENTIONS

Suction only with catheter premeasured to a distance that does not reach to surgical site

EXPECTED OUTCOME

Child does not exhibit evidence of injury to surgical site

NURSING DIAGNOSIS: Anxiety related to inability to swallow, discomfort from surgery

GOAL

Administer comfort measures

INTERVENTIONS

Provide tactile stimulation

Position comfortably postoperatively

Avoid restraints where possible

Administer mouth care

Offer pacifier frequently

*Administer analgesics as prescribed (see Nursing care plan: The child in pain, p. 279)

---

*Dependent nursing action.

EXPECTED OUTCOMES

Child rests calmly, is alert when awake, and engages in non-nutritive sucking

Mouth remains clean and moist

NURSING DIAGNOSIS: Altered family processes related to the child with a physical defect

GOAL

Educate parents in home care

INTERVENTIONS

Teach family

  Positioning

  Signs of respiratory distress

  Signs of contracture—refusal to eat, dysphagia, increased coughing

  Assist in acquiring needed equipment and services

  Care of gastrostomy and esophagostomy when infant has staged surgery, including techniques such as suctioning, care of operative site and/or ostomies, dressing changes, and so on (see Home Care Instructions, p. 564)

EXPECTED OUTCOME

Family demonstrates the ability to provide care to the infant, an understanding of signs of complications, and appropriate actions

See also Nursing care plan: The family of the ill or hospitalized child, p. 254

See also Nursing care plan: The high-risk infant, p. 302

NURSING CARE PLAN
THE INFANT WITH AN ANORECTAL MALFORMATION

A congenital malformation in which the rectum has no outside opening

Low anomaly—Rectum has descended normally through the puborectalis muscle, the internal and external sphincters are present and well developed with normal function, and there is no connection to the gastrointestinal tract; may be anal stenosis with or without an obstructive membrane, frequently with an external fistula to the perineum or vestibule through which meconium is passed.

Intermediate anomaly—Rectum is at or below the level of the puborectalis muscle, the anal dimple and external sphincter are positioned normally, but the anal opening is located anteriorly in the perineum; may be a persistent connection to the gastrointestinal tract.

High anomaly—Rectum ends above the puborectalis muscle; absence of internal and external sphincters and the puborectalis muscle is relatively ineffectual; occurs almost exclusively in males where there is usually a rectourethral fistula; a rectovaginal communication found in females

---

ASSESSMENT

Perform newborn assessment (see p. 10) with special attention to perineal area

Observe for passage of meconium

Observe for ribbonlike stools in older infant or young child who has history of difficult defecation, abdominal distention

Assist with diagnostic procedures—Endoscopy, radiography, renal ultrasound (sometimes)

NURSING DIAGNOSIS: Potential for injury related to inability to evacuate rectum

GOAL

Prevent injury to rectal area

INTERVENTIONS

Avoid taking rectal temperatures preoperatively and postoperatively

Maintain nasogastric suction, if implemented

Maintain scrupulous anal and perineal care

Observe stool patterns to detect normal pattern or abnormality

Position infant side-lying prone with hips elevated or supine with legs suspended at a 90° angle

EXPECTED OUTCOME

Child achieves normal bowel function

NURSING DIAGNOSIS: Altered nutrition: less than body requirements related to inability to feed

GOAL

Provide nourishment

INTERVENTIONS

*Monitor intravenous fluids and/or hyperalimentation as prescribed

Offer nothing by mouth until peristalsis established

Offer pacifier to satisfy non-nutritive sucking needs until bowel elimination achieved (colostomy or rectal reconstruction)

Provide formula or diet for age as soon as peristalsis detected

NURSING DIAGNOSIS: Altered family processes related to child with a defect

GOAL

Prepare family for home care

INTERVENTIONS

Teach care needed for home management
  Rectal dilatation
  Wound care
  Colostomy care (see Home care instructions, p. 564)

EXPECTED OUTCOME

Family demonstrates the ability to provide home care for the infant

See Nursing care plan: The family of the ill or hospitalized child, p. 254

---

*Dependent nursing action.

Hernias

A protrusion of a portion of an organ or organs through an abnormal opening (Table 4-9)

Table 4-9. SUMMARY OUTLINE OF DIAPHRAGMATIC AND ABDOMINAL HERNIAS

Type	Manifestations/diagnostic evaluation	Nursing care

Diaphragmatic
Through foramen of Bochdalek: Protrusion of part of the stomach through an opening in the diaphragm
	Symptoms—mild to severe respiratory distress within a few hours after birth; tachypnea, cyanosis, dyspnea, and severe acidosis
	Breath sounds absent in affected area; bowel sounds may be present
	Rarely asymptomatic
	Diagnosis made by radiographic study
		See Nursing care plan: The high-risk infant and family, p. 302
		Prepare infant for surgical repair
		  Prevent crying
		  Maintain suction, oxygen, and intravenous fluids
		  Place in semi-Fowler position
		  Assist with diagnostic and preoperative procedures
		  *Administer medications
		Postoperative
		  Carry out routine postoperative care and observation
		  Use comfort measures
		  Support parents

Hiatal *(Sliding)* Protrusion of an abdominal structure (usually the stomach) through the esophageal hiatus	Symptoms—dysphagia, failure to thrive, vomiting, neck contortions, frequent unexplained respiratory problems, bleeding, incompetent cardiac sphincter Diagnosis made by fluoroscopy	Be alert to significant signs Carry out routine postoperative care
Abdominal *Umbilical* Soft skin-covered protrusion of intestine and omentum through a weakness in the abdominal wall around the umbilicus	Inspection and palpation of abdomen High incidence in black infants Spontaneous closure by age 1 to 2 years	Discourage use of home remedies, e.g., belly bands, coins Reassure parents of defect's benign nature
Omphalocele Protrusion of intra-abdominal viscera into the base of the umbilical cord	Obvious on inspection Observation for other malformations	Prepare for surgical repair Assist with gradual reduction of abdominal contents in large lesions Keep sac or viscera moist Use overhead warming unit Carry out routine care of intravenous line, nasogastric suction Give nothing by mouth Provide comfort measures *Administer prophylactic antibiotics
Gastroschisis Protrusion of intra-abdominal contents through a defect in the abdominal wall		

*Dependent nursing action.

Unit 4

NURSING CARE OF THE CHILD WITH CARDIOVASCULAR DYSFUNCTION

The cardiovascular system consists of the heart and blood vessels.

NURSING CARE PLAN
THE CHILD WITH CARDIAC DYSFUNCTION

Dysfunction of the heart, congenital or acquired, or the blood vessels

ASSESSMENT

Perform physical assessment with detailed examination of the heart (see p. 44)

See physiologic measurement of pulse and blood pressure, p. 26 and p. 27

Assess general appearance, behavior, and function:

Chest deformities—an enlarged heart sometimes distorts the chest configuration

Unusual pulsations—visible pulsations are seen in some patients

Respiratory excursion—the ease or difficulty of respiration, e.g., tachypnea, dyspnea, presence of expiratory grunt

Clubbing of fingers—is associated with some types of congenital heart disease

Behavior—assuming knee-chest position or squatting is typical of some types of heart disease

Palpation and percussion

Chest—helps discern heart size and other characteristics (such as thrills) associated with heart disease

Abdomen—hepatomegaly and/or splenomegaly may be evident

Peripheral pulses—rate, regularity, and amplitude (strength) may reveal discrepancies

Auscultation

Heart—detect presence of heart murmurs

Heart rate and rhythm—observe for discrepancies between apical and peripheral pulse

Character of heart sounds—reveals deviations in heart sounds and intensity that help localize heart defects

Lungs—may reveal crackles and wheezes

Blood pressure—deviations present in some cardiac conditions, e.g., discrepancies between upper and lower extremities

Assist with diagnostic procedures and tests—Electrocardiography, radiography, echocardiography, fluoroscopy, ultrasonography, angiography, blood analysis (blood count, hemoglobin, packed cell volume, blood gases), cardiac catheterization (see p. 363)

NURSING DIAGNOSIS: Activity intolerance related to imbalance between oxygen supply and demand

GOAL

Reduce cardiac demands and oxygen consumption

INTERVENTIONS

Maintain optimum environmental temperature
Anticipate child's needs
Allow child to assume position of choice
Encourage quiet games and activities
Implement measures to reduce anxiety

EXPECTED OUTCOME

Child rests quietly and exhibits no evidence of distress

NURSING DIAGNOSIS: Decreased cardiac output related to cardiac dysfunction

GOAL

Improve cardiac function

INTERVENTIONS

*Administer medications as prescribed
Avoid activities that create increased demands on the heart (specify)
Allow child to assume position of choice

EXPECTED OUTCOME

Heart rate, volume, and rhythm remain within acceptable limits (specify)

---

*Dependent nursing action.

NURSING DIAGNOSIS: Altered family processes related to a child with a cardiac condition

GOAL

Support family

INTERVENTIONS AND EXPECTED OUTCOMES

See Nursing care plan: The family of the hospitalized child, p. 254
See nursing care plan for specific cardiovascular condition
*Refer family to appropriate support groups and agencies

---

*__American Heart Association,__ 7320 Greenville Ave., Dallas, TX 75231, (214) 373-6300. In Canada: __Canadian Heart Foundation,__ 1 Nicholas St., Suite 1200, Ottawa, Ontario K1N 7B7.

NURSING CARE PLAN
THE CHILD WHO UNDERGOES CARDIAC CATHETERIZATION

A diagnostic procedure in which a radiopaque catheter is inserted through a peripheral blood vessel into the heart.
Right-sided catheterization—The catheter is introduced from a vein (usually the femoral or brachial) into the right atrium.

Left-sided catheterization—The catheter is threaded by way of a systemic artery retrograde into the aorta and left ventricle or, from a right-sided approach, into the left atrium by means of a septal puncture.

Unit 4

1. Preprocedural care

ASSESSMENT

Perform routine physical assessment
Perform cardiac assessment

NURSING DIAGNOSIS: Anxiety and fear related to diagnostic procedure, unfamiliar environment

GOAL

Relieve anxiety

INTERVENTIONS

See Preparation for procedures, p. 211
See Preoperative preparation, p. 267

Provide pacifier for smaller infants if irritable
Provide K-pad or other device for warming small infant
Provide extra diapers for infants

EXPECTED OUTCOME

Child is transported to the cardiac catheterization laboratory with a minimum of distress to child and family

2. Postprocedural care

ASSESSMENT

See postoperative assessment p. 269

Assess:

Vital signs every 15 minutes, with special emphasis on heart rate counted for 1 full minute for evidence of arrhythmias or bradycardia

Blood pressure, especially for hypotension, which may indicate hemorrhage from cardiac perforation or bleeding at the site of initial catheterization

Assess general color and oxygenation by oximetry as prescribed

Pulses, especially below the catheterization site, for equality and symmetry (pulse distal to the site may be weaker for the first few hours after catheterization but should gradually increase in strength)

Temperature and color of the affected extremity, since coolness or blanching may indicate arterial obstruction

Dressing for evidence of bleeding or hematoma formation in the femoral or antecubital area

---

NURSING DIAGNOSIS: Potential for injury related to operative procedure

GOAL

Prevent complications

INTERVENTIONS

Keep leg on operative side as straight as possible
Keep incision and dressing clean and dry
Apply pressure if oozing or bleeding noted
Carry out routine physical assessments
Keep child relatively quiet
Avoid undue excitement

EXPECTED OUTCOMES

Child exhibits no evidence of vein obstruction or bleeding

GOAL

Maintain optimum body temperature

INTERVENTIONS

Provide warmth if infant or child is chilled from exposure during procedure
Avoid either overheating or chilling

EXPECTED OUTCOME

Child's temperature remains within normal range (see inside front cover).

*Administer withheld digitalis and other medications if ordered

---

NURSING DIAGNOSIS: Altered family processes related to a child undergoing a diagnostic procedure

GOAL

Support family

INTERVENTIONS AND EXPECTED OUTCOMES

See Nursing care plan: The family of the ill or hospitalized child, p. 254

See also Nursing care plan: The child in the hospital, p. 246

---

*Dependent nursing action.

NURSING CARE PLAN
THE CHILD WITH CONGENITAL HEART DISEASE

A structural or functional defect of the heart or great vessels present at birth

TYPES OF DEFECTS

Acyanotic defects:

There is no mixing of desaturated (poorly oxygenated venous) blood in the systemic arterial circulation

Caused by (1) left-to-right shunting of blood through an ab-normal opening or (2) obstructive lesions that reduce the flow of blood to various areas of the body

Cyanotic defects:

Desaturated blood is mixed with saturated blood in the systemic arterial circulation, regardless of whether cyanosis is clinically evident

Usually right-to-left shunting of blood through an abnormal opening and/or vessel configuration

---

ASSESSMENT

Perform physical assessment with special emphasis on color, pulse (apical and peripheral), respiration, blood pressure, and examination and auscultation of chest

Take careful health history including evidence of poor weight gain, poor feeding, exercise intolerance, unusual posturing, or frequent respiratory tract infections

Observe child for manifestations of congenital heart disease:

Infants

Cyanosis—generalized, especially mucous membranes, lips and tongue, conjunctiva; highly vascularized areas

Cyanosis during exertion such as crying, feeding, straining, or when immersed in water; peripheral or central

Dyspnea, especially following physical effort such as feeding, crying, straining

Fatigue

Poor growth and development (failure to thrive)

Frequent respiratory tract infections

Feeding difficulties

Hypotonia

Excessive sweating

Syncopal attacks such as paroxysmal hyperpnea, anoxic spells

Older Children

Impaired growth

Delicate, frail body build

Fatigue

Effort dyspnea

Orthopnea

Digital clubbing

Squatting for relief of dyspnea

Headache

Epistaxis

Leg fatigue

See assessment of The child with cardiac dysfunction, p. 362

Unit 4

NURSING DIAGNOSIS: Decreased cardiac output related to structural defect

GOAL

Improve strength and efficiency of the heart

INTERVENTIONS

*Administer digoxin as ordered (see box on p. 268)

EXPECTED OUTCOME

Heart rate and volume indicate satisfactory cardiac output

GOAL

Reduce venous return to the right side of the heart

INTERVENTIONS

Place in knee-chest position or cuddle on shoulder with knees bent (infant)

Direct child to assume squatting position (child)

EXPECTED OUTCOME

Child breathes more easily

NURSING DIAGNOSIS: Activity intolerance related to imbalance between oxygen supply and demand

GOAL

Reduce energy expenditure

INTERVENTIONS

Allow for frequent rest periods

Encourage quiet games and activities

---

*Dependent nursing action.

Caution family to consult with child's cardiologist before taking child on airplane or to a higher altitude

Help the child select activities appropriate to age, condition, and capabilities

Avoid extremes of environmental temperature

EXPECTED OUTCOME

Child determines and engages in activities commensurate with capabilities

---

NURSING DIAGNOSIS: Altered growth and development related to inadequate oxygen and nutrients to tissues; social isolation

GOAL

Promote physical growth

INTERVENTIONS

Provide well-balanced, highly nutritious diet

EXPECTED OUTCOME

Child achieves normal growth (specify)

GOAL

Improve iron-carrying capacity of blood

INTERVENTIONS

*Administer iron preparations as prescribed

Encourage iron-rich foods in the diet

EXPECTED OUTCOME

Child assimilates sufficient iron

GOAL

Avoid social isolation

INTERVENTIONS

Encourage age-appropriate activities

See Nursing care plan: The child with a chronic illness or disability, p. 259

EXPECTED OUTCOME

Child engages in age-appropriate activities

NURSING DIAGNOSIS: Potential for infection related to debilitated physical status

GOAL

Prevent infection

---

*Dependent nursing action.

INTERVENTIONS

Avoid contact with infected persons

Provide for adequate rest

Provide optimum nutrition

EXPECTED OUTCOME

Child remains free of infection

NURSING DIAGNOSIS: Altered family processes related to having a child with a heart condition

See Nursing care plan: The child with a chronic illness or disability, p. 259

GOAL

Reduce family's fears and anxieties

INTERVENTIONS

Discuss with parents their fears regarding child's symptoms, such as pounding heart, cyanotic spells, irritability

EXPECTED OUTCOME

Family discusses their fears and anxieties

GOAL

Help family cope with symptoms of disease

INTERVENTIONS

Encourage family to participate in care of the child while hospitalized

Explore coping strategies with family, such as:

   During dyspneic/cyanotic spell, place child in knee-chest position, with head and chest elevated or over the shoulder

   Keep child warm; encourage rest and sleep

   Decrease child's anxiety by remaining calm

Encourage family to include others in child's care to prevent their own exhaustion

Assist family in determining appropriate physical activity and disciplining methods for child

EXPECTED OUTCOME

Family copes with child's symptoms in a positive way

GOAL

Prepare family for home care of the infant or child

INTERVENTIONS

Teach skills needed for home care

   Administration of medications (see Home Care Instructions, p. 542) (see guidelines for administering digoxin, p. 367)

   Feeding techniques

   Interventions for conserving energy and those directed toward relief of frightening symptoms

   Signs that indicate complications (see p. 368)

   Where and whom to contact for help and guidance

Anticipate need for further information and support

Refer family to local chapter of the American Red Cross for instruction in cardiopulmonary resuscitation (see Home Care instructions, p. 578)

EXPECTED OUTCOMES

Family demonstrates the ability and motivation for home care of the infant

Family members learn cardiopulmonary resuscitation technique

NURSING DIAGNOSIS: Potential for injury (complications) related to cardiac condition and therapies

GOAL

Recognize signs of complications early

INTERVENTIONS

Teach family to recognize signs of complications
  Congestive heart failure (CHF) (p. 365)
  Maintain high index of suspicion regarding digoxin toxicity
    Vomiting (earliest sign)
    Neurologic symptoms (of questionable value with children)
    Bradycardia
    Arrhythmias
    Pulse deficit
  Increased respiratory effort—tachycardia, retraction, grunting, cough, cyanosis
  Hypoxemia—cyanosis, restlessness, tachycardia
  Cerebral thrombosis—compensatory polycythemia (in cyanotic heart disease) is particularly hazardous when child is dehydrated
  Cardiovascular collapse—pallor, cyanosis, hypotonia

EXPECTED OUTCOMES

Family recognizes signs of complications and institutes appropriate action

GOAL

Prepare for diagnostic tests and surgery

INTERVENTIONS

Explain or clarify information presented to family by the practitioner and surgeon
Prepare child and parents for the procedure
Assist with family's decision regarding surgery
Explore feelings regarding palliative or corrective surgery

EXPECTED OUTCOME

Family demonstrates an understanding of tests, surgery, etc. (specify learning and manner of demonstration)

NURSING DIAGNOSIS: Body image disturbance related to having a physical defect

See Nursing care plan: The child with a chronic illness or disability, p. 259

GUIDELINES FOR ADMINISTERING DIGOXIN AT HOME

Give digoxin at regular intervals, usually every 12 hours, such as 8 AM and 8 PM.

Plan the times so that the drug is given *1 hour before* or *2 hours after* feedings.

Use a calendar to mark off each dose that is given or post a reminder, such as a sign on the refrigerator.

Have the prescription refilled *before* the medication is completely used.

Administer the drug carefully by slowly directing it on the side and back of the mouth.

Do not mix it with other foods or fluids, since refusal to consume these results in inaccurate intake of the drug.

If the child has teeth, give water after administering the drug; whenever possible, brush the teeth to prevent tooth decay from the sweetened liquid.

If a dose is missed and more than 4 hours has elapsed, withhold the dose and give the next dose at the regular time; if less than 4 hours has elapsed, give the missed dose.

Do not give a second dose if the child vomits.

Notify the practitioner if more than two consecutive doses have been missed.

Do not increase or double the dose for missed doses.

Notify the practitioner immediately if the child becomes ill.

Keep digoxin in a safe place, preferably a locked cabinet.

In case of accidental overdose of digoxin, call the nearest poison control center immediately.

Modified from Jackson PL: Digoxin therapy at home: keeping the child safe, Am J Maternal Child Nurs 4(2):105-109, 1979.

Unit 4

NURSING CARE PLAN
THE INFANT WITH CONGESTIVE HEART FAILURE

Inability of the heart to pump sufficient blood to meet the metabolic demands of body tissues

ASSESSMENT

Perform physical assessment
Perform cardiac assessment
Take careful health history, especially regarding previous cardiac problems
Observe for manifestations of congestive heart failure:

General
Weakness
Fatigue
Poor feeding
Irritability
Pallor
Duskiness
Cyanosis, especially on exertion

Cardiac
Tachycardia (pulse over 140 in sleeping infants, over 100 in sleeping older children)
Cardiomegaly
Gallop rhythm
Pulsus alternans

Pulmonary
Dyspnea
Costal retractions
Tachypnea
Orthopnea
Cardiac wheezing
Cough
Weak cry
Hoarseness
Gasping
Grunting on expiration

Systemic
Hepatomegaly
Weight gain (edema)
Ascites
Pleural effusions
Distended neck and peripheral veins
Sweating, especially on exertion

Assist with diagnostic procedures and tests—Radiography, electrocardiography
Assess fluid gain or loss
   Weigh daily at same time and on same scale
   Maintain strict intake and output
   Assess for evidence of increased or decreased edema
Monitor cardiac and respiratory function
Assess child for evidence of potassium depletion (see pp. 273-275)

NURSING DIAGNOSIS: Decreased cardiac output related to structural defect, myocardial dysfunction

GOAL

Improve cardiac strength and power

INTERVENTIONS

*Administer digoxin (Lanoxin) as ordered, using established precautions to prevent toxicity
   Make certain dosage is within safe limits
   Ascertain correct preparation for route
   Check dosage with another nurse
   Count apical pulse for 1 full minute prior to giving drug
      Withhold medication and notify the physician if pulse rate is less than 90 to 110 bests per minute (infants) or 70 to 85 (older children), depending on previous pulse readings

Often an ECG rhythm strip is taken to assess cardiac status prior to administration
Ensure adequate intake of potassium
Monitor serum potassium levels (decrease enhances digitalis toxicity)

EXPECTED OUTCOME

Heart beat is strong, regular, and within normal limits for age (see inside front cover)

NURSING DIAGNOSIS: Ineffective breathing pattern related to pulmonary congestion

GOAL

Improve ventilation and oxygen supply

---

*Dependent nursing action.

INTERVENTIONS

Place in inclined posture of 10 to 30 degrees; tilt mattress support of Isolette; place older infant in cardiac chair or infant seat

Avoid any constricting clothing or restraints around abdomen and chest

*Administer oxygen as prescribed

EXPECTED OUTCOME

Respirations remain within normal limits, color is good, and infant rests quietly (see inside front cover for normal variations in respirations)

GOAL

Reduce anxiety

INTERVENTIONS

Employ flexible feeding schedule that reduces fretfulness associated with hunger

Handle child gently

Hold and comfort infant

Employ comfort measures found to be effective in individual cases

Encourage family to provide comfort and solace

*Administer narcotic (morphine sulfate) as prescribed

EXPECTED OUTCOME

Infant rests quietly and breathes easily

NURSING DIAGNOSIS: Fluid volume excess related to fluid accumulation (edema)

GOAL

Help eliminate excess fluid and prevent fluid accumulation

INTERVENTIONS

*Administer diuretics as prescribed

*Feed low-salt formula

    Lonalac (Mead-Johnson)

    Similac PM 60/40 (Ross)

EXPECTED OUTCOME

Infant exhibits evidence of fluid loss—frequent urination, weight loss

---

*Dependent nursing action.

NURSING DIAGNOSIS: Activity intolerance related to imbalance between oxygen supply and demand

GOAL

Reduce cardiac demands and oxygen consumption

INTERVENTIONS

See Nursing care plan: The child with cardiovascular dysfunction, p. 362

Maintain neutral thermal environment for minimal oxidative metabolism

    Place infant in Isolette with servocontrol or under warmer

Maintain in resting state at 10 to 30 degrees

Feed small volumes at frequent intervals (every 2 to 3 hours) using soft nipple with moderately large opening

Implement gavage feeding if infant becomes fatigued before taking an adequate amount

Time nursing activities to disturb infant as little as possible

Implement measures to reduce anxiety

Respond promptly to crying or other expressions of distress

EXPECTED OUTCOME

Infant rests quietly

NURSING DIAGNOSIS: Potential for infection related to reduced body defenses, pulmonary congestion

See Nursing care plan: The child at risk for infection, p. 288

See Nursing care plan: The child with an upper respiratory infection, p. 318

NURSING DIAGNOSIS: Altered family processes related to a child with a life-threatening illness

GOAL

Support family

INTERVENTIONS AND EXPECTED OUTCOMES

See Nursing care plan: The family of the ill or hospitalized child, p. 254

NURSING CARE PLAN
THE CHILD WITH RHEUMATIC FEVER

An inflammatory disease affecting the heart, joints, central nervous system, and subcutaneous tissues

ASSESSMENT

Perform routine physical assessment

Take health history especially regarding evidence of antecedent streptococcus infection

Observe for manifestations of rheumatic fever:

General

Low-grade fever, usually spiking in late afternoon

Unexplained epistaxis

Abdominal pain

Arthralgia without arthritic changes

Weakness

Fatigue

Pallor

Loss of appetite

Weight loss

Specific Manifestations
Carditis

Tachycardia out of proportion to degree of fever

Cardiomegaly

New murmurs or change in preexisting murmurs

Muffled heart sounds

Precardial friction rub

Precordial pain

Changes in ECG (especially prolonged P-R interval)

Migratory polyarthritis

Swollen, hot, red, painful joint(s)

After 1 to 2 days affects different joint(s)

Favors large joints—knees, elbows, hips, shoulders, wrists

Subcutaneous nodes

Nontender swelling

Located over bony prominences

May persist for some time, then gradually resolve

Chorea (St. Vitus dance, Sydenham chorea)

Sudden aimless, irregular movements of extremities

Involuntary facial grimaces

Speech disturbances

Emotional lability

Muscle weakness (can be profound)

Muscle movements exaggerated by anxiety and attempts at fine motor activity; relieved by rest

Erythema marginatum

Erythemous macules with clear center and wavy, well-demarcated border

Transitory

Nonpruritic

Primarily affects trunk and proximal extremities

Assist with diagnostic procedures and tests—Electrocardiography, throat culture, blood analysis for increased erythrocyte sedimentation rate, elevated or rising antistreptolysin-O titer

---

NURSING DIAGNOSIS: Potential for injury related to presence of streptococcal organisms

GOAL

Prevent tissue damage from invasion of streptococci

INTERVENTIONS

*Administer penicillin therapeutically and prophylactically

Teach family to administer penicillin (See Home Care Instructions, p. 542)

Impress on family the importance of compliance with medical regimen

Medication continued throughout childhood

GOAL

Manage complications

INTERVENTIONS

*Administer medications appropriate to complication exhibited by child

Arthritis: See Nursing care plan: The child with juvenile rheumatoid arthritis, p. 455

Carditis: See Nursing care plan: The infant with congestive heart failure, p. 368

Chorea: Sedatives and anticonvulsives

Maintain a quiet environment

Protect from stressful situations

EXPECTED OUTCOME

Child displays minimum or no effects of complications

---

*Dependent nursing action.

*Dependent nursing action.

NURSING DIAGNOSIS: Altered family processes related to an ill and/or hospitalized child

GOAL

Support family

INTERVENTIONS AND EXPECTED OUTCOMES

See Nursing care plan: The family of the ill or hospitalized child, p. 254

See also Nursing care plan: The child in the hospital, p. 246

*Dependent nursing action.

NURSING CARE PLAN
THE CHILD IN CIRCULATORY FAILURE (SHOCK)

A clinical syndrome characterized by prostration and tissue perfusion that is inadequate to meet the metabolic demands of the body, resulting in depressed vital cell function

STAGES OF SHOCK

Compensated shock—Vital organ function is maintained by intrinsic compensatory mechanisms; blood flow is usually normal or increased but generally uneven or maldistributed in the microcirculation.

Uncompensated shock—Efficiency of the cardiovascular system gradually diminishes, until perfusion in the microcirculation becomes marginal despite compensatory adjustments.

Irreversible shock or **terminal shock**—Damage to vital organs such as the heart or brain of such magnitude that the entire organism will be disrupted regardless of therapeutic intervention. Death occurs even if cardiovascular measurements return to normal levels with therapy.

TYPES OF SHOCK

Hypovolemic shock—Reduced circulating blood volume caused by blood loss, plasma loss, intracranial hemorrhage

Distributive shock—Reduced peripheral vascular resistance with an associated increase in venous capacity and pooling causing diminished venous return and cardiac output; caused by anaphylaxis (anaphylactic shock), sepsis (septic shock), loss of neural control (neurogenic shock)

Cardiogenic shock—Decreased cardiac output (not common in children) but caused by congenital heart disease (especially outflow obstruction, systemic-to-pulmonary shunting), inflow or outflow obstruction, primary pump failure, dysrhythmia

ASSESSMENT

Maintain vigilance in situations that predispose to shock (e.g., trauma, burns, overwhelming sepsis, diarrhea, vomiting)
Observe for manifestations of shock:

Early clinical signs
Apprehensiveness
Irritability
Unexplained tachycardia
Normal blood pressure
Narrowing pulse pressure
Thirst
Pallor
Diminished urinary output

Advanced shock
Confusion and somnolence
Tachypnea

Moderate metabolic acidosis
Oliguria
Cool, pale extremities
Decreased skin turgor
Poor capillary filling

Impending cardiopulmonary arrest
Thready, weak pulse
Hypotension
Periodic breathing or apnea
Anuria
Stupor or coma

Monitor vital signs, central venous pressure, intake and output, cardiac function on admission and continuously or very frequently
Assist with diagnostic procedures and tests—Blood count, blood gases, pH, electrocardiography

Unit 4

NURSING DIAGNOSIS: Ineffective breathing pattern related to diminished oxygen needed for impaired tissue perfusion

GOAL

Increase oxygen to lungs

INTERVENTIONS

*Administer oxygen as prescribed
  Position to maintain open airway (e.g., neck in neutral or "sniffing" position)
  Monitor artificial airway and mechanical ventilation (if implemented)

EXPECTED OUTCOME

Lungs are well ventilated

NURSING DIAGNOSIS: Altered tissue perfusion related to reduced blood flow, decreased blood volume, reduced vascular tone

GOAL

Promote venous return and cardiac output

INTERVENTIONS

  Position child flat with legs elevated
*Start (or help start) and monitor intravenous infusion of prescribed fluid and plasma expander
*Administer vasopressor and cardiotonics as prescribed
  Maintain optimum body temperature

---

*Dependent nursing action.

EXPECTED OUTCOME

Child exhibits evidence of improved cardiac output and circulation—pulse, respiration, blood pressure, oxygen saturation, and urinary output within acceptable limits (specify); skin warm, dry, and good color; alert and oriented

NURSING DIAGNOSIS: Altered family processes related to a child in a life-threatening condition

GOAL

Support family

INTERVENTIONS

Keep family informed frequently regarding child's status
Arrange for someone to remain with family and serve as liaison between them and critical care area (if possible)
Allow family to see child as soon as feasible

EXPECTED OUTCOME

Family demonstrates an attitude of assurance that the child is being given needed care
See also: Nursing care plan: The family of the ill or hospitalized child, p. 254

See also:
Nursing care plan for specific disorders producing shock
Nursing care plan: The child in the hospital, p. 246
Nursing diagnosis: Anticipatory grief, p. 306

NURSING CARE OF THE CHILD WITH HEMATOLOGIC DYSFUNCTION

The hematologic system consists of the blood and blood-forming tissues—red bone marrow, lymph nodes, and spleen.

NURSING CARE PLAN
THE NEWBORN WITH HYPERBILIRUBINEMIA

Excessive accumulation of bilirubin in the blood

CLASSIFICATION:

Nonconjugated hyperbilirubinemia—Direct reacting; implies impaired liver function. Type most commonly observed in newborns (see Table 4-7)

Conjugated hyperbilirubinemia—Indirect reacting; implies functioning liver. Usually the result of bile duct obstruction.

ASSESSMENT

Perform newborn assessment (see p. 10)

Observe for manifestations of hyperbilirubinemia:

Jaundice—Yellowish discoloration of skin

Bright yellow or orange—Unconjugated (indirect)

Greenish, muddy yellow—Conjugated (direct)

Intensity of jaundice

Unrelated to degree of bilirubinemia

Determined by serum bilirubin measurements

Hemolytic disease of the newborn:

Jaundice appearing shortly after birth during first 24 hours

Hepatosplenomegaly may be evident

Signs of anemia (notably, marked pallor) in severely affected infants

Assist with diagnostic procedures and tests—Transcutaneous bilirubinometry, serum bilirubin levels, Coombs test (infants of Rh-negative mothers)

Observe for evidence of dehydration (p. 343), hyperthermia

Table 4-10. COMPARISON OF THREE TYPES OF UNCONJUGATED HYPERBILIRUBINEMIA

	Physiologic jaundice	Breast-feeding associated jaundice	Hemolytic disease
Cause	Immature hepatic function plus increased bilirubin load from red blood cell hemolysis	Unknown etiology Early: related to fewer calories consumed by infant before mother's milk established Late: factor in breast milk that inhibits bilirubin conjugation	Blood antigen incompatibility causes hemolysis of large numbers of erythrocytes Liver unable to conjugate and excrete excess bilirubin from hemolysis
Onset	After 24 hours (premature infants, before 48 hours)	Early: 3 to 4 days of age Late: 4 to 5 days	During first 24 hours
Peak	Second to third days	Third week	
Duration	Decline fifth to seventh days	Up to 3 to 12 weeks	
Therapy	Phototherapy	Frequent breast-feeding (early) When bilirubin levels reach 15 to 16 mg/100 ml, temporary discontinuation of breast-feeding for 48 hours (late)	Postnatal: exchange transfusion Prenatal: transfusion (fetus) Prevent sensitization (Rh incompatibility) of Rh-negative mother with RhoGam

Unit 4

NURSING DIAGNOSIS: Potential for injury related to breakdown products of red blood cells in greater number than normal, immature blood-brain barrier

GOAL

Eliminate excess bilirubin

INTERVENTION

*Place infant under phototherapy lamp as prescribed

EXPECTED OUTCOME

Child is exposed to prescribed light source

GOAL

Protect infant during phototherapy

INTERVENTIONS

Shield infant's eyes
  Make certain that lids are closed prior to applying shield
  Check eyes each shift for drainage or irritation
Place infant nude under light, except male genitalia (controversial)
Change position frequently
Monitor body temperature
  Check axillary temperature with reading on servocontrolled unit
Chart duration of therapy, type of lights, distance of lights to infant, use of open or closed bassinet, and shielding of infant's eyes
Avoid the use of oily applications on the skin
Ensure adequate fluid intake to prevent dehydration

EXPECTED OUTCOME

Infant displays no evidence of eye irritation, dehydration, elevated temperature

GOAL

Protect infant during and following exchange transfusion (if appropriate)

INTERVENTIONS

Give infant nothing by mouth prior to procedure (usually for 3-4 hours)
Check donor blood with physician for correct blood group and Rh type
Assist physician during procedure; ensure asepsis
Keep accurate records of amounts of blood infused and withdrawn
Monitor vital signs, especially following infusion of calcium gluconate
Maintain optimal body temperature of infant during procedure (blankets, radiant warmer)
Observe for signs of exchange transfusion reactions
Have resuscitative equipment (supplemental oxygen, airway, manual resuscitation bag, endotracheal tube, and laryngoscope) at bedside
Apply sterile dressing to catheter site

---

*Dependent nursing action.

Check umbilical site for bleeding or infection
Monitor vital signs following transfusion

EXPECTED OUTCOMES

Infant exhibits no signs of adverse effects from transfusion
Vital signs remain within normal limits (see inside front cover for normal variations)
There is no evidence of infection or bleeding at infusion site

---

NURSING DIAGNOSIS: Altered family processes related to child with an adverse physiologic response

GOAL

Provide emotional support to family

INTERVENTIONS

Discontinue phototherapy during family visiting; remove infant's eye shields
Emphasize benign nature of physiologic jaundice
Assure family that skin will regain normal pigmentation
Advise breast-feeding mothers of possibility of prolonged jaundice

EXPECTED OUTCOME

Family demonstrates an understanding of the therapy and prognosis

GOAL

Prepare family for home phototherapy (if prescribed)

INTERVENTIONS

Assess family's understanding of the disorder and the proposed therapy
Instruct family regarding:
  Placement and care of lamp unit
  Proper eye care
    Apply eye patches
    Close lids before applying patches
    Be certain patches fit snugly with no possibility of light leaks
    Remove patches when light is discontinued—During feeding, while family is sleeping
  Taking axillary temperature on infant
    Every 15 minutes for initial hour
    Every 4 hours thereafter while under lights
  Proper positioning while under lamp
    Rotate to expose all areas
    Keep infant nude or dressed in mini-diaper according to unit policy
  Provide increased fluid intake
  Keeping a log of time spent under light, infant's color, feeding patterns, amount of feedings, diaper changes
  Observations for signs of lethargy, change in sleeping pattern, any difficulty arousing infant, changes in stooling or voiding
  Importance of bilirubin tests as prescribed
  See Nursing care plan: The high-risk infant and family, p. 302

EXPECTED OUTCOMES

Family demonstrates the ability to provide home phototherapy for the infant (specify learning and methods of demonstration)

NURSING CARE PLAN
THE CHILD WITH ANEMIA

A condition in which the number of red blood cells and/or the hemoglobin concentration is reduced below normal

ASSESSMENT

Perform physical assessment

Take health history, including careful diet history to identify any deficiencies, evidence of pica—eating clay, ice, paste

Observe for manifestations of anemia:

General manifestations
Muscle weakness
Easy fatigability
    Frequent resting
    Shortness of breath
    Poor sucking (infants)
Pale skin
    Waxy pallor seen in severe anemia

Central nervous system manifestations
Headache
Dizziness
Light-headedness
Irritability
Slowed thought processes
Decreased attention span
Apathy
Depression

Shock (blood loss anemia)
Poor peripheral perfusion
Skin moist and cool
Low blood pressure and central venous pressure
Increased heart rate

Assist with diagnostic tests—Analysis of blood elements

NURSING DIAGNOSIS: Activity intolerance related to generalized weakness, diminished oxygen delivery to tissues

GOAL

Minimize physical exertion

INTERVENTIONS

Anticipate and assist in those activities of daily living that may be beyond child's tolerance

Provide diversional play activities that promote rest and quiet but prevent boredom and withdrawal

Choose appropriate roommate of similar age and interests who requires restricted activity

Plan nursing activities to provide sufficient rest

Assist with activities requiring exertion

EXPECTED OUTCOME

Child plays and rests quietly and engages in activities appropriate to capabilities

GOAL

Increase oxygen to tissues

INTERVENTIONS

Position for optimum air exchange
Administer supplemental oxygen if needed

EXPECTED OUTCOME

Patient breathes easily; respiratory rate and depth normal (see inside front cover)

GOAL

Minimize emotional stress

INTERVENTIONS

Anticipate child's irritability, short attention span, and fretfulness by offering to assist child in activities rather than waiting for request for help

Encourage parents to remain with child

EXPECTED OUTCOME

Child remains calm and quiet

GOAL

Help replace blood elements

INTERVENTIONS

*Administer blood, packed cells, platelets as prescribed (see Table 4-11)

EXPECTED OUTCOME

Child receives the appropriate blood elements without incident

---

*Dependent nursing action

Table 4-11. NURSING CARE OF THE CHILD RECEIVING BLOOD TRANSFUSIONS

Complication	Signs/symptoms	Precautions/nursing responsibilities
Immediate reactions		
Hemolytic reactions—Most severe type, but rare Incompatible blood Intradonor incompatibility in multiple transfusions	Chills Shaking Fever Pain at needle site and along venous tract Nausea/vomiting Sensation of tightness in chest Red or black urine Headache Flank pain Progressive signs of shock and/or renal failure	Positively identify donor and recipient blood types and groups before transfusion is begun; verify with one other nurse or physician Transfuse blood slowly for first 15 to 20 minutes and/or initial 1/5 volume of blood; remain with patient In event of signs or symptoms, stop transfusion immediately, maintain patent intravenous line, and notify physician Save donor blood to re-crossmatch with patient's blood Monitor for evidence of shock Insert urinary catheter and monitor hourly outputs Send sample of patient's blood and urine to laboratory for presence of hemoglobin (indicates intravascular hemolysis) Observe for signs of hemorrhage resulting from disseminated intravascular coagulation (DIC) Support medical therapies to reverse shock
Febrile reactions Leukocyte or platelet antibodies Plasma protein antibodies	Fever Chills	May give acetaminophen for prophylaxis Leukocyte-poor red blood cells are less likely to cause reaction Stop transfusion immediately; report to physician for evaluation
Allergic reactions—Recipient reacts to allergens in donor's blood	Urticaria Flushing Asthmatic wheezing Laryngeal edema	Give antihistamines for prophylaxis to children with tendency toward allergic reactions Stop transfusions immediately Epinephrine for wheezing or anaphylactic reaction
Circulatory overload Too rapid transfusion (even a small quantity) Excessive quantity of blood transfused (even slowly)	Precordial pain Dyspnea Rales Cyanosis Dry cough Distended neck veins	Transfuse blood slowly Prevent overload by using packed red blood cells or administering divided amounts of blood Use infusion pump to regulate and maintain flow rate If signs of overload, stop transfusion immediately Place child upright with feet in dependent position to increase venous resistance
Air emboli—May occur when blood is transfused under pressure	Sudden difficulty in breathing Sharp pain in chest Apprehension	When infusing blood under pressure, normalize pressure before container is empty If air is observed in tubing, clear tubing of air by aspirating air with syringe at the nearest Y connector; disconnect tubing and allow blood to flow until air has escaped only if a Y connector is not available
Hypothermia	Chills Low temperature Irregular heart rate Possible cardiac arrest	Allow blood to warm at room temperature (less than 1 hour) Use an electric warming coil to rapidly warm blood Take temperature if patient complains of chills; if subnormal stop transfusion

Table 4-11. NURSING CARE OF THE CHILD RECEIVING BLOOD TRANSFUSIONS—cont'd

Complication	Signs/symptoms	Precautions/nursing responsibilities
Electrolyte disturbances Hyperkalemia (in massive transfusions or patients with renal problems)	Nausea, diarrhea Muscular weakness Flaccid paralysis Paresthesia of extremities Bradycardia Apprehension Cardiac arrest	Use washed red blood cells or fresh blood if patient at risk
Delayed reactions ***Transmission of infection*** Hepatitis AIDS Malaria Syphilis Bacteria or viruses Other	Signs of infection, e.g., jaundice Toxic reaction: high fever, severe headache or substernal pain, hypotension, intense flushing, vomiting/diarrhea	Blood is tested for HBsAg (hepatitis B), syphilis, and HIV (AIDS); positive units are destroyed. Individuals at risk for carrying certain viruses are deferred from donation Report any sign of infection, and, if occurring during transfusion, stop transfusion immediately, send sample for culture and sensitivity tests, and notify physician
Alloimmunization (antibody formation)	Increased risk of hemolytic, febrile, and allergic reactions	Occurs in patients receiving multiple transfusions Use limited number of donors Observe carefully for signs of reactions
Delayed hemolytic reaction	Destruction of red blood cells and fever 5 to 10 days after transfusion	Observe for posttransfusion anemia and decreasing benefit from successive transfusions

NURSING DIAGNOSIS: Altered nutrition: less than body requirements related to reported inadequate iron intake (less than RDA); knowledge deficit regarding iron rich foods

GOAL

Promote adequate intake of iron-rich foods

INTERVENTIONS

Provide diet counseling to caregiver, especially in regard to
Food sources of iron, e.g., meat, liver, fish, egg yolks, green leafy vegetables, legumes, nuts, whole grains, including iron-fortified infant cereal and dry cereal (see also p. 167)
Feed milk as supplemental food in infant's diet after solids are begun

EXPECTED OUTCOME

Child receives at least minimum daily requirement of iron

GOAL

Increase body iron stores

IMPLEMENTATION

*Administer iron preparations as prescribed
Instruct family regarding correct administration of oral iron preparation
Give in divided doses (specify)
Give between meals
Administer with fruit juice or multivitamin preparation
Do not give with milk or antacids
*Administer the liquid preparation with dropper, syringe, or straw to avoid contact with teeth

EXPECTED OUTCOME

Family relates a diet history that verifies that the child complies with these suggestions
Child is given iron supplement as evidenced by green, tarry stools
Child takes medication appropriately

---

*Dependent nursing action.

NURSING CARE PLAN
THE CHILD WITH SICKLE CELL DISEASE

A hereditary disorder in which normal adult hemoglobin (HgA) is partly or completely replaced by an abnormal hemo- globin (HgS) causing distortion and rigidity of red blood cells under conditions of reduced oxygen tension

ASSESSMENT

Perform physical assessment

Take health history, especially regarding any evidence of sick- ling crisis and history of the disease in family members

Observe for manifestations of sickle cell disease:

General

Growth retardation

Chronic anemia (Hb 6.5 to 8 g/dl)

Delayed sexual maturation

Marked susceptibility to sepsis

Vaso-Occlusive Crisis

Pain in area(s) of involvement

Manifestations related to ischemia of involved areas:

Extremities: painful swelling of hands and feet (sickle cell dactylitis, or "hand-foot syndrome"), painful joints

Abdomen: severe pain resembling acute surgical condition

Cerebrum: stroke, visual disturbances

Chest: symptoms resemble pneumonia, protracted epi- sodes of pulmonary disease

Liver: obstructive jaundice, hepatic coma

Kidney: hematuria

Sequestration Crisis

Pooling of large amounts of blood:

Hepatomegaly

Splenomegaly

Circulatory collapse

Effects of Chronic Vaso-Occlusive Phenomena

Heart: cardiomegaly, systolic murmurs

Lungs: altered pulmonary function, susceptibility to infec- tions, pulmonary insufficiency

Kidneys: inability to concentrate urine, progressive renal failure, enuresis

Genital: priapism (painful constant penile erection)

Liver: hepatomegaly, cirrhosis, intrahepatic cholestasis

Spleen: splenomegaly, susceptibility to infection, functional reduction in splenic activity progressing to autosplenec- tomy

Eyes: intraocular abnormalities with visual disturbances, sometimes progressive retinal detachment and blindness

Extremities: skeletal deformities, especially lordosis and kyphosis, chronic leg ulcers, susceptibility to salmonella osteomyelitis

CNS: hemiparesis, seizures

Assist with diagnostic procedures and tests—Sickle turbidity (Sickledex), hemoglobin electrophoresis

Observe for evidence of complications (crisis)

NURSING DIAGNOSIS: Potential for injury related to abnormal hemoglobin, decreased ambient oxygen, de- hydration

GOAL

Increase tissue oxygenation and prevent sickling

INTERVENTIONS

Explain preventive measures

Avoid strenuous physical exertion

Avoid emotional stress

Prevent infection

Avoid low oxygen environment

EXPECTED OUTCOME

Child avoids situations that reduce tissue oxygenation

GOAL

Promote hydration

INTERVENTIONS

Calculate recommended daily fluid intake and base child's fluid requirements on this *minimum* amount (specify)

Give parents written instructions regarding specific quantity of fluid required

Encourage child to drink

Teach family signs of dehydration (see p. 343)

Stress importance of avoiding overheating as source of fluid loss

EXPECTED OUTCOME

Child drinks an adequate amount of fluid and shows no signs of dehydration

GOAL

Prevent infection

INTERVENTIONS

Stress importance of adequate nutrition, protection from known sources of infection, and frequent medical supervision
Report any sign of infection to physician immediately
Promote compliance with antibiotic therapy
See also: Nursing diagnosis: Potential for infection, (p. 288)

EXPECTED OUTCOME

Child remains free of infection

GOAL

Decrease risks associated with a surgical procedure

INTERVENTIONS

Explain reason for preoperative blood transfusion
Keep child well hydrated
Decrease fear through appropriate preparation
Avoid unnecessary exertion
Promote pulmonary hygiene postoperatively
Use passive range of motion exercises to promote circulation
*Administer oxygen, if prescribed
Monitor for evidence of infection (see p. 288)

EXPECTED OUTCOME

Child undergoes a surgical procedure without crisis

NURSING DIAGNOSIS: Altered family processes related to a child with potentially life-threatening disease

GOAL

Increase understanding of disease

INTERVENTIONS

Teach family and older children characteristics of basic defect and measures to prevent sickling
Stress importance of informing significant health personnel of child's disease
Explain signs of developing crisis, especially fever, pallor, and pain
Reinforce basics of trait transmission
Refer to genetic counseling services

EXPECTED OUTCOME

Child and family demonstrate an understanding of the disease, its etiology, and its therapies

---

*Dependent nursing action.

GOAL

Support family

INTERVENTIONS

*Refer to special organizations and agencies
Refer child to comprehensive sickle cell clinic for ongoing medical care
Be especially alert to family's needs when two or more members are affected

See Nursing care plan: The child with a chronic illness or disability, p. 259

EXPECTED OUTCOMES

Family takes advantage of community services (specify)
Child receives ongoing care from appropriate facility

Sickle cell crisis

NURSING DIAGNOSIS: Altered tissue perfusion related to generalized sickling

GOAL

Increase tissue oxygenation

INTERVENTIONS

†Administer oxygen as prescribed
Promote circulation through passive range of motion exercises

EXPECTED OUTCOME

Child exhibits no evidence of sickling

NURSING DIAGNOSIS: Pain related to tissue anoxia

GOAL

Relieve pain

INTERVENTIONS AND EXPECTED OUTCOMES

See Nursing care plan: The child in pain, p. 279

See also:
Nursing care plan: The child in the hospital, p. 246
Nursing care plan: The family of the hospitalized child, p. 254

---

*A Sickle Cell Home Study Kit For Families is available from the **National Association for Sickle Cell Disease, Inc.,** 4221 Wilshire Blvd., Los Angeles, CA 90010, (800) 321-8453 or (213) 936-7205. Additional resources are **Howard University, Center for Sickle Cell Disease,** 2121 Georgia Ave., N.W., Washington, DC 20059; National Sickle Cell Disease Program, **National Heart, Lung, and Blood Institute,** 9000 Rockville Pike, Bethesda, MD 20205, (301) 496-4000. **Canadian Sickle Cell Society,** 1076 Bathurst St., Suite 305, Toronto, Ontario M5R 3G9.
†Dependent nursing action.

NURSING CARE PLAN
THE CHILD WITH BETA-THALASSEMIA (COOLEY ANEMIA)

An inherited severe, progressive anemia caused by deficient synthesis of hemoglobin

Thalassemia minor or thalassemia trait—Produces a mild microcytic anemia

Thalassemia intermedia—Manifests as splenomegaly and severe anemia

Thalassemia major (Cooley anemia)—Results in anemia of variable severity that is not compatible with life without transfusion support

ASSESSMENT

Perform physical assessment

Obtain family history, especially regarding relatives with evidence of the disease, relatives of Mediterranean heritage

Obtain health history with special concern regarding growth (especially sexual maturation), anemia

Observe for manifestation of β-thalassemia major:

Anemia
Unexplained fever
Poor feeding
Markedly enlarged spleen

Bone changes (older children)
Enlarged head
Prominent frontal and parietal bosses
Prominent malar eminences
Flat or depressed bridge of the nose
Enlarged maxilla
Protrusion of the lip and upper central incisors and eventual malocclusion
Mongoloid appearance of eyes

Other Features
Small stature
Delayed sexual maturation
Bronzed, freckled complexion
Protrusion of the abdomen (hepatosplenomegaly)

With Progressive Anemia
Signs of chronic hypoxia
    Headache
    Precordial and bone pain
    Decreased exercise tolerance
    Listlessness
    Anorexia

Other Symptoms
Frequent epistaxis
Hyperuricemia and gout
Hemochromatosis
Hemosiderosis

Assist with diagnostic procedures and tests—Hematologic studies for blood cell changes, hemoglobin and hematocrit, hemoglobin electrophoresis, serum iron concentration, radiography

NURSING DIAGNOSIS: Potential for injury related to frequent blood transfusions

GOAL

Prevent complications of blood transfusions

INTERVENTIONS

See Nursing care of the child receiving blood transfusion, p. 376
*Administer iron-chelating agent as prescribed
Prepare child and family for splenectomy, if prescribed

EXPECTED OUTCOME

Child exhibits no evidence of complications

*Dependent nursing action

NURSING DIAGNOSIS: Altered family processes related to a child with a chronic, life-threatening disorder

GOAL

Support child and family

INTERVENTIONS

Refer to genetic counseling if requested
Refer to appropriate agencies for support and assistance
See Nursing care plan: The family of the ill or hospitalized child, p. 254

EXPECTED OUTCOMES

Family demonstrates an understanding of the disease and the nature of its transmission

*Family becomes involved with appropriate agencies and support groups

*Cooley's Anemia Foundation, Inc. 105 E. 22nd St., New York, NY 10010; (212) 598-0911. AHEPA Cooley's Anemia Foundation, 136-59 39th Ave., Flushing, NY 11354;
Thalassemia Action Group, 105 E. 22nd St., New York, NY 10010 (212) 598-0911.

See also Nursing care plan: The child with a chronic illness or disability, p. 259
See also Nursing care plan: The child in the hospital, p. 246

NURSING CARE PLAN
THE CHILD WITH HEMOPHILIA

A bleeding disorder caused by a hereditary deficiency of a blood factor essential for coagulation

ASSESSMENT

Perform physical assessment
Take family history, especially regarding evidence of the disease in male relatives
Observe for manifestations of hemophilia:
  Prolonged bleeding anywhere from or in the body
  Hemorrhage from any trauma—loss of deciduous teeth, circumcision, cuts, epistaxis, injections
Excessive bruising—even from a slight injury, such as a fall
Subcutaneous and intramuscular hemorrhages
Hemarthrosis (bleeding into the joint cavities), especially the knees, ankles, and elbows
Hematomas—pain, swelling, and limited motion
Spontaneous hematuria
Assist with diagnostic procedures and tests—Coagulation tests, determination of specific factor deficiency

Unit 4

NURSING DIAGNOSIS: Potential for injury related to hemorrhage

GOAL

Prevent bleeding

INTERVENTIONS

*Prepare and administer intravenous cryoprecipitate or concentrates as needed
Teach home administration of blood factor replacement

EXPECTED OUTCOME

Child has minimal or no bleeding episodes

GOAL

Control bleeding

INTERVENTIONS

Apply pressure to area for 10-15 minutes
Immobilize area

---

*Dependent nursing action.

Elevate site to above level of heart
Apply cold compresses; encourage family to have frozen plastic bags of water prepared in advance

EXPECTED OUTCOME

Child exhibits no evidence of bleeding

GOAL

Decrease risk of injury

INTERVENTIONS

Make environment as safe as possible
Encourage pursuit of intellectual/creative activities
Encourage older child to choose activity but accept responsibility for own safety
Plan with schoolteacher appropriate activity schedule; confer with school nurse regarding severity of bleeding episodes
Discuss with parents appropriate limit-setting patterns
Stress need for oral hygiene using soft toothbrush or available substitute
Discuss diet, especially effect of overweight on hemarthrosis
Advise use of Medic Alert identification in case of emergency
During nursing procedures, especially injections, use local measures to control bleeding

EXPECTED OUTCOME

Child experiences few bleeding episodes

> **NURSING DIAGNOSIS:** Pain related to bleeding into tissues and joints

GOAL

Relieve pain

INTERVENTIONS AND EXPECTED OUTCOME

See Nursing care plan: The child in pain, p. 279

> **NURSING DIAGNOSIS:** Impaired mobility related to effects of hemorrhages into joints and other tissues

GOAL

Prevent crippling effects of joint degeneration

INTERVENTIONS

Use local measures to control bleeding
Institute passive range of motion exercises after acute phase
Exercise unaffected joints and muscles
Consult with physical therapist concerning exercise program
Refer to public health nurse and/or physical therapist for supervision at home
Stress to family serious long-range consequences of hemarthrosis
Support any orthopedic measures in joint rehabilitation
Assess need for pain management to increase ease of mobility

EXPECTED OUTCOME

Bleeding episodes are controlled sufficiently to prevent crippling
See also: Nursing diagnosis: Impaired physical mobility, p. 437

> **NURSING DIAGNOSIS:** Altered family processes related to a child with a serious disease

GOAL

Support family

INTERVENTIONS

Refer for genetic counseling, including identification of carrier offspring, and other female relatives
*Refer to special groups and agencies offering services to families with hemophilia

See also:
Nursing care plan: The family of the ill or hospitalized child, p. 254
Nursing care plan: The child in the hospital, p. 246
Nursing care plan: The child with a chronic illness or disability, p. 259

EXPECTED OUTCOME

Family makes contact with other support groups

***National Hemophilia Foundation,** Soho Bldg, Rm 406, 110 Green St., New York, NY 10012, (212) 219-8180. In Canada: **Canadian Hemophilia Society,** 100 King St. West, Suite 210, Hamilton, Ont. L8P 1A2, (416) 523-6414.

NURSING CARE OF THE CHILD WITH GENITOURINARY DYSFUNCTION

Dysfunction of the genitourinary tract includes that of the kidney proper (renal) or any part of the collecting system: ureters, bladder, and urethra (urinary tract). Dysfunction of the closely related male genital tract is often included in this designation.

NURSING CARE PLAN
THE CHILD WITH URINARY TRACT INFECTION

Bacteriuria with or without signs or symptoms of inflammation in the bladder, kidneys, or both

ASSESSMENT

Perform physical assessment
Take health history
Observe for manifestations of urinary tract infection (UTI):

Newborns May Have
Fever or hypothermia
Sepsis

Children Less Than 2 Years of Age
Failure to thrive
Feeding problems
Vomiting
Diarrhea
Abdominal distention
Jaundice
Frequent or infrequent voiding
Constant squirming
Irritability
Strong-smelling urine
Abnormal stream
Persistent diaper rash

Children Over 2 Years of Age
Enuresis
Daytime incontinence in toilet-trained child
Fever
Strong or foul-smelling urine
Increased frequency of urination

Dysuria
Urinary urgency
Abdominal pain
Costovertebral angle tenderness (flank pain)
Hematuria
Vomiting (preschoolers)

Adolescents
Lower tract infection:
    Frequency
    Painful urination (small amount of turbulent urine)
    Hematuria
    Fever usually absent
Upper tract infection:
    Fever
    Chills
    Flank pain
    Lower tract symptoms
Urine
    Cloudy
    Hazy
    Thick with noticeable strands of mucus and pus
    Unpleasant fishy smell even when fresh

Keep accurate intake and output, observe color and character of urine
Assist with diagnostic tests and procedures—urinalysis, urine culture, tests to rule out structural anomalies (ultrasonography, radiography, intravenous pyelography)

NURSING DIAGNOSIS: Potential for injury related to possibility of kidney damage from chronic infection, knowledge deficit regarding drug administration

GOAL

Help eradicate infective organisms
*Administer antibiotics as prescribed

*Dependent nursing actions.

Teach family to administer medications, especially the importance of continuing the prescribed drug as ordered

EXPECTED OUTCOMES

Child displays no evidence of infection
Family complies with directives

GOAL

Prevent recurrence of infection

Unit 4

INTERVENTIONS

Teach preventive measures to child and family
  Perineal hygiene—wipe from front to back
  Avoid tight clothing or diapers; wear cotton panties rather than nylon
  Check for vaginitis or pinworms, especially if child scratches between legs
  Avoid "holding" urine; encourage child to void frequently, especially before a long trip or other circumstances where toilet facilities are not available
  Empty bladder completely with each void
  Avoid straining at stool
  Encourage generous fluid intake, especially urine acidifying beverages
  Employ play techniques to encourage fluid intake (see p. 276)

EXPECTED OUTCOMES

Child demonstrates good hygiene and preventive practices (specify)
Child drinks an adequate amount of fluid (specify amount)

NURSING DIAGNOSIS: Altered family processes related to a child with a mild disease with a potential for renal damage

GOAL

Support family

INTERVENTIONS

Answer questions and clarify information
Promote follow-up care and management
  Arrange appointments
  Refer to public health agency, if appropriate

EXPECTED OUTCOME

Family exhibits an understanding of the condition
Child receives follow-up care

NURSING CARE PLAN
THE CHILD WITH MINIMAL CHANGE NEPHROTIC SYNDROME

A clinical state characterized by an increased permeability of the glomerular membrane to protein

ASSESSMENT

Perform physical assesment, including extent of edema
Take careful health history, especially relative to recent weight gain, renal dysfunction
Observe for manifestations of nephrotic syndrome:
  Weight gain
  Edema
  Puffiness of face
    Especially around the eyes
    Apparent on arising in the morning
    Subsides during the day
  Abdominal swelling (ascites)
  Respiratory difficulty (pleural effusion)
  Labial or scrotal swelling
  Edema of intestinal mucosal causes:
    Diarrhea
    Anorexia
    Poor intestinal absorption
  Extreme skin pallor (often)
  Irritability

Easily fatigued
Lethargic
Blood pressure normal or slightly decreased
Susceptibility to infection
Urine alterations:
  Decreased volume
  Darkly opalescent
  Frothy
Assist with diagnostic procedures and tests—Urine analysis for protein, casts, and red blood cells; blood analysis for serum protein (total, albumin/globulin ratio, cholesterol), red blood count, serum sodium
Detect evidence of fluid retention
  Assess intake relative to output
    Measure and record intake and output accurately
    Weigh daily (or more often if needed)
  Assess changes in edema
    Measure abdominal girth at umbilicus
    Test urine for specific gravity, albumin
    Collect specimens for laboratory examination

NURSING DIAGNOSIS: Fluid volume excess (total body) related to fluid accumulation in tissues and third spaces

GOAL

Prevent fluid retention

INTERVENTIONS

*Administer steroids (if prescribed as ordered)
*Administer diuretics if ordered
 Limit fluids as indicated

EXPECTED OUTCOME

Child displays no evidence of increased fluid accumulation (specify parameters)

NURSING DIAGNOSIS: Fluid volume deficit (intravascular) related to reduced colloidal osmotic pressure (COP)

GOAL

Assist in raising COP

INTERVENTION

*Administer salt-poor albumin intravenous infusion if ordered

EXPECTED OUTCOME

Child displays no evidence of hypovolemic shock

NURSING DIAGNOSIS: Altered nutrition: less than body requirements related to loss of appetite

GOAL

Provide good nutrition

INTERVENTIONS

Offer nutritious diet (restrict sodium during edema and steroid therapy)
*Administer supplementary vitamins and iron as ordered
 Enlist aid of child, parents, and dietitian in formulation of diet

See also: Nursing care plan: The child with special nutritional needs, p. 277

EXPECTED OUTCOME

Child consumes an adequate diet (specify)

---
*Dependent nursing action.

NURSING DIAGNOSIS: Activity intolerance related to fatigue

GOAL

Conserve energy

INTERVENTIONS

Maintain bed rest initially if severely edematous
Balance rest and activity when ambulatory
Plan and provide quiet activities
Instruct to rest when child begins to feel tired

EXPECTED OUTCOME

Child engages in activities appropriate to capabilities

NURSING DIAGNOSIS: Potential impaired skin integrity related to edema, lowered body defenses

GOAL

Prevent skin breakdown

INTERVENTIONS

Provide meticulous skin care
Cleanse and powder opposing skin surfaces several times per day
Separate opposing skin surfaces with soft cotton
Support edematous organs, such as scrotum
Cleanse edematous eyelids with warm saline wipes
Change position frequently; maintain good body alignment

EXPECTED OUTCOME

Skin displays no evidence of redness or irritation

NURSING DIAGNOSIS: Potential for infection related to diminished body defenses, fluid overload

GOAL

Prevent infection

INTERVENTIONS AND EXPECTED OUTCOMES

See Nursing diagnosis: Potential for infection, p. 288

NURSING DIAGNOSIS: Altered family processes related to a child with a serious disease

GOAL

Support family

INTERVENTIONS AND EXPECTED OUTCOMES

See Nursing care plan: The family of the ill or hospitalized child, p. 254

See also Nursing care plan: The child in the hospital, p. 246

NURSING CARE PLAN
THE CHILD WITH ACUTE POSTSTREPTOCOCCAL GLOMERULONEPHRITIS

A renal disorder characterized by bilateral inflammatory changes in glomeruli that are not caused by infection of the kidney and that follow a streptococcal infection

ASSESSMENT

Initial assessment

Perform physical assessment

Take health history, especially relative to evidence of recent streptococcal infection

Observe for manifestations of acute glomerulonephritis (AGN):
Edema
    Especially periorbital
    Facial edema more prominent in the morning
    Spreads during the day to involve extremities and abdomen
Anorexia
Urine
    Cloudy, smoky brown (resembles tea or cola)
    Severely reduced volume
Pallor
Irritability
Lethargy
Child appears ill
Child seldom expresses specific complaints
Older children may complain
    Headaches
    Abdominal discomfort
    Dysuria
Vomiting not uncommon
Mild to moderately elevated blood pressure

Assist with diagnostic procedures and tests—urinalysis, blood chemistry, antistreptolysin-O, erythrocyte sedimentation rate, C-reactive protein, total serum complement levels, throat culture

Ongoing assessment

Accurate intake and output, appearance of urine
Vital signs, body weight
Observe for signs of complications:
    Report significant deviations of
        Vital signs—blood pressure, pulse, respiration, temperature
        Appearance and volume of urine
        Weight gain relative to size of child
    Report any dyspnea
    Report unusual symptoms
        Vomiting
        Visual disturbances
        Motor disturbances
        Seizure activity
        Severe headache
        Abdominal pain
        Changes in behavior and/or activity level, for example, lethargy, restlessness
Observe for incipient signs of hyperkalemia

NURSING DIAGNOSIS: Fluid volume excess related to compromised regulatory mechanism (kidney)

GOAL

Prevent or control progress of edema

INTERVENTIONS

*Help plan and serve sodium and protein as prescribed
*Limit fluids if ordered

EXPECTED OUTCOME

Child exhibits no evidence of increased fluid retention

*Dependent nursing action.

GOAL

Help reduce blood pressure

INTERVENTIONS

* Administer antihypertensive agents

EXPECTED OUTCOME

Child's blood pressure is within normal limits for age (see inside front cover)

NURSING DIAGNOSIS: Potential for injury related to complications of edema and fluid retention

*Dependent nursing action.

GOAL

Prevent hyperkalemia

INTERVENTIONS

Restrict foods high in potassium during oliguria
Monitor laboratory findings

EXPECTED OUTCOMES

Child exhibits no evidence of hyperkalemia
Serum potassium remains within normal limits

GOAL

Prevent infection

INTERVENTIONS

Avoid contact with infected persons
Keep warm and dry
See Nursing care plan: The child at risk for infection, p. 288

EXPECTED OUTCOME

Child exhibits no evidence of infection

NURSING DIAGNOSIS: Altered family processes related to a child with a serious illness

GOAL

Support family

INTERVENTIONS AND EXPECTED OUTCOMES

See Nursing care plan: The family of the ill or hospitalized child, p. 254

See also Nursing care plan: The child in the hospital, p. 246

NURSING CARE PLAN
THE CHILD WITH ACUTE RENAL FAILURE

An acute condition that results when the kidneys suddenly are unable to excrete urine of sufficient volume or adequate concentration to maintain normal body fluid balance
Causes may be

Prerenal
Hypovolemia
Circulatory insufficiency
Peripheral vasodilation
Increased vascular resistance
Renal arterial occlusion

Renal
Disease of the kidney
Tubular destruction
Vascular
Hypoxic ischemia

Postrenal
Upper tract obstruction
Bladder neck obstruction

ASSESSMENT
Initial assessment

Perform physical assessment
Take careful health history, especially regarding evidence of glomerulonephritis, obstructive uropathy, exposure to or ingestion of toxic chemicals (including heavy metals, carbon tetrachloride, or other organic solvents; nephrotoxic drugs)
Observe for manifestations of acute renal failure (ARF):

Specific
Oliguria
Anuria uncommon (except in obstructive disorders)

Non-specific (may develop)
Nausea
Vomiting
Drowsiness

Edema
Hypertension
Manifestations of underlying disorder or pathology
Assist with diagnostic tests—Urine analysis, blood urea nitrogen, nonprotein nitrogen, creatinine, serum electrolytes, complete blood count, blood gases, specific tests to determine cause of renal failure

Ongoing assessment

Careful monitoring of
Urinary output (insert Foley catheter)
Blood pressure, pulse, and respiration
Cardiac function
Neurologic function
Observe for signs of fluid overload

NURSING DIAGNOSIS: Fluid volume excess related to failure or compromised renal regulatory mechanisms

GOAL

Help remove excess fluid

INTERVENTIONS

*Perform or assist with dialysis (peritoneal dialysis or hemodialysis)

EXPECTED OUTCOME

Child exhibits no evidence of accumulated fluid and waste products

GOAL

Regulate fluid intake

INTERVENTIONS

Administer intravenous or oral fluids as prescribed
See Nursing diagnosis: Fluid volume excess, p. 276

EXPECTED OUTCOME

Child exhibits no evidence of fluid gain

NURSING DIAGNOSIS: Fluid volume deficit related to active fluid loss

GOAL

Replace fluid losses

INTERVENTIONS AND EXPECTED OUTCOMES

See Nursing diagnosis: Fluid volume deficit, p. 276

GOAL

Prevent dehydration

INTERVENTIONS AND EXPECTED OUTCOMES

See Nursing diagnosis: Fluid volume deficit, p. 276

NURSING DIAGNOSIS: Potential for injury related to accumulation of fluid electrolytes and waste products

GOAL

Help remove excess levels of electrolytes and nitrogenous waste

INTERVENTIONS

*Assist with dialysis
*Administer Kayexalate as prescribed
*Provide diet low in protein, potassium, and sodium, if prescribed

---

*Dependent nursing action.

EXPECTED OUTCOME

Child exhibits no evidence of waste product accumulation (hyperkalemia, hypernatremia, etc.)

GOAL

Reduce blood pressure

INTERVENTIONS

*Administer antihypertensives as prescribed
Avoid situations that increase child's anxiety and apprehension
Provide quiet calm environment

EXPECTED OUTCOME

Child's blood pressure remains within acceptable limits (specify)

NURSING DIAGNOSIS: Potential for infection related to diminished body defenses, fluid overload

GOAL

Prevent infection

INTERVENTIONS

Provide aseptic care of intravenous, hyperalimentation, or dialysis sites
*Administer antibiotics if ordered
See Nursing diagnosis: Potential for infection, p. 288

EXPECTED OUTCOME

Child exhibits no evidence of infection

NURSING DIAGNOSIS: Altered family processes related to a child with a life-threatening illness

GOAL

Support family

INTERVENTIONS AND EXPECTED OUTCOMES

See Nursing care plan: The family of the ill or hospitalized child, p. 254

See also Nursing care plan: The child in the hospital, p. 246

---

*Dependent nursing action.

NURSING CARE PLAN
THE CHILD WITH CHRONIC RENAL FAILURE

The diseased kidneys are unable to maintain the chemical composition of body fluids within normal limits under normal conditions

Accumulation of various biochemical substances in the blood that result from diminished renal function produces complications such as:

Retention of waste products, especially the blood urea nitrogen and creatinine

Water and sodium retention, which contributes to edema and vascular congestion

Hyperkalemia of dangerous levels

Metabolic acidosis of a sustained nature because of continual hydrogen ion retention and bicarbonate loss

Calcium and phosphorus disturbances resulting in altered bone metabolism, which in turn causes growth arrest or retardation, bone pain, and deformities known as *renal osteodystrophy*

Anemia caused by hematologic dysfunction including shortened life span of red blood cells, impaired red blood cell production related to decreased production of erythropoietin, prolonged bleeding time, and nutritional anemia

Growth disturbance, probably caused by such factors as poor nutrition, anorexia, and bone demineralization

ASSESSMENT
Initial assessment

Perform routine physical assessment with special attention to measurements of growth parameters

Take health history, especially regarding renal dysfunction, eating behavior, frequency of infections, energy level

Observe for evidence of manifestations of chronic renal failure (CRF):

Early signs:
Loss of normal energy
Increased fatigue on exertion
Pallor, subtle (may not be noticed)
Elevated blood pressure (sometimes)

As the disease progresses:
Decreased appetite (especially breakfast)
Less interest in normal activities
Increased urinary output with compensatory intake of fluid
Pallor more evident
Sallow, muddy appearance of skin

Child may complain of:
Headache
Muscle cramps
Nausea

Other signs and symptoms:
Weight loss
Facial edema
Malaise
Bone or joint pain
Growth retardation
Dryness or itching of the skin
Bruised skin
Sensory or motor loss (sometimes)
Amenorrhea (common in adolescent girls)

Uremic syndrome (untreated):
Gastrointestinal symptoms
Anorexia
Nausea and vomiting
Bleeding tendencies
Bruises
Bloody diarrheal stools
Stomatitis
Bleeding from lips and mouth
Intractable itching
Uremic frost (deposits of urea crystals on skin)
Unpleasant "uremic" breath odor
Deep respirations
Hypertension
Congestive heart failure
Pulmonary edema
Neurologic involvement:
Progressive confusion
Dulled sensorium
Coma (ultimately)
Tremors
Muscular twitching
Seizures

Assist with diagnostic procedures and tests—Urinalysis, complete blood count, blood chemistry, renal biopsy

Ongoing assessment

Take history for new or increasing symptoms

Carry out frequent physical assessments with particular attention to blood pressure, signs of edema, or neurologic dysfunction

Assess psychologic responses to the disease and its therapies

Unit 4

NURSING DIAGNOSIS: Altered nutrition: less than body requirements related to loss of appetite, restricted diet

GOAL

Prevent dietary deficiencies

INTERVENTIONS

Provide foods rich in folic acid and iron
Encourage allowable foods that provide basic nutritional needs
*Administer supplementary iron and vitamins as prescribed
See also Nursing care plan: The child with special nutritional needs, p. 277

EXPECTED OUTCOME

Child shows no evidence of deficiencies

NURSING DIAGNOSIS: Altered growth and development related to restricted diet, chronic illness, chronic anemia

GOAL

Promote physical growth

INTERVENTIONS

Assist child in planning acceptable alternatives for restricted foods

EXPECTED OUTCOME

Child attains maximum growth and development potential

NURSING DIAGNOSIS: Potential for injury related to complications of chronic renal failure

GOAL

Prevent retention of waste products

INTERVENTIONS

Provide diet that reduces excretory demands on kidney
   Limit protein to essential amino acids and no more than required for growth
   Allow no added salt
   Discourage foods high in potassium

EXPECTED OUTCOME

Child consumes an adequate amount of appropriate foods (specify type and amount)

GOAL

Prevent osteodystrophy

---

*Dependent nursing action.

INTERVENTIONS

Restrict protein and phosphorus-containing foods in the diet, especially milk and carbonated beverages
*Administer calcium carbonate (Titralac, Tums)
*Administer alkalizing agents
*Administer supplementary vitamin D

EXPECTED OUTCOME

Child exhibits no evidence of osteodystrophy

GOAL

Prevent or help reduce hypertension

INTERVENTIONS

Monitor fluid intake
Provide low-sodium diet
*Administer diuretics as prescribed
*Administer antihypertensive agents as ordered

EXPECTED OUTCOME

Child's blood pressure remains within acceptable limits (specify)

GOAL

Prevent or help treat anemia

INTERVENTIONS

*Administer supplementary iron
*Administer packed red blood cells periodically as prescribed

EXPECTED OUTCOMES

Child exhibits no evidence of anemia

NURSING DIAGNOSIS: Potential for infection related to diminished body defenses

GOAL

Prevent infection

INTERVENTIONS AND EXPECTED OUTCOMES

See Nursing diagnosis: Potential for infection, p. 288

NURSING DIAGNOSIS: Altered family processes related to having a child with a chronic and potentially life-threatening disease

GOAL

Assist child and family in coping with stresses of the disease

---

*Dependent nursing action.

INTERVENTIONS

Assist parents in diet planning and support their efforts to adjust diet to meet needs of all the members of the family

Provide anticipatory guidance regarding probable and expected events such as symptoms, diet, and effects of medications

Assist parents in decision regarding dialysis and transplantation

Prepare child and family for hemodialysis and/or kidney transplantation

Prepare child and family for home hemodialysis or continuous home peritoneal dialysis

Maintain periodic contact with family

*Refer family to special agencies and support groups

---

*National Kidney Foundation, 2 Park Ave., New York, NY 10016, (212) 889-2210. In Canada: Kidney Foundation of Canada, 4060 Ste. Catherine St. W, Suite 555, Montreal, Quebec H3Z 2Z3. National Association of Patients on Hemodialysis and Transplantation, Inc., 211 E. 43rd St., New York, NY 10017, (212) 867-4486.

EXPECTED OUTCOME

Child and family demonstrate the ability to cope with stresses of illness (specify)

See also:

Nursing care plan: The child with a chronic illness or disability, p. 259

Nursing care plan: The child in the hospital, p. 246

Nursing care plan: The family of the ill or hospitalized child, p. 254

Unit 4

NURSING CARE OF THE CHILD WITH CEREBRAL DYSFUNCTION

Concerns disorders affecting cerebral structure and function

ASSESSMENT

Initial assessment

Take careful history

Family history for evidence of hereditary disease affecting the central nervous system

Health history, especially for clues regarding the cause of dysfunction

Injury or short febrile illness

Encounter with an animal or insect

Ingestion of neurotoxic substances (e.g., plants, drugs)

Inhalation of chemicals

Past illness or known diabetes mellitus

Sudden or progressive alterations in movement (e.g., ataxia, seizures) or mental ability

Headache, nausea, vomiting, double vision, bowel or bladder incontinence in a previously continent child

Unusual behavior, including the nature and frequency

Perform physical assessment with special emphasis on

Neurologic assessment, p. 52

Assessment of cranial nerves, p. 56

Developmental assessment, p. 113

Observe for speed of movement, presence and location of any tremors, twitching, tics, or other unusual movements

Observe gait for evidence of ataxia, spasticity, rigidity, "scissoring"

Note any unusual discharge from body orifices

Note location, extent, and type of any wound

Assess level of consciousness:

Confusion

Failure to comprehend one's surroundings—disorientation relative to time, inability to follow even simple directions, misidentification of persons, short attention span, loss of proper bearings, inability to estimate directions or location, ability to give relevant answers to simple questions (concerning age, location of pain) but inability to give relevant and accurate answers to more complex questions; alert with intact arousal responses

Delirium

Characterized by confusion, agitation, and hyperactivity; marked by illusions, hallucinations, and delusions

Pseudowakeful states

Wakefulness but inability to follow objects or lights, turn eyes toward noise, or speak

Comatose states

Characterized by diminished alertness that extends from somnolence or semistupor to deep coma, a state of unconsciousness from which the patient cannot be aroused, even with powerful stimuli

Infants

Size and shape of the head

Spontaneous activity and postural reflex activity

Sensory responses

Attitude—normal flexed posture, extreme extension, opisthotonos, hypotonia

Symmetry in movement of extremities

Excessive tremulousness or frequent twitching movements

Altered expiratory cycle:

Prolonged apnea

Ataxic breathing

Paradoxic chest movement

Hyperventilation

Skin and hair texture

Distinctive facial features

Presence of a high-pitched, piercing cry

Abnormal eye movements

Inability to suck or swallow

Lip smacking

Asymmetric contraction of facial muscles

Yawning (may indicate cranial nerve involvement)

Muscular activity and coordination

Observe for evidence of increased intracranial pressure:

Tense, bulging fontanel; lack of normal pulsations

Separated cranial sutures

Macewen (cracked-pot) sign

Irritability

High-pitched cry

Increased occipital-frontal circumference (OFC)

Distended scalp veins

Changes in feeding

Cries when held or rocked

"Setting sun" sign

Children

Headache

Nausea

Vomiting—often without nausea

Diplopia, blurred vision

Seizures

Personality and Behavior Signs

Irritability (toddlers), restlessness

Indifference, drowsiness, or lack of interest

Decline in school performance

Diminished physical activity and motor performance

Increased complaints of fatigue, tiredness; increased time devoted to sleep

Significant weight loss possible from anorexia and vomiting

Memory loss if pressure is markedly increased

Inability to follow simple commands

Progression to lethargy and drowsiness

Late Signs

Lowered level of consciousness

Decreased motor response to command

Decreased sensory response to painful stimuli

Alterations in pupil size and reactivity

Sometimes decerebrate or decorticate posturing

Cheyne-Stokes respirations

Papilledema

ASSESSMENT—cont'd

Assist with diagnostic procedures and tests—Lumbar puncture, subdural tap, ventricular puncture, electroencephalography, computed tomography, nuclear brain scan, transillumination, echoencephalography, radiography, magnetic resonance imaging, positron emission transaxial tomography, real time ultrasonography, digital subtraction angiography; blood biochemistry, pH, blood gases, ammonia, glucose, and any special tests

Ongoing assessment (extent of assessment depends on condition)

Monitor vital signs
  Temperature
  Pulse—Rapid, slow, bounding, feeble
  Respirations—Regular or irregular, deep or shallow, pattern of breathing
  Blood pressure—Observe for narrowed pulse pressure, decreased (shock)
Eye movements
  Position of globes—divergence; conjugate deviation; skewed
  Movement of globes—extraocular palsy; nystagmus; fixed gaze
  Pupil size—dilated; pinpoint, unequal
  Pupil reaction—sluggish, absent; different
Motor function
  Voluntary movements of extremities (e.g., purposeful, random)

Changes in muscular tone
Changes in position of body and/or head
Tremor, twitching
Seizure activity (e.g., generalized or local) (see also p. 403)
Signs of meningeal irritation (e.g., nuchal rigidity, opisthotonos)
  Spontaneous—Normal but reduced; involuntary; evoked
  Evoked—Purposeful; reflex withdrawal
  Paresis—Decorticate, decerebrate; any lateralized difference in function
  Crying and speech—Present or absent; conversant or confused; monosyllabic; jargon; type of cry—piercing, difficult to hear
Breath odor—Fruity, foul, fetid, alcohol
Level of consciousness—Easily roused, difficulty in rousing, unable to rouse; roused only with painful stimuli (Table 4-9)
Monitor intracranial pressure device
Monitor central venous pressure device
Monitor fluid intake and output
Weigh daily or as ordered to detect fluid accumulation or reduction
Headache (if information can be elicited)—Presence or absence, type and location, continuous or intermittent
In infants—Measure occipital-frontal circumference
Assess status of fontanel—Size and tension of fontanels

Table 4-12. PEDIATRIC COMA SCALE*

	Score	Over 1 year	Less than 1 year	
Eyes opening	4	Spontaneously	Spontaneously	
	3	To verbal command	To shout	
	2	To pain	To pain	
	1	No response	No response	
		Over 1 year	**Less than 1 year**	
Best motor response	6	Obeys		
	5	Localizes pain	Localizes pain	
	4	Flexion withdrawal	Flexion withdrawal	
	3	Flexion—abnormal (decorticate rigidity)	Flexion—abnormal (decorticate rigidity)	
	2	Extension (decerebrate rigidity)	Extension (decerebrate rigidity)	
	1	No response	No response	
		Over 5 years	**2-5 years**	**0-23 months**
Best verbal	5	Oriented and converses	Appropriate words and phrases	Smiles, coos, cries appropriately
	4	Disoriented and converses	Inappropriate words	Cries
	3	Inappropriate words	Cries and/or screams	Inappropriate crying and/or screaming
	2	Incomprehensible sounds	Grunts	Grunts
	1	No response	No response	No response
Total	3-15			

*Modification of Glasgow Coma Scale.

NURSING CARE PLAN
THE UNCONSCIOUS CHILD

Depressed cerebral function: inability to respond to sensory
    stimuli and have subjective experiences with modification in
    cognition and thus a change in reaction

ASSESSMENT

See neurologic assessment of previous section
Assess state of consciousness (see Table 4-12)

Assist with diagnostic procedures and tests
Perform regular, frequent ongoing neurologic assessments

NURSING DIAGNOSIS: Potential for suffocation (aspiration); ineffective airway clearance related to depressed sensorium, impaired motor function

GOAL

Maintain patent airway

INTERVENTIONS

Position for optimum ventilation
Remove accumulated secretions promptly
Administer care of endotracheal tube or tracheostomy if appropriate; have equipment available for emergency insertion if indicated for respiratory distress
Monitor artificial ventilation

EXPECTED OUTCOME

Airway remains patent

NURSING DIAGNOSIS: Potential for injury related to physical immobility, depressed sensorium, intracranial pathology

GOAL

Minimize intracranial pressure (ICP)

INTERVENTIONS

Elevate head of the bed 15 to 30 degrees
Avoid positions or activities that increase ICP
    Pressure on neck veins
    Flexion or extension of neck
    Head rotation
    Valsalva maneuver
    Painful stimuli
    Respiratory procedures (especially suctioning)

Prevent constipation
Provide
    Quiet, subdued environment
    Pleasant auditory experiences
    Therapeutic touch
    Avoid emotionally stressful conversation (e.g., about pain, condition, prognosis)
*Administer paralyzing agents if prescribed

EXPECTED OUTCOMES

Intracranial pressure remains within safe limits
Child shows no evidence of increased intracranial pressure

GOAL

Prevent cerebral hypoxia

INTERVENTIONS

Position for maximum ventilation
Maintain patent airway
    Position to prevent aspiration: semiprone position; side-lying position
    Aspirate airway as needed
    Insert oral airway if indicated
    Avoid neck hyperextension
Provide oxygen as indicated by objective signs or as ordered
Hyperventilate at prescribed intervals, if ordered
If on mechanical ventilation:
    Monitor for correct settings, proper functioning
    Prepare to provide artificial ventilation in case of ventilatory failure; have manual resuscitation (AMBU) bag at hand
*Administer medications as ordered to prevent cerebral edema and improve cerebral circulation

EXPECTED OUTCOME

Child breathes easily; respirations are within normal limits (see inside front cover)

---

*Dependent nursing action.

GOAL

Prevent cerebral edema

INTERVENTIONS

Elevate head of bed to 15 to 30 degrees
Maintain intravenous fluids as prescribed
*Administer hyperosmolar fluids as prescribed
*Administer corticosteroids as ordered

EXPECTED OUTCOME

Child exhibits no signs of increased intracranial pressure

GOAL

Prevent seizures

INTERVENTIONS

Avoid stimulation that precipitates undesirable responses
*Administer sedatives or anticonvulsants as prescribed
Schedule nursing activities for minimal disturbance

EXPECTED OUTCOME

Child exhibits no seizure activity or undue restlessness and
    agitation

GOAL

Prevent or control hyperthermia

INTERVENTIONS

Remove excess coverings
*Administer antipyretics, if prescribed
Apply and monitor hypothermia blanket if indicated or ordered;
    administer antishivering agents if ordered

EXPECTED OUTCOME

Body temperature remains within safe limits (see inside front
    cover)

GOAL

Prevent respiratory infection

INTERVENTIONS

Turn frequently—at least every 2 hours
Avoid contact with persons with upper respiratory infection
Provide good oral hygiene
Perform chest physiotherapy as prescribed and as tolerated

EXPECTED OUTCOME

Child exhibits no evidence of pulmonary dysfunction

GOAL

Prevent corneal irritation

---

*Dependent nursing action.

INTERVENTIONS

Patch eyes if indicated
Keep lids completely closed
Instill "artificial tears"

EXPECTED OUTCOME

Corneas remain clear and moist

GOAL

Prevent drying and caking of mucous membranes

INTERVENTION

Provide meticulous mouth care

EXPECTED OUTCOME

Mucous membranes remain clean, moist, and free of irritation

GOAL

Protect from physical injury

INTERVENTIONS

Keep siderails up
Pad hard surfaces that may injure extremities during sponta-
    neous or involuntary movement

EXPECTED OUTCOME

Child remains free of physical injury

GOAL

Maintain limb flexibility and functions

INTERVENTIONS

Perform passive range-of-motion exercises
Position to reduce contractures—splint contracting joints if
    needed

EXPECTED OUTCOME

Joints remain flexible and retain full range of motion

NURSING DIAGNOSIS: Potential impaired skin integrity related to immobility, body secretions

GOAL

Maintain skin integrity

INTERVENTIONS

Place child on sheepskin, Egg-crate pad, or other resilient sur-
    face
Change position frequently unless contraindicated by increased
    ICP
Protect pressure points (e.g., trochanter, sacrum, ankle, shoul-
    der, occiput)
Inspect skin surfaces regularly for signs of irritation, redness,
    evidence of pressure

Cleanse skin regularly, at least once daily

Protect skinfolds and surfaces that rub together

Keep clothing and linen clean and dry

Carry out good perineal care under urine collection device

Stimulate circulation by gentle rubbing with lotion or other lubricating substance

Protect lips with cream or ointment

GOAL

Skin remains clean, intact, and free of irritation

> **NURSING DIAGNOSIS:** Feeding, bathing/hygiene, toileting self-care deficits (level 4) related to physical immobility, perceptual and cognitive impairment

GOAL

Ensure adequate nutritional intake

INTERVENTIONS

Provide nourishment in manner suitable to child's condition

Monitor intravenous feedings when ordered

*Feed prescribed formula by means of nasogastric or gastrostomy tube

EXPECTED OUTCOME

Child obtains sufficient nourishment

GOAL

Provide hygienic care

INTERVENTIONS

Bathe daily or more often, if indicated

Dress appropriately

Keep hair combed and styled

EXPECTED OUTCOME

Child appears clean and as well groomed as possible within limitations of condition

GOAL

Provide toileting and ensure adequate elimination

INTERVENTIONS

Provide sufficient liquid intake, unless contraindicated by cerebral edema or if overhydration is a threat

Apply urine collecting device or insert indwelling catheter (if ordered)

Provide proper care of catheter

Use collection appliances, if feasible

Clean skin well after each elimination

Diaper as needed

*Administer stool softener

*Administer suppositories or enema as indicated

---
*Dependent nursing action.

EXPECTED OUTCOMES

Child eliminates sufficient urine (specify)

Bowel is evacuated daily

Child's diaper area remains clean and free of irritation

> **NURSING DIAGNOSIS:** Sensory/perceptual alterations (visual, auditory, kinesthetic, gustatory, tactile, olfactory) related to central nervous system impairment, bed rest

GOAL

Provide sensory stimulation

INTERVENTIONS

Provide tactile stimulation (if it does not evoke undesirable muscle response, e.g., seizures)

Provide auditory stimulation by voice, radio, music box, etc.

Provide visual stimuli appropriate for age

Provide proprioceptive stimulation by rocking, cuddling, etc.

EXPECTED OUTCOMES

Child receives sensory stimulation appropriate to age and condition

Child appears relaxed and rests quietly

> **NURSING DIAGNOSIS:** Altered family processes related to a child hospitalized with a potentially fatal condition or permanent disability

GOAL

Support family

INTERVENTIONS AND EXPECTED OUTCOMES

See Nursing care plan: The family of the ill or hospitalized child, p. 254

GOAL

Assist in child placement, if indicated

INTERVENTIONS

Provide needed information

Answer family's questions; encourage expression of feelings

Refer to persons or agencies for further information and clarification

Support parent's decisions

EXPECTED OUTCOME

Family verbalizes feelings and concerns

NURSING CARE PLAN
THE CHILD WITH A HEAD INJURY

Injury to the cranium and/or its contents

Concussion—Immediate loss of consciousness following head injury

Contusion—Bruising of cerebral tissue—Petechial hemorrhages along superficial aspects of the brain at the site of impact (coup injury) and/or lesion remote from the site of direct trauma (contrecoup injury)

Fractures—Linear, depressed, basilar

ASSESSMENT

See Assessment: The child with cerebral dysfunction, p. 392

Examine head for evidence of injury—Bruises, lacerations, swelling, depression, drainage or bleeding from any orifice

Perform physical assessment of body for evidence of associated injuries

Obtain history of event and subsequent management

Observe for manifestations of head injury:

Minor Injury

May or may not lose consciousness

Transient period of confusion

Somnolence

Listlessness

Irritability

Pallor

Vomiting (1 or more episodes)

Signs of Progression

Altered mental status (e.g., difficulty rousing child)

Mounting agitation

Development of focal lateral neurologic signs

Marked changes in vital signs

Severe Injury

Signs of increased ICP

    Increased head size (infant)

    Bulging fontanel (infant)

Retinal hemorrhage

Extraocular palsies (especially cranial nerve VI)

Hemiparesis

Quadriplegia

Elevated temperature (sometimes)

Unsteady gait (older child)

Papilledema (older child)

Associated Signs

Skin injury (to area of head sustaining injury)

Other injuries (e.g., to extremities)

Observe for additional neurologic data

    Bruises and wounds—Location, extent, type

    Unusual behavior—Note nature and frequency, circumstances related to

    Incontinence (in toilet-trained child)—Bowel, bladder; spontaneous or associated with other phenomena (e.g., seizure activity)

Assist with diagnostic procedures and tests—See assessment for neurologic dysfunction, p. 392

Ongoing assessment

Perform frequent neurologic assessment

Observe level of consciousness

Observe position and movement

Observe for headache

    Young child—Fussy and restless when handled; rolls head from side to side

    Older child—Self-report

Observe for vertigo

    Child assumes a position and vigorously resists efforts to be moved

    Forcible movement causes child to vomit and display spontaneous nystagmus

Observe for seizures (relatively common in head injury)—See p. 403

Observe for drainage from any orifice—Amount and characteristics

Observe for signs of increased intracranial pressure (p. 392)

Unit 4

NURSING DIAGNOSIS: Potential for injury related to head injury

GOAL

Prevent further injury

INTERVENTIONS

Place child on bed rest, head of bed elevated slightly

Implement appropriate safety measures (e.g., siderails up)

    Pad hard surfaces for extremely restless child

    Restrain if needed

Avoid suctioning through nares

Manage associated injuries appropriately (see specific injury)

Offer clear liquids; advance to diet for age as soon as condition permits

EXPECTED OUTCOME

Child exhibits no evidence of complications

NURSING DIAGNOSIS: Altered family processes related to a child with a head injury

GOAL

Prepare family for home care

INTERVENTIONS

Teach family skills needed for home observations (if child is not to be hospitalized); report:
Unusual drowsiness
Deviations in gait, eye movements, coordination
Symptoms such as headache, double vision, nausea
Difficulty rousing from sleep (awaken every 1 to 3 hours during sleep)
Teach skills such as dressing changes

EXPECTED OUTCOME

Family demonstrates the ability to provide needed care (specify skills and method of demonstration)

GOAL

Prepare family for possible posttraumatic symptoms and behaviors

INTERVENTIONS

Inform family of some manifestations of posttraumatic syndrome (see box)

EXPECTED OUTCOME

Family demonstrates an understanding of behaviors the child may exhibit

GOAL

Support family

INTERVENTIONS AND EXPECTED OUTCOMES

See Nursing care plan: The family of the hospitalized child, p. 254

GOAL

Prepare family for long-term care (severe injury)

INTERVENTIONS

*Refer to support groups and agencies specializing rehabilitation and long-term care
Maintain contact with family

EXPECTED OUTCOME

Family contact appropriate agencies

See also Nursing care plan: The unconscious child, p. 394
Observation of seizures, p. 403
Nursing care plan: The child in the hospital, p. 246

---

*__National Head Injury Foundation,__ 333 Turnpike Rd., Southborough, MA 01772, (617) 485-9950. In Canada: __Association for the Rehabilitation for the Brain-Injured,__ 97 Warwick Dr., S.W., Calgary, Alberta T3C 2R5.

SIGNS OF POSTTRAUMATIC SYNDROME

Infants
Pallor
Sweating
Irritability
Sleepiness
May vomit

Children
Behavioral disturbances
    Aggressiveness
    Disobedience
    Withdrawal
    Regression
    Anxiety
Sleep disturbances
Phobias
Emotional lability

Irritability
Altered school performance
Seizures

Adolescents
Headache
Dizziness
Impaired concentration

Structural complications
Hydrocephalus
Focal deficits
    Optic atrophy
    Cranial nerve palsies
    Motor deficits
    Diabetes insipidus
    Aphasia

NURSING CARE PLAN
THE CHILD WITH HYDROCEPHALUS

Excessive accumulation of cerebral spinal fluid (CSF) producing passive dilation of the ventricles

Result of fluid accumulation:

Communicating hydrocephalus—Impaired absorption of CSF within the subarachnoid space

Noncommunicating hydrocephalus—Obstruction to the flow of CSF within the ventricles

ASSESSMENT

Obtain health history, especially regarding a head injury or cerebral infection

Perform physical assessment, especially for evidence of repaired myelomeningocele, occipitofrontal circumference measurement

Observe for manifestations of hydrocephalus:

Infancy, early:

Abnormally rapid head growth

Bulging fontanels (especially anterior) sometimes without head enlargement:

Tense

Nonpulsatile

Dilated scalp veins

Separated sutures

Macewen sign ("cracked-pot" sound) on percussion

Thinning of skull bones

Infancy, later:

Frontal enlargement or "bossing"

Depressed eyes

"Setting sun" sign (sclera visible above the iris)

Pupils sluggish, with unequal response to light

Infancy: general:

Irritability

Lethargy

Infant cries when picked up or rocked and quiets when allowed to lie still

Early infantile reflex acts may persist

Normally expected responses fail to appear

May display:

Change in level of consciousness

Opisthotonos (often extreme)

Lower extremity spasticity

Advanced cases:

Difficulty in sucking and feeding

Shrill, brief, high-pitched cry

Cardiopulmonary embarrassment

Childhood:

Headache on awakening; improvement following emesis or upright posture

Papilledema

Strabismus

Extrapyramidal tract signs (e.g., ataxia)

Irritability

Lethargy

Apathy

Confusion

Often incoherence

Assist with diagnostic procedures—Tomography, echoencephalography, transillumination, ventricular puncture

---

NURSING DIAGNOSIS: Potential for injury related to increased intracranial pressure

GOAL

Prevent increased intracranial pressure

INTERVENTIONS

Carry out postoperative care of shunt as prescribed

Position as prescribed

EXPECTED OUTCOME

Child exhibits no evidence of increased intracranial pressure

NURSING DIAGNOSIS: Potential for infection related to presence of mechanical drainage system

GOAL

Prevent infection

Unit 4

INTERVENTIONS

Provide wound care as prescribed

EXPECTED OUTCOME

Child exhibits no evidence of infection (see p. 288)

NURSING DIAGNOSIS: Potential impaired skin integrity related to pressure areas (especially child with myelomeningocele, see p. 434)

GOAL

Prevent skin breakdown

INTERVENTIONS AND EXPECTED OUTCOME

See The child with integumentary dysfunction, p. 488

NURSING DIAGNOSIS: Altered family processes related to a child with a chronic defect

GOAL

Support family

INTERVENTIONS AND EXPECTED OUTCOMES

See Nursing care plan: The family of the ill or hospitalized child, p. 254

See also:
Nursing care plan: The high-risk infant, p. 302
Nursing care plan: The child with a chronic illness or disability, p. 259

NURSING CARE PLAN
THE CHILD WITH ACUTE BACTERIAL MENINGITIS

Infection of the meninges

ASSESSMENT

Obtain health history, especially regarding a previous infection or injury

Perform physical assessment

Observe for manifestations of bacterial meningitis:

Children and Adolescents
Usually abrupt onset
Fever
Chills
Headache
Vomiting
Alterations in sensorium
Seizures (often the initial sign)
Irritability
Agitation
May develop:
   Delirium
   Aggressive or maniacal behavior
   Drowsiness
   Stupor
   Coma
Nuchal rigidity
   May progress to opisthotonos
Positive Kernig and Brudzinski signs (see p. 54)
Hyperactive but variable reflex responses
Signs and symptoms peculiar to individual organisms:
   Petechial or purpuric rashes (meningococcal infection), especially when associated with a shocklike state
   Joint involvement (meningococcal and *H. influenzae* infection)
   Chronically draining ear (pneumococcal meningitis)

Infants and Young Children
Classic picture rarely seen in children between 3 months and 2 years of age
Fever
Vomiting

Marked irritability
Frequent seizures (often accompanied by a high-pitched cry)
Bulging fontanel
Nuchal rigidity may or may not be present
Brudzinski and Kernig signs are not helpful in diagnosis
   Difficult to elicit and evaluate in the age-group

Neonatal
Extremely difficult to diagnose
Manifestations vague and nonspecific
Well at birth but within a few days begins to look and behave poorly
Refuses feedings
Poor sucking ability
Vomiting or diarrhea
Poor tone
Lack of movement
Poor cry
Full, tense, and bulging fontanel may appear late in course of illness
Neck usually supple

Nonspecific Signs May Be Present
Hypothermia or fever (depending on the maturity of the infant)
Jaundice
Irritability
Drowsiness
Seizures
Respiratory irregularities or apnea
Cyanosis
Weight loss

Assist with diagnostic procedures and tests—Lumbar puncture, spinal fluid examination for glucose, protein, white blood cells

Unit 4

NURSING DIAGNOSIS: Potential for injury related to presence of infection

GOAL

Help eradicate causative organism

INTERVENTION

*Administer antibiotics as prescribed and as soon as possible after admission
Maintain intravenous route for administration of medication

EXPECTED OUTCOME

Child exhibits evidence of diminishing symptoms

NURSING DIAGNOSIS: Potential for infection related to presence of infective organisms

GOAL

Prevent spread of infection

---

*Dependent nursing action

INTERVENTIONS

Place child in isolation for at least 24 hours after initiation of antibiotic therapy
Identify close contacts and high-risk children who might benefit from meningococci vaccinations
See also Nursing care plan: The child at risk for infection, p. 288

EXPECTED OUTCOME

Others do not contract the infection

NURSING DIAGNOSIS: Altered family processes related to a child with a serious illness

GOAL

Support family

INTERVENTIONS AND EXPECTED OUTCOME

See Nursing care plan: The family of the ill or hospitalized child, p. 254
See also Nursing care plan: The unconscious child, p. 394

NURSING CARE PLAN
THE CHILD WITH EPILEPSY

Single or recurrent attacks of loss of consciousness, convulsive movements, or disturbed feelings or behavior associated with excessive neuronal discharges

Convulsion—Involuntary muscular contraction and relaxation

Seizure—A sudden attack; term used to designate a single episode

ASSESSMENT

Obtain health history, especially regarding prenatal, perinatal, and neonatal events; any instances of infection, apnea, colic, or poor feeding; any information regarding previous accidents or serious illnesses

Obtain history of seizure activity including:

Description of child's behavior during attack(s)

Age of onset

Time when seizure occures—Time of day, while awake or during sleep, relationship to meals

Any factors that might have precipitated seizure (e.g., fever, infection), falls that may have caused trauma to the head, anxiety, fatigue, activity (e.g., hyperventilation), environmental events (e.g., exposure to strong stimuli such as bright, flashing lights or loud noises)

Duration, progression, and any postictal feelings or behavior

Perform physical and neurologic assessment

Observe seizure manifestations (see box)

Assist with diagnostic procedures and tests—Electroencephalography, tomography, skull radiography, echoencephalography, brain scan; blood chemistry, serum glucose, blood urea nitrogen, ammonia; specific tests for metabolic disorders

Observe and record child's behavior during a generalized convulsive seizure:

Observe seizure
Describe
Only what is actually observed

Order of events

Duration of seizure

Onset
Significant preseizure events—Bright lights, noise, excitement, emotional outbursts

Behavior

Change in facial expression, such as of fear

Cry or other sound

Stereotyped or automatous movements

Random activity

Position of head, body, extremities

Unilateral or bilateral posturing of one or more extremities

Body deviation to side

Time of onset

Movement
Change of position, if any

Site of commencement—Hand, thumb, mouth, generalized

Tonic phase, if present—Length, parts of body involved

Clonic phase—Twitching or jerking movements, parts of body involved, sequence of parts involved, generalized, change in character of movements

Lack of movement of any extremity

Face
Color change—Pallor, cyanosis, flushing

Perspiration

Mouth—Position, deviating to one side, teeth clenched, tongue bitten, frothing at mouth, flecks of blood or bleeding

Eyes
Position—Straight ahead, deviation upward, deviation outward, conjugate or divergent

Pupils (if able to assess)—Changes in size, equality, reaction to light and accommodation

Respiratory effort
Presence and length of apnea

Presence of stertor

Other
Involuntary urination

Involuntary defecation

Observe postictally
Method of termination

State of consciousness—Unresponsiveness, drowsiness, confusion

Orientation to time, place, persons, and so on

Sleeping but able to be aroused

Motor ability

Any change in motor power

Ability to move all extremities

Any paresis or weakness

Ability to whistle (if appropriate to age)

Speech—Changes, peculiarities, type and extent of any difficulties

Sensations

Complaint of discomfort and pain

Any sensory impairment of hearing, vision

Recollection of preseizure sensations, warning of attack

Awareness that attack was beginning

Promote rest

Make child comfortable

Allow child to rest after seizure

Reduce sensory stimuli

Record length of postictal sleep

Notify physician if seizure is followed by other seizures in rapid succession or if duration of seizure is excessive

Reduce anxiety

Provide calm, relaxed atmosphere

Unit 4

SEIZURE MANIFESTATIONS

I. Partial Seizures

Simple Partial Seizures

Characterized by:

 Localized motor symptoms

 Somatosensory, psychic, autonomic symptoms

 Combination of these

 Abnormal discharges remain unilateral

Manifestations:

 Aversive seizure (most common motor seizure in children)

  Eye or eyes and head turn away from the side of the focus

  Awareness of movement or loss of consciousness

 Sylvan seizure

  Tonic-clonic movements involving the face

  Salivation

  Arrested speech

  Most common during sleep

 Jacksonian march (rare in children)

  Orderly, sequential progression of clonic movements beginning in a foot, hand, or face and moving or "marching" to adjacent body parts

Special Sensory Seizures

Characterized by various sensations, including:

 Numbness, tingling, prickling, paresthesia, or pain originating to one area (e.g., face or extremities) and spreading to other parts of the body

 Visual sensations or formed images

 Motor phenomena such as posturing or hypertonia

 Uncommon in hildren under 8 years of age

Complex Partial Seizures (psychomotor seizures)

Observed more often in children from 3 years through adolescence

Characterized by:

 Period of altered behavior

 Amnesia for event (no recollection of behavior)

 Inability to respond to environment

 No loss of consciousness during attack

 Drowsiness or sleep usually follows seizure

 Confusion and amnesia may be prolonged

 Complex sensory phenomena

  Most frequent sensation—Strange feeling in the pit of the stomach that rises toward the throat

  Often accompanied by:

   Odd or unpleasant odors or tastes

   Complex auditory or visual hallucinations

   Ill-defined feelings of elation or strangeness (e.g., deja vu, a feeling of familirity in a strange environment)

  Small children may emit a cry or attempt to run for help

  May be strong feelings of fear and anxiety, distorted sense of time and self

 Patterns of motor behavior:

  Stereotypic

  Similar with each subsequent seizure

  May suddenly cease activity, appear dazed, stare into space, become confused and apathetic, and become limp or stiff or display some form of posturing

May be confused

May perform purposeless, complicated activities in a repetitive manner (automatisms), such as walking, running, kicking, laughing, or speaking incoherently, most often followed by postictal confusion or sleep

Rarely manifests auras such as rage or temper tantrums

Aggressive acts uncommon during seizure

II. Generalized Seizures

Tonic-Clonic Seizures (traditionally known as grand mal)

Most common and most dramatic of all seizure manifestations

Occur without warning

Tonic phase: lasts approximately 10 to 20 seconds

Manifestations:

 Eyes roll upward

 Immediate loss of consciousness

 If standing, falls to floor or ground

 Stiffens in generalized, symmetric tonic contraction of entire body musculature

 Arms usually flexed

 Legs, head, and neck extended

 May utter a peculiar piercing cry

 Apneic, may become cyanotic

 Increased salivation

Clonic phase: lasts about 30 seconds but can vary from only a few seconds to a half hour or longer

Manifestations:

 Violent jerking movements as the trunk and extremities undergo rhythmic contraction and relaxation

 May foam at the mouth

 May be incontinent of urine and feces

As attack ends, movements become less intense, occur at longer intervals, then cease entirely

Status epilepticus; series of seizures at intervals too brief to allow the child to regain consciousness between the time one attack ends and the next begins

 Requires emergency intervention

 Can lead to exhaustion, respiratory failure, and death

Postictal state:

 Appears to relax

 May remain semiconscious and difficult to rouse

 May awaken in a few minutes

 Remains confused for several hours

 Poor coordination

 Mild impairment of fine motor movements

 May have visual and speech difficulties

 May vomit or complain of severe headache

 When left alone, usually sleeps for several hours

 On awakening is fully conscious

 Usually feels tired and complains of sore muscle and headache

 No recollection of entire event

SEIZURE MANIFESTATION—cont'd

Absence Seizures (traditionally called *petit mal* or *lapses*)

Characterized by:
  Brief loss of consciousness
  Minimal or no alteration in muscle tone
  May go unrecognized because little change in child's behavior
  Abrupt onset; suddenly develops 20 or more attacks daily
  Attack often mistaken for inattentiveness or daydreaming
  Attacks can be precipitated by hyperventilation, hypoglycemia, stresses (emotional and physiologic), fatigue, or sleeplessness

Manifestations:
  Brief loss of consciousness
  Appear without warning or aura
  Usually last about 5 to 10 seconds
  Slight loss of muscle tone may cause child to drop objects
  Able to maintain postural control; seldom falls
  Minor movements such as lip smacking, twitching of eyelids or face, or slight hand movements
  Not accompanied by incontinence
  Amnesia for episode
  May need to reorient self to previous activity

Atonic and Akinetic Seizures (also known as *drop attacks*)

Characterized by:
  Onset usually between 2 and 5 years of age
  Sudden, momentary loss of muscle tone and postural control
  Attacks recur frequently during the day, particularly in the morning hours and shortly after awakening

Manifestations:
  Loss of tone causes child to fall to floor violently
    Unable to break the fall by putting out hand
    May incur a serious injury to the face, head, or shoulder
  Loss of consciousness only momentary

Myoclonic Seizures

A variety of convulsive episodes
May be isolated as benign essential myoclonus
May occur in association with other seizure forms

Characterized by:
  Sudden, brief contractures of a muscle or group of muscles
  Occur singly or repetitively
  No loss of consciousness or postictal state
  May or may not be symmetric

Infantile Spasms

Also called: infantile myoclonus, massive spasms, hypsarrhythmia, salaam attacks, or infantile myoclonic spasms
Most commonly occur between 3 and 12 months of age
Twice as common in males as in females
Child may have numerous seizures during the day without postictal drowsiness or sleep
Outlook for normal intelligence poor

Manifestations:
  Possible series of sudden, brief, symmetric, muscular contractions
    Head flexed, arms extended, and legs drawn up
    Eyes may roll upward or inward
    May be preceded or followed by a cry or giggling
    May or may not be loss of consciousness
    Sometimes flushing, pallor, or cyanosis
  Infants who are able to sit but not stand:
    Sudden dropping forward of the head and neck with trunk flexed forward and knees drawn up—The "salaam" or "jackknife" seizure
  Less often: alternate clinical forms observed
    Extensor spasms rather than flexion of arms, legs, and trunk and head nodding
    Lightning attacks involving a single, momentary, shock-like contraction of the entire body

---

NURSING DIAGNOSIS: Potential for injury related to sudden and unexpected loss of consciousness

GOAL

Prevent physical injury during seizure

INTERVENTIONS

Protect child during a seizure
  Do not attempt to restrain child or use force
  If child is standing or sitting in wheelchair at beginning of attack, ease child down so that he will not fall; when possible, place cushion or blanket under child
  Do not put anything in child's mouth
  Loosen restrictive clothing
  Prevent child from hitting hard or sharp objects that might cause injury during uncontrolled movements
  Remove object(s)
  Pad object(s)
  Move furniture out of way
  Allow seizure to end without interference
Educate parents and child regarding appropriate activities for the child
  Age-appropriate
  Avoid contact sports
  Avoid situations that pose a danger during a seizure (climbing trees, play apparatus)
  Provide companionship during permissible activities such as swimming, bicycling
Educate teachers and other persons who are associated with the child regarding correct behavior during a seizure

EXPECTED OUTCOME

Child exhibits no evidence of physical injury

GOAL

Prevent or control seizure activity

INTERVENTIONS

*Administer anticonvulsants

Teach family the administration of medications (see Home Care Instructions, p. 542)

Stress importance of complying with therapeutic regimen

Avoid situations that are known to precipitate a seizure, for example, blinking lights, emotional stress

EXPECTED OUTCOME

Child remains free of seizure activity

GOAL

Prevent complications from medication

INTERVENTIONS

Be aware of and teach family to recognize unfavorable reactions to medications

Encourage periodic physical and laboratory assessment to determine possible deviations from normal findings

EXPECTED OUTCOME

Child and family demonstrate an understanding of possible unfavorable responses to medications and the appropriate intervention (specify)

---

*Dependent nursing action.

NURSING DIAGNOSIS: Altered family processes related to a child with a chronic illness

GOAL

Support family

INTERVENTIONS

See Nursing diagnosis: Altered family processes, p. 261

*Refer to special support groups and agencies

EXPECTED OUTCOMES

Family becomes involved with special group

See also: Nursing care plan: The child with a chronic illness or disability, p. 259

Nursing care: See Nursing care plan: The unconscious child, p. 394

---

*Epilepsy Foundation of America,** 4351 Garden City Drive, Landover, MD 20785, (301) 459-3700. In Canada: **Epilepsy Canada,** 2099 Alexandre De Seve, Bureau 27, Montreal, Quebec H2L 4R8.

NURSING CARE OF THE CHILD WITH METABOLIC DYSFUNCTION

NURSING CARE PLAN
THE CHILD WITH DIABETES MELLITUS

A disorder involving primarily carbohydrate metabolism and characterized by a deficiency (relative or absolute) of the hormone insulin

Idiopathic DM can be classified into two major groups and one newly described type:

Insulin-dependent (IDDM), or **type I**—Characterized by catabolism and the development of ketosis in the absence of insulin replacement therapy; onset is typically in childhood and adolescence but can be at any age

Non-insulin-dependent (NIDDM), or **type II**—Appears to involve resistance to insulin action and defective glucose-mediated insulin secretion; onset is usually after age 40, and there appears to be considerable heterogeneity; affected persons may or may not require daily insulin injections

Maturity-onset diabetes of youth (MODY)—Transmitted as an autosomal-dominant disorder in which there is formation of structurally abnormal insulin that has decreased biologic activity

ASSESSMENT

Perform physical assessment

Obtain family history, especially regarding other members who have diabetes

Obtain health history, especially relative to weight loss, frequency of drinking and voiding, increased appetite, diminished activity level, behavior changes, and other manifestations of diabetes mellitus as follows:

The three polys (cardinal signs of diabetes)
  Polyphagia
  Polyuria
  Polydipsia
IDDM
  Weight loss
  Child may start bed-wetting
  Irritability and "not himself"
  Shortened attention span
  Lowered frustration tolerance
  Appears overly tired
  Dry skin
  Blurred vision
  Sores that are slow to heal

  Flushed skin
  Headache
NIDDM
  Overweight
  Fatigue
  Frequent infections
Child will exhibit:
  Hyperglycemia
    Elevated blood glucose
    Glucosuria
  Diabetic ketosis
    Ketones as well as glucose in urine
    No noticeable dehydration
  Diabetic ketoacidosis
    Dehydration
    Electrolyte imbalance
    Acidosis
Perform or assist with diagnostic procedures and tests—Fasting blood sugar, serum insulin levels, urine for ketones

Unit 4

NURSING DIAGNOSIS: Potential for injury related to insulin deficiency

GOAL

Replace insulin deficit

INTERVENTIONS

Obtain serum glucose level
*Administer insulin as prescribed
Understand the action of insulin
    Understand the differences in composition, time of onset, and duration of action for the various insulin preparations
Employ correct techniques when preparing and administering insulin
    Subcutaneous injection
    Rotation of sites

EXPECTED OUTCOME

Child demonstrates reduced blood glucose levels

NURSING DIAGNOSIS: Potential for injury related to hypoglycemia

GOAL

Elevate blood glucose level

INTERVENTIONS

Recognize signs of hypoglycemia (Table 4-10, p. 410)
    Be particularly alert at times when blood gluclose levels are lowest
    Test for glucose
Offer readily absorbed carbohydrates, such as orange juice, hard candy, or milk
Follow with complex carbohydrate, such as bread or cracker
*Administer glucagon, if prescribed

EXPECTED OUTCOME

Child ingests an appropriate carbohydrate
Child displays no evidence of hypoglycemia

NURSING DIAGNOSIS: Knowledge deficit (diabetes management) related to care of a child with newly diagnosed diabetes mellitus

GOAL

Educate parents and child regarding diabetic management

INTERVENTIONS

Select methods, vocabulary, and content appropriate to the level of the learner
Allow 3 or 4 days for family and child to begin to adjust to the initial impact of the diagnosis

---

*Dependent nursing action.

Select an environment conducive to learning
Allow ample time for the education process
Restrict length of teaching sessions
    Child—15-20 minutes
    Parents—45-60 minutes
Involve all senses and employ a variety of teaching strategies
Provide pamphlets or other supplementary materials

EXPECTED OUTCOME

Child and/or family display attitudes conducive to learning

GOAL

Teach child and family nature of the disease

INTERVENTIONS

Provide information regarding the pathophysiology of diabetes and the function and actions of insulin and glucagon in relation to caloric intake
Answer questions and clarify misconceptions
Explain function and expected effects of procedures and tests

EXPECTED OUTCOME

Child and/or family demonstrate an understanding of the disease and its therapy (specify indicators)

GOAL

Teach child and family meal planning

INTERVENTIONS

Enlist the services of a dietitian
Emphasize the relationship between normal nutritional needs and the disease
Become familiar with the family's food preferences
Teach or reinforce the learners' understanding of the basic food groups and the diet plan prescribed (e.g., exchange diet)
Help the child and family estimate food weights by volume
Suggest low-carbohydrate snack items
Guide family in assessing the labels of food products for carbohydrate content
Teach or reinforce an understanding of the concept of exchanges
Relate carbohydrate equivalents to familiar foods
Retain cultural patterns and family preferences as much as possible

EXPECTED OUTCOME

Child and/or family demonstrate an understanding of diet planning and food selection (specify indicators)

GOAL

Teach characteristics of and administration of insulin

INTERVENTIONS

Teach child and family the characteristics of the insulins prescribed for the child
Teach the proper mixing of insulins and acceptable substitutions (when the familiar brand is unavailable)
Teach injection procedure
    Impress upon the learners that the procedure will be a routine part of the child's life

Involve caregivers and the child, if old enough
Teach basic techniques using an orange or similar item
See Home Care Instructions, p. 547
Use demonstration and return demonstration techniques on another before injecting the child
Help families and child work out a set rotational pattern
Teach proper care of insulin and equipment
Teach management of continuous infusion pump (if used)

EXPECTED OUTCOMES

Child and/or family demonstrate an understanding of insulin, its various forms, and action (specify indicators)
Child and/or family demonstrate injection technique correctly
Child and/or family develop a rotation plan
Child and/or family demonstrate correct use of pump and care of injection site

GOAL

Teach blood glucose testing

INTERVENTIONS

Teach:
    Blood glucose monitoring and/or use of equipment selected for use
    Interpretation of results
    Care and maintenance of equipment

EXPECTED OUTCOME

Child and/or family demonstrate the correct use of the glucose monitoring equipment

GOAL

Teach urine testing

INTERVENTIONS

Teach:
    All methods of urine testing and interpretation of results
    Proper care of test materials and equipment

EXPECTED OUTCOME

Child and/or family demonstrate urine testing and interpretation

GOAL

Teach importance of hygiene

INTERVENTIONS

Emphasize the importance of personal hygiene
Encourage regular dental care and yearly ophthalmologic examinations
Teach proper care of cuts and scratches
Teach proper foot care

EXPECTED OUTCOME

Child and family demonstrate an understanding of the importance of proper hygiene

GOAL

Teach importance of exercise

INTERVENTIONS

Arrange for occupational therapy program that includes physical activity
Work with child, family, and others (e.g., coaches) to help plan a home exercise program
Reiterate practitioner's instructions regarding adjustment of food and/or insulin to meet the child's activity pattern; reinforce with examples

EXPECTED OUTCOME

Child and family helps child outline and carry out a regular exercise program

GOAL

Teach child and family recognition and management of hyperglycemia and hypoglycemia

INTERVENTIONS

Instruct learners in how to recognize signs of hyperglycemia and hypoglycemia (especially hypoglycemia)
Explain the relationship of insulin needs to illness, activity, and intense emotion (either positive or negative)
Teach how to adjust food, activity and insulin at times of illness and during other situations that alter blood sugar levels
Suggest carrying source of carbohydrate, such as sugar cubes or hard candy, in pocket or handbag
Instruct parents and child in how to treat hypoglycemia with food, simple sugars, or glucagon

EXPECTED OUTCOME

Child and family demonstrate an understanding of the signs and management of a hypoglycemic reaction (specify)

GOAL

Teach importance of identification

INTERVENTIONS

Encourage the acquisition of a means of identification, such as an identification bracelet, that explains the child's condition in case of emergency

EXPECTED OUTCOME

Family acquires and child wears identification bracelet

GOAL

Teach record keeping

INTERVENTIONS

Help child and family to design a form for keeping records of:
    Insulin administered
    Blood and urine tests
    Food intake
    Marked variation in exercise
    Illness

EXPECTED OUTCOME

Family and child keep an accurate record of insulin administration, glucose testing, etc.

GOAL

Facilitate self-management

INTERVENTIONS

Encourage honesty in recording, such as eating a forbidden candy bar

Encourage independence in applying the concepts learned in teaching sessions

Instruct when to seek assistance from medical personnel

EXPECTED OUTCOME

Child takes responsibility for management of disease commensurate with age and capabilities

NURSING DIAGNOSIS: Body image disturbance related to biologic changes, insulin dependency

GOAL

Promote positive body image

INTERVENTIONS AND EXPECTED OUTCOMES

See Nursing diagnosis: Body image disturbance, p. 265

GOAL

Promote positive adjustment to the disease

INTERVENTIONS AND EXPECTED OUTCOMES

See Nursing diagnosis: Body image disturbance, p. 265

NURSING DIAGNOSIS: Altered family processes related to situational crisis (child with a chronic disorder)

See also Nursing care plan: The child with a chronic illness or disability, p. 259

Table 4-13. COMPARISON BETWEEN MANIFESTATIONS OF HYPOGLYCEMIA AND HYPERGLYCEMIA

Variable	Hypoglycemia	Hyperglycemia
Onset	Rapid (minutes)	Gradual (days)
Mood	Labile, irritable, nervous, weepy	Lethargic
Mental status	Difficulty concentrating, speaking, focusing, coordinating	Dilled sensorium Confused
Inward feeling	Shaky feeling, hunger Headache Dizziness	Thirst Weakness Nausea/vomiting Abdominal pain
Skin	Pallor Sweating	Flushed Signs of dehydration
Mucous membranes	Normal	Dry, crusty
Respirations	Shallow	Deep, rapid (Kussmaul)
Pulse	Tachycardia	Less rapid, weak
Breath odor	Normal	Fruity, acetone
Neurologic	Tremors Late: hyperflexia, dilated pupils, convulsion	Diminished reflexes Paresthesia
Ominous signs	Shock, coma	Acidosis, coma
Blood:		
Glucose	Low: below 60 mg/dl	High: 250 mg/dl or more
Ketones	Negative	High/large
Osmolarity	Normal	High
pH	Normal	Low (7.25 or less)
Hematocrit	Normal	High
HCO_3	Normal	Less than 20 mEq/L
Urine:		
Output	Normal	Polyuria (early) to oliguria (late)
Sugar	Negative	High
Acetone	Negative	High

NURSING CARE PLAN
THE CHILD WITH KETOACIDOSIS

Acidosis accompanied by an accumulation of ketones in the body, resulting from faulty carbohydrate metabolism

ASSESSMENT

See Nursing care plan: The child with diabetes mellitus, p. 407
Be alert to signs of acidosis, especially in children with known diabetes mellitus
  Signs of dehydration
  Abdominal pain
  Vomiting
  Fever
  Deep, labored (Kussmaul) respirations
  Acetone breath
  Somnolence or coma
  Cherry-red lips
Observe for evidence of precipitating factors such as infection, stress, or omission of insulin injections
Perform or assist with diagnostic procedures and tests—Blood glucose measurements, serum electrolytes, pH, urinalysis

Ongoing assessment

Monitor intravenous infusion
Attach to cardiac monitor
Insert Foley catheter and monitor urinary output
Assess vital signs frequently
  Pulse quality and rate
  Depth and rate of respirations
  Blood pressure
  Temperature
Monitor blood glucose levels every 1-2 hours as ordered
Monitor urine glucose and acetone every 1-2 hours if ordered
Monitor mental status, level of consciousness
Monitor serum electrolytes, pH, glucose, and blood gases
Monitor urine glucose, acetone, specific gravity, and volume frequently
Assess degree of shock, if present, and implement therapeutic measures
Observe for signs of complications such as cerebral edema, hyperkalemia, or kypokalemia

NURSING DIAGNOSIS: Potential for injury related to unconsciousness secondary to cerebral dysfunction, metabolic imbalance

GOAL

Correct hyperglycemia

INTERVENTIONS

*Administer insulin intravenously and subcutaneously as prescribed

EXPECTED OUTCOME

Child's blood glucose levels are within normal limits

GOAL

Replace fluid and electrolyte losses and correct acidosis

INTERVENTIONS

*Administer fluids as prescribed or in manner dictated by child's condition
*Administer electrolytes as prescribed
*Administer sodium bicarbonate if prescribed

EXPECTED OUTCOMES

Child's electrolytes and pH are within normal limits
Child exhibits evidence of good hydration

GOAL

Manage associated problems

INTERVENTIONS

Carry out therapeutic regimen as prescribed for infection if present
Implement appropriate care for the child who is unconscious (p. 394)

EXPECTED OUTCOME

Child exhibits no evidence of complications

---
*Dependent nursing action

NURSING CARE OF THE CHILD WITH NEOPLASTIC DISEASE

NURSING CARE PLAN
THE CHILD WITH CANCER

A neoplasm characterized by the uncontrolled growth of anaplastic cells that tend to metastasize to distant body parts

ASSESSMENT

Perform physical assessment

Obtain health history with special attention to vague complaints (e.g., fatigue, pain in a limb, night sweating, lack of appetite, headache, and general malaise), any evidence of a lingering disorder, parental concerns

Assist with diagnostic procedures and tests—Blood and urine examination, radiology, lumbar puncture, imaging techniques, biopsy, bone marrow aspiration

Assess family's coping capabilities and support system(s)

See also nursing care plans for specific cancers

NURSING DIAGNOSIS: Potential for injury related to malignant process

GOAL

Help eradicate malignancy

INTERVENTIONS

*Administer chemotherapeutic agents as prescribed

Assist with radiotherapy as ordered

Assist with procedures for administration of chemotherapeutic agents (e.g., lumbar puncture for intrathecal administration)

Prepare child and family for surgical procedure

See also Nursing care plan: The child undergoing chemotherapy or radiotherapy, p. 413

EXPECTED OUTCOMES

Child achieves a remission from disease

NURSING DIAGNOSIS: Pain related to physiologic effects of neoplasia

GOAL

Relieve pain

INTERVENTIONS

Assess need for pain management (see p. 279)

During terminal stage, appreciate that pain control is necessary component of physical and emotional care

Avoid excessive noise or light

Place all commodities within easy reach

Use gentle, minimal physical manipulation

Avoid pressure (bedclothes, sheets) on painful areas

Experiment with using heat or cold on painful areas (use cautiously because of easy skin breakdown)

Whenever possible, make use of procedures that minimize discomfort, such as a venous access device (Broviac catheter, implanted port), or Ommaya reservoir

Change position frequently; if difficult for child, coordinate with pain relief from analgesics

Avoid pressure on bony prominences or painful sites (water bed, bean bag chair, flotation mattress); ensure good body alignment

Evaluate effectiveness of pain relief with degree of alertness vs sedation

Implement appropriate nonpharmacologic pain reduction techniques

*Administer analgesics as prescribed

Avoid aspirin or any of its compounds

*Administer drugs on preventive schedule

Monitor effectiveness of therapy on pain assessment record (p. 281)

See also Nursing care plan: The child in pain, p. 279

EXPECTED OUTCOME

Child rests quietly, exhibits no evidence of discomfort, verbalizes no complaints of discomfort

---

NURSING DIAGNOSIS: Altered nutrition: less than body requirements related to loss of appetite

---

*Dependent nursing action.

*Dependent nursing action

GOAL

Stimulate appetite

INTERVENTIONS

Encourage parents to relax; stress legitimate nature of loss of appetite

Allow child *any* food tolerated; plan to improve quality of food selections when appetite increases

Stress expected increase in appetite from steroids

Take advantage of any hungry period; serve small "snacks"

Fortify foods with nutritious supplements, such as powdered milk or commercial supplements

Allow child to be involved in food preparation and selection

Make food appealing

Remember usual food practices of children in each age-group, such as food jags in toddlers or normal occurrence of physiologic anorexia

Assess family for additional problems (e.g., use of food by child as a control mechanism if appetite does not improve despite improved physical status)

See also Nursing care plan: The child with special nutritional needs, p. 277

EXPECTED OUTCOME

Child consumes adequate amounts of appropriate foods

NURSING DIAGNOSIS: Potential activity intolerance related to anemia, reduced energy and fatigue

GOAL

Promote rest and reduce fatigue

INTERVENTIONS

Allow child to monitor own activity

Encourage rest periods throughout day and at least 8 to 10 hours of sleep at night

EXPECTED OUTCOME

Child engages in activites according to ability

NURSING DIAGNOSIS: Fear related to diagnostic tests, procedures, and treatments

GOAL

Reduce fear related to diagnostic procedures and tests

INTERVENTIONS

Explain procedure carefully at the child's level of understanding

Explain what will take place and what the child will feel, see, and hear

Use recall of each step as method of distraction

Explain responsibility of child, e.g., need to remain motionless during test and/or radiotherapy

Provide the child with some means for involvement with the procedure (e.g., holding a piece of equipment, such as bandage, tape), counting with the operator, answering questions, etc.

Implement distracting techniques and pain reduction techniques as indicated (see Nursing care plan: The child in pain, p. 279)

See also Preparing children for procedures, p. 211

EXPECTED OUTCOMES

Child readily responds to verbal directives

Child repeats information accurately

NURSING DIAGNOSIS: Fear related to diagnosis and prognosis

See Nursing care plan: The child who is terminally ill or dying, p. 292

NURSING DIAGNOSIS: Altered family processes related to having a child with a life-threatening disease

GOAL

Prepare family for diagnostic/therapeutic procedures

INTERVENTIONS

Explain reason for each test and procedure

Whenever possible, make use of procedures that minimize discomfort, such as a venous access device (Broviac catheter, implanted port), or Ommaya reservoir

Explain reason for radiotherapy

Explain operative procedure honestly (if appropriate)

Avoid overemphasis on benefits, which may not be evident for several days postoperatively

See also Preparation for procedures, p. 211

EXPECTED OUTCOME

Child and family demonstrate understanding of procedures (specify learnings and manner of demonstration)

GOAL

Support family

INTERVENTIONS

Teach parents about disease process

Explain all procedures that will be done to child

Schedule time for family to be together, without interruptions from staff

Help family plan for future, especially toward helping child live a normal life

Encourage family to discuss feelings regarding child's course prior to diagnosis and his prospects for survival

Discuss with family how they will tell child about outcome of surgery and need for additional treatment (if appropriate)

Refer to local chapter of American Cancer Society or other organizations

EXPECTED OUTCOMES

Family demonstrates knowledge of child's disease and treatments (specify methods of learning and evaluation)

Family expresses feelings and concerns and spends time with child

See also:
Nursing care plan: The child in the hospital, p. 246
Nursing care plan: The family of the ill or hospitalized child, p. 254

NURSING DIAGNOSIS: Anticipatory grief related to perceived potential loss of a child

GOAL

Help family face possibility of child's death

INTERVENTIONS

Provide consistent contact with family
Clarify, refocus, and supply information as needed
Help family plan care of child, especially at terminal stage (e.g., extent of extraordinary lifesaving measures)

Provide or help arrange for hospice care if family desires
Arrange for spiritual support in accordance with family's beliefs and/or affiliations

EXPECTED OUTCOMES

Family remains open to counseling and nursing contacts
Family and child discuss their fears, concerns, needs, and desires at terminal stage
Family investigates hospice care
Appropriate religious representative is contacted (specify)

GOAL

Support family

INTERVENTIONS AND EXPECTED OUTCOMES

See Nursing care plan: The child who is terminally ill or dying, p. 292

NURSING CARE PLAN
THE CHILD UNDERGOING CHEMOTHERAPY OR RADIOTHERAPY

Destruction of neoplastic cells by pharmacologic agents or radiation produces variable responses in normal tissues

See Tables 4-11 and 4-12.

ASSESSMENT

Perform physical assessment
See also Nursing care plan: The child with cancer, p. 412
Observe for signs of complications of therapies—Infection, hemorrhage, anemia
Observe for signs of problems related to chemo- or radiotherapy—Nausea and vomiting, anorexia, mucosal ulceration,

neuropathy (weakness and numbing of extremities resulting in difficulty walking or fine hand movement, footdrop, jaw pain, postirradiation somnolence), hemorrhagic cystitis (burning on urination, frequency), alopecia, moon face, mood changes
Assist with diagnostic procedures and tests—Blood and urine examination, neurologic examination, radiography

---

NURSING DIAGNOSIS: Potential for infection related to depressed body defenses

GOAL

Minimize risk of infection

INTERVENTIONS

Place child in private room
Advise all visitors and staff to practice handwashing
Screen all visitors and staff for signs of infection

Use scrupulous aseptic technique for all invasive procedures
Evaluate child for any potential sites of infection (needle punctures, mucosal ulceration, minor abrasions, dental problems)
Provide nutritionally complete diet for age
*Administer antibiotics as prescribed

EXPECTED OUTCOMES

Child does not come in contact with infected persons or contaminated articles
Child consumes diet appropriate for age (specify)

*Dependent nursing action.

NURSING DIAGNOSIS: Potential for injury (hemorrhage, hemorrhagic cystitis) related to interference with cell proliferation

GOAL

Prevent hemorrhage

INTERVENTIONS

Use all measures to prevent infection, especially in ecchymotic areas
Use local measures to stop bleeding
Restrict strenuous activity that could result in accidental injury
Involve child in responsibility for limiting activity when platelet count drops
* Administer platelets as prescribed

EXPECTED OUTCOME

Child exhibits no evidence of bleeding

GOAL

Prevent hemorrhagic cystitis

INTERVENTIONS

Observe for signs (burning and pain or urination)
Give liberal (3000 ml/m²/day) fluid intake
Encourage frequent voiding, including during nighttime

EXPECTED OUTCOMES

Child voids without discomfort
No hematuria present

GOAL

Prevent or reduce the effects of anemia

INTERVENTIONS AND EXPECTED OUTCOME

See Nursing care plan: The child with anemia, p. 375

NURSING DIAGNOSIS: Impaired skin integrity related to administration of chemotherapeutic agents, immobility

GOAL

Prevent skin breakdown

INTERVENTIONS AND EXPECTED OUTCOME

See Nursing diagnosis: Impaired skin integrity, p. 490

GOAL

Reduce undesirable effects of therapy

---

*Dependent nursing action.

INTERVENTIONS

Suggest and/or implement measures to reduce discomfort from radiotherapy
Select loose-fitting clothing over irradiated area to minimize additional irritation
Protect area from sunlight and sudden changes in temperature (avoid ice packs, heating pads)

EXPECTED OUTCOME

Child and family comply with suggestions (specify)

NURSING DIAGNOSIS: Potential fluid volume deficit related to nausea and vomiting

GOAL

Prevent vomiting

INTERVENTIONS

*Administer initial dose of antiemetic prior to onset of nausea and vomiting
*Administer antiemetic around the clock for as long as nausea and vomiting typically last
Avoid foods with strong odors

EXPECTED OUTCOME

Child retains food and fluid

NURSING DIAGNOSIS: Altered mucous membranes related to administration of chemotherapeutic agents

GOAL

Prevent or reduce effects of oral ulceration

INTERVENTIONS

Inspect mouth daily for oral ulcers; avoid oral temperatures
Institute meticulous oral hygiene as soon as a drug is used that causes oral ulcers
Use soft-sponge toothbrush, cotton-tipped applicator, or gauze-wrapped finger
Administer frequent (at least every 4 hours and after meals) mouthwashes (normal saline)
Apply local anesthetics to ulcerated areas before meals and as needed
Serve bland, moist, soft diet
Encourage fluids; use a straw to help bypass painful areas
Report evidence of ulcers to practitioner
Avoid juices containing ascorbic acid, lemon swabs, and hot or cold food
*Administer anti-infective medication as ordered

EXPECTED OUTCOME

Mucous membranes remain intact
Ulcers show evidence of healing

---

*Dependent nursing action.

Unit 4

GOAL

Prevent or reduce effects of rectal ulceration

INTERVENTIONS

Wash perianal area after each bowel movement

Use warm sitz baths or tub baths as frequently as necessary for comfort

Apply protective skin barriers (transparent film dressings, occlusive ointment) to perineal area

Expose ulcerated area to warm heat to hasten healing

Observe for constipation resulting from child's voluntary refusal to defecate or from chemotherapy

Avoid rectal temperatures and suppositories

Record bowel movements; use stool softener to prevent constipation; may need stimulants for evacuation

EXPECTED OUTCOMES

Rectal mucosa remains clean and intact

Ulcerated areas heal without complications

Child has regular bowel movements

NURSING DIAGNOSIS: Impaired physical mobility related to neuromuscular impairment (neuropathy)

GOAL

Reduce effects of peripheral neuropathy

INTERVENTIONS

Encourage ambulation when child is able

Alter activity to prevent accidents if weakness occurs, including school attendance

Use footboard to prevent footdrop

Provide fluids and soft foods to lessen chewing movements

EXPECTED OUTCOME

Child ambulates without incident or difficulty

NURSING DIAGNOSIS: Body image disturbance related to loss of hair, moon face, debilitation

GOAL

Help child and family cope with hair loss

INTERVENTIONS

Introduce idea of wig prior to hair loss

Administer good scalp hygiene

Provide adequate covering during exposure to sunlight, wind, or cold

Suggest keeping thin hair clean, short, and fluffy to camouflage partial baldness

Stress that hair begins to regrow in 3-6 months and may be a slightly different color or texture

Stress that alopecia during a second treatment with same drug may be much less severe

Encourage good hygiene, grooming, and sex-appropriate items to enhance appearance, such as wig, scarves, hats, makeup, attractive, sex-appropriate clothing

EXPECTED OUTCOMES

Child verbalizes concern regarding hair loss

Child helps determine methods to reduce effects of hair loss and applies these methods

Child appears clean, well-groomed, and attractively dressed

GOAL

Promote adjustment to altered facial appearance

INTERVENTIONS

Encourage rapid reintegration with peers to lessen contrast of changed facial appearance

Stress that this reaction is temporary

Evaluate weight gain carefully (in weight gain resulting from administration of steroids, extremities remain thin)

Encourage visits from friends before discharge to prepare child for reactions and questions

Encourage early and consistent interaction with peers

EXPECTED OUTCOMES

Family demonstrates understanding of consequences of therapies

Child resumes former activities and relationships within capabilities

GOAL

Encourage expression of feelings

INTERVENTIONS

Provide opportunities for child to discuss feelings and concerns

Provide materials for nonverbal expression (e.g., play, art)

EXPECTED OUTCOME

Child expresses feelings regarding altered body in words, play, art (specify)

NURSING DIAGNOSIS: Diversional activity deficit related to restricted environment (private room)

GOAL

Provide diversion

INTERVENTIONS

Provide age-appropriate toys that can be properly cleaned

Involve child life specialist or other supportive services in planning diversional activities

See also Nursing diagnosis: Diversional activity deficit, p. 264

EXPECTED OUTCOMES

Child engages in activities appropriate for age and interests

Suitable toys are provided

NURSING DIAGNOSIS: Altered family processes related to a child undergoing therapy

GOAL

Prepare family for side effects and/or complications of chemotherapy or radiotherapy

INTERVENTIONS

Advise family of expected therapy side effects vs toxicities; clarify which demand medical evaluation (mucosal ulceration, hemorrhagic cystitis, peripheral neuropathy, evidence of infection or dehydration)

Reassure family that such reactions are not caused by return of cancer cells

Interpret prognostic statistics carefully, realizing family's temporary need to interpret them as they see necessary

Prepare family for expected mood changes from steroids

Interpret mood changes based on drugs or reactions to disease/treatment

EXPECTED OUTCOMES

Family demonstrates knowledge of instructions (specify methods of learning and evaluation)

Family demonstrates an understanding of behavior changes

GOAL

Support child during treatment for myelosuppression

INTERVENTIONS

Explain reason for antibiotics and/or transfusions, particularly why platelets are reserved for acute, uncontrolled bleeding episodes

Observe for signs of transfusion reaction (see Table 4-11)

Record approximate time for hemostasis to occur after administration of platelets

EXPECTED OUTCOME

Child demonstrates understanding of procedures and tests (specify method and learnings)

GOAL

Prepare family for home care

INTERVENTIONS

Teach preventive measures at discharge (handwashing and isolation from crowds)

Stress importance of isolating child from any known cases of chickenpox or other childhood diseases; work with school nurse and physician to determine optimum time for school reattendance

EXPECTED OUTCOME

Family demonstrates the ability to provide home care for the child

See also Nursing care plan: The child with cancer, p. 412

Table 4-14. SUMMARY OF CHEMOTHERAPEUTIC AGENTS USED IN THE TREATMENT OF CHILDHOOD CANCERS*

Agent/administration	Side effects and toxicity	Comments and specific nursing considerations
Alkylating agents		
Mechlorethamine (nitrogen mustard, Mustargen) IV, IT‡	N/V§ (½-8 hours later) (severe) BMD‖ (2-3 weeks later) Alopecia Local phlebitis	Vesicant†
Cyclophosphamide (Cytoxan, CTX,¶ Endoxan) PO, IV, IM‡	N/V (3-4 hours later) (severe at high doses) BMD (10-14 days later) Alopecia Hemorrhagic cystitis Severe immunosuppression Stomatitis (rare) Hyperpigmentation Transverse ridging of nails Infertility	BMD has platelet-sparing effect Give dose early in day to allow adequate fluids afterward Force fluids before administering drug and for 2 days after to prevent chemical cystitis; encourage frequent voiding even during night Warn parents to report signs of burning on urination or hematuria to practitioner
Chlorambucil (Leukeran) PO	N/V (mild) BMD (7-14 days later) Diarrhea Dermatitis Less commonly may be hepatotoxicity	Usually slow onset of side effects; side effects related to high doses
Antimetabolites		
Cytosine arabinoside (Ara-C, Cytosar, Cytarabine, arabinosyl cytosine) IV, IM, SC,‡ IT	N/V (mild) BMD (7-14 days later) Mucosal ulceration Immunosuppression Hepatitis (usually subclinical)	Crosses blood-brain barrier Use with caution in patients with hepatic dysfunction
5-Azacytidine (5-AzaC) IV	N/V (moderate) BMD (7-14 days later) Diarrhea	Infuse slowly via IV drip to decrease severity of N/V
Mercaptopurine (6-MP, Purinethol) PO	N/V (mild) Diarrhea Anorexia Stomatitis BMD (4-6 weeks later) Immunosuppression Dermatitis Less commonly may be hepatic dysfunction	6-MP is an analog of xanthine; therefore allopurinol (Zyloprim) delays its metabolism and increases its potency, necessitating a lower dose (⅓ to ¼) of 6-MP
Methotrexate (MTX, Amethopterin) PO, IV, IM, IT May be given in conventional doses (mg/m²) or high doses (g/m²)	N/V (severe at high doses) Diarrhea Mucosal ulceration (2-5 days later) BMD (10 days later) Immunosuppression Dermatitis	Side effects and toxicity are dose related Potency and toxicity increased by reduced renal function, salicylates, sulfonamides, and aminobenzoic acid; avoid use of these substances, such as aspirin

*Table includes principal drugs used in the treatment of childhood cancers. Several other conventional and investigational chemotherapeutic agents may be employed in the treatment regimen.

†Vesicants (sclerosing agents) can cause severe cellular damage if even minute amounts of the drug infiltrate surrounding tissue. Only nurses experienced with chemotherapeutic agents should administer vesicants. These drugs must be given through a free-flowing intravenous line. The infusion is stopped *immediately* if any sign of infiltration (pain, stinging, swelling, or redness at needle site) occurs. Interventions for extravasation vary, but each nurse should be aware of the institution's policies and implement them at once.

‡IV, intravenous; IT, intrathecal; PO, by mouth; IM, intramuscular; SC, subcutaneous.

§N/V, nausea and vomiting. Mild = <20% incidence; moderate = 20% to 70% incidence; severe = >75% incidence.

‖BMD, bone marrow depression.

¶Abbreviations stand for chemical compound.

Table 4-14. SUMMARY OF CHEMOTHERAPEUTIC AGENTS USED IN THE TREATMENT OF CHILDHOOD CANCERS—cont'd

Agent/administration	Side effects and toxicity	Comments and specific nursing considerations
Antimetabolites—cont'd		

	Photosensitivity
	Alopecia (uncommon)
	Toxic effects include
	  Hepatitis (fibrosis)
	  Osteoporosis
	  Nephropathy
	  Pneumonitis (fibrosis)
	Neurologic toxicity with IT use—pain at injection site, meningismus (signs of meningitis without actual inflammation), especially fever and headache; potential sequelae—transient or permanent hemiparesis, convulsions, dementia, and death
		High dose therapy:
		  Citrovorum factor (folinic acid or leucovorin) decreases cytotoxic action of MTX; used as an antidote for overdose and to enhance normal cell recovery following high-dose therapy; avoid use of vitamins containing folic acid during MTX therapy unless prescribed by physician
		IT therapy:
		  Drug *must* be mixed with preservative-free diluent
		  Report signs of neurotoxicity immediately

6-Thioguanine (6-TG, Thioguan) PO	N/V (mild)
	BMD (7-14 days later)
	Stomatitis
	Rarely
	  Dermatitis
	  Photosensitivity
	  Liver dysfunction
		Side effects are unusual

Plant alkaloids		
Vincristine (Oncovin) IV	Neurotoxicity—paresthesia (numbness), ataxis, weakness, foot drop, hyporeflexia, constipation (adynamic ileus), hoarseness (vocal cord paralysis), abdominal, chest, and jaw pain, mental depression Fever N/V (mild) BMD (minimal; 7-14 days later) Alopecia	Vesicant Report signs of neurotoxicity because may necessitate cessation of drug Individuals with underlying neurologic problems may be more prone to neurotoxicity Monitor stool patterns closely; administer stool softener Excreted primarily by liver into biliary system; administer cautiously to anyone with biliary disease
Vinblastine (Velban) IV	Neurotoxicity (same as for vincristine but less severe) N/V (mild) BMD (especially neutropenia; 7-14 days later) Alopecia	Same as for vincristine
VP-16-213 (Etoposide, VePesid)	N/V (mild to moderate) BMD (7-14 days later) Alopecia Hypotension with rapid infusion Bradycardia Diarrhea (infrequent) Stomatitis (rare) May reactivate erythema of irradiated skin (rare) Allergic reaction with anaphylaxis possible	Give slowly via IV drip with child recumbent Have emergency drugs available at bedside*

*Emergency drugs include oxygen and parenteral preparations of epinephrine 1:1000, diphenhydramine or similar antihistamine, aminophylline, corticosteroids, and vasopressors.
Continued.

Table 4-14 SUMMARY OF CHEMOTHERAPEUTIC AGENTS USED IN THE TREATMENT OF CHILDHOOD CANCERS—cont'd

Agent/administration	Side effects and toxicity	Comments and specific nursing considerations
Antibiotics		
Actinomycin-D (Dactinomycin, Cosmegen, ACT-D) IV	N/V (2-5 hours later) (moderate) BMD (especially platelets; 7-14 days later) Immunosuppression Mucosal ulceration Abdominal cramps Diarrhea Anorexia (may last few weeks) Alopecia Acne Erythema or hyperpigmentation of previously irradiated skin Fever Malaise	Vesicant Enhances cytotoxic effects of radiation therapy but increases toxic effects May cause serious desquamation of irradiated tissue

Doxorubicin (Adriamycin, Doxyrubicin) IV	N/V (moderate)
	Stomatitis
	BMD (7-14 days later)
	Fever, chills
	Local phlebitis
	Alopecia
	Cumulative-dose toxicity includes
	   Cardiac abnormalities
	   ECG changes
	   Heart failure
		Vesicant (extravasation may *not* cause pain)
		Use only sterile distilled water as a diluent
		Observe for any changes in heart rate or rhythm and signs of failure
		Cumulative dose must not exceed 550 mg/m^2
		Warn parents that drug causes urine to turn red (for up to 12 days after administration); this is normal, not hematuria

Daunorubicin (Daunomycin, Rubidomycin) IV	Similar to doxorubicin	Similar to doxorubicin

Bleomycin (Blenoxane) IV, IM, SC	Allergic reaction—fever, chills, hypotension, anaphylaxis
	Fever (nonallergic)
	N/V (mild)
	Stomatitis
	Cumulative dose effects include
	   Skin—rash, hyperpigmentation, thickening, ulceration, peeling, nail changes, alopecia
	   Lungs—Pneumonitis with infiltrate that can progress to fatal fibrosis
		Should give test dose (SC) before therapeutic dose administered
		Have emergency drugs* at bedside
		Hypersensitivity occurs with first one to two doses
		May give acetaminophen before drug to reduce likelihood of fever
		Concentration of drug in skin and lungs accounts for toxic effects

Hormones		
Corticosteroids (prednisone most frequently used; many proprietary names such as Meticorten, Deltasone, Paracort) PO; also IM or IV but rarely used	For short-term use, no acute toxicity Usual side effects are mild: moon face, fluid retention, weight gain, mood changes, increased appetite, gastric irritation, insomnia, susceptibility to infection	Explain expected effects, especially in terms of body image, increased appetite, and personality changes Monitor weight gain Recommend moderate salt restriction Administer with antacid and early in morning (sometimes given every other day to minimize side effects) May need to disguise bitter taste (crush tablet and mix with syrup, jam, ice cream or other highly-flavored substance; use ice to numb tongue before administration; place tablet in gelatin capsule if child can swallow it) Observe for potential infection sites; usual inflammatory response and fever are absent

*Emergency drugs include oxygen and parenteral preparations of epinephrine 1:1000, diphenhydramine or similar antihistamine, aminophylline, corticosteroids, and vasopressors.

Table 4-14 SUMMARY OF CHEMOTHERAPEUTIC AGENTS USED IN THE TREATMENT OF CHILDHOOD CANCERS—cont'd

Agent/administration	Side effects and toxicity	Comments and specific nursing considerations
Hormones—cont'd		
	Long-term effects of chronic steroid administration are mood changes, hirsutism, trunk obesity (buffalo hump), thin extremities, muscle wasting and weakness, osteoporosis, poor wound healing, bruising, potassium loss, gastric bleeding, hypertension, diabetes mellitus, growth retardation	All of above; in addition, encourage foods high in potassium (bananas, raisins, prunes, coffee, chocolate) Test stools for occult blood Monitor blood pressure Test blood for sugar and urine for acetone Observe for signs of abrupt steroid withdrawal: flulike symptoms, hypotension, hypoglycemia, shock
Enzymes		

L-asparaginase (Elspar) IV, IM	Allergic reactions (including anaphylactic shock)
	Fever
	N/V (mild)
	Anorexia
	Weight loss
	Arthralgia
	Toxicity—
	   Liver dysfunction
	   Hyperglycemia
	   Renal failure
	   Pancreatitis
		Have emergency drugs at bedside*
		Record signs of allergic reaction, such as urticaria, facial edema, hypotension, or abdominal cramps
		Check weight daily
		Normally, BUN and ammonia levels rise as a result of drug—not evidence of liver damage
		Check urine for sugar and blood amylase

Nitrosoureas		
Carmustine (BCNU) IV Lomustine (CCNU) PO	N/V (2-6 hours later) (severe) BMD (3-4 weeks later) Burning pain along IV infusion (usually due to alcohol diluent) BCNU—flushing and facial burning on infusion	Prevent extravasation; contact with skin causes brown spots Oral form—give 4 hours after meals when stomach is empty Reduce IV burning by diluting drug and infusing slowly via IV drip Crosses blood-brain barrier
Other agents		

Hydroxyurea (Hydrea) PO	N/V (mild)
	Anorexia
	Less commonly
	   Diarrhea
	   BMD
	   Mucosal ulceration
	   Alopecia
	   Dermatitis
		Must be given cautiously in patients with renal dysfunction

Procarbazine (Matulane) PO	N/V (moderate)
	BMD (3-4 weeks later)
	Lethargy
	Dermatitis
	Myalgia
	Arthralgia
	Less commonly
	   Stomatitis
	   Neuropathy
	   Alopecia
	   Diarrhea
		Central nervous system depressants (phenothiazines, barbiturates) enhance central nervous system symptoms
		Monoamine oxidase (MAO) inhibition sometimes occurs; therefore all other drugs are avoided unless medically approved; red wine, fava beans, and broad bean pods are avoided

Unit 4

Table 4-14. SUMMARY OF CHEMOTHERAPEUTIC AGENTS USED IN THE TREATMENT OF CHILDHOOD CANCERS—cont'd

Agent/administration	Side effects and toxicity	Comments and specific nursing considerations
Dacarbazine (DTIC-Dome) IV	N/V (especially after first dose) (severe) BMD (7-14 days later) Alopecia Flulike syndrome Burning sensation in vein during infusion (not extravasation)	Vesicant (less sclerosive) Must be given cautiously in patients with renal dysfunction Decrease IV rate or use warm moist towels on IV site to decrease burning
Cisplatin (Platinol) IV	Renal toxicity (severe) N/V (1-4 hours later) (severe) BMD (mild, 2-3 weeks later) Ototoxicity Neurotoxicity (similar to that for vincristine) Electrolyte disturbances, especially hypomagnesium, hypocalcemia, hypokalemia, and hypophosphatemia Anaphylactic reactions may occur	Renal function (creatinine clearance) must be assessed before giving drug Must maintain hydration before and during therapy (specific gravity of urine is used to assess hydration) Mannitol may be given IV to promote osmotic diuresis and drug clearance Monitor intake and output Monitor for signs of ototoxicity (e.g., ringing in ears) and neurotoxicity; report signs immediately; ensure that routine audiogram is done before treatment for baseline and routinely during treatment Do not use aluminum needle; reaction with aluminum decreases potency of drug Monitor for signs of electrolyte loss; i.e. hypomagnesium—tremors, spasm, muscle weakness, lower extremity cramps, irregular heartbeat, convulsions, delirium Have emergency drugs at bedside*

*Emergency drugs include oxygen and parenteral preparations of epinephrine 1:1000, diphenhydramine or similar antihistamine, aminophylline, coricosteroids, and vasopressors.

Unit 4

Table 4-15. EARLY SIDE EFFECTS OF RADIOTHERAPY

Site/effects	Nursing interventions	Site/effects	Nursing interventions
Gastrointestinal tract		**Skin**	
Nausea/vomiting	Give antiemetic on regular schedule Measure amount of emesis to prevent dehydration	Alopecia (within 2 weeks; begins to regrow by 3-6 months)	Introduce idea of wig Stress necessity of scalp hygiene and need for head covering in cold weather
Anorexia	Encourage fluids and foods best tolerated, usually light, soft diet Monitor weight loss	Dry or moist desquamation	Do not refer to skin changes as a "burn" (implies use of too much radiation) Keep skin clean Wash daily, using soap sparingly
Mucosal ulceration	Use frequent mouthwashes and oral hygiene to prevent mucositis		Do not remove skin marking for radiation fields Avoid exposure to sun
Diarrhea	Can be controlled with antispasmodics and kaolin pectin preparations Observe for signs of dehydration		For dryness, apply lubricant For desquamation, consult physician for skin hygiene and care
Potential effects: Pancreatitis Parotitis Loss of taste	May need analgesics to relieve discomfort Combat severe dryness of mouth with oral hygiene and liquid diet	**Head** Nausea/vomiting Alopecia Potential effects Parotitis Loss of taste Xerostomia (dry mouth)	Same as for gastrointestinal tract Regular dental care, fluoride treatments
		Urinary bladder Rarely cystitis	More likely to occur with concomitant use of cyclophosphamide Encourage liberal fluid intake and frequent voiding
		Bone marrow Myelosuppression	Institute bleeding and infection precautions Observe for signs of anemia

Unit 4

NURSING CARE PLAN
THE CHILD WITH LEUKEMIA

A progressive, malignant disease of the blood-forming organs, characterized by distorted proliferation and development of leukocytes and their precursors in the blood and bone marrow

Acute lymphoblastic leukemia (ALL)—Lymphatic, lymphocytic, lymphoblastic, lymphoblastoid leukemia

Acute nonlymphoid (myelogenous) leukemia (ANLL, AML)—Granulocytic, myelocytic, monocytic, myelogenous, and monoblastic, monomyeloblastic

ASSESSMENT

Perform physical assessment

Obtain health history, especially relative to early evidence of possible leukemia (see Nursing care plan: The child with cancer—Assessment, p. 412)

Observe for manifestations of leukemia (Table 4-16)

Assist with diagnostic procedures and tests—Blood examination, lumbar puncture, bone marrow aspiration, biopsy

Observe for evidence of complications—Bleeding, ulceration, central nervous system manifestations

See Nursing care plan: The child with cancer, p. 412

See Nursing care plan: The child undergoing chemotherapy or radiotherapy p. 414

NURSING DIAGNOSIS: Altered family processes related to having a child with leukemia

GOAL

Prepare child and family for diagnostic procedures

INTERVENTIONS

See preparation for procedures, p. 211

Explain basic elements of blood to provide foundational information for tests and therapies

Encourage older children and parents to learn meaning of various blood values

Explain bone marrow aspiration and lumbar puncture with step-by-step approach

EXPECTED OUTCOME

Family demonstrates understanding of procedures (specify learning and manner of demonstration)

GOAL

Arrange for additional support

INTERVENTIONS

See Nursing diagnosis: Altered family processes, p. 261

Refer family to community agencies and support groups

EXPECTED OUTCOME

Family acquires needed support

*American Cancer Society, 1599 Clifton Rd., NE, Atlanta, GA 30329, (404) 329-7617. Leukemia Society of America, Inc., 211 East 43rd Street, New York, NY 10017. Candelighters, Suite 1001, 1901 Pennsylvania Ave. NW, Washington, D.C. 20006, (202) 659-5139. In Canada: Canadian Cancer Society, 77 Bloor St. West, Suite 1702, Toronto, ONT M55 3A1 (416) 961-7223.

Table 4-16. PATHOLOGY AND RELATED CLINICAL MANIFESTATIONS OF LEUKEMIA

Organ or tissue	Consequences	Manifestations
Bone marrow dysfunction	Decreased RBC—anemia	Pallor, fatigue
	Neutropenia—infection	Fever
	Decreased platelets—bleeding tendencies	Hemorrhage (petechiae)
	Invasion of bone marrow—bone weakness; invasion of periosteum	Tendency to fractures
		Pain
Reticuloendothelial system:		
Liver	Infiltration, enlargement, eventual fibrosis	Hepatomegaly
Spleen		Splenomegaly
Lymph glands		Lymphadenopathy
CNS		
Meninges	Increased intracranial pressure, ventricular enlargement	Severe headache
		Vomiting
		Irritability, lethargy
		Papilledema
		Eventual coma
	Meningeal irritation	Pain
		Stiff neck and back
Hypermetabolism	Cell deprivation of nutrients by invading cells	Muscle wasting
		Weight loss
		Anorexia
		Fatigue

NURSING CARE PLAN
THE CHILD WITH A BRAIN TUMOR

Neoplasm orignating from nerve cells, neuroepithelium, glia, cranial nerves, blood vessels, pineal gland, or hypophysis

ASSESSMENT

Perform physical assessment

Perform neurologic assessment with special attention to ocular signs (see p. 292), level of consciousness (see p. 292), cranial nerve function (especially nerves V through X) (see p. 56), coordination, signs of increased intracranial pressure (see p. 392)

Observe for signs of dehydration (*sunken* fontanel is *not* a sign, since it usually remains bulging because of increased intracranial pressure)

Observe for manifestations of brain tumor:

Headache
Recurrent and progressive
In frontal or occipital areas
Worse on arising, less during day
Intensified by lowering head and straining, such as during bowel movement, coughing, sneezing

Vomiting
With or without nausea or feeding
Progressively more projectile
More severe in morning
Relieved by moving about and changing position

Neuromuscular changes
Incoordination or clumsiness
Loss of balance (use of wide-based stance, falling, tripping, banging into objects)
Poor fine motor control
Weakness
Hyporeflexia or hyperreflexia
Positive Babinski sign
Spasticity
Paralysis

Behavioral changes
Irritability
Decreased appetite
Failure to thrive
Fatigue (frequent naps)
Lethargy
Coma

Cranial nerve neuropathy
Cranial nerve involvement varies according to tumor location
Most common signs
 Head tilt
 Visual defects (nystagmus, diplopia, strabismus, episodic "greying out" of vision, and visual field defects)

Vital sign disturbances
Decreased pulse and respiration
Increased blood pressure
Decreased pulse pressure
Hypothermia or hyperthermia

Other signs
Seizures
*Cranial enlargement
*Tense, bulging fontanel at rest
Nuchal rigidity
Papilledema (edema of optic nerve)

Measure head circumference daily on child with open sutures
Assess child's physical capabilities
Observe intervals of sleep and wakefulness; observe level of activity when awake: if child sleeps for a long interval, assess ease of arousal
Assess mental functioning by asking simple questions (name, age, residence)
Assist with diagnostic procedures and tests—Tomography, magnetic resonance imaging, angiography, electroencephalography, lumbar puncture (sometimes), biopsy (during surgery)

*Present only in infants and young children

© 1990 The CV Mosby Co. All rights reserved.

1. Preoperative care

See also Nursing care plan: The child undergoing surgery: preoperative care, p. 267

NURSING DIAGNOSIS: Potential for injury related to altered neurologic functioning

GOAL

Protect from injury

INTERVENTIONS

Have seizure precautions at bedside
Maintain siderails on bed
Assist with ambulation

EXPECTED OUTCOME

Child remains free of injury

NURSING DIAGNOSIS: Pain related to increased intracranial pressure

GOAL

Relieve pain

INTERVENTIONS

Provide pain relief with environmental manipulation (dimly lit room, no noise, no sudden movement)
*Administer analgesics as prescribed; observe for side effects that may mask level of consciousness and/or depress respiratory center
See Nursing care plan: The child in pain (p. 279)

EXPECTED OUTCOME

Child exhibits minimum evidence of discomfort

GOAL

Prevent increasing intracranial pressure

INTERVENTIONS

Prevent constipation to avoid straining at stool
*Administer stool softeners as prescribed
Prevent coughing or sneezing
See Nursing diagnosis: Potential for injury, Minimize intracranial pressure p. 394

EXPECTED OUTCOME

Child exhibits no evidence of increased intracranial pressure

---

*Dependent nursing action.

NURSING DIAGNOSIS Sensory-perceptual alterations (visual, auditory, kinesthetic, gustatory, tactile, olfactory) related to interference with reception, transmission, and/or integration of sensory input

GOAL

Help compensate for sensory-perceptual deficits

INTERVENTIONS

See Nursing care plan: The child with visual impairment, p. 458
See Nursing care plan: The child with hearing impairment, p. 463
Stimulate appetite with attractively served meals
    Provide preferred foods
    See Nursing care plan: The child with special nutritional needs, p. 277
Assist child to orient to time and space, especially when ambulating
Keep daily records of signs and symptoms to assess child's physical capabilities and to assist family in adjusting to insidious or acute deterioration

EXPECTED OUTCOME

Child adjusts to sensory-perceptual deficits

NURSING DIAGNOSIS: Altered family processes related to having a child with a serious illness

GOAL

Prepare child and family for diagnostic/operative procedures

INTERVENTIONS

Explain reason for each test and radiotherapy
Explain responsibility of the child, for example, need to remain motionless during test and/or radiotherapy
Explain operative procedure honestly
    Avoid overpreparation
    Avoid overemphasis on positive benefits, which may not be evident for several days postoperatively
Arrange for child and parents to visit special intensive care unit where the child will be postoperatively
Explain to child common experiences after surgery, for example, may be very sleepy, have a headache, and must remain quiet
See also Preparation for procedures, p. 211
See Nursing care plan: The child with cancer, p. 412

EXPECTED OUTCOMES

Family demonstrates an understanding of tests and procedures (specify learnings and manner of demonstration)
Child and family visit the ICU
Child and family demonstrate an understanding of information presented (specify information and manner of demonstration)

GOAL

Prepare child's scalp for surgery for brain tumor

INTERVENTIONS

Prepare child and parents for head shaving (may be done in OR after anesthesia)
  If done in room or while awake:
    Provide absolute privacy
    Allow child to look into mirror at different stages to lessen shock of total baldness, unless this increases anxiety
  Provide an attractive covering (lacy nightcap or baseball cap)
  Save long hair by braiding it first
  Shave head carefully to avoid skin cuts, which can become infected
  Cleanse scalp as prescribed
Prepare child and parents for the large dressing; may help to show a picture or wrap gauze around a doll's head

EXPECTED OUTCOME

Head is shaved with a minimum of distress to child and family

2. Postoperative care

See Nursing care plan: The child undergoing surgery: postoperative care, p. 267

NURSING DIAGNOSIS: Potential for injury related to intracranial trauma

GOAL

Position for minimal stress on operative site

INTERVENTIONS

*Consult with surgeon regarding positioning, which may differ from the following:
  Infratentorial—Position child flat and on either side, not on back; neck is usually slightly extended to prevent strain on sutures
  Supratentorial—Elevate head usually above level of heart; do not lower head unless ordered by physician
  Post sign above bed noting exact position of head
  Turn child cautiously to maintain proper position

EXPECTED OUTCOMES

Minimal stress is applied to operative site
Child remains in desired position

GOAL

Maintain integrity of dressings

INTERVENTIONS

Observe dressings for drainage
  Reinforce with sterile gauze pads but do not remove bandage
  Circle area of drainage to note further seepage
  Report evidence of clear fluid (cerebrospinal fluid) immediately
Restrain child's hands as necessary to preserve intact dressing

---

*Dependent nursing action.

EXPECTED OUTCOME

Dressing remains intact

GOAL

Prevent hyperthermia

INTERVENTIONS

Place hypothermia blanket on bed prior to child's return to room
View any temperature elevation as potential sign of infection

EXPECTED OUTCOME

Temperature remains within acceptable limits (specify)

GOAL

Prevent fluid overload or dehydration

INTERVENTIONS

Check gag and swallowing reflexes before offering clear oral fluids
  Stop oral fluids if vomiting occurs
Calculate all fluids very carefully to prevent overload

EXPECTED OUTCOME

Child exhibits no signs of fluid overload or dehydration

GOAL

Prevent eye damage

INTERVENTIONS

Apply ice compresses to eyes for short intervals to relieve edema
Keep eyes closed or apply eye dressings
May need to instill normal saline eye drops to prevent corneal ulceration if blink reflex is depressed

EXPECTED OUTCOME

Eyes remain clear with no evidence of irritation

NURSING DIAGNOSIS: Altered family processes related to a child with critical surgery for a life-threatening disease

GOAL

Support family

INTERVENTIONS

Help family plan for future, especially toward helping child live a normal life
Encourage family to discuss feelings regarding child's course prior to diagnosis and prospects for survival
Discuss with family how they will tell the child about the outcome of surgery and need for additional treatment
Help family plan a realistic activity schedule
  Resumption of school attendance

Unit 4

Limited or modified physical activity (for example, may have to wear a helmet to protect the skull until it is completely healed)

Encourage to pursue academic goals

Help child prepare for questions from peers regarding "brain surgery," hair loss, or any residual neurologic deficit

Provide continuing support for family through comprehensive oncology clinic and/or community nursing service

EXPECTED OUTCOMES

Family discusses feelings and concerns

Family devises a realistic activity schedule

Child and family employ safety devices (specify)

Child attends school with reasonable regularity (specify)

Family receives continuing support (specify type and amount)

See also:

Nursing care plan: The child in the hospital, p. 246

Nursing care plan: The family of the ill or hospitalized child, p. 254

Nursing care plan: The child with a chronic illness or disability, p. 259

See specific disability resulting from therapy

NURSING CARE PLAN
THE CHILD WITH A BONE TUMOR

Neoplasm of the bone

Osteosarcoma (osteogenic sarcoma)—tumor arising from

bone-forming mesenchyme

Ewing sarcoma—tumor arising from bone marrow

ASSESSMENT

Perform physical assessment

Observe for manifestations of bone tumors:

Pain localized at affected site

May be severe or dull

Often relieved by position of flexion

Frequently brought to attention when child

Limps

Curtails own physical activity

Is unable to hold heavy objects

Examine affected area for functional status, signs of inflammation, size of mass, regional lymph node involvement, and any

evidence of systemic involvement (see Assessment of the child with cancer, p. 412)

Obtain health history, especially regarding pain (clues to duration and rate of tumor growth)

Assist with diagnostic procedures and tests—Radiography, tomography, radioisotope bone scan, needle or surgical bone biopsy, lung tomography, other tests for differential diagnosis, bone marrow aspiration (Ewing sarcoma)

OSTEOSARCOMA

1. Preoperative care

See Nursing care plan: The child undergoing surgery: preoperative care p. 267

NURSING DIAGNOSIS: Anticipatory grieving related to prospect of loss of limb

---

GOAL

Prepare child and family for possible amputation or limb salvage procedure

INTERVENTIONS

Employ straightforward honesty

Avoid disguising diagnosis with terms such as "infection"

Emphasize lack of alternatives

Answer questions regarding information presented by surgeon and clarify any misconceptions

Avoid overwhelming child or parents with too much information

Be available and willing to listen and to talk to child and parents about their concerns

Allow for and encourage expression of feelings

EXPECTED OUTCOMES

Family and child express feelings regarding the potential loss

Family and child readily discuss concerns and ask appropriate questions

GOAL

Help child adjust to impending loss

INTERVENTIONS

Allow child time and opportunity to go through grief process

Introduce, but do not elaborate on, information regarding need for chemotherapy

Reserve extensive discussion of chemotherapy and rehabilitation until after surgery

Allow for expression of feelings regarding the loss and the undesirable effects of chemotherapy

Assist child to cope with side effects

Encourage independence

EXPECTED OUTCOME

Child expresses feelings about impending change in life-style

2. Postoperative care

See Nursing care plan: The child undergoing surgery, p. 269

> **NURSING DIAGNOSIS:** Impaired physical mobility related to amputation of lower extremity

GOAL

Administer postoperative care

INTERVENTIONS

Employ appropriate stump care according to limb involved

EXPECTED OUTCOME

Stump remains free of infection and/or irritation

GOAL

Assist with managing loss of limb

INTERVENTIONS

Assist with early ambulation and use of temporary prosthesis

Arrange for, carry out, or supervise physical therapy as prescribed

Arrange for preparation of permanent prosthesis

Teach use of auxilliary appliances such as wheelchair or crutches

EXPECTED OUTCOME

Child and family adjust to loss of limb

> **NURSING DIAGNOSIS:** Body image disturbance related to loss of limb

GOAL

Assist child to adjust to disability

INTERVENTIONS

Encourage visits from friends before discharge to prepare child for reactions and questions

Encourage early and consistent interaction with peers

Assist child to become adept in use of appliances

Assist child to select clothing to camouflage prosthesis

Encourage good hygiene, grooming, and sex-appropriate items to enhance appearance, such as wig (for hair loss from antimetabolites), makeup, attractive, sex-appropriate clothing

EXPECTED OUTCOMES

Child resumes former contacts and activities commensurate with limitations

Child appears clean, well-groomed, and attractively dressed

> **NURSING DIAGNOSIS:** Altered family processes related to having a child with a lifelong disability, traumatic therapy

GOAL

Support parents

INTERVENTIONS

Allow parents to express their feelings and concerns

Interpret the child's emotional reactions, such as depression, expressions of anger and hostility

EXPECTED OUTCOME

Parents verbalize feelings and concerns

GOAL

Begin preparation for supplemental therapies and their effects

INTERVENTIONS

See Preparation for procedures, p. 211

Impress on child importance of therapy

Explain probable side effects of antimetabolites

EXPECTED OUTCOME

Parents and child demonstrate an attitude of understanding of therapies and their side effects

GOAL

Prepare for discharge

INTERVENTIONS

Answer questions regarding posthospital care

Teach parents skills and give information necessary for home care

Teach stump care, if appropriate, to parents and child, if child is old enough to assume some responsibility

Assess home for environmental handicaps (such as stairs), accessibility of school, and so on

Arrange for and emphasize importance of maintaining physical therapy regimen

Arrange for acquisition of needed supplies such as dressings, crutches, wheelchair in addition to prosthesis

Encourage family to allow child to live as normal a life as possible

Refer to appropriate agencies and groups to facilitate care and adjustment such as the American Cancer Society, parent groups (see p. 424)

Maintain contact with family

Refer to agencies for aid and assist family to prepare environment

EXPECTED OUTCOMES

Child and family demonstrate skills needed for home care (specify)

Child and family demonstrate an understanding of therapeutic regimen

Child attends school with reasonable regularity (specify)

Family receives continuing support (specify type and amount)

See also:
Nursing care plan: The child with a chronic illness or disability, p. 259
Nursing care plan: The child in the hospital, p. 246
Nursing care plan: The family of the ill or hospitalized child p. 254
See Nursing care plan: The child with cancer, p. 412
See Nursing care plan: The child undergoing chemotherapy or radiotherapy, p. 414

NURSING CARE PLAN
THE CHILD WITH WILMS TUMOR

A malignant neoplasm of the kidney composed of embryonal elements

---

ASSESSMENT

Perform physical assessment

Obtain health history, especially related to parental observation of increased abdominal girth (e.g., clothes fit tighter)

Observe for manifestations of Wilms tumor:
    Abdominal swelling or mass
        Firm
        Nontender
        Does not extend beyond midline
    Hematuria (less than ¼ of cases)
    Anemia secondary to hemorrhage within the tumor
        Pallor
        Anorexia
        Lethargy
    Hypertension (occasionally)
    Weight loss
    Fever

Manifestations resulting from compression of tumor mass

Secondary metabolic alterations from tumor or metastasis

If metastasis, symptoms of lung involvement:
    Dyspnea
    Cough
    Shortness of breath
    Chest pain (sometimes)

Assist with diagnostic procedures and tests—Ultrasound, tomography of chest and abdomen, blood analysis, kidney function tests to determine function of unaffected kidney, liver function tests to detect evidence of metastasis

---

NURSING DIAGNOSIS: Potential for injury related to presence of encapsulated tumor

GOAL

Prevent rupture of tumor capsule preoperatively

INTERVENTIONS

Avoid palpating abdomen
Post signs at head of bed stating the above

EXPECTED OUTCOME

Tumor remains encapsulated

NURSING DIAGNOSIS: Altered family processes related to having a child with a life-threatening illness

GOAL

Prepare child and family for the surgery

INTERVENTIONS

See Nursing care plan: The child undergoing surgery, p. 267
Prepare family for large incision and dressing
Prepare family for anticipated postoperative therapies and their probable effects

EXPECTED OUTCOME

Family demonstrates an understanding of the disorder, therapies, and expected outcomes (specify knowledge and manner of demonstration)

See also:
Nursing care plan: The child in the hospital, p. 246
Nursing care plan: The family of the ill or hospitalized child, p. 254
Nursing care plan: The child with cancer, p. 412
Nursing care plan: The child undergoing chemotherapy or radiotherapy, p. 414

NURSING CARE OF THE CHILD WITH NEUROMUSCULAR DYSFUNCTION

Disorders in which the site of origin is located in the brain or spinal cord

Pyramidal—Those fibers that extend from the cortex, come together in the medulla, cross from one side to the other, then extend down the cord to synapse with anterior horn motor neurons

Extrapyramidal—Complex network of motor neurons that comprise relays between motor areas of the cortex, basal ganglia, thalamus, cerebellum, and brainstem.

Motor neurons:

Upper motor (pyramidal) neurons—Those that extend from the brain to a synapse in the anterior horn of the spinal cord

Lower motor neurons—Those that extend from the anterior horn cells to the myoneural junction at the muscle site

ASSESSMENT

See Neurologic assessment, p. 52
See Assessment of reflexes, p. 55
Observe for manifestations of upper and lower neuron involvement (see box)

Assist with diagnostic procedures and tests—Electromyography, nerve conduction velocity measurement, muscle biopsy, serum enzyme measurements (e.g., creatine phosphokinase, aldolase, serum glutamic-oxalacetic transaminase, lactic dehydrogenase)

MANIFESTATIONS OF UPPER AND LOWER NEURON INVOLVEMENT

UPPER MOTOR NEURON SYNDROME

Spastic paralysis in muscle groups below lesion (reflex arcs below lesion are intact)

Hyperreflexia with tendon reflexes exaggerated, Babinski reflex present

No wasting of muscle mass because of increased muscle tone

Flexion contractures and spasms of muscle groups below lesion level common

No skin or tissue changes

LOWER MOTOR NEURON SYNDROME

Flaccid paralysis caused by muscle atonia (reflex arcs are permanently damaged)

Reflex with associated muscle response absent

Marked atrophy of atonic muscle

Fasciculations (local twitching of muscle groups) common
No flexor spasms

Loss of hair
Skin and tissue changes
Cornified nails

Unit 4

NURSING CARE PLAN
THE CHILD WHO IS PARALYZED

Loss or impairment of sensation and/or motor function—classified by etiology, muscle tone, distribution, or parts of the body affected

Paraplegia—Paralysis in two extremities, usually the legs and lower part of the body

Quadriplegia, or **tetraplegia**—Paralysis of four extremities

Hemiplegia—Paralysis of one side of the body

Flaccid paralysis—Paralysis with loss of muscle tone

Spastic paralysis—Paralysis with involuntary contraction of one or more muscles with associated loss of muscular function

ASSESSMENT

See previous section
See Neurologic assessment, p. 52
See Assessment of reflexes, p. 55
Observe for manifestations of paralysis:
  Loss of sensation and/or motor function in affected areas
    Limpness
    Loss of pinprick sensation in tested area
    Loss of position or vibration sense in tested area

Constipation
Loss of anal sphincter control
Change in urinary patterns; enuresis
Assist with diagnostic procedures and tests—Perform or assist
  with extensive neurologic examination including, determining level of injury, residual sensory or motor function (if any),
  autonomic function

Unit 4

NURSING DIAGNOSIS: Impaired physical mobility related to nerve damage

See Nursing diagnosis: Impaired physical mobility, p. 437

NURSING DIAGNOSIS: Potential for injury related to
paralysis, immobility

GOAL

Prevent physical injury

INTERVENTIONS

Implement and maintain safety devices according to degree of
  dysfunction (specify)
Employ correct techniques for moving, transporting, and otherwise manipulating paralyzed body part(s)

EXPECTED OUTCOME

Child remains free of physical injury

GOAL

Prevent circulatory complications

INTERVENTIONS

Monitor peripheral pulses and skin temperature
Ensure frequent position changes
Wrap legs in elastic bandage or stockings to decrease pooling
  when in upright position
Perform range of motion exercises
Encourage child to be as active as condition and restrictive
  devices allow
*Administer peripheral sympathetic stimulating agents if ordered

EXPECTED OUTCOME

Peripheral circulation remains good as evidenced by color, capillary filling

GOAL

Prevent disuse syndrome in unaffected parts

INTERVENTIONS

See Nursing diagnosis: Impaired physical mobility, p. 437

EXPECTED OUTCOME

Child uses unaffected parts

GOAL

Prevent contracture deformities

INTERVENTIONS

Maintain correct body alignment
Perform range of motion, active, passive, and stretching exer-
  cises
Employ joint splints and braces as indicated

EXPECTED OUTCOMES

Joints remain flexible
Child exhibits no evidence of contractures

GOAL

Prevent complications of bone demineralization

INTERVENTIONS

Handle extremities carefully when turning and positioning
Ensure adequate fluid intake
Acidify urine (ascorbic acid, apple juice, cranberry juice)
Use upright posture on tilt table daily
*Administer calcium-mobilizing drugs if ordered

EXPECTED OUTCOMES

Child develops no fractures
Serum calcium remains within normal limits

GOAL

Prevent or minimize hip and lower extremity deformity

INTERVENTIONS

Carry out passive range-of-motion exercises
Carry out muscle stretching when indicated
Carry out exercises with care to avoid fracturing fragile bones
Maintain hips in slight to moderate abduction to prevent dis-
  location

*Dependent nursing action

*Dependent nursing action.

EXPECTED OUTCOME

Lower extremities maintain flexibility

NURSING DIAGNOSIS: Potential impaired skin integrity related to immobility

See Nursing diagnosis: Potential impaired skin integrity, p. 490

NURSING DIAGNOSIS: Potential for infection related to neuromuscular impairment, immobility

GOAL

Prevent upper respiratory tract infection

INTERVENTIONS

Maintain interventions that facilitate respiratory efforts
Change position frequently
Carry out percussion, vibration, and drainage (or suction) as necessary
Encourage coughing and deep breathing
Avoid contact with infected persons
Observe for signs of acute respiratory distress

EXPECTED OUTCOMES

Lungs remain clear
Respirations remain within normal limits (specify) (see inside front cover for normal variations)

GOAL

Facilitate respiratory efforts

INTERVENTIONS

Place in position that promotes chest expansion and diaphragm excursion
Ensure good body alignment when in sitting or standing position
Avoid restriction of chest or abdominal musculature
Supply torso support to promote chest expansion

EXPECTED OUTCOME

Child exhibits no evidence of hypoventilation

GOAL

Prevent urinary tract infection

INTERVENTIONS

Implement bladder training in appropriate children
Administer urinary antiseptics if ordered
Catheterize for severe retention
Teach self-catheterization to appropriate children (paraplegia)

EXPECTED OUTCOME

Child does not develop urinary tract infection

NURSING DIAGNOSIS: Constipation related to neuromuscular impairment

GOAL

Prevent constipation

INTERVENTIONS

*Administer stool softeners as prescribed
Provide bowel training

EXPECTED OUTCOME

Child evacuates bowel daily

NURSING DIAGNOSIS: Sexual dysfunction related to inability to feel sexual stimuli, inability to attain and/or maintain an erection

GOAL

Help attain sexual gratification

INTERVENTIONS

Teach touch approach
Teach alternative methods for sexual gratification
Refer to qualified sex therapist for long-term sexual adjustment

EXPECTED OUTCOME

Patient achieves some type of sexual gratification

NURSING DIAGNOSIS: Altered family processes related to a child with a physical disability

GOAL

Support family

INTERVENTIONS AND EXPECTED OUTCOMES

See Nursing diagnosis: Altered family processes, p. 261

See also:
Nursing care plan: The child with chronic illness or disability, p. 259
Nursing care plan: The child in the hospital, p. 246
Nursing care plan: The family of the ill or hospitalized child, p. 254
Nursing care plan: The child who is immobilized, p. 439

---

*Dependent nursing action.

Unit 4

Quadriplegia:
Special needs

NURSING DIAGNOSIS: Ineffective breathing pattern related to diaphragmatic paralysis

GOAL

Facilitate respirations

INTERVENTIONS

See Nursing care plan: The child at risk for infection, p. 288
Monitor ventilatory device
Teach "frog breathing" techniques
Change and maintain tracheostomy as needed (if the patient has a tracheostomy)

EXPECTED OUTCOMES

Lungs are well aerated
Child "breathes" for short periods without mechanical ventilation

NURSING DIAGNOSIS: Ineffective thermoregulation related to absence of sweating, dilated blood vessels

GOAL

Maintain optimum body temperature

INTERVENTIONS

Regulate environmental temperature to maintain optimum body temperature
Add or remove clothing and blankets according to body temperature

EXPECTED OUTCOME

Child maintains optimum body temperature (see inside front cover)

NURSING DIAGNOSIS: Dysreflexia related to autonomic nerve dysfunction

GOAL

Eliminate precipitating stimulus

INTERVENTIONS

Recognize autonomic dysreflexia (manifested by flushed face, sweating on forehead, pupillary constriction, marked hypertension, headache, bradycardia)
Rule out other causes (e.g., orthostatic hypotension)
Identify precipitating factor (e.g., constipation, full bladder)
Correct cause (e.g., empty bladder or bowel)

EXPECTED OUTCOME

Symptoms of autonomic dysreflexia are relieved

NURSING CARE PLAN
THE INFANT WITH MYELOMENINGOCELE

Hernial protrusion of a saclike cyst of meninges, spinal fluid, and a portion of the spinal cord with its nerves through a bony defect in the vertebral column
Other terms used to describe spinal defects:
  Myelodysplasia—All-inclusive term that refers to defective development of any part of the spinal cord; usually used to describe abnormalities without gross superficial defects
  Spinal dysraphia or **spina bifida**—Defect in closure of the vertebral column with varying degrees of tissue protrusion through the bony cleft

Spina bifida occulta—Fusion failure of posterior vertebral arches without accompanying herniation of spinal cord or meninges; usually not visible externally
Spina bifida cystica—Defect in closure with external saccular protrusion through the bony spine with varying degrees of nerve involvement
Meningocele—Form of spina bifida cystica; consists of a saclike cyst of meninges filled with spinal fluid

ASSESSMENT

Perform physical assessment
Observe for manifestations of myelomeningocele:
  Visible sac
  Sensory disturbances usually parallel motor dysfunction
    Below second lumbar vertebra
      Flaccid, areflexic partial paralysis of lower extremities
      Varying degrees of sensory deficit
      Overflow incontinence with constant dribbling of urine
      Lack of bowel control
      Rectal prolapse (sometimes)
    Below third sacral vertebra
      No motor impairment

May be saddle anesthesia with bladder and anal sphincter paralysis
Joint deformities (sometimes produced in utero)
  Talipes valgus or varus contractures
  Kyphosis
  Lumbosacral scoliosis
  Hip dislocations
Perform or assist with neurologic examination to determine level of motor and sensory impairment
Inspect myelomeningocele for any changes in appearance, for example, abrasions, tears, signs of infection
Observe for signs that indicate hydrocephalus, see p. 399
Assist with diagnostic procedures and tests—Radiography, tomography

---

NURSING DIAGNOSIS: Potential for infection related to presence of infective organisms, nonepithelialized meningeal sac, paralysis

GOAL

Prevent local infection

INTERVENTIONS

Position infant to prevent contamination from urine and stool
Cleanse myelomeningocele carefully with sterile saline
Apply sterile dressings; moisten with sterile solution as ordered (saline, silver nitrate, antibiotic)
*Administer antibiotics as ordered
Administer similar care of operative site postoperatively

EXPECTED OUTCOME

Meningeal sac remains clean, intact, and exhibits no evidence of infection

GOAL

Prevent urinary tract infection

INTERVENTIONS

Avoid urethral contamination with stool
See also Nursing care plan: The child with urinary tract infection, p. 383

EXPECTED OUTCOME

Child remains free of urinary tract infection

---

*Dependent nursing action.

NURSING DIAGNOSIS: Potential for trauma related to delicate spinal lesion

GOAL

Prevent local trauma

INTERVENTIONS

Handle infant carefully
Place infant in prone position or side-lying position, if permitted
Apply protective devices to sac, if prescribed
Modify routine nursing activities, for example, feeding, making bed, comforting activities

EXPECTED OUTCOME

Meningeal sac remains intact

NURSING DIAGNOSIS: Potential impaired skin integrity related to paralysis, continual dribbling of urine and feces

GOAL

Prevent skin irritation

INTERVENTIONS

Change diapers as soon as soiled, if diapered
Keep perianal area clean and dry
See also Nursing diagnosis: Potential impaired skin integrity, p. 490

EXPECTED OUTCOME

Perianal area remains clean and dry; no evidence of irritation

See also:
Nursing care plan: The child with a chronic illness or disability, p. 259
Nursing care plan: The child in the hospital, p. 246
Nursing care plan: The family of the ill or hospitalized child, p. 254

Unit 4

NURSING CARE PLAN
THE CHILD WITH CEREBRAL PALSY

Impaired muscle control resulting from a nonprogressive abnormality in the pyramidal motor system

Clinical classification of cerebral palsy:

Spastic—May involve one side, both sides

Hypertonicity with poor control of posture, balance, and coordinated motion

Impairment of fine and gross motor skills

Active attempts at motion increase abnormal postures and overflow of movement to other parts of the body

Dyskinetic—Abnormal involuntary movement

Athetosis—Characterized by slow, wormlike, writhing movements that usually involve all extremities, the trunk, neck, facial muscles, and tongue

Involvement of the pharyngeal, laryngeal, and oral muscles causes drooling and dysarthria (imperfect speech articulation)

Involuntary movements may take on choreoid (involuntary, irregular, jerking movements) and dystonic (disordered muscle tone) manifestations that increase in intensity under emotional stress and around adolescence

Ataxic

Wide-based gait

Rapid repetitive movements performed poorly

Disintegration of movements of the upper extremities when the child reaches for objects

Mixed-type—Combination of spasticity and athetosis

Rigid, tremor, and atonic—uncommon types

Deformities

Lack of active movement

ASSESSMENT

Perform physical assessment

Obtain health history, especially relative to prenatal and perinatal factors and circumstances surrounding birth that predispose to fetal anoxia

Observe for manifestations of cerebral palsy, especially those related to attainment of developmental milestones:

Delayed gross motor development

A universal manifestation

Delay in all motor accomplishments

Increases as growth advances

Abnormal motor performance

Very early preferential unilateral hand use

Abnormal and asymmetric crawl

Standing or walking on toes

Uncoordinated or involuntary movements

Poor sucking

Feeding difficulties

Persistent tongue thrust

Alterations of muscle tone

Increased or decreased resistance to passive movements

Opisthotonic postures (exaggerated arching of back)

Feels stiff on handling or dressing

Difficulty in diapering

Rigid and unbending at the hip and knee joints when pulled to sitting position (an early sign)

Abnormal postures

Maintains hips higher than trunk in prone position with legs and arms flexed or drawn under the body

Scissoring and extension of legs and with the plantar flexed in supine position

Persistent infantile resting and sleeping posture

Arms abducted at shoulders

Elbows flexed

Hands fisted

Reflex abnormalities

Persistence of primitive infantile reflexes

Obligatory tonic neck reflex at any age

Nonpersistence beyond 6 months of age

Persistence or hyperactivity of the Moro, plantar, and palmar grasp reflexes

Hyperreflexia, ankle clonus, and stretch reflexes elicited on many muscle groups on fast passive movements

Associated disabilities (may or may not be present)

Subnormal learning and reasoning (mental retardation)

Seizures

Impaired behavioral and interpersonal relationships

Sensory impairment (vision, hearing)

Assist with diagnostic procedures and tests if indicated—Electroencephalography, tomography, screening for metabolic defects, serum electrolyte values

Perform developmental, hearing, or visual tests as indicated (See Unit 1)

Unit 4

NURSING DIAGNOSIS: Impaired physical mobility related to neuromuscular impairment

GOAL

Establish locomotion

INTERVENTIONS

Encourage sitting, crawling, and walking at appropriate ages
Carry out therapies that strengthen and improve control
Assist child in using reciprocal leg motion when learning to walk
Provide incentives to locomote
Ensure adequate rest before attempting locomotion activities
Incorporate play that encourages desired behavior
Employ aids that facilitate locomotion such as parallel bars, crutches
Prepare child and family for surgical procedures if indicated
See also Nursing diagnosis: Potential for injury. Prevent deformity

EXPECTED OUTCOME

Child acquires locomotion within capabilities (specify)

NURSING DIAGNOSIS: Potential for injury related to physical disability, neuromuscular impairment, perceptual and cognitive impairment

GOAL

Prevent physical injury

INTERVENTIONS

Provide safe physical environment
    Padded furniture
    Siderails on bed
    Sturdy furniture that does not slip
    Avoid scatter rugs and polished floors
Select toys appropriate to age and physical limitations
Encourage sufficient rest
Use restraints when child is in chair or vehicle
Provide child who is prone to falls with protective helmet and enforce its use
Institute seizure precautions for susceptible child
*Administer anticonvulsant drugs as prescribed

EXPECTED OUTCOME

Family provides a safe environment for the child (specify)
Child is free of injury

GOAL

Prevent deformity

INTERVENTIONS

Apply and correctly use braces
Carry out and teach family to perform stretching exercises

---

*Dependent nursing action

Employ appropriate range of motion exercises
Perform preoperative and postoperative care for child who requires corrective surgery

EXPECTED OUTCOME

Child benefits from appropriate preventive measures (specify measures and child's expected response)

NURSING DIAGNOSIS: Fatigue related to increased energy expenditure

GOAL

Ensure balanced diet

INTERVENTIONS

Provide extra calories to meet energy demands of increased muscle activity
Monitor weight gain
Provide vitamin, mineral, and/or protein supplements if eating habits are poor
Devise aids and techniques to facilitate feeding

EXPECTED OUTCOMES

Child eats a balanced diet
Weight remains within acceptable limits (specify)

GOAL

Promote relaxation

INTERVENTIONS

Maintain a well-regulated schedule that allows for adequate rest and sleep periods
Be alert for evidence of fatigue, which tends to aggravate symptoms

EXPECTED OUTCOME

Child is sufficiently rested

GOAL

Promote general health

INTERVENTIONS

Ensure regular routine health maintenance
    Physical assessment
    Dental care
    Immunizations

EXPECTED OUTCOMES

Child receives regular health assessments (specify schedule) (see p. 152)
Child receives appropriate immunizations (specify) (see p. 176) and dental care (specify) (see p. 182)

Unit 4

NURSING DIAGNOSIS: Impaired verbal communication

GOAL

Facilitate communication

INTERVENTIONS

Enlist the services of a speech therapist early
Talk to child slowly
Use articles and pictures to reinforce speech
Employ feeding techniques that help facilitate speech such as using lips, teeth, and various tongue movements
Teach and use nonverbal communication methods to dysarthritic child who would benefit, e.g., Blissymbols
Help family acquire electronic equipment to facilitate nonverbal communication (e.g., typewriter, microcomputer with voice synthesizer)

EXPECTED OUTCOME

Child is able to communicate needs to caregivers (specify desired communication and means of accomplishment)

NURSING DIAGNOSIS: Bathing/hygiene, dressing/grooming, feeding, toileting self-care deficits related to physical disability

See:
Nursing diagnosis: Bathing/hygiene self-care deficit, p. 468
Nursing diagnosis: Dressing/grooming self-care deficit, p. 468
Nursing diagnosis: Feeding self-care deficit, p. 468
Nursing diagnosis: Toileting self-care deficit, p. 468

NURSING DIAGNOSIS: Body image disturbance related to perception of disability

GOAL

Promote a positive body image

INTERVENTIONS

Capitalize on child's assets and provide compensation for liabilities
Praise child for accomplishments and "near" accomplishments such as partial completion of a task
Plan activities and goals *with* the child
See also Nursing diagnosis: Body image disturbance, p. 265

EXPECTED OUTCOME

Child exhibits behaviors that indicate positive body image (specify)

NURSING DIAGNOSIS: Altered family processes related to a child with a lifelong disability

GOAL

Support family

INTERVENTIONS

See Nursing diagnosis: Altered family processes, p. 261
*Refer to special support group(s) and agencies

EXPECTED OUTCOMES

See Nursing care plan (above)
Family contacts special support group

See also:
Nursing care plan: The child with a chronic illness or disability, p. 259
Nursing care plan: The child with mental retardation impairment, p. 466
Nursing care plan: The child with impaired vision, p. 458
Nursing care plan: The child with impaired hearing, p. 463

***United Cerebral Palsy Association,** 7 Penn Plaza, Ste. 804, New York, NY 10001, (800) USA-1UCP. In Canada, the **Canadian Cerebral Palsy Association,** 40 Dundas St., Suite 222, P.O. Box 110, Toronto, Ontario M5G2C2, (416) 979-7923.

Unit 4

NURSING CARE OF THE CHILD WITH MUSCULOSKELETAL DYSFUNCTION

Disorders involving the bones, muscles, and joints of the body

NURSING CARE PLAN
THE CHILD WHO IS IMMOBILIZED

Immobilization is a major therapy for injuries to soft tissues,
long bones, ligaments, vertebrae, and joints

ASSESSMENT
Assess for evidence of the physical effects of immobilization in
Table 4-17.
Assess for evidence of the following psychologic responses to
immobilization:
  Immobility deprives the child of:
    A means of communication, expression, and impulse con-
    trol
    A natural outlet for feelings
    A means of stress reduction
  Immobility restricts the amount and variety of environmental
  stimuli:
    Decrease in tactile input
    Restricted limbs transmit less than normal sensation
    Proprioception impaired

Decreased sensorimotor activity
May feel isolated, bored, and forgotten
May express anger and aggression inappropriately
Restlessness
Prolonged immobilization can produce:
  Difficulty in problem solving
  Difficulty in concentrating on activities
  Egocentrism (older children)
  Sluggish intellectual and psychomotor responses
  Decreased communication
  Increased fantasizing
  Depression
  Regression—Greater reliance on others

Unit 4

Table 4-17. PRIMARY AND SECONDARY PHYSICAL EFFECTS OF IMMOBILIZATION*

Primary effects	Secondary effects	Primary effects	Secondary effects
Muscular system		Venous stasis	Pulmonary emboli and/or thrombi
Decreased muscle strength, tone, and endurance	Decreased venous return and decreased cardiac output	Dependent edema	Tissue breakdown and susceptibility to infection
	Decreased metabolism and need for oxygen	**Respiratory system**	
	Decreased exercise tolerance	Decreased need for oxygen	Altered oxygen—Carbon dioxide exchange and metabolism
	Bone demineralization		
Disuse atrophy and loss of muscle mass	Catabolism	Decreased chest expansion and diminished vital capacity	Diminished oxygen intake Dyspnea and inadequate arterial oxygen saturation; acidosis
	Loss of strength		
Loss of joint mobility	Contractures, ankylosis of joints	Poor abdominal tone and distention	Interference with diaphragmatic excursion
Weak back muscles	Secondary spinal deformities	Mechanical or biochemical secretion retention	Hypostatic pneumonia
Weak abdominal muscles	Impaired respiration		Bacterial and viral pneumonia
Skeletal system			Atelectasis
Bone demineralization—osteoporosis, hypercalcemia	Negative calcium balance	Loss of respiratory muscle strength	Poor cough Upper respiratory infection
	Pathologic fractures	**Gastrointestinal system**	
	Calcium deposits	Distention caused by poor abdominal muscle tone	Interference with respiratory movements
	Extraosseous bone formation, especially at hip, knee, elbow, and shoulder	No specific primary effect	Difficulty in feeding in prone position; gravitation effect on feces through ascending colon or weakened smooth muscle tone may cause constipation
	Renal calculi		
Negative calcium balance	Life-threatening electrolyte imbalance		
Metabolism			Anorexia
Decreased metabolic rate	Slowing of all systems	**Urinary system**	
	Decreased food intake	Alteration of gravitational force	Difficulty in voiding in prone position
Negative nitrogen balance	Decline in nutritional state	Impaired ureteral peristalsis	Urinary retention in calyces and bladder
	Impaired healing		Infection
Hypercalcemia	Electrolyte imbalance		Renal calculi
Decreased production of stress hormones	Decreased physical and emotional coping capacity	**Integumentary system**	
		No specific primary effect	Decreased circulation and pressure leading to tissue injury
Cardiovascular system			
Decreased efficiency of orthostatic neurovascular reflexes	Inability to adapt readily to upright position		Difficulty with personal hygiene
	Pooling of blood in extremities in upright posture		
Diminished vasopressor mechanism	Orthostatic hypotension with syncope—Hypotension, decreased cerebral blood flow, tachycardia		
Altered distribution of blood volume	Decreased cardiac workload		
	Decreased exercise tolerance		

*Not all problems will apply in every situation.

NURSING DIAGNOSIS: Impaired physical mobility related to mechanical restrictions, physical disability (specify level)

GOAL

Provide mobilization (if appropriate)

INTERVENTIONS

Transport child by gurney, stroller, wagon, bed, or other conveyance from confines of room

EXPECTED OUTCOME

Child moves from confines of room

GOAL

Promote autonomy

INTERVENTIONS

Provide mobilizing devices (braces, crutches, wheelchair)
Assist with acquisition of specialized equipment
Instruct in use of equipment
Encourage activities that require mobilization
Allow as much freedom of movement as possible and encourage normal activities

EXPECTED OUTCOMES

Child moves about without assistance
Child engages in activities appropriate to limitations and developmental level

NURSING DIAGNOSIS: Potential impaired skin integrity related to immobility, therapeutic appliances

See Nursing diagnosis: Potential for impaired skin integrity, p. 490

NURSING DIAGNOSIS: Potential for trauma related to impaired mobility

GOAL

Prevent falls

INTERVENTIONS

Teach correct use of mobilizing devices and/or apparatus
Assist with moving and/or ambulating as needed
Remove hazards from environment (specify)
Modify environment as needed (specify)
Keep call button within reach
Keep siderails up at all times
Assist child to use bathroom or commode if possible

EXPECTED OUTCOME

Child remains free of injury

GOAL

Prevent other injuries (specify)

INTERVENTIONS

Implement safety measures appropriate to child's developmental age (specify)

EXPECTED OUTCOME

Child exhibits no signs of injury

NURSING DIAGNOSIS: Body image disturbance related to immobilization, mechanical appliances

See Nursing diagnosis: Body image disturbance, p. 265

NURSING DIAGNOSIS: Altered family processes related to a child with disability

GOAL

Support family

INTERVENTIONS AND EXPECTED OUTCOMES

See Nursing diagnosis: Altered family processes, p. 261

See also:
Nursing care plan: The child in the hospital, p. 246
Nursing care plan: The family of the ill or hospitalized child, p. 254

Unit 4

NURSING CARE PLAN
THE CHILD WITH A FRACTURE

A fracture is a break in the continuity of a bone caused when the resistance of the bone yields to a stress force exerted on it

Complete fracture—Fracture fragments are separated

Incomplete fracture—Fracture fragments remain attached

Simple, or **closed fracture**—Fracture does not produce a break in the skin

Open, or **compound fracture**—Fractures with an open wound through which the bone is or has protruded

Complicated fracture—Bone fragments cause damage to other organs or tissues (e.g., lung or bladder)

Comminuted fracture—Small fragments of bone are broken from fractured shaft and lie in surrounding tissue (very rare in children)

Most frequent fractures in children:

Bends—A child's flexible bone can be bent 45 degrees or more before breaking. However, if bent, the bone will straighten slowly, but not completely, to produce some deformity but without the angulation that exists when the bone breaks. Bends occur more commonly in the ulna and fibula, often associated with fractures of the radius and tibia.

Buckle fracture—Compression of the porous bone produces a *buckle,* or *torus,* fracture. This appears as a raised or bulging projection at the fracture site. Torus fractures occur in the most porous portion of the bone near the metaphysis (the portion of the bone shaft adjacent to the epiphysis) and are more common in young children.

Greenstick fracture—Occurs when a bone is angulated beyond the limits of bending. The compressed side bends and the tension side fails, causing an incomplete fracture similar to the break observed when a green stick is broken.

Complete fracture—Divides the bone fragments. They often remain attached by a periosteal hinge, which can aid or hinder reduction.

ASSESSMENT

Obtain history of event, previous injury, experience with health personnel

Observe manifestations of fracture:

Signs of injury
  Generalized swelling
  Pain or tenderness
  Diminished functional use of affected part

May be bruising

Severe muscular rigidity

Crepitus (grating sensation at fracture site)

Assess for location of fracture—Observe for deformity, instruct child to point to painful area

Assess for circulation and sensation distal to fracture site

Assist with diagnostic procedures and tests—Radiography, tomography

Unit 4

1. The child in a cast

Categories of casts:
Upper extremity cast—Immobilizes wrist and/or elbow
Lower extremity cast—Immobilize ankle and/or knee
Spinal and cervical casts—Immobilizes the spine
Spica cast—Immobilizes hip and knee

Casting materials:
Plaster of Paris—Cotton tape permeated with calcium sulfate crystals that interlock as tape dries (tepid water–activated)
Synthetic:
Polyester/cotton tape permeated with polyurethane resin (cool water–activated)
Knitted fiberglass tape with polyurethane resin (tepid water–activated or photoactivated)
Knitted thermoplastic polyester fabric (hot water–activated)

ASSESSMENT OF CASTED EXTREMITY(S)

Monitor cardiovascular status
Monitor peripheral pulses
Blanch skin on extremity distal to fracture to ascertain adequate circulation to the part
Feel cast for tightness; cast should allow insertion of fingers between skin and cast after it has dried
Assess for increase in
Pain
Swelling
Coldness
Cyanosis
Assess finger or toe movement and sensation
Request child to move fingers or toes
Observe for spontaneous movement in children who are unable to respond to requests
Report signs of impending circulatory impairment immediately
Instruct child to report any feelings of numbness or tingling

Check temperature (plaster cast):
Chemical reaction in cast drying process, which generates heat
Water evaporation, which causes heat loss
Inspect skin for irritation or pressure areas
Inspect inside cast for items that a small child may place there
Observe for signs of infection
Check for drainage
Smell cast for foul odor
Feel cast for "hot spots" indicating infection under the cast
Be alert to increased temperature, lethargy, and discomfort
Observe for respiratory impairment (spica cast)
Assess child's chest expansion
Observe respiratory rate
Observe color and behavior
Assess for evidence of bleeding (surgical open reduction)
Outline area of bleeding; assess for increase
Assess need for pain medication (p. 279)

Unit 4

NURSING DIAGNOSIS: Potential for injury related to presence of cast, tissue swelling, possible nerve damage

GOAL

Prevent circulatory impairment

INTERVENTIONS

Elevate casted extremity
Place leg cast on pillows, making certain that leg is well supported and that there is no pressure on heel
Elevate arm on pillows or support in stockinette sling suspended from intravenous infusion pole—either in bed or during ambulation; triangular arm sling is adequate for lesser elevation and support

EXPECTED OUTCOME

Toes/fingers are warm, pink, sensitive, and demonstrate brisk capillary filling

GOAL

Maintain cast integrity

INTERVENTIONS

Handle damp cast with palms of hands; avoid indenting the cast with fingertips (plaster cast)
Cover rough edges of cast with adhesive "petals"
Do not allow weight bearing until cast is completely dry—even if weight-bearing device is attached
Change position of child in body cast or hip spica cast periodically (small child can be managed easily; adolescent may require one or two persons; eventually children become very adept at moving themselves)
Do *not* use abduction stabilizer bar between legs of hip spica as handle for turning
Position with buttocks lower than shoulders during toileting to prevent urine from flowing under cast at the back; body can be supported on pillows
Protect rim of cast around perineal area of body cast with plastic film to prevent soiling during toileting
Use plastic-backed disposable diaper with edges tucked underneath rim of cast for infants and small children who are not toilet trained or who are prone to "accidents"; a sanitary napkin can also be used if waterproof material is placed between pad and cast
Caution against activities that might cause physical damage to cast

Remove soiled areas of cast with damp cloth and small amount of white, low-abrasive cleanser; do not cover soiled areas with shoe polish or paint

EXPECTED OUTCOME

Cast dries evenly and remains clean and intact

GOAL

Prevent physical injury

INTERVENTIONS

Keep a clear path for ambulation
    Remove toys, hazardous floor rugs, pets, or other items over which the child might stumble
Teach to use crutches appropriately if lower limb fracture
    The crutches should fit properly, have a soft rubber tip to prevent slipping, and be well padded at the axilla

EXPECTED OUTCOME

Child remains free of injury

NURSING DIAGNOSIS: Pain related to physical injury

GOAL

Provide comfort

INTERVENTIONS

See Nursing care plan: The child in pain, p. 279
Position for comfort; use pillows to support dependent areas
Alleviate itching underneath cast by alcohol swabs; cool air blown from Asepto syringe, fan, or hair dryer (on low or cool setting); or scratching or rubbing the unaffected extremity
Avoid using powder or lotion under cast, since these substances have tendency to "ball" and produce irritation

EXPECTED OUTCOMES

Child exhibits no evidence of discomfort
Minor discomforts are eased

NURSING DIAGNOSIS: Potential impaired skin integrity related to cast

GOAL

Prevent skin irritation

INTERVENTIONS

Make certain that all edges are smooth and free from irritating projections; trim and/or pad as necessary; petal cast edges if needed
Do not allow the child to put anything inside the cast
    Keep small items that might be placed inside the cast away from small children
Caution older children not to place items under cast
Keep exposed skin clean and free of irritants

EXPECTED OUTCOME

Skin remains intact with no evidence of irritation

NURSING DIAGNOSIS: Impaired physical mobility related to musculoskeletal impairment

GOAL

Maintain muscle use of unaffected areas

INTERVENTIONS

Encourage to ambulate as soon as possible
Support casted arm in sling
Teach use of mobilizing devices such as crutches for casted leg (walking device is applied when weight bearing allowed)
Encourage child with an ambulation device to ambulate as soon as general condition allows
Provide and encourage use of muscles in play activities and diversions
Carry out range of motion exercises of unaffected limbs, if paralyzed

EXPECTED OUTCOMES

Unaffected extremities maintain good muscle tone
Child engages in activities appropriate to his age and condition

---

NURSING DIAGNOSIS: Altered family processes related to child with a physical injury

GOAL

Educate family for home care

INTERVENTIONS

Teach cast care and management
    Observe the extremities (fingers or toes) for any evidence of swelling; discoloration (darker or lighter than a comparable extremity), or foul odor and contact the health professional if noted.
    Check movement of the visible extremities frequently.
    Keep the casted extremity elevated on pillows or similar support for the first day, or as directed by the practitioner.
    Follow physician's orders regarding any restriction of activities.
    Restrict strenuous activities for the first few days.
        Engage in quiet activities but encourage use of muscles.
        Move the joints above and below the cast on the affected extremity.
    Encourage frequent rest for a few days keeping the injured extremity elevated while resting.
    Avoid allowing the affected limb to hang down for any length of time.
        Keep an injured upper extremity elevated (e.g., in a sling) while upright.
        Elevate a lower limb when sitting and avoid standing for too long.
Help family plan suitable activities
Help family in problem solving of modification of clothing to fit over casted area

Help family devise supportive devices and modification of furniture for positioning (such as pillows, pads, and so on)

Help family in problem solving of means of transporting child including use of appropriate car restraints

EXPECTED OUTCOMES

Family demonstrates cast care

Family provides appropriate care of cast and seeks assistance when needed

NURSING DIAGNOSIS: Fear related to cast application and removal

GOAL

Support child during cast application

INTERVENTIONS

Explain what will take place and what the child can do to help

See also Preparation for procedures, p. 211

EXPECTED OUTCOME

Child submits to casting with minimal distress and cooperates during procedure

GOAL

Support child during cast removal

INTERVENTIONS

Explain procedure

  Noise of the saw

  Tickling sensation from vibration

  Unlikelihood of injury from procedure

Demonstrate safety of equipment

Provide reassurance

EXPECTED OUTCOME

Child cooperates throughout procedure

2. The child in traction

Purposes of traction for reduction of fractures:

To fatigue the involved muscle and reduce muscle spasm so that bones can be realigned

To position the distal and proximal bone ends in desired re-alignment to promote satisfactory bone healing

To immobilize the fracture site until realignment has been achieved and sufficient healing has taken place to permit casting or splinting

Other uses for traction:

To provide rest for an extremity

To help prevent or improve contracture deformity

To correct a deformity

To treat a dislocation

To allow preoperative or postoperative positioning and alignment

To provide immobilization of specific areas of the body

To reduce muscle spasms (rare in children)

Traction is applied by:

Manual traction—Traction applied to the body part by the hand placed distally to the fracture site. Nurses frequently provide manual traction during cast application.

Skin traction—Pull applied directly to the skin surface and indirectly to the skeletal structures. The pulling mechanism is attached to the skin with adhesive material or an elastic bandage. Both types are applied over soft, foam-backed traction straps to distribute the traction pull.

Skeletal traction—Pull applied directly to the skeletal structure by a pin, wire, or tongs inserted into or through the diameter of the bone distal to the fracture.

See Figs. 4-1 to 4-7 for various types of traction

ASSESSMENT OF TRACTION

Check desired line of pull and relationship of distal fragment to proximal fragment

 Check whether fragment is being directed upward, adducted, or abducted

Check function of each component

 Position of bandages, frames, splints

 Ropes: In center tract of pulley, taut, no fraying, knots tied securely

 Pulleys

  In original position on attachment bar; have not slid from original site

  Wheels freely movable

 Weights

  Correct amount of weight

  Hanging freely

  In safe location

Check bed position—Head or foot elevated as directed for desired amount of pull and countertraction

Assess child's behavior to determine if traction causes pain or discomfort

Skin traction

 Replace nonadhesive straps and/or Ace bandage on skin traction *when permitted* and/or absolutely necessary, but make certain that traction on limb is maintained by someone during procedure

 Assess bandages to ascertain if they are correctly applied (diagonal or spiral), not too loose or too tight, which could cause slippage and malalignment of traction

Skeletal traction

 Check pin sites frequently for signs of bleeding, inflammation, or infection

 Check pin screws to be certain that screws are tight in metal clamp that attaches traction apparatus to pin

Note pull of traction on pin; pull should be even

Observe for correct body alignment with emphasis on alignment of shoulders, hip, and leg(s)

Check after child has moved

Assess circular dressings for excessive tightness

Assess restraining devices

 Make certain that they are not too loose or too tight

 Remove periodically and check for pressure areas

Note if any tightness, weakness, or contractures are developing in uninvolved joints and muscles

Note any neurovascular changes, such as

 Color in skin and nail beds

 Alterations in sensation

 Alterations in motor ability

NURSING DIAGNOSIS: Potential for injury related to immobility and traction apparatus

GOAL

Prevent complications

INTERVENTIONS

Encourage deep breathing frequently with maximal inspiratory chest expansion

Apply restraints when indicated

Maintain correct angles at joints

Carry out passive, active, or active-with-resistance exercises of uninvolved joints

Take measures to correct or prevent further development of deformity such as applying foot plate to prevent footdrop

*Cleanse and dress pin sites on skeletal traction as ordered

*Apply topical antiseptic or antibiotic daily as ordered

Cover ends of pins with protective cord or padding to prevent child's being scratched by pin

Do not remove skeletal traction or adhesive traction straps on skin traction

Understand purpose of traction

Understand function of traction in each specific situation

*Administer stool softeners as indicated

*Administer rectal suppository or mild laxative if indicated

Make certain that child ingests sufficient amount of calcium-rich foods

---

*Dependent nursing action.

EXPECTED OUTCOMES

Circulation in extremities remains satisfactory; movement, good color, sensation present
Child exhibits no signs of complications

NURSING DIAGNOSIS: Pain related to physical injury

GOAL

Relieve pain
See Nursing care plan: The child in pain, p. 279

NURSING DIAGNOSIS: Potential impaired skin integrity related to immobility, traction apparatus

GOAL

Prevent skin breakdown

INTERVENTIONS

Provide sheepskin, Egg crate, or alternating pressure mattress underneath hips and back
Make total body skin checks for redness or breakdown, especially over areas that receive greatest pressure
Wash and dry skin at least twice daily
Stimulate circulation with gentle massage over pressure areas
Change position at least every 2 hours to relieve pressure, if possible

EXPECTED OUTCOME

Skin remains clean and intact with no evidence of irritation

NURSING DIAGNOSIS: Impaired physical mobility (specify level) related to musculoskeletal impairment

GOAL

Maintain limb function

INTERVENTIONS

Provide apparatus (e.g., overhead trapeze) and encourage child in activities that provide exercise for uninvolved muscles and joints

EXPECTED OUTCOME

Joints remain flexible; muscles retain tone

NURSING DIAGNOSIS: Fear related to discomfort, unfamiliar apparatus

GOAL

Decrease anxiety and gain cooperation

INTERVENTIONS

Explain traction apparatus to child
Explain to child what nursing care will be
Determine with child ways to participate in own care
Make certain that child knows how to call for help
Provide assurance that the child will not be left totally helpless

EXPECTED OUTCOME

Child cooperates throughout procedures

GOAL

Relieve discomfort

INTERVENTIONS

Use pads, pillows, and rolls to position for comfort
See also Nursing care plan: The child in pain, p. 279

EXPECTED OUTCOMES

Child plays and interacts readily
Child exhibits no signs of discomfort

NURSING DIAGNOSIS: Bathing/hygiene, feeding, dressing/grooming, toileting self-care deficits related to impaired mobility

GOAL

Promote maximum self-help

INTERVENTIONS

Devise means to facilitate self-help in daily activities
Assist with self-care activities where needed, for example, bathe inaccessible parts, make food easy to eat without assistance, provide grooming

EXPECTED OUTCOME

Child assists with self-care activities—Feeds self, washes reachable areas, attends to grooming within child's capabilities (specify)

GOAL

Facilitate elimination

INTERVENTIONS

Determine child's words for elimination needs
Provide privacy
Use fracture pan for bowel movements and voiding for females
Check frequency and consistency of bowel movements
Adjust fluid and food intake according to stools, for example, increase fluids, fruits, grains for constipation

EXPECTED OUTCOMES

Elimination is managed with minimum difficulty
Child has regular bowel movements

See also:
Nursing care plan: The child in the hospital, p. 246
Nursing care plan: The family of the ill or hospitalized child, p. 254

Unit 4

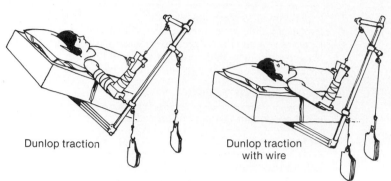

Dunlop traction

Dunlop traction with wire

Fig. 4-1. Dunlop traction.

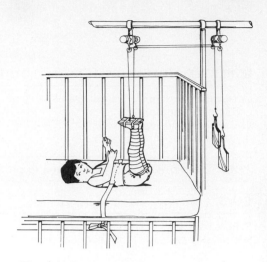

Fig. 4-2. Bryant traction.

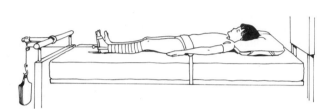

Fig. 4-3. Buck extension traction.

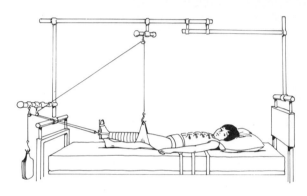

Fig. 4-4. Russell traction.

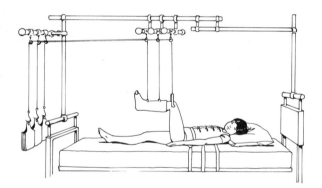

Fig. 4-5. Ninety-degree–ninety-degree traction.

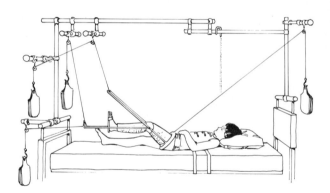

Fig. 4-6. Balance suspension with Thomas ring splint and Pearson attachment.

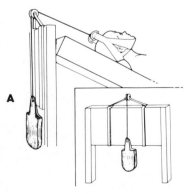

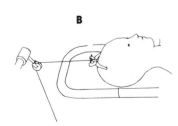

B

Fig. 4-7. Cervical traction. **A,** With chin strap. **B,** With Crutchfield tongs.

Figs. 4-1 to 4-7 (Redrawn from Hilt NE and Schitt EW: Pediatric orthopedic nursing, St. Louis, 1975, The CV Mosby Co.

NURSING CARE PLAN
THE CHILD WITH CONGENITAL HIP DYSPLASIA (CONGENITAL DISLOCATED HIP)

Malformations of the hip with various degrees of deformity that are present at birth

Acetabular dysplasia (or preluxation)—The mildest form, in which there is neither subluxation nor dislocation. The femoral head remains in the acetabulum.

Subluxation—The femoral head loses contact with the acetabulum and is displaced posteriorly and superiorly over the fibrocartilaginous rim. The femoral head remains in contact with the acetabulum, but a stretched capsule and ligamentum teres cause the head of the femur to be partially displaced.

Dislocation—The femoral head loses contact with the acetabulum and is displaced posteriorly and superiorly over the fibrocartilaginous rim

ASSESSMENT

Perform physical assessment
Observe for manifestations of congenital hip dysplasia:

Infant: (see p. 449)
Shortening of limb on affected side (Galeazzi sign, Allis sign)
Restricted abduction of hip on affected side
Unequal gluteal folds (infant prone)
Positive Ortolani test

Older infant and child:
Affected leg shorter than the other
Telescoping or piston mobility of joint
The head of the femur can be felt to move up and down in buttock when the extended thigh is pushed first toward the child's head and then pulled distally

Trendelenburg sign
When the child stands first on one foot and then on the other (holding onto a chair, rail, or someone's hands) bearing weight on the affected hip, the pelvis tilts downward on the normal side instead of upward as it would with normal stability
Prominent greater trochanter
Greater trochanter prominent and appears above a line from the anterior superior iliac spine to the tuberosity of the ischium
Marked lordosis (bilateral dislocations)
Waddling gait (bilateral dislocations)
Repeat hip inspection at every postnatal well-baby check for undetected or overlooked signs
Assist with diagnostic procedures and tests—Radiography, sonography
Assess corrective device for proper application and/or maintenance

NURSING DIAGNOSIS: Impaired physical mobility (level 3) related to immobilizing device

GOAL

Facilitate mobilization

INTERVENTIONS

Improve means of transportation for child
Devise self-mobilization equipment

EXPECTED OUTCOME

Child moves about environment

NURSING DIAGNOSIS: Potential for injury related to presence of corrective device, immobility

GOAL

Prevent physical injury

INTERVENTIONS

Modify handling techniques to avoid injury
Modify furniture and equipment to accommodate corrective device
*Acquire car seat especially designed for child in corrective device

*Available from Jerome Koziatek and Associates, Inc., 190 W. Boston Rd., Hinkley, OH 44233-9631. Directions for modification of several standard, government-approved car seats available from Automobile Safety for Children Program, James Whitcomb Riley Hospital for Children, Indiana School of Medicine, 702 Barnhill Drive, P-121, Indianapolis, IN 46223.

Unit 4

Teach family correct application of corrective device or cast care (see p. 443)

EXPECTED OUTCOME

Child remains free of injury

NURSING DIAGNOSIS: Altered family processes related to child with physical defect

GOAL

Support family

INTERVENTIONS

Assist family with problem-solving regarding care and child development
See also applicable portions of Nursing care plan: The child with a chronic illness or disability, p. 259

EXPECTED OUTCOME

Family members cope with disability and maintain corrective device properly

NURSING DIAGNOSIS: Altered growth and development related to immobilization

GOAL

Facilitate developmental achievement of locomotion

INTERVENTIONS

Provide mobilizing devices for older infant or child
Place infant prone on floor to promote locomotion
Provide opportunities for locomotion commensurate with developmental stage as soon as corrective device is removed.

EXPECTED OUTCOME

Child achieves locomotion following removal of appliance

NURSING CARE PLAN
THE CHILD WITH CONGENITAL CLUBFOOT

A common deformity in which the foot is twisted out of its normal shape or position
Described according to position of the ankle and foot:
  Talipes varus—An inversion or a bending inward
  Talipes valgus—An eversion or bending outward
  Talipes equinus—Plantar flexion in which toes are lower than heel

Talipes calcaneus—Dorsiflexion, in which toes are higher than heel
Talipes equinovarus—Composite deformity in which the foot is pointed downward and inward in varying degrees of severity

ASSESSMENT

Perform physical assessment
Determine if deformity can be passively corrected or is fixed

NURSING DIAGNOSIS: Potential for injury related to cast or other device

GOAL

Prevent physical injury
See Nursing care plan: The child in a cast, p. 443
See Nursing diagnosis: Impaired, physical mobility, p. 437

NURSING DIAGNOSIS: Altered family processes related to a child with a physical disability

GOAL

Support family

INTERVENTIONS AND EXPECTED OUTCOMES

See also Nursing care plan: The child with a chronic illness or disability, p. 259

NURSING CARE PLAN
THE CHILD WITH LEGG-CALVÉ-PERTHES DISEASE (COXA PLANA)

Progressive degeneration or ischemic necrosis of the capitular epiphysis (head) of the femur

Stage I: Aseptic necrosis or infarction of the femoral capital epiphysis with degenerative changes producing flattening of the upper surface of the femoral head—the *avascular stage.*

Stage II: Capital bone absorption and revascularization with fragmentation (vascular resorption of the epiphysis) that gives a mottled appearance on radiographs—the *fragmentation, or revascularization, stage.*

Stage III: New bone formation, which is represented on radiographs as calcification and ossification or increased density in the areas of radiolucency; this filling-in process appears to take place from the periphery of the head centrally—the *reparative stage.*

Stage IV: Gradual reformation of the head of the femur without radiolucency and, it is hoped, to a spherical form—the *regenerative stage.*

ASSESSMENT

Perform physical assessment
Observe for manifestations of coxa plana:
  Insidious onset
  Intermittent appearance of limp on affected side
  Pain:
    Soreness or aching
    In hip, along entire length of thigh, or in vicinity of knee
    Most evident on rising or at end of a long day

Usually accompanied by joint dysfunction and limited range of motion
Stiffness
Point tenderness over hip capsule
External hip rotation (late sign)
Assist with diagnostic procedures and tests—Radiography, tomography
Assess corrective device for proper application, evidence of irritation

---

NURSING DIAGNOSIS: Potential for injury related to musculoskeletal impairment, unaccustomed use of appliance

GOAL

Prevent physical injury

INTERVENTIONS

Evaluate environment for possible hazards to mobilization; modify for safety
Instruct child in correct use of crutches or other mobilization assisting device
See also Nursing diagnosis: Impaired physical mobility, p. 437

EXPECTED OUTCOME

Child ambulates without injury

GOAL

Maintain alignment of head of femur in acetabulum

INTERVENTIONS

Supervise application and/or use of
  Non-weight-bearing devices—abduction brace, cast (see p. 443), harness sling
  Abduction-ambulation braces or casts

Instruct child and family regarding what constitutes non-weight-bearing, for example, no standing or kneeling on affected leg
Provide correct traction care, if employed

EXPECTED OUTCOMES

Child demonstrates correct and safe use of immobilizing device
Child and family demonstrate correct application and maintenance of corrective device
Family demonstrates an understanding of correct non-weight-bearing activities
Caregiver demonstrates an understanding of traction care

NURSING DIAGNOSIS: Altered family processes related to child with temporary but extended disability

GOAL

Provide ongoing and follow-up care

INTERVENTIONS

Assist family in coping with the child and therapy
Refer to appropriate health agencies and so on, as indicated by family's needs
Enlist cooperation of school personnel

EXPECTED OUTCOMES

Family copes with child's therapy with little or no difficulty
School personnel support child

NURSING CARE PLAN
THE CHILD WITH OSTEOMYELITIS

Infection of bone

ASSESSMENT

Perform physical assessment

Obtain health history, especially regarding any penetrating wound, surgery, infection elsewhere in body, or physical injury

Observe for manifestations of acute osteomyelitis:

General:
History of trauma to affected bone (frequent)
Child appears very ill
Irritability
Restlessness
Elevated temperature
Rapid pulse
Dehydration

Local:
Tenderness
Increased warmth
Diffuse swelling over involved bone
Involved extremity painful, especially on movement
Involved extremity held in semiflexion
Surrounding muscles tense and resist passive movement

Assist with diagnostic procedures and tests—Radiography, tomography, scintigraphy, blood culture, WBC, erythrocyte sedimentation rate

NURSING DIAGNOSIS: Potential for infection related to presence of organisms, vulnerable tissues

GOAL

Prevent spread of infection and promote healing

INTERVENTIONS

* Administer antibiotics as prescribed
Wound care
  Maintain asepsis
  * Cleanse area as ordered, including irrigation if prescribed
  * Apply appropriate medication, wound packing, and so on, as ordered
  Dress wound according to instructions
Maintain immobilization with
  Positioning
  Devices such as casts, splints, traction (p. 443 and p. 446)
Perform wound irrigations as prescribed

Ensure a nutritious diet
Maintain integrity and sterility of venous access

EXPECTED OUTCOME

Wound heals without complications

NURSING DIAGNOSIS: Pain related to infectious process

See Nursing care plan: The child in pain, p. 279

NURSING DIAGNOSIS: Altered family processes related to a child with an acute illness

See Nursing care plan: The family of the ill or hospitalized child, p. 254

See also Nursing care plan: The child in the hospital, p. 246

---
*Dependent nursing action.

---
*Dependent nursing action.

NURSING CARE PLAN
THE CHILD WITH STRUCTURAL SCOLIOSIS

A lateral curvature of the spine usually associated with a rotary deformity

---

ASSESSMENT

Perform physical assessment

Observe for manifestations of scoliosis (see p. 50)
Assist with diagnostic procedures—Radiography

NURSING DIAGNOSIS: Potential for injury related to unaccustomed brace

GOAL

Prevent injury

INTERVENTIONS

Assess environment for hazards
Teach safety precautions such as using hand rail on stairways and avoiding slippery surfaces
Help develop safe methods of mobilization

EXPECTED OUTCOME

Child remains free of injury related to wearing brace

GOAL

Help child adjust to restricted movement

INTERVENTIONS

Demonstrate alternative modes of accomplishing tasks such as getting in and out of bed, dressing
Help devise alternatives for restricted activities and coping with awkwardness

EXPECTED OUTCOME

Child demonstrates appropriate adaptation to corrective device (specify)

NURSING DIAGNOSIS: Potential impaired skin integrity related to corrective device

GOAL

Prevent skin irritation and breakdown

INTERVENTIONS

Examine skin surfaces in contact with brace for signs of irritation
Implement corrective action to treat or prevent skin breakdown

EXPECTED OUTCOME

Skin remains clean with no evidence of irritation

NURSING DIAGNOSIS: Body image disturbance related to perception of defect in body structure

GOAL

Assist in physical adjustment to appliance

INTERVENTIONS

Attempt to determine source of any discomfort
Refer to orthotist for needed adjustment and service
Assist with plan for personal hygiene
Help in selection of appropriate apparel to wear over brace and footwear to maintain proper balance
Reinforce teaching regarding removal and reapplication of appliance
Investigate any complaints of discomfort

EXPECTED OUTCOMES

Brace fits well and produces no discomfort
Child complies with directions for wear and care of brace
Child is well-groomed and wears attractive attire

GOAL

Promote positive body image

INTERVENTIONS

Encourage child to discuss feelings about wearing brace
Emphasize positive aspects and eventual outcome

EXPECTED OUTCOMES

Child verbalizes feelings and concerns
Child plans in terms of long-range goals as well as short-range ones

See also Nursing care plan: The child with a chronic illness or disability, p. 259

Unit 4

Surgical therapy for structural scoliosis

Harrington instrumentation—Implantation of metal rods by way of clips to hold the vertebrae and bone fragments for permanent fusion; child immobilized on a Stryker frame following surgery

Luque segmental instrumentation—A flexible L-shaped metal rod fixed by wires to the bases of the spinous processes; patient can walk within a few days and no postoperative immobilization necessary

Dwyer instrumentation—A titanium cable through cannulated screws transfixed to each vertebra; child cared for in bed following surgery

Zielke procedure—Combinatin of Harrington and Dwyer procedures

Cotrel-Dubousset procedure—A form of bilateral segmental fixation that uses two knurled rods and multiple hooks

---

ASSESSMENT (Preoperative)

See Nursing care plan: The child undergoing surgery: Preoperative care, p. 267

Assess status of child with progressive traction application

  See Nursing care plan: The child in traction, p. 446

  Assess peripheral nerves both proximally and distay to curvature

  Assess cranial nerves and deep tendon reflexes in extremities

  Assess urinary output

ASSESSMENT (Postoperative)

Perform postoperative assessments of circulation, vital signs, wound

Perform neurologic assessment, especially of extremities

Postoperative care

See Nursing care plan: The child undergoing surgery: Postoperative care, p. 269

NURSING DIAGNOSIS: Potential for injury related to surgery

GOAL

Promote active movement

INTERVENTIONS

Encourage child to exercise by contracting and relaxing thigh and calf muscles periodically

See also Nursing diagnosis: Impaired physical mobility, p. 437

EXPECTED OUTCOME

Child maintains optimum movement of lower extremities

GOAL

Prevent injury to surgical repair

INTERVENTIONS

Place on Stryker frame for care (Harrington instrumentation)

Maintain proper body alignment; avoid twisting movements

Logroll with care when moving child

Keep flat for 12 hours before logrolling (Luque procedure)

  Beginning activity—Have child roll from side-lying to sitting position

Walk slowly with aid of safety belt and walker; unassisted ambulation allowed by sixth day

Assist with physical therapy and range of motion exercises

EXPECTED OUTCOME

Child attains ambulation without injury

GOAL

Prevent abdominal distention (from paralytic ileus)

INTERVENTIONS

* Insert and maintain nasogastric suction

Assess for returning bowel function (e.g., bowel sounds)

EXPECTED OUTCOME

Child exhibits no evidence of bowel distention

NURSING DIAGNOSIS: Pain related to surgical procedure

GOAL

Relieve pain

See Nursing care plan: The child in pain, p. 279

INTERVENTIONS

*Administer opioids around the clock until pain can be controlled with nonopioids

Consider patient-controlled analgesia for child able to follow instructions

NURSING OUTCOME

Child exhibits evidence of only minimum discomfort

---

*Dependent nursing action.

NURSING DIAGNOSIS: Altered patterns of urinary elimination related to surgical procedure, loss of blood, and renal hypoperfusion

GOAL

Faciliate urinary elimination

INTERVENTIONS

*Insert indwelling catheter

EXPECTED OUTCOME

Urinary bladder remains empty

GOAL

Promote urinary output

INTERVENTIONS

Maintain intravenous infusion (see p. 229)

EXPECTED OUTCOME

Child has a sufficient urinary output

─────────

*Dependent nursing action.

NURSING DIAGNOSIS: Impaired physical mobility related to spinal surgery and instrumentation

See Nursing diagnosis: Impaired physical mobility, p. 437

NURSING DIAGNOSIS: Altered family processes related to a child with a physical disability

GOAL

Support family
*Refer family to support groups and agencies

EXPECTED OUTCOME

Family members avail themselves of services

See also:
Nursing care plan: The child in the hospital, p. 246
Nursing care plan: The family of the ill or hospitalized child, p. 254
Nursing care plan: The child with a chronic illness or disability, p. 259

─────────

***National Scoliosis Foundation, Inc.** 93 Concord Ave., P.O. Box 547, Belmont, MA 02178, (617) 489-0880. **Scoliosis Association, Inc.** P.O. Box 51353, Raleigh, NC 27609, (919) 846-2639. Recommended publication: *Scoliosis: A Handbook for Parents.* The book can be purchased by sending $1.00 to the Scoliosis Research Society, 222 S. Prospect, Suite 127, Park Ridge, IL 60068.

Unit 4

NURSING CARE PLAN
THE CHILD WITH JUVENILE RHEUMATOID ARTHRITIS

Inflammatory disease of joints with an unknown inciting agent
Three major disease courses:
Systemic onset—Involves few joints

Pauciarticular—Involves few joints, usually fewer than five
Polyarticular—Simultaneous involvement of four or more joints

ASSESSMENT

Perform physical assessment
Obtain health history, especially regarding symptoms related to illness and joint involvement
Observe for manifestations of juvenile rheumatoid arthritis (JRA):
Involved joints:
　Stiffness
　Swelling
　Tenderness
　Painful to touch or relatively painless
　Warm to touch (seldom red)
　Loss of motion

Characteristic morning stiffness or "gelling" on arising in the morning or after inactivity
Extraarticular manifestations:
　Systemic onset—Fever, malaise, myalgia, rash, pleuritis or pericarditis adenomegaly, splenomegaly, hepatomegaly
　Pauciarticular—Chronic or acute iridocyclitis, mucocutaneous lesions, sacroiliitis
　Polyarticular—Possible low-grade fever, malaise, weight loss, rheumatoid nodules, vasculitis
Assist with diagnostic procedures and tests—WBC, ESR, tests for rheumatoid factors (not usually of value in children), antinuclear antibodies, radiography, joint aspiration

NURSING DIAGNOSIS: Pain related to joint inflammation

See Nursing care plan: The child in pain, p. 279

GOAL

Reduce inflammation

INTERVENTIONS

*Administer anti-inflammatory drugs

EXPECTED OUTCOMES

Child exhibits no evidence of discomfort
Joints indicate no evidence of inflammation

GOAL

Relieve pain

INTERVENTIONS

Provide heat to painful joints by way of
    Tub baths, including whirlpool
    Paraffin baths
    Warm moist pads
    Soaks
Maintain preventive schedule of drug administration
Avoid overexercising painful, swollen joints
See Nursing care plan: The child in pain, p. 279

EXPECTED OUTCOME

Child is able to move with minimum discomfort

NURSING DIAGNOSIS: Impaired physical mobility related to discomfort

GOAL

Preserve joint function

INTERVENTIONS

Carry out or supervise physical therapy regimen
    Muscle strengthening exercises
    Joint mobilization exercises
Apply splints, sandbags, if needed, to maintain position and reduce flexion deformity
Lie flat in bed with joints extended
Use prone position frequently with no pillow, or a very thin one
Incorporate therapeutic exercises in play activities
    Swimming
    Throwing a ball
    Hanging from monkey bar
    Riding tricycle or bicycle
Supervise and encourage activities of daily living
Encourage child's natural tendency to be active

---

*Dependent nursing action

EXPECTED OUTCOMES

Joint flexibility improves in relation to baseline findings
Child develops no contractures
Child engages in activities suitable to his interests, capabilities, and developmental level

NURSING DIAGNOSIS: Bathing/hygiene, dressing/grooming, feeding, toileting self-care deficits related to discomfort, immobility

GOAL

Perform activities of daily living

INTERVENTIONS

Encourage maximum independence
Provide and/or help devise methods to facilitate independent functioning
    Select clothes for convenience in putting on and fastening
    Modify utensils (spoons, toothbrush, comb, and so on) for easier grasp
    Elevate toilet seat, if needed
    Install handrails for convenience and safety (hallways, bathroom)
Teach application of splints (when able) and encourage responsibility for their use

EXPECTED OUTCOME

Child is involved in self-help to maximum capabilities

GOAL

Conserve energy

INTERVENTIONS

Schedule regular periods for sleep and rest, especially during acute flare-ups

EXPECTED OUTCOME

Child engages in appropriate activities with undue fatigue

NURSING DIAGNOSIS: Altered family processes related to a child with a chronic illness

GOAL

Support family

INTERVENTIONS AND EXPECTED OUTCOMES

*Refer family to special support group(s) and agencies

See also Nursing care plan: The child with a chronic illness or disability, p. 259

***Arthritis Foundation** and the **American Juvenile Arthritis Foundation,** 1314 Spring Street, N.W. Atlanta, GA 30309, (404) 872-7100. In Canada, the **Arthritis Society,** 250 Bloor St. East, Suite 401, Toronto, Ontario M4W 2P2.

NURSING CARE PLAN
THE CHILD WITH DUCHENNE MUSCULAR DYSTROPHY

Inherited disorder characterized by gradual degeneration of muscle fibers

ASSESSMENT

Perform physical assessment

Obtain family history, especially regarding evidence of the disorder in relatives

Obtain health history

Observe for manifestations of Duchenne muscular dystrophy:
  Waddling gait
  Lordosis
  Frequent falls
  Gower sign (child turns onto side or abdomen, flexes knees to assume a kneeling position, then with knees extended gradually pushes torso to an upright positin by "walking" the hands up the legs)
  Enlarged muscles (especially thighs and upper arms)

Feel unusually firm or woody on palpation

Later stages
  Profound muscular atrophy

Mental deficiency (common)
  Mild (about 20 IQ points below normal)
  Frank mental deficit present in 25% of cases

Complications
  Contracture deformities of hips, knees, and ankles
  Disuse atrophy
  Obesity

Assess child's physical capabilities

Assist with diagnostic procedures and tests—Serum enzyme measurements (creatine phosphokinase, aldolase, glutamic-oxaloacetic transaminase), electromyography, muscle biopsy

NURSING DIAGNOSIS: Impaired physical mobility related to muscle weakness

GOAL

Promote independent functioning

INTERVENTIONS

Help child and family design a program that affords maximum independence and reduces predictable and preventable disabilities

Help child develop self-help skills (e.g. easily fastened clothing, utensils)
  Modify clothing for wheelchair wear, fit over contracted limbs
  Help family modify the environment to facilitate self-help

Encourage in maintaining outside interests and activities

EXPECTED OUTCOME

Child achieves maximum independence (specify behaviors)

GOAL

Prevent deformities

INTERVENTIONS

Carry out physical therapy program

Help family modify activities during times of illness

Help family acquire needed equipment to promote mobility

EXPECTED OUTCOME

Child's deformity is minimal (specify)

NURSING DIAGNOSIS: Altered family processes related to a child with a disability

GOAL

Support family

INTERVENTIONS

See Nursing diagnosis: Altered family processes, p. 261
*Refer to support groups and special supplementary services and agencies
Refer family to genetic counseling services

EXPECTED OUTCOME

See Nursing diagnosis above
Family becomes involved with support group(s)

NURSING DIAGNOSIS: Anticipatory grieving related to a child with a potentially terminal disability

See Nursing diagnosis: Anticipatory grieving, p. 306

See also:
Nursing care plan: The child with a chronic illness or disability, p. 259
Nursing care plan: The child who is terminally ill or dying, p. 292

*Muscular Dystrophy Association of America, Inc., 810 Seventh Ave., New York, NY 10019, (212) 586-0808. In Canada the Muscular Dystrophy Association of Canada, 150 Eglinton Ave. East, Suite 400, Toronto, Ontario M4P 1E8.

NURSING CARE OF THE CHILD WITH SENSORY OR COGNITIVE IMPAIRMENT

Sensory and cognitive impairment includes problems of children with impaired vision and hearing and children with mental retardation

NURSING CARE PLAN
THE CHILD WITH IMPAIRED VISION

Visual loss that cannot be corrected with regular prescription lenses

Classification of visual impairment:

School vision (partially sighted)—Visual acuity between 20/70 and 20/200

Legal blindness—Visual acuity of 20/200 or less and/or visual field of 20 degrees or less in the better eye

See also Table 4-15

ASSESSMENT

Perform physical assessment with special emphasis on assessment of the eyes (p. 34)

See Vision screening, p. 124

Obtain health history, especially relative to illness or injury that may have contributed to visual impairment; include prenatal history

Obtain family history for diseases or defects with known hereditary predisposition

At birth assess neonate's response to a bright, shiny object; observe for signs associated with congenital blindness

Check for strabismus (lack of binocularity); refer to ophthalmologist for evaluation if malalignment persists past 2 to 3 months of age

Test for visual acuity as soon as child is cooperative (sometimes by age 2 years)

Advise parents of Home Eye Test for Preschoolers, which is available from National Society to Prevent Blindness*

Observe for signs or behaviors that indicate eye problems (see below); include questions regarding behavioral indications of vision impairment in health histories

Assume responsibility as school nurse for follow-up care of children who require corrective lenses or other types of treatments, such as patching

Stress to parents importance of continued periodic eye examinations, since child's eyesight may change significantly in a short period of time.

Observe eye for manifestations of visual impairment:

Congenital blindness

Does not follow a moving light

No orientation response to visual stimuli

Does not initiate eye-to-eye contact with caregiver

Constant nystagmus

Fixed pupils

Marked strabismus

Slow lateral movements

Refractive errors

Rubs eyes excessively

Tilts head or thrusts head forward

Has difficulty in reading or other close work

Holds books close to eyes

Writes or colors with head close to table

Clumsy; walks into objects

Blinks more than usual or is irritable when doing close work

Is unable to see objects clearly

Does poorly in school, especially in subjects that require demonstration, such as arithmetic

Dizziness

Headache

Nausea following close work

Strabismus

Squints eyelids together or frowns

Has difficulty in focusing from one distance to another

Inaccurate judgment in picking up objects

Unable to see print or moving objects clearly

Closes one eye to see

Tilts head to one side

If combined with refractive errors, may see any of above

Diplopia

Photophobia

Dizziness

Headache

Cross-eye

*500 E. Remington Rd., Schaumburg, IL 60173 (800) 331-2020

ASSESSMENT—cont'd

Glaucoma

Mostly seen in acquired types—Loses peripheral vision

May bump into objects that are not directly in front of child

Sees halos around objects

May complain of mild pain or discomfort (severe pain, nausea, vomiting if sudden rise in pressure)

Redness

Excessive tearing (epiphora)

Photophobia

Spasmodic winking (blepharospasm)

Corneal haziness

Enlargement of eyeball (buphthalmos)

Cataract

Gradually less able to see objects clearly

May lose peripheral vision

Nystagmus (with complete blindness)

Gray opacities of lens

Strabismus

Absence of red reflex

NURSING DIAGNOSIS: Altered growth and development related to sensory-perceptual alterations (visual)

GOAL

Promote development and independence

INTERVENTIONS

Provide visual-motor activities for infant (sitting in chair or swing, holding head up, standing, crawling, or grasping for objects)

Provide an environment that fosters familiarity and security; arrange furniture to allow safe ambulation; place identifying markers to denote steps or other dangerous areas

Enroll child in special programs for the blind as soon as possible to learn independent skills, braille reading and writing, and navigational skills (cane method, sighted guide, or guide dog)

Encourage participation in active play

Discuss need for experimenting with active play in safe environment and with other children

EXPECTED OUTCOMES

Infant or child engages in appropriate activities for level of development (specify)

Child demonstrates an attitude of security in the environment

GOAL

Provide opportunities for play/socialization

INTERVENTIONS

Talk to child about the environment

Guide family to selection of play material that encourages motor development and stimulates the sense of hearing and touch

Discuss with family how play for blind children differs from that of sighted children

Encourage family to initiate play activities and teach child how to use toys

Assess adequacy of environmental stimulation if blindisms are present

Use behavior modification to discourage blindisms

Discuss importance of consistent limit setting in helping child learn acceptable behavior and tolerate frustration

Discuss with child's family possible opportunities for socialization

See Nursing diagnosis: Altered growth and development, p. 261

EXPECTED OUTCOME

Parents engage in appropriate activities with the blind child and have realistic expectations for the child

---

NURSING DIAGNOSIS: Altered family processes related to diagnosis of blindness in a child

See Nursing diagnosis: Altered family processes, p. 261

GOAL

Assist family in adjusting to child's loss of sight

INTERVENTIONS

Anticipate the usual grief reactions to loss

Stress to family (and older child) that such feelings are normal and that grief takes time to resolve

Help family gain a realistic concept of child's disability and abilities

Encourage formal rehabilitation as soon as realistically feasible

Assist family in orienting newly blind child to environment and in making immediate surroundings safe to encourage ambulation

Listen to family's concerns regarding the child's visual loss

*Refer to community agencies and support groups

---

*Commissions for the Blind; local schools for the blind; **American Foundation for the Blind, Inc.,** 15 W. 16th St., New York, NY 10011, (212) 620-2000; **National Federation of the Blind,** 1800 Johnson St., Baltimore, MD 21230; **National Association for Parents of the Visually Impaired, Inc.,** P.O. Box 562, Camden, NY, 13316, (315) 245-3442; **National Association for Visually Handicapped,** 22 West 21st St., New York, NY 10010, (212) 889-3141; **American Council of the Blind,** 1010 Vermont Ave., NW, Washington, DC 20005, (800) 424-8666 or (202) 393-3666. In Canada: **Canadian National Institute for the Blind,** 1931 Bayview Ave., Toronto, Ontario, M4G 4C8; **Low Vision Association of Canada,** 145 Adelaide St. West, Toronto, Ontario M5H 3H4; **Blind Organization of Ontario,** 597 Parliament St., Suite B-3, Toronto, Ontario M4X 1W3.

EXPECTED OUTCOMES

Parents express their feelings and concerns regarding loss of sight

Parents demonstrate an understanding of the child's disability and its implications

GOAL

Promote parent-child attachment

INTERVENTIONS

Help parents identify clues other than eye contact from the infant that signify communication with them

Encourage parents to discuss their feelings regarding lack of visual contact or smiling from the child

Stress that lack of such responses is not an indication of child's rejection or dislike of parents

Demonstrate by own example acceptance of the child

Emphasize positive abilities or attributes

Encourage parents in their attempts to promote child's development

EXPECTED OUTCOME

Parents and child exhibit a positive relationship

NURSING DIAGNOSIS: Potential for injury related to environmental hazards, noncompliance with therapeutic plan

---

GOAL

Prevent defects of vision

INTERVENTIONS

Provide prophylactic eye care at birth

Administer oxygen cautiously to premature infant

Periodically screen all children from birth through adolescence for visual impairment

Participate in immunization programs for children

Teach safety regarding common causes of eye injuries

Stress importance of good eye care—use of proper lighting, avoidance of excessive close work, proper rest and nutrition, and yearly eye examinations

See guidelines for preventing eye injuries in box, p. 461, that follows

EXPECTED OUTCOME

Healthy child does not acquire visual defect

GOAL

Prevent complications from eye trauma

INTERVENTIONS

Prevent further injury by instituting appropriate emergency care (see box, p. 461)

Avoid any implication of guilt

Reassure parent and child; avoid giving false reassurance; apprise them of each step of treatment, especially if therapy interferes with vision (patching eyes)

EXPECTED OUTCOME

Child exhibits no evidence of complications

GOAL

Prevent complications from infection

INTERVENTIONS

Teach family correct procedure for instilling ophthalmic preparations (always in conjunctival cul-de-sac); see Home Care Instructions, p. 555

Ensure proper dosage by holding dropper vertically, slowly closing the lids, and having child rotate the eyeball for even distribution

Wipe excess medication for inner canthus outward to prevent contamination of contralateral eye

Emphasize regular administration of drug for entire term of therapy to completely eradicate infection

EXPECTED OUTCOME

Family complies with instructions and performs procedures correctly (specify)

GOAL

Prevent complications of eye defects

INTERVENTIONS

Encourage compliance with corrective therapies

Strabismus:

Discuss with school-age child necessity of patch in preserving vision; allow child to verbalize feelings regarding altered facial appearance; help overcome visual difficulties imposed by seeing with weaker eye (favorable seating in school, large-print books, and additional time to complete assignments)

Teach parents correct procedures for instilling anticholinesterase drugs

Refractive errors:

For secure fit of glasses, use ones with rounded temporal pieces or attach elastic strap to handles and around back of head

Include older child in selection of frames

Encourage parents to compare value of more expensive attractive frames and inducement for wearing them against cost

If glasses are recommended for continuous wearing, discuss possibility of temporary removal for special occasions

Encourage use of protective shields during contact sports

Stress improvement in visual acuity as reason for wearing glasses

Discuss feasibility of contact lenses with selected families

Know procedures for care, insertion, and removal of lens; teach these to parents and older children

EXPECTED OUTCOMES

Child and family comply with therapy and perform procedures correctly

Child wears corrective lenses and cares for equipment correctly

See also Nursing care plan: The child with a chronic illness or disability, p. 259

GUIDELINES FOR PREVENTING EYE INJURIES

Infants and toddlers

Avoid any toys with long pointed handles, such as a pinwheel on a stick

Keep pointed instruments and tools out of reach (e.g., scissors, knives, screwdrivers, rulers, pencils, sticks)

Do not allow child to *walk* or *run* with any pointed object in the hand (e.g., spoon, lollipop, toothbrush)

Keep child away from play of older children and adults that involves projectile activities (throwing a ball, golf, target shooting, swings)

Stress importance of fire safety and poison protection in preventing thermal/chemical burns to eye

Shield child's eyes when in direct sunlight

Preschoolers

Supervise use of sharp or pointed objects, especially scissors

Teach proper use of pointed objects, such as toy guns or scissors, namely, to always point them *away* from their face or from anyone else at close range

Teach child to walk carefully (never run) while carrying any sharp or pointed object

Keep child away from projectile activities

Begin teaching respect for firearms

Avoid playing with mirror where it can reflect sun

School-age children and adolescents

Teach proper use and respect for potentially dangerous equipment such as power tools (flying objects from them), firearms, firecrackers where legally permitted, and racquet sports

Stress use of eye protection when riding motorcycles or using equipment such as power saws or chemistry sets

Teach to open soda bottles with screw cap pointing away from face

Encourage safe use of curling iron

Advise them of danger of excessive sunlight (ultraviolet burns)

Warn to never look directly at the sun even with sunglasses; avoid using mirror in sunlight

Monitor duration of wear of contact lens to prevent corneal scratching and possible scarring

EMERGENCY CARE OF EYE INJURY

Foreign object

Examine eye for presence of a foreign body (evert upper lid to examine upper eye)

Remove a freely movable object with pointed corner of gauze pad lightly moistened with water

Do not irrigate eye or attempt to remove a penetrating object (see below)

Caution child against rubbing eye

Chemical burns

Irrigate eye copiously with tap water for 20 minutes

Evert upper lid to flush thoroughly

Hold child's head with eye under tap of running lukewarm water

Allow child to rest with eyes closed

Keep room darkened

Refer to an ophthalmologist

Ultraviolet burns

If skin is burned, patch both eyes (make sure lids are completely closed); secure dressing with Kling bandages wrapped around head rather than tape

Allow child to rest with eyes closed

Refer to an ophthalmologist

Hematoma ("black eye")

Use a flashlight to check for gross hyphema (visible fluid meniscus across iris; more easily seen in light-colored than brown eyes)

Apply ice for first 24 hours to reduce swelling if no hyphema is present

Refer to an ophthalmologist if hyphema is present

Penetrating injuries

Never remove an object that has penetrated eye

Follow strict aseptic technique in examining eye

Observe for:

    Aqueous or vitreous leaks (fluid leaking from point of penetration)

    Hyphema

    Shape and equality of pupils, reaction to light

    Prolapsed iris (not perfectly circular)

Apply a Fox shield if available (not a regular eye patch)

Maintain bed rest with child in 30-degree Fowler position

Apply patch over unaffected eye to prevent bilateral movement

Caution child against rubbing eye

Refer to ophthalmologist

Unit 4

Table 4-18. TYPES OF VISUAL IMPAIRMENT

Defect	Description	Pathophysiology	Treatment
Refractive errors			
Myopia (near-sightedness)	Ability to see objects clearly at close range but not at a distance	Results from eyeball that is too long, causing image to fall in front of retina	Corrected with biconcave lenses that focus rays on retina
Hyperopia (hypermetropia or farsightedness)	Ability to see objects clearly at a distance Because of accommodative ability, child can usually see objects at all ranges Most children normally hyperopic until about 7 years of age	Results from eyeball that is too short, causing image to focus beyond retina	If correction is required, use convex lenses to focus rays on retina
Astigmatism	Unequal curvatures in refractive apparatus	Results from unequal curvatures in cornea or lens that cause light rays to bend in different directions	Corrected with special lenses that compensate for refractive errors
Anisometropia	Different refractive strengths in each eye	May develop amblyopia as weaker eye is used less	Treated with corrective lenses, preferably contact lenses, to improve vision in each eye so they work as a unit
Amblyopia (lazy eye)	Reduced visual acuity in one eye	Results when one eye does not receive sufficient stimulation Each retina receives different images, resulting in diplopia (double vision) Brain accommodates by suppressing less intense image Visual cortex eventually does not respond to visual stimulation with loss of vision in that eye	Preventable if primary visual defect, such as anisometropia or strabismus, begins before 6 years of age
Strabismus (squint or crosseye)	Malalignment of eyes Esotropia-inward deviation of eye Exotropia-outward deviation of eye	May result from muscle imbalance or paralysis, poor vision, or as congenital defect Since visual axes not parallel, brain receives two images, and amblyopia can result	Treatment depends on cause of strabismus May involve occlusion therapy (patching stronger eye) to increase visual stimulation to weaker eye Early diagnosis essential to prevent vision loss
Cataracts	Opacity of crystalline lens	Prevents light rays from entering eye and refracting them on retina	Requires surgery to remove cloudy lens and replacement of lens (contact or prescription glasses) Must be treated early to prevent blindness from amblyopia
Glaucoma	Increased intraocular pressure	Congenital type results from defective development of some component related to flow of aqueous humor Increased pressure on optic nerve causes eventual atrophy and blindness	Requires surgical treatment (goniotomy) to open outflow tracts May need more than one operation

NURSING CARE PLAN
THE CHILD WITH IMPAIRED HEARING

Classification of complete or partial loss of hearing

Hearing impairment—Disability that may range in severity from mild to profound

Deaf—Hearing disability precludes successful processing of linguistic information through audition, with or without a hearing aid

Hard-of-hearing—Residual hearing, with a hearing aid, sufficient to enable successful processing of linguistic information through audition

Types of hearing loss

Conductive (middle-ear)—Interference with transmission of sound to the middle ear; mainly involves interference with intensity of sound

Sensorineural (perceptive or nerve deafness)—Involves damage to the inner ear structures or consequences of acquired conditions (e.g., infections, ototoxic drugs, exposure to excessive noise); sounds are distorted, severely affecting discrimination and comprehension

Mixed conductive-sensorineural—Interference with transmission of sound in the middle ear and along neural pathways; frequently results from recurrent otitis media and its complications

Central auditory imperception—All hearing losses that do not demonstrate defects in the conductive or sensorineural structures

ASSESSMENT

Perform physical assessment; note any associated anomalies (e.g., low-set ears)

See assessment of the ears p. 36

Obtain family history, especially regarding members with hearing impairment

Prenatal and perinatal history, especially regarding illness or drugs during gestation, type and duration of delivery, Apgar score, hypoxia

Health history, especially regarding immunizations, serious illnesses, seizures, high fever, ototoxic drugs, ear infection

History of responses to auditory stimuli, previous audiometric testing

History of motor development, self-care, adaptive behaviors, socialization, behaviors (e.g., temper tantrums, vibratory stimulation, stubbornness), recent behavioral/personality changes

Observe for manifestations of hearing impairment:

Infants

Lack of startle or blink reflex to a loud sound

Failure to be awakened by loud environmental noises

Failure to localize a source of sound by 6 months of age

Absence of babble or inflections in voice by age 7 months

General indifference to sound

Lack of response to the spoken word; failure to follow verbal directions

Response to loud noises as opposed to the voice

Children

Use of gestures rather than verbalization to express desires, especially after age 15 months

Failure to develop intelligible speech by age 24 months

Monotone quality, unintelligible speech, lessened laughter

Vocal play, head banging, or foot stamping for vibratory sensation

Yelling or screeching to express pelasure, annoyance (tantrums), or need

Asking to have statements repeated or answering them incorrectly

Responding more to facial expression and gestures than verbal explanation

Avoidance of social interaction; often puzzled and unhappy in such situations, prefers to play alone

Inquiring, sometimes confused facial expression

Suspicious alertness, sometimes interpreted as paranoia, alternating with cooperation

Frequently stubborn because of lack of comprehension

Irritable at not making self understood

Shy, timid, and withdrawn

Often appears "dreamy," "in a world of his own," or markedly inattentive

Perform or assist with audiometry testing, auditory evoked potential testing, tympanometry, auditory acuity measurements

Unit 4

Table 4-19. CLASSIFICATION OF HEARING LOSS BASED ON SYMPTOM SEVERITY

Hearing level (dB)	Effect
Slight—<30 (hard of hearing)	Has difficulty in hearing faint or distant speech Usually is unaware of hearing difficulty Likely to achieve in school but may have problems No speech defects
Mild to moderate—30-55 (hard of hearing)	Understands conversational speech at 3 to 5 feet but has difficulty if speech faint or not facing speaker May have speech difficulties
Marked—55-70 (hard of hearing)	Unable to understand conversational speech unless loud Considerable difficulty with group or classroom discussion Requires special speech training
Severe—70-90 (deaf)	May hear a loud voice if nearby May be able to identify loud environmental noises Can distinguish vowels but not most consonants Requires speech training
Profound—>90 (deaf)	May hear only loud sounds Requires extensive speech training

NURSING DIAGNOSIS: Sensory-perceptual alterations (auditory) related to hearing impairment

GOAL

Maximize residual hearing

INTERVENTIONS

Help family investigate reliable hearing aid dealers
Discuss types of hearing aids and their proper care
Teach child how to regulate hearing aid for maximum benefit
Help child focus on all sounds in the environment and talk about them
For older child, discuss methods of camouflaging the aid to make it less conspicuous

EXPECTED OUTCOME

Child acquires and uses hearing aid

NURSING DIAGNOSIS: Impaired verbal communication related to inability to hear auditory cues

GOAL

Promote communication process

INTERVENTIONS

Encourage family to attend the rehabilitation program in order to continue learning in the home; encourage them to learn sign language
Teach language that serves a useful purpose
Encourage use of language and books in the home
Encourage spontaneous language but correct speech impairments

EXPECTED OUTCOMES

Family continues communication practices in the home environment
Family provides stimulation to the child

GOAL

Facilitate lipreading

INTERVENTIONS

Test child for visual problems that may interfere with learning to lipread or use sign language
Teach family and others involved with child (e.g., teacher) behaviors that facilitate lipreading:
    Attract child's attention before speaking; use light touch to signal speaker's presence
    Stand close to child
    Face child directly or move to a 45-degree angle
    Stand still; do not walk back and forth or turn away to point or look elsewhere
    Establish eye contact and show interest
    Speak at eye level and with good lighting on speaker's face
    Be certain nothing interferes with speech patterns, such as chewing food or gum
    Speak clearly and with a slow and even rate
    Use facial expression to assist in conveying messages
    Keep sentences short
    Do not repeat if child does not understand the words; rephrase message

EXPECTED OUTCOMES

Child communicates with others in manner taught (specify)
Persons communicating with child use good communication techniques

NURSING DIAGNOSIS: Altered growth and development related to defective communication

GOAL

Facilitate communication

INTERVENTION

See above

GOAL

Promote independence and development

INTERVENTIONS

Help family transfer normal child-rearing practices to this child
Emphasize importance of attaining independence in self-care
Provide child with devices that foster independence (hearing ear dog, special signaling aids for telephone or door bell)
Discuss importance of discipline and limit setting

EXPECTED OUTCOME

Child performs activities of daily living appropriate to level of development

GOAL

Provide opportunities for play and socialization

INTERVENTIONS

Guide family in selection of toys that maximize visual and tactile senses, as well as residual hearing
Encourage child to participate in group activities
Help child follow group discussion by pointing out the speaker and arranging the group in a semicircle
Help child develop friendships among hearing and deaf peers
Help child achieve a sense of security in ability to compete with peers

EXPECTED OUTCOME

Child engages in activities appropriate to developmental level

GOAL

Encourage education within a regular classroom

INTERVENTIONS

Discuss with teacher ways of communicating effectively with child (such as through facilitating lipreading)
Promote socialization with classmates

EXPECTED OUTCOME

Child attends school regularly

NURSING DIAGNOSIS: Potential for injury related to environmental hazards, infection

GOAL

Prevent hearing loss

INTERVENTIONS

Infancy
  Encourage immunization at appropriate age administration of ototoxic drugs
  Prevent ear infection; detect early
Childhood
  Assess hearing ability of children who are receiving ototoxic antibiotics
  Promote compliance with treatment regimens for otitis media
  Discuss with parents measures to prevent otitis media
  Evaluate auditory ability of children prone to chronic ear or respiratory problems
  Assess sources of excessive noise in child's environment; institute appropriate measures to decrease sound levels (turn music lower, use ear protection)
  Participate in immunization program for children

EXPECTED OUTCOMES

Infant or child does not develop hearing loss
Child is not exposed to excess noise levels
Child is properly immunized

NURSING DIAGNOSIS: Altered family processes related to diagnosis of deafness of a child

GOAL

Assist the family in adjusting to child's loss of hearing

INTERVENTIONS

Anticipate the usual grief reaction to loss
Help family deal with any guilt feelings regarding previous responses to child when true nature of the problem was unknown
Help family realize extent of child's disability and its tremendous influence on speech and language development
Discuss advantages and limitations of amplifying devices with different types of hearing loss
Encourage formal rehabilitation as soon as possible

EXPECTED OUTCOMES

Family expresses feelings and concerns regarding the child's loss of hearing
Family demonstrates an understanding of the implications of hearing loss
Family becomes involved in programs

GOAL

Provide emotional support

Unit 4

INTERVENTIONS

Be available to the family for assistance

Encourage family members to discuss their feelings regarding the disability

Stress child's abilities rather than disability

Become familiar with techniques used for communication if following the family on a long-term basis

*Refer family to appropriate community agencies for medical, psychiatric, educational, vocational, or financial assistance

Involve parents in local parent groups for deaf children

---

*John T. Tracy Clinic, 806 West Adams Blvd., Los Angeles, CA 90007, (213) 748-5481; Alexander Graham Bell Association for the Deaf, 3417 Volta Place, NW, Washington, DC 20007, (202) 337-5220 or (Voice/TTY). American Society of Deaf Children, 814 Thayer Ave., Silver Spring, MD, (301) 585-5400 or (Voice/TDD). In Canada: Canadian Hearing Society, 271 Spadina Rd., Toronto, Ontario M5R 2V3. Information about hearing aids is available from the National Hearing Aid Society, 20361 Middlebelt Rd., Livonia, MI 48152; 1-800-521-5247 (in Michigan, 1-313-478-2610).

EXPECTED OUTCOMES

Family expresses feelings and concerns about the disability and its ramifications

Family members avail themselves of available resources

GOAL

Promote parent-child attachment

INTERVENTIONS

Help family identify clues other than verbal ones that signify infant's communication with them

Encourage family to stimulate child with visual and tactile cues

Stress importance of continuing to talk to child even though child may not hear their voices

EXPECTED OUTCOME

Parents and child demonstrate a positive relationship

See also Nursing care plan: The child with a chronic illness or disability, p. 259

NURSING CARE PLAN
THE CHILD WITH MENTAL RETARDATION

Significant subaverage general functioning existing concurrently with deficits in adaptive behavior and manifested during the developmental period (between conception and age 18 years)*

General intellectual functioning—Results of various individually administered general intelligence tests

Significantly subaverage intellectual functioning—An intelligence quotient (IQ) of approximately 70 or below

Adaptive behavior—Effectiveness or degree with which individuals meet the standards of personal independence and social responsibility expected for age and cultural group

See Table 4-20 for classification of mental retardation

ASSESSMENT

Perform physical assessment

Perform developmental assessment

Obtain family history, especially regarding mental retardation and hereditary disorders in which mental retardation is a feature (e.g., phenylketonuria, tuberous sclerosis, neurofibromatosis)

Obtain health history for evidence of

Prenatal, perinatal, or postnatal trauma or physical injury

Prenatal maternal infection (e.g., rubella) or intoxication (e.g., chronic alcoholism, drug consumption)

Inadequate nutrition

Deprived environment

Psychiatric disorders (e.g., autism)

Infections, especially those involving the brain (e.g., meningitis, encephalitis, measles) or a high body temperature

Assist with diagnostic tests—Chromosome analysis, metabolic dysfunction, radiography, tomography, electroencephalography

Perform or assist with intelligence tests—Stanford-Binet, Wechsler Intelligence Scale for Children

Perform or assist with testing of adaptive behaviors—Vineland Social Maturity Scale, American Association of Mental Retardation Adaptive Behavior Scale

Observe for early manifestations of mental retardation:

Nonresponsiveness to contact

Poor eye contact during feeding

Diminished spontaneous activity

Decreased alertness to voice or movement

Irritability

Slow feeding

---

*American Association on Mental Retardation (AAMR).

Table 4-20. CLASSIFICATION OF MENTAL RETARDATION

Level (IQ)*	Preschool (birth-5 years)— maturation and development	School age (6-21 years)— training and education	Adult (21 years and older)— social and vocational adequacy
Mild—50-55 to approximately 70	Often not noticed as retarded by casual observer but is slower to walk, feed self, and talk than most children; follows same sequence in development as normal children	Can acquire practical skills and useful reading and arithmetic to a third- to sixth-grade level with special education; can be guided toward social conformity; achieves mental age of 8 to 12 years	Can usually achieve social and vocational skills adequate to self-maintenance; may need occasional guidance and support when under unusual social or economic stress; can adjust to marriage but not childrearing
Moderate—35-40 to 50-55	Noticeable delays in motor development, especially in speech; responds to training in various self-help activities	Can learn simple communication, elementary health and safety habits, and simple manual skills; does not progress in functional reading or arithmetic; achieves mental age of 3 to 7 years	Can perform simple tasks under sheltered condition; participates in simple recreation; travels alone in familiar places; usually incapable of self-maintenance
Severe—20-25 to 35-40	Marked delay in motor development; little or no communication skills; may respond to training in elementary self-help, for example, self-feeding	Usually walks, barring specific disability; has some understanding of speech and some response; can profit from systematic habit training; achieves mental age of toddler	Can conform to daily routines and repetitive activities; needs continuing direction and supervision in protective environment
Profound—below 20-25	Gross retardation; minimal capacity for functioning in sensori-motor areas; needs total care	Obvious delays in all areas of development; shows basic emotional responses; may respond to skillful training in use of legs, hands, and jaws; needs close supervision; achieves mental age of young infant	May walk; needs complete custodial care; has primitive speech; usually benefits from regular physical activity

*Based on classification from American Association on Mental Deficiency.

NURSING DIAGNOSIS: Altered growth and development related to impaired cognitive functioning

GOAL

Promote optimum development

INTERVENTIONS

Involve child and family in an early infant stimulation program (Table 4-21)

Assess child's developmental progress at regular intervals; keep detailed records to distinguish subtle changes in functioning

Help family set realistic goals for child

Encourage learning of self-care skills as soon as child achieves readiness

Reinforce self-care activities

Encourage family to investigate special day-care programs and educational classes as soon as possible

Emphasize that child has same needs as other children, e.g., play, discipline, social interaction

Prior to adolescence, counsel child and parents regarding physical maturation, sexual behavior, marriage, and family

Encourage optimum vocational training

EXPECTED OUTCOMES

Child and family are actively involved in infant stimulation program

Family applies concepts and continues activities in home care of child

Child performs activities of daily living at optimum capacity

Family investigates educational programs

Appropriate limit setting, recreation, and social opportunities are provided

Adolescent issues are explored and implemented as appropriate

Unit 4

NURSING DIAGNOSIS: Bathing/hygiene self-care deficit related to cognitive impairment

GOAL

Promote self-care skills

INTERVENTIONS

Provide bathing and hygiene as needed
Encourage child to assist with care to his/her maximum capability
Teach handwashing, teeth brushing, and other hygienic behaviors as early as possible; repeat teaching

EXPECTED OUTCOME

Child assists with bathing and hygienic care to his/her fullest capacity

NURSING DIAGNOSIS: Dressing/grooming self-care deficit related to cognitive impairment

GOAL

Promote self-help

INTERVENTIONS

See Table 4-22 on Infant stimulation program for self-dressing
See Table 4-23 on Infant stimulation program for self-grooming

EXPECTED OUTCOME

Child assists with self-care to his/her maximum potential

NURSING DIAGNOSIS: Feeding self-care deficit related to cognitive impairment

GOAL

Promote self-feeding

INTERVENTIONS

See Table 4-24 on Infant stimulation program for self-feeding

EXPECTED OUTCOME

Child feeds self

NURSING DIAGNOSIS: Toileting self-care deficit related to cognitive impairment

GOAL

Promote self-toileting

INTERVENTIONS

See Table 4-25 on Child stimulation program for self-toileting

EXPECTED OUTCOME

Child manages toileting to his/her optimum capabilities

NURSING DIAGNOSIS: Altered family processes related to having a child with mental retardation

GOAL

Support family at time of diagnosis

INTERVENTIONS

Inform family as soon as possible after birth
Have both parents present at informing conference
Give family written information about the condition, when possible (e.g., a specific syndrome or disease)
Discuss with family members benefits of home care vs institutionalization; allow them opportunities to investigate all residential alternatives before making a decision
Encourage family to meet other families with a similarly affected child
Refrain from giving definitive answers about the degree of retardation; stress the potential learning abilities of retarded children, especially with early stimulation
Demonstrate acceptance of infant through own behavior
Emphasize normal characteristics of child
Encourage family members to express their feelings and concerns

EXPECTED OUTCOMES

Family expresses feelings and concerns regarding the birth of a child with mental retardation and its implications
Family members make realistic decisions based on their needs and capabilities
Family members demonstrate acceptance of child

GOAL

Help family prepare for future care of child

INTERVENTIONS

As child grows older, discuss with parents options to home care, especially as parents near retirement or old age
Help family investigate residential settings other than institutionalization
Encourage family to include affected member in planning and to continue meaningful relationships after placement
Refer to agencies that provide support and assistance

EXPECTED OUTCOMES

Family identifies realistic goals for future care of child
Family avails themselves of supportive services

See also Nursing care plan: The child with a chronic illness or disability, p. 259

Unit 4

Table 4-21. INFANT STIMULATION PROGRAM FOR GROSS MOTOR DEVELOPMENT

Normal age of achievement (months)	Behavior	Activity*
Birth	Assumes flexed position, kicks, has dance reflex	Exercise limbs several times each day Place child in flexed position; encourage movement such as kicking Hold child upright with feet touching a flat surface to stimulate dance reflex
3-4	Holds head erect	Hold child prone; encourage to raise head Place child supine and pull up by arms; encourage to raise head forward Place child in sitting position, hold head erect, gradually release support on sides of head to learn muscle control If child holds head erect, tilt child to one side to learn balance Support child in sitting position with head erect; if head falls forward, attract child's attention to encourage to look up
4-5	Rolls over—prone to supine	Place child prone but slightly lying on one side; place hand on hip and push down while pulling up on the ipsilateral arm; encourage child to push with arm underneath body; gradually encourage child to use free arm to push self over completely
5-6	Rolls over—supine to prone	Place child supine, cross one leg over the other, and gently push child to one side; reduce assistance as child learns to roll alone Roll child over and over
8	Sits up unsupported	Place child in sitting position but supported several times each day Support child in sitting position; gently tilt to one side to learn balance Place child in sitting position with the back against a wall; kneel in front of child and encourage leaning away from the wall to learn balance Sit child on floor with knees in an Indian position; place child's hands on floor to balance self Use same Indian position, kneel down in front of child, and gently push child to one side to practice righting self Sit child on large beach ball with feet flat on the floor; sway child from side to side to regain balance
9-10	Goes from sitting to standing position	Sit child on a low stool or chair with feet firmly placed on floor; place a towel around the chest and gently pull up to standing position; help child sit down again; gradually reduce assistance Place child in crib or playpen and in sitting position; encourage to get up to reach an object
10	Crawls	Place child on abdomen; encourage child to come forward by moving an object away Place child over a large, rolled towel that is high enough to allow hands to rest on the floor; encourage bearing weight on hands; straighten arms to increase weight bearing Use same position but with small towel so that elbows and lower arms rest on floor; encourage to lift up or come forward slightly; press down on child's shoulders to stimulate effort to maintain this position When bearing weight on hands, place rolled towel or beach ball under child's chest to stimulate getting on all fours; gently support around the waist and pull child up; release assistance as bears more weight Lay child across beach ball; roll forward, backward, and to each side to stimulate balance in either direction

Modified from Gregory P: Pediatr Nurs 1(4):23-29, 1975.

*With each activity the parent continues the actual behavior with a verbal command and praises the child for each increment in motor development, as well as for cooperation and/or signs of enjoyment.   *Continued.*

Unit 4

Table 4-21. INFANT STIMULATION PROGRAM FOR GROSS MOTOR DEVELOPMENT—cont'd

Normal age of achievement (months)	Behavior	Activity*
	Stands with support	Play wheelbarrow; hold at hips and let child walk forward on hands; as child bears more weight, hold by feet and let child move forward Encourage "walking like a bear" (last step before walking); stand child upright, support at the hips, and have child lean forward or gently push over to bear weight on hands; encourage to walk in this position and to straighten up If child resists standing, place child upright with back against the wall, grasp the knees, and manually straighten the legs; as child controls legs, reduce the amount of assistance While child is in crib or playpen, place in standing position and holding onto railing While child is in standing position, holding your hands, encourage to bear weight and "jump" up and down
10-12	Stands alone for short periods	With child in standing position, release support for a moment to encourage standing alone
12-14	Walks with support	Hold both of child's hands in front of you and guide in walking; gradually hold only one hand Encourage child to cruise around furniture and push a chair or carriage
14	Walks alone	Place child in standing position in front of you; reach out to child but do not provide support; encourage to walk forward Hold by one hand; release your grasp while child is walking

Table 4-22. INFANT STIMULATION PROGRAM FOR SELF-DRESSING

Normal age of achievement (months)	Behavior	Activity
15	Cooperates by extending arm or leg	Give child verbal directions ("Put your hands over your head") and assist child in procedure; gradually give only verbal command
18	Takes off mittens, hat, or socks	Demonstrate taking off article of clothing; then give only verbal command Use loose-fitting socks
	Unzips	Place child's finger on zipper head; assist to pull it down; gradually reduce assistance until child can do it on verbal command
	Tries to put on shoes	Begin with having child extend foot, put open shoe or slipper in child's hand, and demonstrate getting it over toes; demonstrate how to push foot into shoe and hit the sole with the hand to make sure heel is inside; demonstrate "stepping into" shoes Use oversized shoes at first
21	Undresses	Demonstrate step-by-step procedure, for example, pants: pull down pants to child's ankles, have child pull them off, then pull down to knees, then hips, and last, have child pull them from waist For shirt: unbutton shirt, pull off shoulders and one arm, have child pull off other arm, then pull off shoulders only and have child do both arms

Table 4-22. INFANT STIMULATION PROGRAM FOR SELF-DRESSING—cont'd

Normal age of achievement (months)	Behavior	Activity
24	Removes shoes	Loosen shoes completely; demonstrate taking them off by pushing from heel; take them off partway, have child do rest; gradually have child do it by self Demonstrate untying shoe by placing two beads or bells at the ends of the laces, grasping each, and pulling the bow out; have child first pull one string with parent until gradually can do both un-aided
	Helps in dressing	Use same technique as for learning to cooperate with undressing (15 months) and self-undressing (21 months) Concentrate on putting the clothes on first and fastening them later Sew tabs or colorful appliques on shirts and pants to indicate front or back Practice buttoning with large buttons; use front-fastening clothes

Table 4-23. INFANT STIMULATION PROGRAM FOR SELF-GROOMING

Normal age of achievement (months)	Behavior	Activity
14	Brushes teeth mainly with help	Establish a routine (after each meal and before bedtime) Demonstrate toothbrushing to child on yourself Use small toothbrush with minute amount of pleasant-tasting toothpaste (preferably containing fluoride) Use a mirror for child to observe procedure Place toothbrush in child's hand and assist in brushing Teach child how to rinse toothbrush and mouth
18	Helps with bath	Explain to child what you are doing ("I am washing my face.") Give child washcloth and soap, guide hand to imitate your action; gradually reduce assistance
24	Washes hands with help	Demonstrate procedure Place child by sink with a stool so bowl can be reached easily Regulate water, give child soap, help rub soap on hands, rinse, and dry; gradually reduce assistance
	Helps with washing hair	Place child's hands in hair while lathering scalp; show child the bubbles on hands and use a mirror for child to observe shampooing; as child learns to rub scalp, gradually reduce assistance During rinse, give child a towel to hold over the eyes Give child a large-toothed comb for hair; guide child's hand in learning to comb own hair
30-36	Brushes teeth alone (but with parents' assistance and supervision)	Demonstrate placing paste on toothbrush Encourage child to brush own teeth using "any direction" method Reinforce any previously learned skills Remind child to brush according to set routine Begin visits to the dentist (if not begun sooner)
36	Washes hands alone	Place all utensils within easy reach Regulate water for child (safety measure against burning) Teach child to turn off faucets Reinforce all previously learned skills When child has sense of responsibility concerning danger (hot), teach how to regulate water and check the temperature each time

Unit 4

Table 4-24. INFANT STIMULATION PROGRAM FOR SELF-FEEDING

Normal age of achievement (months)	Behavior	Activity
Birth	Has sucking, rooting, and swallowing reflexes	Gently stroke around child's lips and mouth to stimulate puckering in order to strengthen lip muscles if sucking is weak Maintain in midline and slightly flexed
1	Is able to take food from a spoon	Press spoon on the tongue to stimulate jaw closure; press gently above the thyroid cartilage to stimulate swallowing; after spoon is withdrawn, close the mouth by pushing up on the mandible; wipe excess food from the lips in one stroke to prevent disrupting the normal closing and swallowing sequence Introduce pureed foods of different tastes and textures
4-5	Can approximate cup to lips	Offer small amounts of formula from a cup Place hands on lower jaw to provide better lip closure
5-6	Can use fingers to bring food to mouth	Give child dry toast, zwieback, pretzel, or cracker Dip fingers into food and bring hand to child's lips Place food in child's hand and gradually make child reach for it if not used to voluntarily grasping objects
6-7	Is able to chew solids	Introduce soft foods that require some chewing (cooked carrots, baked meats, baked potato, cheese, and so on) Place a small piece of food on the back molar area to stimulate chewing
8-9	Holds a spoon and plays with it during feeding	Give child a small spoon at feeding time Reinforce any attempts at self-feeding (putting spoon in mouth, in food, and so on) Improvise appropriate utensil if child has difficulty in holding spoon
9	Holds own bottle Finger feeds	Place the bottle in child's hands and bring it to the mouth; gradually release your hand Fill it only partway with milk or use a small (4-ounce) bottle Purchase a special nipple with a straw attached that draws milk from the bottom of the bottle if child is unable to tilt the bottle Give firmly cooked food cut into small pieces
12	Drinks from a cup with much spilling	Give child a cup, beginning with the same procedure as for a bottle
15	Drinks from a cup with less spilling	Use a wide, unbreakable cup with two handles Introduce a straw if child is unable to lift a cup; to initiate sucking liquid up the straw, fill the straw with juice, cover the top end with your finger, place the bottom end in child's mouth, and gradually release your finger to let the fluid in when child makes sucking movements Wean child gradually from one bottle at a time, eliminating the nighttime one last
18	Uses a spoon with much spilling	Give child a spoon, a bowl, and "sticky" food (applesauce or mashed potatoes) Guide child's hand toward the bowl and then into mouth if child is unwilling to feed self; gradually fade out the assistance Anchor the bowel to the table if child has poor motor coordination

Table 4-24. INFANT STIMULATION PROGRAM FOR SELF-FEEDING—cont'd

Normal age of achievement (months)	Behavior	Activity
24	Holds cup in one hand Uses spoon with little spilling	Give a small-diameter cup that is easily grasped with one hand; add small amount of liquid
36	Begins to use fork; holds it in fist	Give a small-handled and short-pronged fork Guide the hand to pierce the food if child is reluctant
48	Eats with fork held with fingers	Continue encouraging use of fork
72-84	Uses knife	Encourage "spreading" with knife, followed by cutting tender foods Introduce knife and fork cutting

Table 4-25. CHILD STIMULATION PROGRAM FOR SELF-TOILETING

Normal age of achievement (years)	Behavior	Activity

1-2½	Is able to
	  Sit unsupported
	  Walk and stand alone
	  Walk alone backward/forward
	  Balance well
	  Climb onto a chair
	  Retain urine for at least 2 hours
		Assess physical behaviors that indicate readiness for training; begin after most signs are evident
		Begin bowel training before bladder training
		Record approximate schedule of evacuation
		Place on potty-chair at regular intervals (upon awakening, after meals, before bedtime)
		Stay with child while on potty-chair (usually 5-20 minutes)
		Keep potty-chair in bathroom
		Use training pants rather than diapers; whenever possible, leave diapers off child to experienced feeling of voiding without clothing

	Recognizes urge to let go and hold on Is able to communicate this sensation to parent Has desire to please parent by voluntarily controlling elimination	Assess psychologic readiness for toileting Point out when diapers are wet or dry Use consistent words or gestures to indicate need for elimination Praise for success Avoid punishment or excessive pressure
3 (may be as long as 5 years)	Stays dry during night	Take to toilet just before bedtime Do not offer excessive fluids before bedtime
	Seats self on toilet	When child is trained, gradually reduce use of potty-chair for regular toilet If needed, keep small stool by toilet for climbing onto seat (sitting with legs facing tank reduces feeling of "falling in")
3-3½	Voids standing up (male)	Use imitation of watching father (or other male) Provide small stool for easy access to toilet May need to direct stream initially
	Washes/dries hands with supervision	Turn on faucets for child; provide small stool Make hygiene routine part of toileting

Continued.

Unit 4

Table 4-25. CHILD STIMULATION PROGRAM FOR SELF-TOILETING—cont'd

Normal age of achievement (years)	Behavior	Activity
3½-4	Attempts to wipe self but is unsuccessful	Offer toilet paper Teach correct procedure from front to back
	Undresses/dresses self	Uses clothing that is easy to manage (elastic waist pants, dress)
	Flushes toilet	Remind to flush toilet after elimination
	Completely cares for self at toilet, including wiping and handwashing	Encourage independence

NURSING CARE PLAN
THE CHILD WITH DOWN SYNDROME

A congenital defect characterized by varying degrees of mental retardation and associated physical defects

Also known as Trisomy 21

ASSESSMENT

Perform physical assessment

Perform developmental assessment

Obtain family history, especially relative to mother's age or any similarly affected child in the family

Observe for manifestations of Down syndrome:

Physical Characteristics (most frequently observed)

Small rounded skull with a flat occiput

Inner epicanthal folds and oblique palpebral fissures (upward, outward slant of the eyes)

Small nose with a depressed bridge (saddle nose)

Protruding, sometimes fissured, tongue

Hypoplastic mandible (makes tongue appear large)

High-arched palate

Short, thick neck

Hypotonic musculature (protruding abdomen, umbilical hernia)

Hyperflexible and lax joints

Simian line (transverse crease on the palmar side of the hand; see Fig. 1-7, p. 30)

Broad, short, and stubby hands and feet

Intelligence

Varies from severely retarded to low normal intelligence

Generally within mild to moderate range

Social Development

May be 2 to 3 years beyond mental age, especially during early childhood

Congenital Anomalies (increased incidence)

Most common is congenital heart disease

Other defects include:

Renal agenesis

Duodenal atresia

Hirschsprung disease

Tracheoesophageal fistula

Hip subluxation

Instability of the first and second cervical vertebrae (atlantoaxial instability)

Sensory Problems (frequently associated)

Conductive hearing loss (very common)

Strabismus *eyes crossed*

Myopia *nearsighted*

Nystagmus *involuntary rhythmic movements of eyes*

Cataracts

Conjunctivitis

Growth and Sexual Development

Growth in both height and weight reduced; obesity common

Sexual development delayed, incomplete, or both

Males infertile; females can be fertile

Premature aging common; lowered life expectancy

Assist with diagnostic tests—Chromosome analysis

Unit 4

NURSING DIAGNOSIS: Potential for infection related to hypotonia, increased susceptibility to respiratory infection

GOAL

Prevent respiratory infection

INTERVENTIONS

Teach the parents postural drainage and percussion
Stress importance of changing child's position frequently, especially sitting posture
Encourage use of cool-mist vaporizer
Teach suctioning of nares
Stress importance of good mouth care (follow feedings with clear water)

EXPECTED OUTCOME

Child exhibits no evidence of infection or respiratory distress

NURSING DIAGNOSIS: Impaired swallowing related to hypotonia, large tongue, cognitive impairment

GOAL

Minimize feeding difficulties in infancy

INTERVENTIONS

Suction nares before each feeding
Schedule small frequent feedings; allow child to rest during feedings
Feed solid food by pushing it to back and side of mouth; use long, straight-handled infant spoon
Point out to family that tongue thrust does not indicate refusal of food
Calculate caloric needs to meet energy requirements; base intake on height and weight, not chronologic age
Monitor height and weight at regular intervals
Provide sufficient fiber and fluids to prevent constipation

EXPECTED OUTCOMES

Infant consumes an adequate amount of food for age and size (specify)
Family reports satisfactory feeding
Infant gains weight in accordance with standard weight tables

NURSING DIAGNOSIS: Altered family processes related to having a child with Down syndrome

See Nursing care plan: The child with mental retardation, p. 466
See Nursing care plan: The child with a chronic illness or disability, p. 259

GOAL

Prepare family for care of asssociated defect(s) (specify)

INTERVENTIONS

See Nursing care plan: The child with congenital heart disease, p. 365
See Nursing care plan: The child with acute respiratory infection, p. 318
*Refer family to community agencies and support groups

EXPECTED OUTCOME

Family is able to cope with the care needed by the specific health problem (specify)

GOAL

Provide support

INTERVENTIONS

Refer to genetic counseling services if indicated and/or desired
Refer to organizations and parent groups designed for families with Down syndrome

EXPECTED OUTCOME

Family avails themselves of support groups

NURSING DIAGNOSIS: Potential for injury (physical) related to parental age factors

GOAL

Prevent Down syndrome

INTERVENTIONS

Discuss with high-risk women risks of giving birth to child with Down syndrome
Encourage all pregnant women at risk (over age 35, family history of Down syndrome, or previous birth of child with Down syndrome) to consider amniocentesis during twelfth to sixteenth week of pregnancy to rule out Down syndrome in fetus
Discuss option of elective abortion with women who are carrying an affected fetus
Discuss with parents of adolescent children with Down syndrome the possibility of conception in a female and the need for contraceptive methods

EXPECTED OUTCOMES

Pregnant women at risk seek evaluation for Down syndrome
Families demonstrate an understanding of options available to them
Families of an affected female child seek contraceptive advice

*__National Down Syndrome Society,__ 141 Fifth Ave., Suite 75, New York, NY 10010 (1-800-221-4602) or (212) 460-9330; __National Down Syndrome Congress,__ 1800 Dempster, Park Ridge, IL 60068 (1-800-232-6372) or (312) 823-7550; __Association for Children with Down Syndrome, Inc.,__ 2616 Martin Ave., Bellmore, Long Island, NY 11710, (516) 221-4700.

Unit 4

NURSING CARE OF THE CHILD WITH A COMMUNICABLE DISEASE

Any disease transmitted from one person or animal to another person directly by contact with body substances of affected persons, or indirectly via substances or inanimate objects, or via vectors

NURSING CARE PLAN
*THE CHILD WITH A COMMUNICABLE DISEASE**

An illness caused by a specific infectious agent or its toxic products through a direct or indirect mode of transmission of that agent from a reservoir

ASSESSMENT

Perform physical assessment
Obtain history of exposure to disease and history of current illness
Observe for manifestations characteristic of each disease:
Type, configuration, and distribution of lesions
Type and characteristics of associated manifestations

See Table 4-26, which describes the major communicable diseases of childhood
Assist with diagnostic procedures—Collection of specimens

*Nursing care plan: The child with pediculosis capitis, p. 495
Selected bacterial infections, p. 498

NURSING DIAGNOSIS: Potential for infection related to susceptible host and infectious agents

GOAL

Prevent disease

INTERVENTIONS

Operate under a high index of suspicion for children who are susceptible to infectious diseases
Identify high-risk children to whom communicable disease may be fatal; in case of an outbreak, advise parents to confine child to the home
Participate in public education regarding prophylactic immunizations, method of spread of communicable diseases, proper preparation and handling of food and water supplies, and control of animal vectors in regard to reservoirs of disease (not a factor in childhood communicable disease but in other infectious illness such as malaria)
Participate in immunization programs or screening programs to identify streptococcal infections

EXPECTED OUTCOME

Susceptible children do not contract the disease

GOAL

Prevent spread of disease

INTERVENTIONS

Institute appropriate precautions (see p. 291)
Make referral to public health nurse when necessary to ensure appropriate procedures in the home
Work with families to ensure compliance with therapeutic regimens
Identify close contacts who may require prophylactic treatment (specific immune globulin or antibiotics)
Report disease to local health department

EXPECTED OUTCOME

Infection remains confined to original source

GOAL

Prevent complications

INTERVENTIONS

Ensure compliance with therapeutic regimen (bed rest, antibiotics, adequate hydration)
Institute seizure precautions if febrile convulsions are a possibility

Monitor temperature; unexpected elevations may signal an infection

Attend to good body hygiene

Ensure adequate hydration with small frequent sips of water or favorite drinks and soft, bland foods (gelatin, pudding, ice cream, soups); feed again after vomiting; observe for signs of hydration

EXPECTED OUTCOME

Child exhibits no evidence of complications such as infection or dehydration

---

NURSING DIAGNOSIS: Potential impaired skin integrity related to child's propensity to scratch

GOAL

Prevent scratching

INTERVENTIONS

Keep nails short and clean

Apply mittens or elbow restraints

Dress in lightweight, loose, and nonirritating clothing

Cover affected areas (long sleeves, pants, one-piece outfit)

Bathe in cool water with no soap or apply cool compresses

Apply soothing lotions

Avoid exposure to heat or sun

EXPECTED OUTCOME

Skin remains intact

NURSING DIAGNOSIS: Pain related to skin lesions, malaise

GOAL

Relieve discomfort

INTERVENTIONS

Keep mucous membranes moist with use of cool-mist vaporizer, gargles, and lozenges

Apply petrolatum to chapped lips or nares

Cleanse eyes with physiologic saline solution

Keep skin clean (change bedclothes and linens at least daily)

Administer oral hygiene

Assess need for pain medication (p. 279)

Employ nonpharmacologic pain reduction techniques (p. 286)

*Administer analgesics, antipyretics and antipruritic medication as needed

EXPECTED OUTCOMES

Skin and mucous membranes are clean and free of irritants

Child exhibits minimal evidence of discomfort (specify)

---

*Dependent nursing action.

NURSING DIAGNOSIS: Impaired social interaction related to isolation from peers

GOAL

Prepare child for restriction of activities

INTERVENTIONS

Explain reason for confinement and use of any special precautions

Allow child to play with gloves, mask, and gown (if used)

EXPECTED OUTCOME

Child demonstrates understanding of restrictions

GOAL

Promote social interaction

INTERVENTIONS

Always introduce self to child; allow to see face before donning protective clothing, if required

Provide diversionary activity

Encourage parents to remain with child during hospitalization

Help child view restrictions as challenging rather than a solely negative experience

Encourage contact with friends via telephone (in hospital can use intercom between room and nurse's station)

EXPECTED OUTCOME

Child engages in suitable activities and interactions

NURSING DIAGNOSIS: Altered family processes related to child with an acute illness

GOAL

Provide emotional support

INTERVENTIONS

Reinforce family's effort to carry out plan of care

Provide assistance when necessary, such as visiting nurse to help with home care

Keep family aware of child's progress

Stress rapidity of recovery in most cases

Prepare child's peers for altered physical appearance, such as with chickenpox

EXPECTED OUTCOMES

Family continues to comply with expectations

Peers accept child

Unit 4

Table 4-26. COMMUNICABLE DISEASES OF CHILDHOOD

Unit 4

Disease

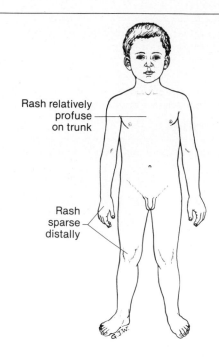

Rash relatively profuse on trunk

Rash sparse distally

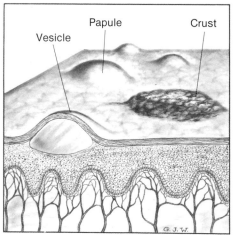

Vesicle   Papule   Crust

CHICKENPOX
Agent: varicella zoster
Source: primary secretions of respiratory tract of infected persons; to a lesser degree skin lesions (scabs not infectious)
Transmission: direct contact, droplet spread, and contaminated objects
Incubation period: 2 to 3 weeks, commonly 13 to 17 days
Period of communicability: probably 1 day before eruption of lesions (prodromal period) to 6 days after first crop of vesicles when crusts have formed

DIPHTHERIA
Agent: *Corynebacterium diphtheriae*
Source: discharges from mucous membranes of nose and nasopharynx, skin, and other lesions of infected person
Transmission: direct contact with infected person, a carrier, or contaminated articles
Incubation period: usually 2 to 5 days, possibly longer
Period of communicability: variable; until virulent bacilli are no longer present (identified by three negative cultures); usually 2 weeks but as long as 4 weeks

ERYTHEMA INFECTIOSUM (FIFTH DISEASE)
Agent: parovirus B19 (PV)
Source: infected persons
Transmission: Unknown; possibly respiratory secretions and blood
Incubation period: 6 to 14 days, maybe as long as 20 days
Period of communicability: uncertain; most outbreaks subside in 1 to 2 months

EXANTHEMA SUBITUM (ROSEOLA)
Agent: probably virus
Source: unknown
Transmission: unknown (virtually limited to children between 6 months and 2 years of age)
Incubation period: unknown
Period of communicability: unknown

Clinical manifestations	Therapeutic management/complications	Nursing considerations

Prodromal stage: slight fever, malaise, and anorexia for first 24 hours; rash highly pruritic; begins as macule, rapidly progresses to papule and then vesicle (surrounded by erythematous base, becomes umbilicated and cloudy, breaks easily and forms crusts); all three stages (papule, vesicle, crust) present in varying degrees at one time
Distribution: centripetal, spreading to face and proximal extremities but sparse on distal limbs
Constitutional signs and symptoms: elevated temperature from lymphadenopathy, irritability from pruritus
	Specific: none
	Supportive: Diphenhydramine hydrochloride or antihistamines to relieve itching; skin care to prevent secondary bacterial infection
	Complications:
	  Secondary bacterial infections (abscesses, cellulitis, pneumonia, sepsis)
	  Encephalitis
	  Varicella pneumonia
	  Hemorrhagic varicella (tiny hemorrhages in the vesicles and numerous petechiae in the skin)
	  Reye syndrome (possibly related to aspirin)
		Maintain *strict* isolation in hospital
		Isolate child in home until vesicles have dried (usually 1 week after onset of disease) and isolate high-risk children from infected children
		Administer skin care: give bath and change clothes and linens daily; administer topical application of calamine lotion; keep child's fingernails short and clean; apply mittens if child scratches
		Lessen pruritus; keep child occupied
		Remove loose crusts that rub and irritate skin
		Teach child to apply pressure to pruritic area rather than scratch it
		If older child, reason with child regarding danger of scar formation from scratching
		Avoid use of aspirin

Varies according to anatomic location of pseudomembrane
Nasal: resembles common cold, serosanguineous mucopurulent nasal discharge without constitutional symptoms; may be frank epistaxis
Tonsillar/pharyngeal: malaise; anorexia; sore throat; low-grade fever; pulse increased above expected for temperature within 24 hours; smooth, adherent, white or gray membrane; lymphadenitis possibly pronounced (bull's neck); in severe cases, toxemia, septic shock, and death within 6 to 10 days
Laryngeal: fever, hoarseness, cough, with or without previous signs listed; potential airway obstruction, apprehensive, dyspneic retractions, cyanosis
	Antitoxin (usually intravenously); preceded by skin or conjunctival test to rule out sensitivity to horse serum
	Antibiotics (penicillin or erythromycin)
	Complete bed rest (prevention of myocarditis)
	Tracheostomy for airway obstruction
	Treatment of infected contacts and carriers
	Complications:
	  Myocarditis (second week)
	  Neuritis
		Maintain *strict* isolation in hospital
		Participate in sensitivity testing; have epinephrine available
		Administer antibiotics; observe for signs of sensitivity to penicillin
		Administer *complete* care to maintain bed rest
		Use suctioning as needed
		Regulate humidity for optimum liquefaction of secretions
		Observe respirations for signs of obstruction

Rash appears in three stages:
I—erythema on face, chiefly on cheeks, "slapped face" appearance; disappears by 1 to 4 days
II—about 1 day after rash appears on face, maculopapular red spots appear, symmetrically distributed on upper and lower extremities; rash progresses from proximal to distal surfaces and may last a week or more
III—rash subsides but reappears if skin is irritated or traumatized (sun, heat, cold, friction)
	None necessary
	Complications:
	  Self-limited arthritis and arthralgia
	  May result in fetal death if mother infected during pregnancy
		Reassure parents regarding benign nature of condition in affected child
		Precautions for infected pregnant women of child not necessary
		Place hospitalized child (immunosuppressed or with aplastic crises) suspected of PV infection on respiratory and contact isolation
		Pregnant women: need not be excluded from work-place where PV infection; should not care for patients with aplastic crises; low risk of fetal death to those in contact with affected children

Persistent high fever for 3 to 4 days in child who appears well Precipitous drop in fever to normal with appearance of rash **Rash:** discrete rose-pink macules or maculopapules appearing first on trunk, then spreading to neck, face, and extremities; nonpruritic, fades on pressure, lasts 1 to 2 days **Associated signs and symptoms:** cervical/postauricular lymphadenopathy, injected pharynx, cough, coryza	Non specific Antipyretics to control fever Anticonvulsives for child with history of febrile seizures **Complications:** Febrile seizures	Teach parents measures for lowering temperature (antipyretic drugs) If child is prone to seizures, discuss appropriate precautions Reassure parents regarding benign nature of illness

Continued.

Table 4-26. COMMUNICABLE DISEASES OF CHILDHOOD—cont'd

Disease

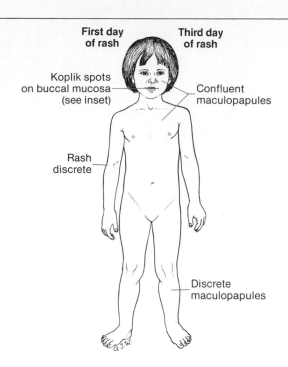

First day of rash · Third day of rash

Koplik spots on buccal mucosa (see inset)

Confluent maculopapules

Rash discrete

Discrete maculopapules

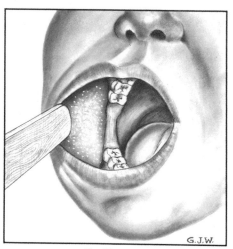

Koplik spots

MEASLES (RUBEOLA)

Agent: virus

Source: respiratory tract secretions, blood, and urine of infected person

Transmission: usually by direct contact with droplets of infected person

Incubation period: 10 to 20 days

Period of communicability: from 4 days before to 5 days after rash appears but mainly during prodromal (catarrhal) stage

MUMPS

Agent: virus

Source: saliva of infected persons

Transmission: direct contact with or droplet spread from an infected person

Incubation period: 14 to 21 days

Period of communicability: most communicable immediately before and after swelling begins

PERTUSSIS (WHOOPING COUGH)

Agent: *Bordetella pertussis*

Source: discharge from respiratory tract of infected persons

Transmission: direct contact or droplet spread from infected person; indirect contact with freshly contaminated articles

Incubation period: 5 to 21 days, usually 10

Period of communicability: greatest during catarrhal stage before onset of paroxysms and may extend to fourth week after onset of paroxysms

Clinical manifestations	Therapeutic management/complications	Nursing considerations
Prodromal (catarrhal) stage: fever and malaise, followed in 24 hours by coryza, cough, conjunctivitis, Koplik spots (small, irregular red spots with a minute, bluish white center first seen on the buccal mucosa opposite the molars 2 days before rash; symptoms gradually increase in severity until second day after rash appears, when they begin to subside **Rash:** appears 3 to 4 days after onset of prodromal stage, begins as erythematous maculopapular eruption on face and gradually spreads downward; more severe in earlier sites (appears confluent) and less intense in later sites (appears discrete); after 3 to 4 days assumes brownish appearance, and fine desquamation occurs over areas of extensive involvement **Constitutional signs and symptoms:** anorexia, malaise, generalized lymphadenopathy	**Supportive:** bed rest during febrile period; antipyretics Antibiotics to prevent secondary bacterial infection in high-risk children **Complications:** Otitis media Pneumonia Bronchiolitis Obstructive laryngitis and laryngotracheitis Encephalitis	Isolation until fifth day of rash; if hospitalized, institute respiratory precautions Maintain bed rest during prodromal stage; provide quiet activity **Fever:** instruct parents to administer antipyretics; avoid chilling; if child is prone to seizures, institute appropriate precautions (fever spikes to 40° C [104° F] between fourth and fifth days) **Eye care:** dim lights if photophobia present; clean eyelids with warm saline solution to remove secretions or crusts; keep child from rubbing eyes; examine cornea for signs of ulceration **Coryza/cough:** use cool mist vaporizer; protect skin around nares with layer of petrolatum; encourage fluids and soft bland foods **Skin care:** keep skin clean; use tepid baths as necessary
Prodromal stage: fever, headache, malaise, and anorexia for 24 hours, followed by "earache" that is aggravated by chewing **Parotitis:** by third day, parotid gland(s) (either unilateral or bilateral) enlarges and reaches maximum size in 1 to 3 days; accompanied by pain and tenderness **Other manifestations:** submaxillary and sublingual infection, orchitis, and meningoencephalitis	**Symptomatic and supportive:** analgesics for pain and antipyretics for fever Intravenous fluid may be necessary for child who refuses to drink or vomits because of meningoencephalitis **Complications:** Sensorineural deafness Postinfectious encephalitis Myocarditis Arthritis Hepatitis Epididymo-orchitis Sterility (extremely rare in adult males)	Isolation during period of communicability; institute respiratory precautions during hospitalization Maintain bed rest during prodromal phase until swelling subsides Give analgesics for pain; if child is unwilling to chew medication, use elixir form Encourage fluids and soft, bland foods; avoid foods requiring chewing Apply hot or cold compresses to neck, whichever is more comforting To relieve orchitis, provide warmth and local support by means of tight-fitting underpants (stretch bathing suit works well)
Catarrhal stage: begins with symptoms of upper respiratory infection, such as coryza, sneezing, lacrimation, cough, and low-grade fever; symptoms continue for 1 to 2 weeks, when dry, hacking cough becomes more severe **Paroxysmal stage:** cough that most commonly occurs at night consists of a series of short, rapid coughs followed by a sudden inspiration that is associated with a high-pitched crowing sound or "whoop"; during paroxysms cheeks become flushed or cyanotic, eyes bulge, and tongue protrudes; paroxysm may continue until a thick mucous plug is dislodged; vomiting frequently follows an attack; stage generally lasts 4 to 6 weeks, followed by convalescent stage	Antimicrobial therapy (such as erythromycin) Administration of pertussis-immune globulin **Supportive treatment:** hospitalization required for infants, children who are dehydrated, or those who have complications Bed rest Increased oxygen intake and humidity Adequate fluids Intubation possibly necessary **Complications:** Pneumonia (usual cause of death) Atelectasis Otitis media Convulsions Hemorrhage (subarachnoid, subconjunctival, epistaxis) Weight loss and dehydration Hernia Prolapsed rectum	Isolation during catarrhal stage; if hospitalized, institute respiratory precautions Maintain bed rest as long as fever is present Keep child occupied during the day (interest in play is associated with fewer paroxysms) Reassure parents during frightening episodes of whooping cough Provide restful environment and reduce factors that promote paroxysms (dust, smoke, sudden change in temperature, chilling, activity, excitement); keep room well ventilated Encourage fluids; offer small amount of fluids frequently; refeed child after vomiting Keep child in Croupette with high humidity; suction gently but often to prevent choking on secretions Observe for signs of airway obstruction (increased restlessness, apprehension, retractions, cyanosis) Involve public health nurse if child is cared for at home

Unit 4

Continued.

Table 4-26. COMMUNICABLE DISEASES OF CHILDHOOD—cont'd

Disease

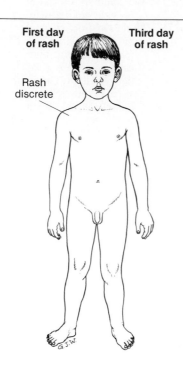

First day
of rash

Third day
of rash

Rash
discrete

POLIOMYELITIS

Agent: enteroviruses, 3 types; type 1—most frequent cause of paralysis, both epidemic and endemic, type 2—least frequently associated with paralysis, type 3—second most frequent in association with paralysis

Source: feces and oropharyngeal secretions of infected persons, especially young children

Transmission: direct contact with persons with apparent or inapparent active infection; spread is via fecal-oral and pharyngeal-oropharyngeal routes

Incubation period: usually 7 to 14 days, with range of 5 to 35 days

Period of communicability: not exactly known; virus is present in throat and feces shortly after infection and persists for about 1 week in throat and 4 to 6 weeks on feces

RUBELLA (GERMAN MEASLES)

Agent: virus

Source: primarily nasopharyngeal secretions of person with apparent or inapparent infection; virus also present in blood, stool, and urine

Transmission: direct contact and spread via infected person; indirectly via articles freshly contaminated with nasopharyngeal secretions, feces, or urine

Incubation period: 14 to 21 days

Period of communicability: 7 days before to about 5 days after appearance of rash

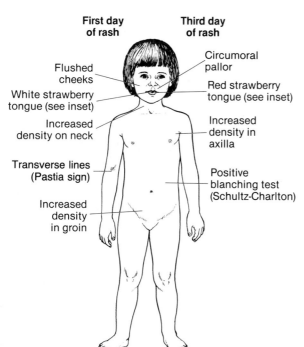

First day
of rash

Third day
of rash

Flushed
cheeks

Circumoral
pallor

White strawberry
tongue (see inset)

Red strawberry
tongue (see inset)

Increased
density on neck

Increased
density in
axilla

Transverse lines
(Pastia sign)

Positive
blanching test
(Schultz-Charlton)

Increased
density
in groin

SCARLET FEVER

Agent: group A β-hemolytic streptococci

Source: usually from nasopharyngeal secretions of infected persons and carriers

Transmission: direct contact with infected person or droplet spread; indirectly by contact with contaminated articles, ingestion of contaminated milk or other food

Incubation period: 2 to 4 days, with range of 1 to 7 days

Period of communicability: during incubation period and clinical illness approximately 10 days; during first 2 weeks of carrier phase, although may persist for months

First day

Third day

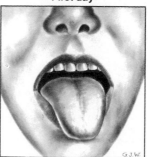

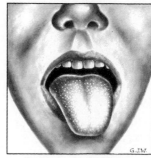

White strawberry tongue

Red strawberry tongue

Clinical manifestations	Therapeutic management/complications	Nursing considerations

May be manifest in three different forms:
Abortive or inapparent—fever, uneasiness, sore throat, headache, anorexia, vomiting, abdominal pain; lasts a few hours to a few days
Nonparalytic—same manifestations as abortive but more severe, with pain and stiffness in neck, back, and legs
Paralytic—initial course similar to nonparalytic type, followed by recovery and then signs of central nervous system paralysis
	No specific treatment, including antimicrobials or gamma globulin
	Complete bed rest during acute phase
	Assisted respiratory ventilation in case of respiratory paralysis
	Physical therapy for muscles following acute stage
	Complications:
	  Permanent paralysis
	  Respiratory arrest
	  Hypertension
	  Kidney stones from demineralization of bone during prolonged immobility
		Maintain complete bed rest
		Administer mild sedatives as necessary to relieve anxiety and promote rest
		Participate in physiotherapy procedures (use of moist hot packs and range of motion exercises)
		Position child to maintain body alignment and prevent contractures or decubiti; use footboard
		Encourage child to move; administer analgesics for maximum comfort during physical activity
		Observe for respiratory paralysis (difficulty in talking, ineffective cough, inability to hold breath, shallow and rapid respirations); report such signs and symptoms to physician; have tracheostomy tray at bedside

Prodromal stage: absent in children, present in adults and adolescents; consists of low-grade fever, headache, malaise, anorexia, mild conjunctivitis, coryza, sore throat, cough, and lymphadenopathy; lasts for 1 to 5 days, subsides 1 day after appearance of rash **Rash:** first appears on face and rapidly spreads downward to neck, arms, trunk, and legs; by end of first day body is covered with a discrete, pinkish red maculopapular exanthema; disappears in same order as it began and is usually gone by third day **Constitutional signs and symptoms:** occasionally low-grade fever, headache, malaise, and lymphadenopathy	No treatment necessary other than antipyretics for low-grade fever and analgesics for discomfort **Complications:** Rare (arthritis, encephalitis, or purpura); most benign of all childhood communicable diseases; greatest danger is teratogenic effect on fetus	Reassure parents of benign nature of illness Employ comfort measures as necessary Isolate child from pregnant women

Prodromal stage: abrupt high fever, pulse increased out of proportion to fever, vomiting, headache, chills, malaise, abdominal pain
Enanthema: tonsils enlarged, edematous, reddened, and covered with patches of exudate; in severe cases appearance resembles membrane seen in diphtheria; pharynx is edematous and beefy red; during first 1 to 2 days tongue is coated and papillae become red and swollen (white strawberry tongue); by the fourth or fifth day white coat sloughs off, leaving prominent papillae (red strawberry tongue); palate is covered with erythematous punctate lesions
Exanthema: rash appears within 12 hours after prodromal signs; red pinhead-sized punctate lesions rapidly become generalized but are absent on the face, which becomes flushed; rash is more intense in folds of joints; by end of the first week desquamation begins, which may be complete by 3 weeks or longer
	Treatment of choice is a full course of penicillin (or erythromycin in penicillin-sensitive children); fever should subside 24 hours after beginning therapy
	Antibiotic therapy for newly diagnosed carriers (nose or throat cultures positive for streptococci)
	Supportive measures: bed rest during febrile phase, analgesics for sore throat
	Complications:
	  Otitis media
	  Peritonsillar abscess
	  Sinusitis
	  Rheumatic fever
	  Glomerulonephritis
		Institue respiratory precautions until 24 hours after initiation of treatment
		Ensure compliance with oral antibiotic therapy (intramuscular benzathine penicillin G [Bicillin] may be given if parents' reliability in giving oral drugs is questionable)
		Maintain bed rest during febrile phase; provide quiet activity during convalescent period
		Relieve discomfort of sore throat with analgesics, gargles, lozenges, antiseptic throat sprays (Chloraseptic), and inhalation of cool mist
		Encourage fluids during febrile phase; avoid irritating liquids (citrus juices) or rough foods; when child is able to eat, begin with soft diet
		Advise parents to consult physician if fever persists after beginning therapy
		Discuss procedures for preventing spread of infection

NURSING CARE PLAN
THE CHILD WITH INFECTIOUS MONONUCLEOSIS

An acute, self-limiting infectious disease presumed to be of viral origin and characterized by an increase in the mononuclear elements in the blood

ASSESSMENT

Perform physical assessment
Observe for manifestations of infectious mononucleosis:

Early
Headache
Malaise
Fatigue
Chilliness
Low-grade fever
Loss of appetite
Puffy eyes

Full-blown disease
Cardinal features
  Fever
  Sore throat
  Cervical adenopathy

Common features
  Splenomegaly (may persist for several months)
  Palatine petechiae
  Macular eruption (especially on trunk)
  Exudative pharyngitis/tonsillitis
  Hepatic involvement to some degree, often associated with jaundice

Obtain health history, especially regarding possible recent exposure to the disease
Assist with diagnostic tests—Blood analysis, heterophil antibody test, and rapid specific tests (e.g., Monospot, slide test, 5-minute enzyme immunoassay)

NURSING DIAGNOSIS: Fatigue related to infectious process

GOAL

Promote rest

INTERVENTIONS

Help child and family determine appropriate activities according to symptoms and interests
Encourage bed rest for marked fatigue
Encourage youngster to regulate activities according to own tolerance

EXPECTED OUTCOME

Youngster engages in activities as tolerated and rests sufficiently (specify amount)

NURSING DIAGNOSIS: Pain (mild) related to sore throat, malaise

GOAL

Relieve discomfort

INTERVENTIONS

*Administer analgesics as indicated
Provide hot or cool gargles for throat discomfort
Promote rest

EXPECTED OUTCOME

Child exhibits minimum or no evidence of discomfort

NURSING DIAGNOSIS: Altered family processes related to a child with a potentially serious illness

GOAL

Support family

INTERVENTIONS AND EXPECTED OUTCOME

See Nursing diagnosis: Altered family processes, p. 261

*Dependent nursing action.

NURSING CARE PLAN
THE CHILD WITH A SEXUALLY TRANSMITTED DISEASE

A contagious disease usually acquired by sexual intercourse or other genital contact

ASSESSMENT

Perform physical assessment
Observe for physical evidence of sexually transmitted disease (STD) (see box)
Obtain health history, especially relative to sexual activity, including names of contacts

Assist with diagnostic procedures and tests—Smears, blood and urine analyses, specimens for smears and cultures, blood serology

SEXUALLY TRANSMITTED DISEASES

Gonorrhea	Male: urethritis—dysuria with profuse yellow discharge, frequency, urgency, nocturia Female: cervicitis (postpubertal)—may be associated with discharge, dysuria, dyspareunia; vulvovaginitis (prepubertal)		Pruritus and edema of external genitalia; foul-smelling, greenish vaginal discharge; sometimes postcoital bleeding May be asymptomatic, especially in males
Chlamydia	Male: meatal erythema, tenderness, itching, dysuria, urethral discharge Female: mucopurulent cervical exudate with erythema, edema, congestion	Candidiasis, or moniliasis	Edema and erythema of vulva and thick white, cheesy vaginal discharge May be satellite lesions on groin, thighs, and buttocks Cutaneous lesions on penis May be asymptomatic
Syphilis	Primary stage: chancre—a hard, painless, red, sharply defined lesion with indurated base, raised border, eroded surface, and scanty yellow discharge; usually located on penis, vulva, or cervix Secondary stage: systemic influenza-like symptoms and lymphadenopathy, rash; usually appears 1 to 3 weeks after healing of chancre	Human papilloma virus	Genital warts, which can be randomly located on any part of the genitalia, perineum, perianal area, thighs, or buttocks; in females can extend to include the cervix
Herpes progenitalis	Small (usually painful) vesicles on genital area, buttocks, and thighs; itching usually initial symptom; when vesicles break, shallow, circular, extremely painful lesions remain	Acquired immuno deficiency syndrome	See p. 486

NURSING DIAGNOSIS: Potential for injury related to presence of infection in the reproductive system

GOAL

Prevent extension of infection

INTERVENTIONS

*Administer appropriate antibiotic as prescribed

EXPECTED OUTCOME

Youngster exhibits no evidence of infection

NURSING DIAGNOSIS: Potential for infection related to sexual contact with affected person

*Dependent nursing action.

GOAL

Prevent infection

INTERVENTIONS

Provide sex education to young people, which includes information about sexually transmitted diseases
   Clinical manifestations
   Treatment available and where obtained
   Dispel myths associated with mode of transmission
Refer suspected or confirmed cases for treatment
Locate sexual contacts of affected youngsters and refer for examination and treatment
Encourage use of condoms or other barriers in sexually active youngsters

EXPECTED OUTCOME

Others do not contract the disease

VD Hotline 1-800-277-8922.

NURSING CARE PLAN
THE CHILD WITH ACQUIRED IMMUNE DEFICIENCY SYNDROME (AIDS)

A disease caused by the human immunodeficiency virus (HIV), which produces a generalized disturbance that involves all four major components of the immune mechanism

ASSESSMENT

Perform physical assessment
Obtain history relative to risk factors for AIDS in children:
   Maternal factors:
      Intravenous drug use
      Maternal promiscuity
      Diagnosis of AIDS in the mother
      Haitian or central African origin
   High-risk groups:
      Intravenous drug abusers
      Recipients of multiple transfusions
      Sexual partners of risk group and members
      Sexually active homosexual males
      Bisexual males
Observe for manifestations of AIDS in children:
   Failure to thrive
  *Recurrent bacterial infections
     Pneumonitis
     Otitis media
  *Parotitis (often chronic)

*Unique to pediatric AIDS.

Persistent oral candidiasis
Hepatosplenomegaly
Neurologic features
   Seizures
   Truncal ataxia
   Cognitive deficits
Observe for manifestations of congenital AIDS in infants of high-risk mothers:
   Dysmorphic features (Marion and others, 1986)
      Microcephaly
      Progressive loss of developmental milestones
      Hypertelorism
      Prominent, boxlike forehead
      Mild obliquity of eyes
      Flattened nasal bridge
      Long palpebral fissures with blue sclerae
      Short nose with flattened columella
      Well-formed, triangular philtrum
      Prominent upper vermilion border

NURSING DIAGNOSIS: Potential for infection related to risk factors for AIDS

GOAL

Prevent AIDS

INTERVENTIONS

Educate children and youth regarding the prevention of transmission of AIDS

Attempt to discourage youth from engaging in intimate sexual contacts (especially casual contacts), including homosexual pairings

Educate sexually active youth regarding use of condoms to minimize exposure to genital mucous membranes and secretions

Educate intravenous drug users regarding dangers of sharing needles and IV equipment (if unable to prevent IV drug use)

Check all blood products for evidence of AIDS testing before administration

EXPECTED OUTCOME

Children and youth do not contract AIDS infection

GOAL

Prevent transmission of disease to others

INTERVENTIONS

See above

Implement and carry out Universal Precautions for prevention of infection, especially body substance isolation (see p. 289)

Place restrictions on behaviors and contacts for affected children who bite or who do not have control of their bodily secretions

EXPECTED OUTCOME

Others do not acquire the disease

NURSING DIAGNOSIS: Potential for infection related to depressed immune response

GOAL

Prevent infections

INTERVENTIONS

See Nursing care plan: The child at risk for infection, p. 288

*Administer medications as prescribed

Maintain a clean environment

*Administer appropriate immunizations as prescribed

EXPECTED OUTCOME

Child remains free of infection

*Dependent nursing action.

NURSING DIAGNOSIS: Body image disturbance related to having a dreaded disease

GOAL

Promote a positive body image

INTERVENTIONS AND EXPECTED OUTCOME

See Nursing diagnosis: Altered body image, p. 265

GOAL

Encourage a positive attitude in others toward affected child

INTERVENTIONS

Educate health personnel regarding risks and safeguards in relationships with affected children

Become involved in educating the public regarding AIDS
  In schools
  In communities at large

Promote a positive attitude from peers and other persons toward the affected child through education and example

EXPECTED OUTCOME

Child engages in positive interpersonal interactions

NURSING DIAGNOSIS: Altered family processes related to having a child with a dreaded and life-threatening disease

GOAL

Support family

INTERVENTIONS AND EXPECTED OUTCOMES

See Nursing care plan: The family of the ill or hospitalized child, p. 254

NURSING DIAGNOSIS: Anticipatory grief related to having a child with a potentially fatal illness

See Nursing diagnosis: Anticipatory grief, p. 306
AIDS hotline: 1-800-342-AIDS
In Canada: AIDS Information Line, 1-800-972-2437

See also:
Nursing care plan: The child with pediculosis capitis, p. 495
Selected bacterial infections, p. 498

Unit 4

NURSING CARE OF THE CHILD WITH A DISORDER MANIFEST IN THE SKIN

Skin lesions originate from:
Contact with injurious agents (e.g., infectious organisms, toxic chemicals, physical trauma)
Hereditary factors

Some external factor that produces a reaction in the skin (e.g., allergens)
Systemic disease of which the lesions are a cutaneous manifestation (e.g., measles, lupus erythematosus, nutritional deficiency disease)

NURSING CARE PLAN
THE CHILD WITH A DISORDER AFFECTING THE SKIN

A condition that causes alteration in the appearance and/or function of the skin

---

ASSESSMENT

Perform physical assessment with special regard for skin manifestations:

Erythema—Reddened area caused by increased amounts of oxygenated blood in the dermal vasculature

Ecchymoses—Pinpoint tiny and sharply circumscribed spots in the superficial layers of the epidermis

Petechiae—Localized red or purple discolorations caused by extravasation of blood into dermis and subcutaneous tissues

Primary lesions—Skin changes produced by internal or external environmental changes (see box)

Secondary lesions—Skin changes that result from alteration in the primary lesions, such as those caused by rubbing, scratching, medication, or involution and healing (see box)

Describe distribution pattern of lesion (e.g., extensor surfaces, creases, exposed areas, entire body, diaper area)

Describe configuration and arrangement of any lesions (e.g., discrete, grouped or clustered, annular [ringed], confluent, linear, diffuse)

Describe any associated characteristics such as temperature, moisture, texture, elasticity, and hardness of skin in general or in area of lesion(s)

Observe for evidence of subjective manifestations associated with lesions (e.g., pruritis, pain or tenderness, burning, prickling, stinging, crawling, anesthesia, hyperesthesia, hypesthesia, or hypoesthesia; constant or intermittent; aggravated by specific activity or circumstance)

Observe for evidence of aggravating factor (e.g., foreign body such as a sliver, insect barb, cactus spine), presence of insect (e.g., chiggers, fleas, ticks, mites)

Obtain health history for previous skin reactions, allergies, diseases associated with skin manifestations

Obtain recent history for onset, possible precipitating events, and course of development. Possible precipitating factors include exposure to infectious disease, contact with chemicals, plants, animals, insects, sunshine, allergenic clothing or toys (e.g., wool), metals, topical applications (e.g., soaps, makeup, lotions, bath salts), excess heat or cold, wooded areas, beach

Obtain a nutrition history, especially regarding foods known to be allergenic

Assist with diagnostic procedures—Skin testing, microscopic examination of scrapings, biopsy, culture, cytodiagnosis, patch testing, blood tests

PRIMARY SKIN LESIONS

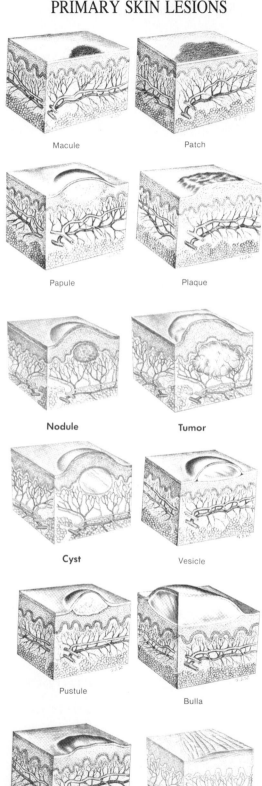

Flat circumscribed area of color change (red, brown, purple, white, tan); less than 1 cm in diameter; nonpalpable
Example: Freckle, nevus, measles, flat mole

Small, circumscribed, firm, elevated, discoloration (red, pink, tan, brown, bluish); less than 1 cm in diameter; the more superficial it is, the more distinct are the borders
Example: Wart, ringworm, milia, pigmented nevi

Solid, circumscribed, firm elevation; round or ellipsoid; located deep in dermis or subcutaneous tissue
Example: Dermatofibroma, dermoid cyst, lipoma

Elevated, circumscribed, palpable, encapsulated semisolid or fluid-filled mass in dermis or subcutaneous tissue
Example: Epidermoid cyst, sebaceous cyst

Vesicle filled with pus; may or may not be caused by infection
Example: Acne, impetigo, folliculitis

Elevated, round or flat topped, irregularly shaped; transient, changing; variable diameter; pale pink in color
Example: Insect bites, urticaria

Flat, circumscribed, irregularly shaped, discoloration; nonpalpable; greater than 1 cm in diameter
Example: Mongolian spot, vitiligo, port-wine stain

Flattened, raised, firm, surface area relatively large in relation to height; greater than 1 cm in diameter
Example: Psoriasis

Elevated, solid; may or may not be clearly demarcated; greater than 1 cm in diameter; and deeper than nodule
Example: Cavernous hemangioma, neoplasm

Small (less than 1 cm in diameter), superficial circumscribed elevation; contains serous or blood-tinged fluid
Example: Chicken pox, herpes, poison ivy

Fluid-filled vesicle greater than 1 cm in diameter; a large vesicle; bleb; blister
Example: Second-degreee burn, bullous impetigo

Loss of superficial epidermis, linear or punctate
Example: Scratch, abrasion

Macule   Patch

Papule   Plaque

Nodule   **Tumor**

Cyst   Vesicle

Pustule   Bulla

Wheal   **Lichenification**

Unit 4

SECONDARY SKIN LESIONS

Mound of flaky, dead, cornified tissue shed from the skin; irregular shape; variable thickness and diameter; dry or oily; silver, white, or tan color
Example: Psoriasis, ringworm

Dried masses of serum, pus, dead skin, and debris that can be found surmounting any lesion; slightly elevated; brown, black, tan, or straw-colored
Example: Impetigo, scab, eczema

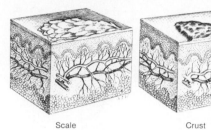

Scale   Crust

Irregularly shaped, concave, excavation with loss of epidermis and dermis; variable size; exudative; red or reddish blue
Example: Decubiti

Deep linear split through epidermis into dermis; small; deep; red
Example: Chapping, tinea pedis

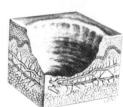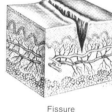

Ulcer   Fissure

Permanent thick to thin fibrous tissue that replaces damaged corium by production and deposition of collagen; irregular shape; red, pink, or white; atrophic or hypertrophic
Example: Vaccination, healed wound, abrasion, laceration

Rough, thickened, and hardened epidermis with accentuated skin markings
Example: Result of chronic dermatitis, such as eczema

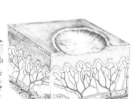

Scar   **Excoriation**

> **NURSING DIAGNOSIS:** Impaired skin integrity related to environmental agents, somatic factors, immunologic deficit

GOAL

Promote healing

INTERVENTIONS

Carry out therapeutic regimens as prescribed or support and assist parents in carrying out treatment plan
*Administer topical treatments and applications
*Administer systemic medications, if ordered

Prevent secondary infection and autoinoculation
Encourage rest
Reduce external stimuli that aggravate condition
Encourage well-balanced diet
Administer skin care and general hygiene measures

EXPECTED OUTCOME

Affected area exhibits signs of healing

> **NURSING DIAGNOSIS:** Potential impaired skin integrity related to pressure, immobility, therapeutic appliances

GOAL

Prevent skin irritation or breakdown

---

*Dependent nursing action.

INTERVENTIONS

Place child on sheepskin, Egg-crate pad, or other resilient surface

Change position frequently

Protect pressure points, for example, trochanter, sacrum, ankle, shoulder, occiput

Inspect skin surfaces regularly for signs of irritation, redness, evidence of pressure

Eliminate mechanical factors causing pressure, friction, or irritation

Maintain meticulous skin cleanliness

Stimulate circulation by gentle rubbing with lotion or other lubricating substance

EXPECTED OUTCOME

Skin remains clean and intact with no evidence of irritation

> **NURSING DIAGNOSIS:** Potential impaired skin integrity related to mechanical trauma, body secretions, increased susceptibility to infection

GOAL

Maintain skin integrity

INTERVENTIONS

Keep skin clean and dry; cleanse skin at least once daily

Inspect total skin area frequently for evidence of irritation or breakdown

Protect skinfolds and surfaces that rub together

Keep clothing and linen clean and dry

Apply protective lotion to areas where excoriation is most likely—anal and perineal areas, knees, elbows, ankles, chin, and so on

Carry out good perineal care under urine collection device, when applicable

Keep suture line dry, especially in areas subject to moisture (e.g., mouth, perineum)

EXPECTED OUTCOME

Skin remains clean, dry, and free of irritation

GOAL

Prevent secondary infection

INTERVENTIONS

Maintain careful handwashing before handling affected child

Wear surgical gloves when handling or dressing affected parts if indicated by nature of lesion

Teach child and family hygienic care and medical asepsis

Devise methods to prevent secondary infection of lesion in small or uncooperative children

    Keep nails short and clean

    Apply mittens or elbow restraints

    Dress in one-piece outfit with long sleeves and legs

EXPECTED OUTCOME

Skin lesions remain confined to primary sites

GOAL

Protect healthy skin surface

INTERVENTIONS

Teach and impress on child importance of keeping hands away from lesion(s)

Help child determine ways of preventing autoinoculation

Devise means for keeping small or uncooperative children from spreading infection to other areas

Protect healthy skin from maceration by keeping it dry

EXPECTED OUTCOME

Healthy skin remains clean and intact

> **NURSING DIAGNOSIS:** Potential for infection related to presence of infective organisms

GOAL

Prevent spread of infection to self and others

INTERVENTIONS

Implement universal precautions (see p. 289)

Isolate affected child from susceptible individuals if indicated

Maintain careful handwashing after caring for child

Avoid unnecessary close contact with affected child during infective stage of disease

Use correct technique for disposal of dressings, solutions, and other fomites in contact with lesion(s)

Teach and reinforce positive habits of hygienic care

EXPECTED OUTCOMES

Infection remains confined to primary site

Child and family comply with preventive measures

> **NURSING DIAGNOSIS:** Potential impaired skin integrity related to allergenic factors

GOAL

Prevent occurrence and/or recurrence

INTERVENTIONS

Avoid or reduce contact with agents or circumstances known to precipitate skin reaction

Teach child to recognize agents or circumstances that produce reaction

EXPECTED OUTCOME

Child avoids precipitating agents

> **NURSING DIAGNOSIS:** Altered oral mucous membranes related to dehydration, nothing by mouth, mouth breathing

Unit 4

GOAL

Prevent drying and caking of oral mucous membranes

INTERVENTIONS

Administer special mouth care while fluids by mouth are restricted

Moisten mouth with gauze pledgets, mist spray, or ice (if permitted)

Apply lip balm, petroleum jelly, or other protective substance to lips

EXPECTED OUTCOME

Mucous membranes remain moist and clean

NURSING DIAGNOSIS: Pain related to skin lesions, pruritis

GOAL

Relieve discomfort

INTERVENTIONS

Avoid or reduce external stimuli that aggravate discomfort, such as clothing and bed linen

Implement other appropriate nonpharmacologic pain reduction techniques (p. 286)

*Apply soothing treatments and topical applications as ordered

*Administer medications to relieve discomfort and/or restlessness and irritability

See Nursing care plan: The child in pain, p. 279

EXPECTED OUTCOME

Child remains calm and exhibits no evidence of discomfort

NURSING DIAGNOSIS: Body image disturbance related to perception of appearance

---

GOAL

Promote a positive self-image

INTERVENTIONS

Encourage child to express feelings about personal appearance and perceived reactions of others

See Nursing diagnosis: Body image disturbance, p. 265

EXPECTED OUTCOME

Child verbalizes feelings and concerns

GOAL

Provide tactile contact

---

*Dependent nursing action.

INTERVENTIONS

Hold child

   Remember that there is no substitute for the stimulation and comfort of human contact

Touch and caress unaffected area

EXPECTED OUTCOMES

Child exhibits signs of comfort

Child responds positively to tactile stimulation

GOAL

Support child

INTERVENTIONS

Teach self-care where appropriate

Involve child in planning treatment schedules

Support and encourage child in efforts to deal with multiple problems that may be associated with disorder, including discomfort, rejection, discouragement, and feelings of self-revulsion

Encourage child to maintain usual activities

EXPECTED OUTCOMES

Child collaborates in determining means for improving appearance

Child maintains customary activities and relationships

NURSING DIAGNOSIS: Altered family processes related to having a child with a severe skin condition (e.g., eczema, psoriasis, ichthyosis)

GOAL

Support family

INTERVENTIONS

Teach family skills needed to carry out therapeutic program

Inform family of expected and unexpected results of therapy and a course of action to follow

Help devise special techniques to carry out therapy

Be aware of overprotectiveness and restrictiveness, which can stifle child's emotional growth

Allow and encourage family members, particularly the one who cares for the child most of the time, to express negative feelings, such as anger, frustration, and perhaps guilt

Stress that negative feelings are normal, acceptable, and expected but that they must have an outlet in order for family members to remain healthy

Encourage family in efforts to carry out plan of care

Provide assistance when appropriate

Refer to agencies and services that assist with social, financial, and medical problems

EXPECTED OUTCOMES

Family demonstrates necessary skills (specify)

NURSING CARE PLAN
THE CHILD WITH ATOPIC DERMATITIS (ECZEMA)

A superficial inflammatory process involving primarily the epidermis

ASSESSMENT

Perform physical assessment with special emphasis on characteristics and distribution of skin manifestations

Obtain family history for evidence of skin lesions, atopy

Obtain health history, especially relative to previous involvement, environmental or dietary factors associated with present and previous exacerbations

Observe for manifestations of eczema:

Distribution of lesions:
Infantile form—Generalized, especially cheeks, scalp, trunk, and extensor surfaces of extremities
Childhood form—Flexural areas (antecubital and popliteal fossae, neck), wrists, ankles, and feet
Preadolescent and adolescent form—Face, sides of neck, hands, feet, face, and antecubital and popliteal fossae (to a lesser extent)

Appearance of lesions:
Infantile form
Erythema
Vesicles
Papules
Weeping
Oozing
Crusting
Scaling
Often symmetrical
Childhood form
Symmetrical involvement
Clusters of small erythematous or flesh-colored papules or minimally scaling patches
Dry and may be hyperpigmented
Lichenification (thickened skin with accentuation of creases)

Keratosis pilaris (follicular hyperkeratosis) common
Adolescent/adult form
Same as childhood manifestations
Dry, thick lesions (lichenified plaques) common
Confluent papules

Other manifestations
Intense itching
Unaffected skin dry and rough
Black children likely to exhibit more papular and/or follicular lesions than white children
May exhibit one or more of the following:
Lymphadenopathy, especially near affected sites
Increased palmar creases (many cases)
Atopic pleats (extra line or groove of lower eyelid)
Prone to cold hands
Pityriasis alba (small, poorly defined areas of hypopigmentation)
Facial pallor (especially around nose, mouth, and ears)
Bluish discoloration beneath eyes ("allergic shiners")
Increased susceptibility to unusual cutaneous infections (especially viral)
Personality traits often associated with eczema:
Active
Restless
Irritable
Aggressive
Frequently precocious and bright

Observe lesions for type, distribution, and evidence of secondary infection

Perform or assist with diagnostic procedures—Skin testing, elimination diet

Unit 4

NURSING DIAGNOSIS: Impaired skin integrity related to eczematous lesions

GOAL

Promote healing and relieve pruritis

INTERVENTIONS

*Carry out prescribed therapeutic regimen
  Dry method:
    Bathe infrequently
    Cleanse skin with nonlipid, hydrophilic agent (e.g., Cetaphil)
  Wet method:
    Bathe frequently, up to 4 times per day
    Follow immediately with application of lubricant
    Use no soap or very mild soap (e.g., Neutrogena, Lowila, Dove)
    Provide oil or oilated oatmeal baths, if prescribed
    Avoid showers
    *Apply hydrating preparations as prescribed
*Provide hypoallergenic diet as prescribed

EXPECTED OUTCOME

Child appears comfortable and rests and plays quietly

GOAL

Relieve itching

INTERVENTIONS

Eliminate any woolen or rough garment or furry stuffed toys; nylon garments promote sweating
Launder all clothes or bedsheets in mild detergent and rinse very well
Provide colloid bath (e.g., cornstarch in warm water) for temporary relief at bedtime
Apply cool compresses if needed
*Administer oral antihistamines, if prescribed
*Administer mild sedative, if prescribed

EXPECTED OUTCOME

Child does not scratch and rests or plays quietly

GOAL

Provide hygienic care without aggravating lesions

INTERVENTIONS

Administer good personal hygiene—Cleansing method as prescribed; no bubble bath, bath oil, perfume, or powder
Dress in loose-fitting, one-piece, long-sleeve and long-pants outfit (if appropriate for weather conditions)

EXPECTED OUTCOME

Child is clean, well groomed, and exhibits no evidence of irritation

*Dependent nursing action.

GOAL

Prevent or minimize scratching

INTERVENTIONS

Keep fingernails and toenails short and clean
Wrap hands in soft cotton gloves or stockings; pin to shirt cuff
Avoid overheating, high humidity, and perspiration
Use elbow restraints when absolutely necessary, but allow supervised periods of unrestricted movement
Encourage exposure to ultraviolet light, but avoid sunburn

EXPECTED OUTCOME

Affected areas remain free of irritation

GOAL

Promote rest

INTERVENTIONS

Plan meals, baths, medications, and treatments around nap or bedtime
Make child as comfortable as possible before sleep to enhance restfulness (for example, give sedation and then bathe before bedtime)

EXPECTED OUTCOME

Child receives an adequate amount of rest for age

NURSING DIAGNOSIS: Altered family processes related to child's discomfort and lengthy therapy

GOAL

Prepare family for home care

INTERVENTIONS

Encourage play activities that are suitable to skin condition and child's developmental age
Demonstrate proper procedure for dilution of soaks and applying wet dressings
Suggest applying dressings at quiet times when child is well rested and has received medication for itching

EXPECTED OUTCOME

Family demonstrates correct performance of procedures (specify procedures)

GOAL

Assist parents in avoiding causative allergens

INTERVENTIONS

Avoid any furry, hairy stuffed toys or dolls
> Avoid play materials that contain allergens (e.g., wheat-based paste or finger paint)
> Provide kinesthetic, moving toys, large toys, which require less fine motor skills if hands are covered, and quiet musical or visual toys

Stress reason for hypoallergenic diet or removal of inhalants, especially that positive results are not immediate (see guidelines for allergy-proofing the house, p. 330)

Give written list of foods restricted as well as those allowed

Identify hidden sources of allergenic foods, such as milk, wheat, and eggs

Assess home environment *before* suggesting ways to eliminate inhalants

Make public health referral for long-term home care follow-up

EXPECTED OUTCOME

Family eliminates irritating substances from diet and environment of child

See also Nursing diagnosis: Altered family processes

NURSING CARE PLAN
THE CHILD WITH PEDICULOSIS CAPITIS

Infestation of the scalp by *Pediculus humanis capitis* (head lice)

ASSESSMENT

Perform physical assessment

Inspect scalp for evidence of nits or nit cases at base of hair shaft
> Systematically spread hair with two tongue depressors or popsicle sticks

Observe for:
> Any movement that indicates a louse
> Nits as evidenced by whitish oval specks adhering to hair shaft
> Empty nit cases appearing as translucent oval specks

Distinguish nits from dandruff by adherent nature: dandruff falls off hair readily

---

NURSING DIAGNOSIS: Potential impaired skin integrity related to insect bites, scratching

GOAL

Eradicate lice and nits

INTERVENTIONS

Apply, or teach family to apply, pediculicide shampoo or rinse
> Follow directions described on label of pediculicide
> Read directions several times in quiet environment before application
> Make child as comfortable as possible during procedure
>> Playing "beauty parlor" adds a dimension of fun as well as providing eye safety
>> Use plastic drape to prevent drug getting on other body parts
>> Instruct child to shut eyes tightly during application; if irritation occurs, flush well with tepid water
> Do not use hair dryer
> Use fine-tooth comb on dry or slightly damp hair to remove empty nit cases

Launder washable items of clothing and linens in hot water and dry in dryer on hot setting for at least 20 minutes

Soak combs, brushes, and other hair utensils in pediculicide shampoo or lotion for 1 hour or in boiling water for 10 minutes. (Some advocate placing nonwashable, noncleanable items in a tightly closed plastic bag that remains sealed for 14 days.)

Vacuum mattresses and upholstered furniture carefully; pediculosis sprays are not recommended

EXPECTED OUTCOME

Inspection of scalp reveals no evidence of lice or nits

GOAL

Prevent infestation/reinfestation

INTERVENTIONS

Caution children against sharing combs, hats, caps, scarves, coats, or other items used on or near the hair

Explain or reinforce explanation of the condition and its mode of transmission

Treat any family member with evidence of infestation

Stress importance of second application of pediculicide or shampoo
*Contact community agencies for suggestions for reducing epidemics

EXPECTED OUTCOME

Child does not become infected with organism

NURSING DIAGNOSIS: Body image disturbance related to infestation

GOAL

Reassure child and family

*National Pediculosis Association, P.O. Box 149, Newton, MA 02161 (617) 449-6487.

INTERVENTIONS

Allay child's feelings of shame and embarrassment
Reassure family that anyone can get pediculosis with no association with age, cleanliness, socioeconomic level
Caution family against cutting child's hair or shaving head as treatment or punishment (cutting long hair may help with removal of nit cases)

EXPECTED OUTCOME

Child accepts therapy with no evidence of self-consciousness

NURSING CARE PLAN
THE ADOLESCENT WITH ACNE

An inflammatory process involving the pilosebaceous follicles of the face, neck, shoulders, back, and upper chest

ASSESSMENT

Perform physical assessment
Obtain family history and health history
Observe for manifestations of acne:
  Noninflamed
    Comedones—Compact masses of keratin, lipids, fatty acids, and bacteria that dilate the follicular duct producing

Closed comedones or "whiteheads"
Open comedones or "blackheads"
Inflamed
  Papules
  Pustules
  Nodules
  Cysts

NURSING DIAGNOSIS: Impaired skin integrity related to excretions/secretions

GOAL

Reduce lesions

INTERVENTIONS

Teach child and family to:
*Express comedones periodically as prescribed
  Blackheads—By direct pressure with comedone extractor
  Whiteheads—Nick gently and superficially with No. 11 blade before extrusion
*Apply medication (e.g., retinoic acid) as prescribed

*Dependent nursing action.

EXPECTED OUTCOME

Lesions are expressed without difficulty

NURSING DIAGNOSIS: Potential impaired skin integrity related to presence of secretions, presence of infective organisms

GOAL

Prevent inflammation and scarring

INTERVENTIONS

Carefully cleanse skin with soap and water prior to expression of comedones

Caution against using excessive pressure in comedone expression

Express limited number of comedones each day

*Apply peeling agent(s) as prescribed

Teach correct cleansing techniques and medical asepsis

Caution against too vigorous scrubbing to prevent skin damage

Impress the importance of following instructions, such as using only prescribed preparations and appliances

Instruct about shampooing, hairstyling, and the selection and use of cosmetics

Instruct in proper care of equipment used for therapy

*Administer oral corticosteroids and assist with intralesion injections of the drug

*Administer antibiotics as prescribed

Stress to those on retinoic acid therapy the importance of avoiding exposure to sun; apply sunscreen for protection

Prepare adolescent for surgical procedure(s)

Assist with incision and drainage of cystic or pustular lesions

Prepare adolescent for and assist with x-ray therapy

EXPECTED OUTCOME

Lesions heal with minimum scarring

GOAL

Reduce number of lesions

INTERVENTIONS

Avoid oily applications to the skin

Shampoo hair and scalp frequently (if prescribed)

Style hair off the forehead

Avoid use of cosmetic preparations, if possible; otherwise avoid oil-base products

Avoid face contact with other areas of the body, for example, chin resting on hands, lying with face on arm

*Administer estrogens (in selected female cases)

EXPECTED OUTCOME

Adolescent uses appropriate precautions

GOAL

Promote general health

INTERVENTIONS

Encourage adequate rest and moderate exercise

Help adolescent plan a well-balanced diet

Help adolescent find mechanisms to reduce emotional stress

Implement measures to correct constipation (if it exists)

Assess for any foci of infection and initiate measures to eliminate them

Eliminate any given food the adolescent has found that aggravates the symptoms

EXPECTED OUTCOME

Adolescent complies with general hygiene measures

---

*Dependent nursing action.

NURSING DIAGNOSIS: Body image disturbance related to perception of facial lesions

GOAL

Educate the adolescent

INTERVENTIONS

Dispel myths regarding the etiology of the condition

Reassure adolescent regarding unfounded fears

Provide accurate information regarding the disease process and the therapy to be implemented

EXPECTED OUTCOME

Adolescent demonstrates an understanding of etiology of lesions

GOAL

Obtain medical treatment

INTERVENTIONS

Be alert to cues that the adolescent wants to discuss the skin problem

Broach the subject of therapy for the adolescent with obvious skin lesions

Suggest an understanding dermatologist who is sympathetic to the special needs of the adolescent

Discourage self-treatment with over-the-counter preparations

EXPECTED OUTCOMES

Adolescent discusses feelings and concerns

Adolescent complies with suggestions

GOAL

Encourage self-care

INTERVENTIONS

Re-emphasize importance of cleanliness and medical asepsis

Provide written instructions, including the cause of the lesions and the therapeutic regimen outlined

Motivate the adolescent to assume responsibility for following through on instructions

Instruct in the technique of comedo extraction and other therapeutic and hygienic measures

Discourage mirror gazing and "picking" at lesions

EXPECTED OUTCOME

Adolescent assumes responsibility for care of skin lesions and complies with preventive measures

GOAL

Support the adolescent

INTERVENTIONS

Allow the adolescent to express feelings about the disorder, its effect on appearance, and the length of time required for therapy

Unit 4

Provide positive reinforcement for compliance

Encourage maintenance of normal activities and interaction with peers

Explore job opportunities and after-school interests with the adolescent

Emphasize the positive aspects, such as the self-limited nature of the disorder, the efficacy of therapy, and improvement in appearance

Assist adolescent in selection of grooming and other items to enhance appearance

EXPECTED OUTCOME

Adolescent discusses feelings and concerns regarding appearance and identifies positive aspects of appearance

NURSING DIAGNOSIS: Altered family processes related to the child with a troublesome skin problem

GOAL

Obtain cooperation and understanding of family

INTERVENTIONS

Explain the disorder and therapy prescribed

Caution the family against nagging about compliance

Teach family the technique of comedo extraction

Explain the nature of the adolescent personality and the effect the disorder has on self-image and identity formation

EXPECTED OUTCOME

Family demonstrates an understanding of the adolescent's skin problem and shows a supportive attitude

Selected skin infections

BACTERIAL INFECTIONS

Disorder/organism	Manifestations	Treatment	Comments
Impetigo contagiosa—*Streptococcus, Staphylococcus*	Begins as a reddish macule Becomes vesicular Ruptures easily, leaving superficial, moist erosion Tends to spread peripherally in sharply marginated irregular outlines Exudate dries to form heavy, honey-colored crusts Pruritus common Systemic effects: minimal or asymptomatic	Careful removal of undermined skin, crusts, and debris by softening with 1:20 Burow solution compresses Topical application of bactericidal ointment Systemic administration of oral or parenteral antibiotics (penicillin) in severe or extensive lesions	Tends to heal without scarring unless secondary infection Autoinoculable and contagious Very common in toddler, preschooler
Pyoderma—*Staphylococcus, Streptococcus*	Deeper extension of infection into dermis Tissue reaction more severe Systemic effects: fever, lymphangitis	Soap and water cleansing Wet compresses Bathing with antibacterial soap as prescribed Topical antibiotics	Autoinoculable and contagious May heal with or without scarring
Folliculitis (pimple), furuncle (boil), carbuncle (multiple boils)—*Staphylococcus aureus*	Folliculitis: infection of hair follicle Furuncle: larger lesion with more redness and swelling at a single follicle Carbuncle: more extensive lesion with widespread inflammation and "pointing" at several follicular orifices Systemic effects: malaise, if severe	Skin cleanliness Local warm moist compresses Topical application of antibiotic agents Systemic antibiotics in severe cases Incision and drainage of severe lesions, followed by wound irrigations with antibiotics or suitable drain implantation	Autoinoculable and contagious Furuncle and carbuncle tend to heal with scar formation A lesion should *never* be squeezed
Cellulitis—*Streptococcus, Staphylococcus, Haemophilus influenzae*	Inflammation of skin and subcutaneous tissues with intense redness, swelling, and firm infiltration Lymphangitis "streaking" frequently seen Involvement of regional lymph nodes common May progress to abscess formation Systemic effects: fever, malaise	Oral or parenteral antibiotics Rest and immobilization of both affected area and child Warm moist compresses to area	Hospitalization may be necessary for child with systemic symptoms Otitis media may be associated with facial cellulitis

Unit 4

VIRAL INFECTIONS

Disorder/organism	Manifestations	Treatment	Comments
Verruca (warts)	Small, benign tumors Usually well-circumscribed, gray or brown, elevated firm papules with a roughened, finely papillomatous texture Occur anywhere but usually appear on exposed areas such as fingers, hands, face, and soles May be single or multiple Asymptomatic	Not uniformly successful Local destructive therapy, individualized according to location, type, and number—surgical removal, electrocautery, curettage, cryotherapy (liquid nitrogen), caustic solutions (lactic acid and salicylic acid in flexible collodion, retinoic acid, salicylic acid plasters), radiographic treatment Hypnotherapy may be effective	Common in children Tend to disappear spontaneously Course unpredictable Most destructive techniques tend to leave scars Autoinoculable Repeated irritation will cause to enlarge Destructive technique tends to leave scars, which may cause problems with walking
Verruca plantaris (plantar wart)	Located on plantar surface of feet and, because of pressure, are practically flat; may be surrounded by a collar of hyperkeratosis	Apply caustic solution to wart, wear foam insole with hole cut to relieve pressure on wart; soak 20 min after 2-3 days. Repeat until wart comes out	
Herpes simplex virus type I (cold sore, fever blister) Herpes simplex virus type II (genital)	Grouped, burning, and itching vesicles on inflammatory base, usually on or near mucocutaneous junctions (lips, nose, genitals, buttocks) Vesicles dry, forming a crust, followed by exfoliation and spontaneous healing in 8-10 days May be accompanied by regional lymphadenopathy	Avoidance of secondary infection Burow solution compresses during weeping stages No topical therapy has proved to be effective in preventing recurrences Oral antiviral (Acyclovir) for initial infection or to reduce severity in reccurrance	Heal without scarring unless secondary infection Aggravated by corticosteroids Positive psychologic effect from treatment May be fatal in children with depressed immunity
Varicella Zoster virus (herpes zoster; shingles)	Caused by same virus that causes varicella (chickenpox) Virus has affinity for posterior root ganglia, posterior horn of spinal cord, and skin; crops of vesicles usually confined to dermatome following along course of affected nerve Usually preceded by neuralgic pain, hyperesthesias, or itching May be accompanied by constitutional symptoms	Symptomatic Analgesics for pain Mild sedation sometimes helpful Local moist compresses Drying lotions may be helpful Ophthalmic variety: systemic corticotropin (ACTH) and/or corticosteroids	Pain in children usually minimal Postherpetic pain does not occur in children Chickenpox may follow exposure; isolate affected child from other children in a hospital or school May occur in children with depressed immunity; can be fatal
Molluscum contagiosum; caused by a pox virus	Flesh-colored papules with a central caseous plug (umbilicated) Usually asymptomatic	Cases in well children resolve spontaneously in about 18 months Treatment reserved for troublesome cases Curettage or cryotherapy	Common in school-age children Spread by skin including contact autoinoculation and fomite-to-skin contact

DERMATOPHYTOSES (RINGWORM)

Disorder/organism	Manifestations	Treatment	Comments
Tinea capitis—*Microsporum audouini, M. canis, Trichophyton tonsurans*	Lesions in scalp but may extend to hairline or neck Characteristic configuration of scaly, circumscribed patches and/or patchy, scaling areas of alopecia Generally asymptomatic, but severe, deep inflammatory reaction may occur that manifests as boggy, encrusted lesions (kerions) Pruritic Diagnosis: microscopic examination of scales	Oral griseofulvin Oral ketoconazole for difficult cases Selenium sulfide shampoos Topical antifungal agents, e.g., clotrimazole, haloprogin, miconazole; treatment extended for weeks or months—even after subjective symptoms subside	Person-to-person transmission Animal-to-person transmission *M. audouini* transmitted from one human being to another directly or from personal items; *M. canis* usually contracted from household pets, especially cats Rarely, permanent loss of hair Atopic individuals more susceptible
Tinea corporis—*Trichophyton, rubrum Microsporum Canis, T. Mentagrophytes Epiclemophyton*	Generally round or oval, erythematous scaling patch that spreads peripherally and clears centrally; may involve nails (tinea unguium); Usually unilateral Diagnosis: direct microscopic examination of scales	Oral griseofulvin Local application of antifungal preparation such as tolnaftate, haloprogin, miconazole, clotrimazole; apply 1 inch beyond periphery of lesion; continue application 1 to 2 weeks after no sign of lesion	Usually of animal origin from infected pets Majority of infections in children caused by *M. canis* and *M. audouini*
Tinea cruris ("jock itch")—*Epidermophyton floccosum, T. rubrum, T. Mentographytes*	Skin response similar to tinea corporis Localized to medial proximal aspect of thigh and crural fold; may involve scrotum in males Pruritic Diagnosis: same as for tinea corporis	Local application of tolnaftate liquid Wet compresses or sitz baths may be soothing	Rare in preadolescent children Health education regarding personal hygiene

Tinea pedis ("athlete's foot")—*E. floccosum, T. rubrum, T. interdigitale*	On intertriginous areas between toes or on plantar surface of feet
	Lesions vary:
	  Maceration and fissuring between toes
	  Patches with pinhead-sized vesicles on plantar surface
	Pruritic
	Diagnosis: direct microscopic examination of scrapings
		Oral griseofulvin
		Local applications of tolnaftate liquid and antifungal powder containing tolnaftate
		Acute infections: compresses or soaks followed by application of glucocorticoid cream
		Elimination of conditions of heat and perspiration by clean, light socks and well-ventilated shoes; avoidance of occlusive shoes
			Most frequent in adolescents and adults; rare in children but see an increase with wearing of plastic shoes
			Transmission to other individuals rare despite general opinion to contrary
			Ointments not successful

Candidiasis (moniliasis)—*Candida albicans*	Grows in chronically moist areas Inflamed area with white exudate, peeling, and easy bleeding Pruritic Diagnosis: characteristic appearance	Nystatin and clotrimazole for oral, enteric, and cantaneous infections	Common form of diaper dermatitis Oral form common in infants, and children who are immunosuppressed

SYSTEMIC MYCOSES

Disorder/organism	Skin manifestations	Systemic manifestations	Treatment	Comments
Actinomycosis—*Actinomyces israelii*	Deep-seated granulomatous nodules and subcutaneous abscesses that drain as chronic fistulas, especially in jaw or neck	General health not affected	Penicillin or other antibiotics Incision and wide debridement of lesions	Access frequently through a carious tooth or mucous membranes of mouth Uncommon in children Noninfectious
North American blastomycosis—*Blastomyces dermatitidis*	Chronic granulomatous lesions and microabscesses in any part of body Initial lesion is a papule; undergoes ulceration and peripheral spread	Pulmonary symptoms, such as cough, chest pain, weakness, and weight loss May have skeletal involvement, with bone destruction and formation of cutaneous abscesses	Intravenous administration of amphotericin B	Usual portal of entry is lungs Source of infection unknown Noninfectious Pulmonary involvement may be mild and self-limiting and require no treatment Progressive disease often fatal
Cryptococcosis—*Cryptococcus neoformans (Torula histolytica)*	Usually on face; acneiform, firm, nodular, painless eruption	Central nervous system (CNS) manifestations; headache, dizziness, stiff neck, and signs of increased intracranial pressure Low-grade fever, mild cough, lung infiltration	Intravenous amphotericin B; may be administered intrathecally for CNS involvement, 5-flurocytosine for meningitis Excision and drainage of local lesions	Acquired by inhalation of dust but may enter through skin Prognosis serious Noninfectious Increased incidence in persons receiving corticosteroids with lymphoreticular malignancies, or type II diabetes
Histoplasmosis—*Histoplasma capsulatum*	Not distinctive or uniform but most appear as punched-out or granulomatous ulcers	General systemic symptoms may include pallor, diarrhea, vomiting, irregular spiking temperature, hepatosplenomegaly, and pulmonary symptoms Any tissue of body may be involved with related symptoms	Intravenous amphotericin B for severe cases Oral ketoconazole	Organism cultured from soil, especially where contaminated with fowl droppings Fungus enters through skin or mucous membranes of mouth and respiratory tract Endemic in Mississippi and Ohio River valleys Disseminated diseases most common in infants and children
Coccidioidomycosis (valley fever)—*Coccidioides immitis*	Erythema nodosum Erythema multiforme Erythematous maculopapular rash	Primary lung disease usually asymptomatic May be sign of acute febrile illness Disseminated disease is very serious	Intravenous amphotericin B Intravenous miconazole (synthetic imidazole) Intravenous miconazole plus oral ketoconazole for CNS involvement Surgical resection of persistent pulmonary cavities	Inhalation of aerospores from soil Endemic in southwestern United States Usually resolves spontaneously Increased incidence in dark-skinned races (Filipino, black, Mexican, Asian)

Unit 4

Skin lesions caused by animal or insect contacts

SKIN LESIONS CAUSED BY INSECT BITES AND STINGS

Mechanism/characteristics	Manifestations	Management
Insect bites—flies, gnats, mosquitoes, fleas		
Mechanism: Foreign protein in insects' saliva introduced when skin penetrated for a blood-sucking meal Distribution: Almost everywhere—fleas, mosquitoes, ants Suburbs and rural areas—bees Urban areas—hornets, wasps, yellow jackets	Hypersensitivity reaction Papular urticaria Firm papules; may be capped by vesicles or excoriated Little or no reaction in nonsensitized person	Treatment: Administer antipruritic agents and baths Administer antihistamines Prevent secondary infection Prevention: Avoid contact Remove focus, such as treating furniture, mattresses, carpets, and pets, where insects may live Apply insect repellent when exposure is anticipated
Chiggers—harvest mite		
Mechanism: Creeps into skin pores and hair follicles to feed Manifestations: Erythematous papules Intense itching	Same as insect bites May require systemic steroids for extensive bites	Insects favor warm areas of body, especially intertriginous areas and areas covered with clothing Avoid contact, especially in areas of tall grass and underbrush Apply insect repellent when exposure is anticipated
Hymenoptera stings—bees, wasps, hornets, yellow jackets, fire ants		
Mechanism: Injection of venom through stinging apparatus Venom contains histamine, allergenic proteins, and often a spreading factor, hyaluronidase Severe reactions caused by hypersensitivity and/or multiple stings Hypersensitive children should wear identifying tag to indicate allergy and therapy needed; family should keep emergency medication and be taught its administration	Local reaction: small red area, wheal, itching, and heat Systemic reactions: may be mild to severe, including generalized edema, pain, nausea and vomiting, confusion, respiratory embarrassment, and shock	Treatment: Scrape off stinger carefully if present Cleanse with soap and water Apply cool compresses or ice packs Apply common household product (e.g., lemon juice, paste made with aspirin, baking soda, or Adolph's Meat Tenderizer) Elevate involved extremity Administer antihistamines Severe reactions: administer epinephrine, corticosteroids; treat for shock Prevention: Teach child to wear shoes, to avoid wearing bright clothing or perfumed grooming products that might attract the insect, and to avoid places where the insect may be contacted

SKIN LESIONS CAUSED BY ARACHNIDS

Mechanism/characteristics	Manifestations	Management
Black widow spider		
Mechanism:	Mild sting at time of bite	Treatment:
Venom injected through a clawlike appendage; has neurotoxic action	Area becomes swollen, painful, and erythematous	Cleanse wound with antiseptic
Characteristics:	Dizziness, weakness, and abdominal pain	Apply ice packs
Spider is recognized by red or orange hourglass-shaped marking on underside	May produce delirium, paralysis, convulsions, and (if large amount of venom absorbed) death	Antivenin
Avoids light and bites in self-defense		Muscle relaxant, such as calcium gluconate
		Analgesics and/or sedatives
		Prevention:
		Teach children to avoid places that harbor the spider (e.g., woodpiles)
Brown recluse spider		
Mechanism:	Mild sting at time of bite	Treatment:
Venom injected via fangs	Transient erythema followed by bleb or blister; mild to severe pain in 2-8 hours; purple, star-shaped area in 3-4 days; necrotic ulceration in 7-14 days	Local application of cool compresses
Venom contains powerful necrotoxin		Antibiotics
Characteristics:		Corticosteroids
Spider is fawn to dark brown and recognized by fiddle-shaped mark on head	Systemic reactions may include fever, malaise, restlessness, nausea and vomiting, and joint pain	Relief of pain
Shy; bites only when annoyed or surprised	Generalized petechial eruption	Wound may require skin graft
Prefers dark areas where seldom disturbed	Wounds heal with scar formation	Some advocate early excision of necrotic area and surrounding tissue
		Prevention:
		Teach children to avoid possible nesting sites (e.g., woodpiles)
Scorpions		
Mechanism:	Intense local pain, erythema, numbness, burning, restlessness, vomiting	Treatment:
Sting by means of hooked caudal stinger that discharges venom	Ascending motor paralysis with convulsions, weakness, rapid pulse, excessive salivation, thirst, dysuria, pulmonary edema, coma, and death	Delay absorption of venom by application of tourniquets for 10-15 minutes; apply cold with ice packs or submerge in cold water
Venom of more venomous species contains hemolysins, endotheliolysins, and neurotoxins		Administration of antivenin
Characteristics:	Some species produce only local tissue reaction with swelling at puncture site (distinctive)	Surveillance in PICU
Usual habitat is southwestern United States	Symptoms subside in a few hours	Prevention:
	Deaths occur among children under 4 years of age, usually in first 24 hours	Teach children to avoid possible nesting sites
Ticks		
Mechanism:	Tick usually attached to skin, head embedded	Treatment:
In process of sucking blood, head and mouth parts are buried in skin	Produce firm, discrete, intensely pruritic nodules at site of attachment	Grasp tick with fingers protected by gloves or tissues as close as possible to point of attachment
Characteristics:	May cause urticaria or persistent localized edema	Pull straight up with steady, even pressure
Feed on blood of mammals		Remove any remaining part (e.g., head) with sterile needle
Significant in humans because of pathologic organism carried		Cleanse wounds with soap and disinfectant
May be vectors of various infectious diseases, such as Rocky Mountain spotted fever, Q fever, tularemia, relapsing fever, Lyme disease, tick paralysis		If bare hands touch tick during removal, wash hands thoroughly with soap and water
Must attach and feed 1-2 hours to transmit disease		Prevention:
Usual habitat is very wooded area		Teach children to avoid areas where prevalent
		Inspect skin (especially scalp) after being in wooded areas

Unit 4

DISORDERS TRANSMITTED BY ARTHROPODS

Disorder/organism/host	Manifestations	Management	Comments
Edemic typhus—*R. mooseri* Arthropod: rat fleas, or lice Transmission: flea bite; inhaling or ingesting flea excreta Mammal source: rats	Headache, arthralgia, backache followed by fever; may last 9-14 days Maculopapular rash after 1-8 days of fever begins in trunk and spreads to periphery; rarely involves face, palms, soles	Control; eliminate rat reservoir, insect vectors, or both Treatment: Supportive Tetracycline Chloramphenical	Fairly common in U.S. Shorter duration than epidemic typhus Mild, seldom fatal illness Difficult to distinguish from epidemic typhus
Epidemic typhus—*R. prowazekii* Arthropod: body louse Transmission: infected feces into broken skin Mammal source: humans	Abrupt onset of chills, fever, diffuse myalgia, headache, malaise Maculopapular rash becomes petechial 4 to 7 days later spreading from trunk outward	Control: immediate destruction of vectors Treatment: Tetracycline or chloramphenicol	Patient should be isolated until deloused See discussion on p. 495 for management of pediculosis Excreta from infected lice also in dust—disinfect patient's clothing, bedding, and possessions with DDT and wash in hot water
Lyme disease—Spirochete *Borrelia burgdorferi* Arthropod: tick Transmission: tick bite Mammal source: rodents, deer	Stage 1: tick bite Stage 2: erythema chronicum migrans, papule at bite site progresses to large circumferential ring with a raised edematous doughnutlike border Stage 3: systemic involvement—cardiac, neurologic, musculoskeletal	Control: protection from tick bite by proper wearing apparel, tick repellent Treatment: Antibiotics Supportive	Regional distribution: Northeast (Massachusetts to Maryland); Midwest (Wisconsin, Minnesota); West (California, Oregon)
Rickettsialpox—*R. akari* Arthropod: mouse mite Transmission: mite Mammal source: house mouse	Maculopapular rash following primary lesion at site of bite, fever, chills, headache	Control: eradication of rodent reservoir and mite vector Treatment: Tetracycline or chloramphenicol Supportive	Self-limited nonfatal disease Endemic in New York City Found in many cities in U.S.
Rocky Mountain spotted fever—*R. rickettsii* Arthropod: tick Transmission: tick bite Mammal source: wild rodents; dogs	Gradual onset: fever, malaise, anorexia, myalgia Abrupt onset: rapid temperature elevation, chills, vomiting, myalgia, severe headache Maculopapular or petechial rash primarily on extremities (ankles and wrists) but may spread to other areas	Control: protection from tick bite by proper wearing apparel, tick repellent Treatment: Tetracycline or chloramphenicol Vigorous supportive therapy	Usually self-limited in children Onset in children may resemble any infectious disease Severe disease rare in children Children and dogs should be inspected regularly if they play in wooded areas See previous box for management of ticks
Scabies Arthropod: *Sarcoptes scabiei* Transmission: mite burrows into stratum cornium and lays eggs Mammal source: human contact	Severe pruritis Lesions in interdigital, axillary-cubital, popliteal, inguinal areas Children: minute grayish brown, threadlike lesion (mite burrows); black dot at end (mite); located primarily on hands and feet Infants: eczematous eruption; located primarily on feet and ankles	Control: destruction Treatment: scabicide applied to cool, dry skin; leave on for recommended time (usually 4 hours)	Employ methods to treat all members of household

Miscellaneous skin disorders

Disease/causative agent	Local manifestations	Management	Comments
252rUrticaria—usually allergic response to drugs or infection	Development of wheals Vary in size and configuration and tend to appear quickly, spread irregularly, and fade within a few hours May be constant or intermittent, sparse or profuse, small or large, discrete or confluent May be acute, chronic, or recurrent in acute attacks	Local soothing and antipruritic applications Antihistamines Epinephrine or ephedrine Cortisone or corticotropin (ACTH) in severe cases Severe upper respiratory involvement may require tracheostomy	Known etiologic agents should be avoided May be accompanied by malaise, fever, lymphadenopathy Severe cases may involve mucous membranes, internal organs, and joints Obstruction to air passages constitutes medical emergency
Psoriasis—unknown; hereditary predisposition may be triggered by stress	Round, thick, dry, reddish patches covered with coarse, silvery scales over trunk and extremities; first lesions commonly appear in scalp; facial lesions more common in children than adults Affected cells proliferate at a much more rapid rate than normal cells	Exposure to sunlight, ultraviolet light Topical corticosteroids Tar derivatives Trihydroxyanthracine Keratolytic agents (salicylic acid) Psoralin—ultraviolet A (PUVA)* Emolients may provide relief	Uncommon in children under age 6 yrs Persons are otherwise healthy individuals Coal tar and psoralin act synergistically with ultraviolet light Keratolytic agents enhance absorption of corticosteroids Humidifiers may help in winter
Intertrigo—mechanical trauma and aggravating factors of excessive heat, moisture, and sweat retention	Red, inflamed, moist, partially denuded, marginated areas, the shape of which is determined by location Appear where opposing skin surfaces rub together, such as intergluteal folds, groin, neck, and axilla Hyperhydrosis and obesity are often factors	Affected areas kept clean and dry Skin folds kept separated with a generous supply of non-medicated powder Area exposed to air and light Remove excess clothing	A form of diaper irritation Prevent recurrence by keeping susceptible areas clean and dry Frequently associated with overheating from too much clothing
Erythema multiforme (Stevens-Johnson syndrome)—unknown; associated with ingestion of some drugs; often follows upper respiratory infection	Erythematous papular rash Lesions enlarge by peripheral expansion; develop central vesicle Involves most skin surfaces except scalp May extend to mucous membranes, especially oral, ocular, and urethral	Symptomatic and supportive Maintain adequate fluid intake (oral or IV), calorie, and protein Cutaneous hygiene Appropriate treatment of complications Diligent monitoring of urine volume and specific gravity, hemoglobin and hematocrit, serum electrolyte levels, total body weight	Rash often preceded by fever and malaise Complications include renal failure and severe eye disease Respiratory involvement in a number of cases Self-limiting, but recovery may extend for weeks; skin lesions subside without scarring; mucous membrane lesions may persist for months Recurrence rate 20%; mortality as high as 10%
Neurofibromatosis—inherited disorder	Café-au-lait spots, pigmented nevi, axillary freckling Slow-growing cutaneous and subcutaneous neurofibromas	Symptomatic treatment of associated manifestations, e.g., speech defects, seizures, skeletal defects (scoliosis, kyphosis), learning disabilities Surgical removal of troublesome tumors	Autosomal-dominant inheritance pattern High mutation rate

*Use with caution.

Unit 4

NURSING CARE PLAN
THE CHILD WITH THERMAL BURNS

Destruction of skin by thermal, chemical, electric, or radioactive agents

Burn severity criteria:

Minor Burns

Partial-thickness burns of less than 15% of body surface

Full-thickness burns of less than 2% of body surface

Moderate Burns

Partial-thickness burns of 15% to 25% of body surface

Full-thickness burns of less than 10% of body area, except in small children and when the burns involve critical areas, such as the face, hands, feet, or genitalia

Major or Critical Burns

Burns complicated by respiratory tract injury

Partial-thickness burns of 25% total area or greater

Burns of face, hands, feet, or genitalia, even if they appear to be partial thickness

Full-thickness burns of 10% of body surface or greater

Any child younger than 2 years of age, unless the burn is very small and very superficial

Electric burns that penetrate

Deep chemical burns

Respiratory tract damage

Burns complicated by fractures or soft tissue injury

Burns complicated by concurrent illness, such as obesity, diabetes, epilepsy, and cardiac and renal diseases

ASSESSMENT

Initial assessments

Assess respiratory status

Assess for extent of burn injury based on percentage of body surface area involved

Children from birth to age 5 years (Fig. 4-8)

Older children (Fig. 4-9)

Assess for depth of burn injury

Superficial (first-degree) burns—Involves epidermis

Dry red surface

Blanches on pressure and refills

Painful

Partial-thickness (second-degree) burns

Blistered, moist

Mottled pink or red

Red blanches on pressure and refills

Very painful

Full-thickness (third-degree) burns

Tough, leathery

Dull, dry surface

Brown, tan, red, or black

Does not blanch on pressure

Little pain, but surrounded by painful partial-thickness burns

Assess for evidence of associated injuries

Check eyes for injury or irritation

Check nasopharynx for edema or redness

Check for singed hair, including nasal hair

Assess for other injuries (e.g., bruises, fractures, internal injuries)

Observe for evidence of respiratory distress

Assess need for pain medication

Weigh child on admission; take vital signs

Assess level of consciousness (See p. 392)

Obtain history of burn injury, especially time of injury, nature of burning agent, duration of contact, if injury occurred in an enclosed area, any medication given

Obtain pertinent history relative to preburn condition—Weight, preexisting illnesses, any allergies

Assist with diagnostic procedures and tests—Blood count, urinalysis, wound cultures, hematocrit

Ongoing assessments

Monitor vital signs, including blood pressure

Measure intake and output

Monitor intravenous infusion; observe for evidence of overhydration

Assess circulation of areas peripheral to burns

Assess for evidence of healing, stability of temporary cover or graft, infection

Observe for evidence of complications—Pneumonia, wound sepsis, Curling (stress) ulceration, central nervous system dysfunction (hallucinations, personality changes, delirium, seizures, alterations in sensorium), hypertension

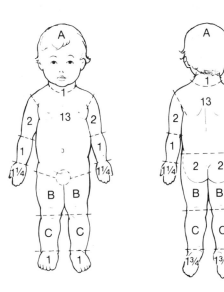

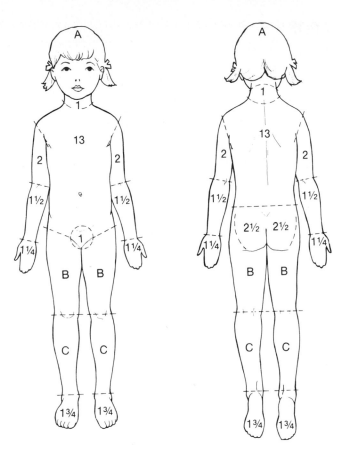

Management and rehabilitative phases of burn care

NURSING DIAGNOSIS: Impaired skin integrity related to thermal injury

GOAL

Facilitate wound healing

INTERVENTIONS

Shave hair from wound and area immediately surrounding burn, if needed

Thoroughly cleanse wound and surrounding skin; debride of devitalized tissues

Keep child from scratching and picking at wound
   Provide distraction
   Older child: explain reasons
   Young child: apply restraining devices as needed
   Maintain care in handling wound to avoid damaging epithelializing and granulating tissues
   Offer high-calorie, high-protein meals and snacks
   Prevent infection
*Administer supplementary vitamins and minerals—vitamins A, B, and C and zinc sulfate

EXPECTED OUTCOME

Wound heals without evidence of damage or inflammation

GOAL

Protect graft area

---

*Dependent nursing action.

INTERVENTIONS

Position for minimal disturbance of graft site
Restrain if necessary

EXPECTED OUTCOME

Skin graft remains intact

NURSING DIAGNOSIS: Pain related to skin trauma, therapies

GOAL

Relieve pain

INTERVENTIONS

Assess need for pain medication (see p. 279)
Position for comfort
Employ appropriate nonpharmacologic pain-reduction techniques (see p. 286)
*Administer analgesics as needed

EXPECTED OUTCOME

Child exhibits only minimum evidence of pain

---

*Dependent nursing action.

Unit 4

GOAL

Prevent pain

INTERVENTIONS

Avoid touching or moving painful areas
Reduce irritation, for example, avoid drafts, movement
Anticipate need for pain medication and administer before onset of pain

EXPECTED OUTCOME

Child exhibits only minimum evidence of pain

NURSING DIAGNOSIS: Potential for infection related to denuded skin, presence of pathogenic organisms

GOAL

Control bacterial growth on wound

INTERVENTIONS

Implement and maintain isolation precautions according to unit policy
Maintain careful handwashing by members of staff and visitors
Wear clean or sterilized gown, cap, mask, and sterile gloves when handling wound area
Avoid injury to crust and eschar
Avoid patient contact with persons who have upper respiratory or skin infection
Cover wound and/or patient according to protocol of unit
Administer good oral hygiene
*Apply prescribed topical antimicrobial preparation and dressings (if ordered) to wound
Obtain wound cultures three times per week to ascertain any increase in wound flora

EXPECTED OUTCOMES

Possible sources of infection are eliminated
Wound displays minimum or no evidence of infection

NURSING DIAGNOSIS: Altered nutrition: less than body requirements related to increased catabolism, loss of appetite

GOAL

Maintain adequate nutrition and prevent nitrogen loss

INTERVENTIONS

Provide high-calorie, high-protein meals and snacks

EXPECTED OUTCOME

Child maintains a positive nitrogen balance—no weight loss

GOAL

Stimulate appetite

---

*Dependent nursing action

INTERVENTIONS

Encourage oral feeding (see p. 277)
Provide foods child likes
Allow self-help
Provide meals when child is most likely to eat well
Provide attractive meals and surroundings
Provide companionship at meals
Employ "contract" with older children

EXPECTED OUTCOMES

Child consumes a sufficient amount of nutrients (specify)
Child interacts with other children

NURSING DIAGNOSIS: Impaired physical mobility (specify level) related to pain, impaired joint movement

GOAL

Promote optimum functioning (physical)

INTERVENTIONS

Carry out range of motion exercises
Encourage mobility if child is unable to move extremities
Ambulate as soon as feasible
Splint involved joints at night and rest periods
Encourage and promote self-help activities
Administer analgesia before painful activity (e.g., physical therapy)

EXPECTED OUTCOME

Joints remain flexible with maximum functional capacity

GOAL

Minimize scar formation

INTERVENTIONS

Position in functional attitude for minimum deformity and optimum function
Apply splints as ordered and designed
Wrap healing tissue with elastic bandage or dress in elastic garments as ordered
Carry out physical therapy

EXPECTED OUTCOME

Wound heals with minimum scar formation; joints remain flexible and functional

---

NURSING DIAGNOSIS: Body image disturbance related to perception of appearance and mobility

GOAL

Meet emotional needs

INTERVENTIONS

Convey positive attitude toward child

Encourage parents to visit
Encourage as much independence as condition allows
Arrange for continued schooling
Promote peer contact where possible

EXPECTED OUTCOMES

Child accepts efforts of family and caregivers
Child engages in activities with others according to age and
  capabilities

GOAL

Help build positive body image

INTERVENTIONS

Explore feelings concerning physical appearance
Discuss feelings about returning to home and family, school,
  and friends
Provide reinforcement of positive aspects of appearance and
  capabilities
Point out evidence of healing
Discuss aids that camouflage disfigurement
  Wigs
  Clothing, for example, turtleneck sweaters
  Makeup
Provide recreational and diversional activities
Promote constructive thinking in child

EXPECTED OUTCOMES

Child discusses feelings and concerns regarding appearance and
  perceived reactions of others
Child verbalizes positive suggestions for adjusting to appearance

GOAL

Promote self-care

INTERVENTIONS

Assist with self-care activities as needed
Encourage self-care according to capabilities
Begin early in hospitalization to discuss "going home"
Accept regressive behavior where appropriate
Help child develop independence and self-help capabilities
See Nursing diagnosis: Body image disturbance, p. 265

EXPECTED OUTCOMES

Child verbalizes and otherwise demonstrates interest in going
  home
Child engages in self-help activities

NURSING DIAGNOSIS: Altered family processes related to situational crisis (child with a serious injury)

GOAL

Prepare family for discharge

INTERVENTIONS

Teach wound care to caregiver
Discuss diet, rest, and activity
Explore attitudes toward child's reentry into the family
Explore family's concept regarding child's capabilities and the
  possible restrictions and freedom they will allow
Help family set realistic goals for themselves, child, and other
  family members
Help family acquire needed equipment and supplies

EXPECTED OUTCOMES

Family demonstrates an understanding of the needs of the child
  and the impact his condition will have on them
Family sets realistic goals for selves, child, and others

GOAL

Participate in follow-up care

INTERVENTIONS

Coordinate team management of child and family
Arrange for return visits
Assess needs of family
Arrange for referral to agencies based on need assessment
Collaborate with school nurse to help with child's reintegration
  into school and the world of peers
Visit school to prepare teacher and peers, if possible

EXPECTED OUTCOMES

Family maintains contact with health providers
Child attends school regularly and interacts with age-mates

See also:
Nursing care plan: The child in the hospital, p. 246
Nursing care plan: The family of the ill or hospitalized child, p.
  254

Unit 4

NURSING CARE OF THE CHILD WITH PSYCHOPHYSIOLOGIC DYSFUNCTION

Those disorders in which psychologic dysfunction plays a role

NURSING CARE PLAN
THE CHILD WITH NONORGANIC FAILURE TO THRIVE

Failure to thrive is a deviation from an established growth pattern in a child under 3 years of age

Nonorganic failure to thrive—Caused by factors unrelated to organic dysfunction and most often the result of psychosocial factors, especially relationships between the child and the primary caregiver, usually the mother

ASSESSMENT

Perform physical assessment—especially growth

Obtain detailed history—especially feeding behaviors

Observe for evidence of parental maladaptive behaviors toward infant:

Persistent ambivalence or negative feelings about the fetus and the pregnancy during the prenatal period

Makes no plans for obtaining basic infant supplies

Appears indifferent to infant at time of delivery; may appear sad or angry; is expressionless

Makes no effort to establish eye-to-eye contact with infant

Handles infant only when necessary

Does not talk to infant

Makes few or no spontaneous movements with infant

Asks few questions about care

Sees infant as ugly, fat, or unattractive

Displays disgust with infant's drooling and sucking sounds; is revolted by infant's body fluids

Annoyed with diaper changing

Perceives infant's odor as revolting

Holds infant with little support to head and body

Holds infant away from body during feeding or props bottle for feeding; seldom cuddles infant

Does not coo or talk to infant

Refers to infant in an impersonal manner

Develops inappropriate responses to infant's needs, such as leaving infant in one place for long periods, leaving child alone in room, overfeeding or underfeeding, overstimulating or understimulating infant, forcing or refusing eye contact, bouncing or tickling infant when infant is fatigued

Cannot discriminate between infant's signals for hunger, comfort, rest, body contact

Is convinced the infant has a defect or disease even when reassured to the contrary

Makes negative statements regarding parenting role

Believes the infant is judging him/her and efforts as an adult

Believes the infant does not love him/her

Develops paradoxical attitudes and behaviors toward the infant

Assess infant's feeding behaviors, temperament

Assess family for marital stress, physical or mental illness, death or illness in a previous child, alcoholism, drug use, financial crises

Determine if pregnancy was planned or unplanned, any disturbing events associated with pregnancy or delivery of the child

Perform developmental tests

Assist with diagnostic procedures and tests, including those to rule out organic disease

Observe for evidence of parental characteristics such as:

History of maternal deprivation as a child

Low self-esteem; feelings of inadequacy

Desire for dependency

Loneliness, isolation

Limited support system

Multiple life crises and stress

NURSING DIAGNOSIS: Altered growth and development related to socially restricted environment (infant deprivation), physical neglect

GOAL

Provide a nurturing environment for the hospitalized child

INTERVENTIONS

Apply primary care concepts to ensure continuity of care with a minimum number of caregivers

Provide gentle, confident, and loving handling

Perform physical care with as much holding, rocking, and cuddling as the child will respond to

Encourage eye-to-eye contact

Employ consistent schedule in meeting child's needs for food, hygiene, care, and rest

Assign a foster grandparent or child life specialist to child

Provide sensory stimulation and play appropriate to the child's developmental level

EXPECTED OUTCOME

Child displays a positive response to interventions (e.g., social smile)

NURSING DIAGNOSIS: Altered nutrition: less than body requirements related to deprivation of necessities, emotional deprivation

GOAL

Make feeding a priority goal

INTERVENTIONS

Provide unlimited feedings of a regular diet for the age of the child (preferably foods to which the child is accustomed)

Avoid interruption of feedings with other activities, such as laboratory examinations or radiography

Keep accurate record of intake to ensure ingestion of calculated daily calories

Weigh daily and record to ascertain weight gain

EXPECTED OUTCOME

Child gains 1 to 2 ounces per day (minimum)

GOAL

Introduce a positive feeding environment

INTERVENTIONS

Assign one nurse for feeding

Maintain calm, even temperament; be persistent

Provide a quiet, unstimulating environment

Hold young child for feeding

Maintain eye-to-eye contact with child

Talk to child by giving appropriate directions and praise for eating

Follow the child's rhythm of feeding

Establish a structural routine and follow it consistently

EXPECTED OUTCOME

Infant responds positively to feeding practices (specify)

NURSING DIAGNOSIS: Altered parenting related to (specify, e.g., knowledge deficit, poverty)

GOAL

Reduce parental anxiety and provide education

INTERVENTIONS

Welcome parents and encourage, but do not push, them to become involved in the child's care

Teach parents about the child's physical care, developmental skills, and emotional needs through example, not lecture

Afford parents the opportunity to discuss their lives and feelings toward the child

Supply emotional nurturance without encouraging dependency

Promote parents' self-esteem and confidence by praising their achievements with the child

Prepare parents for adjustments with anticipatory guidance

EXPECTED OUTCOME

Parents demonstrate the ability to provide appropriate care to the child

GOAL

Prepare for discharge

INTERVENTIONS

Assess home environment and relationships

Continue interventions begun in the hospital

Establish a consistent contact system through public health nurse

Establish an infant stimulation program

Provide for stress-relieving services to the family

Refer to appropriate agencies for assistance with financial, social, mental health, or other family needs

EXPECTED OUTCOMES

Child exhibits continued weight gain appropriate for age

Family follows through on programs and activities

Unit 4

NURSING CARE PLAN
THE CHILD WHO IS MALTREATED

Child maltreatment is a broad term that includes intentional physical abuse or neglect, emotional abuse or neglect, or sexual abuse of children, usually by an adult

Physical abuse—The deliberate infliction of physical injury

Physical neglect—Omission of a direct act or behavior that has a detrimental effect on the child's physical and/or psychologic development

Emotional abuse—The deliberate attempt to destroy or significantly impair a child's self-esteem or competence

Emotional neglect—Failure to meet the child's needs for affection, attention, and emotional nurturance

Sexual abuse—Contacts or interactions between a child and an adult when the child is being used for the sexual stimulation of that adult or another person

ASSESSMENT

Perform physical assessment with special attention to manifestations of potential abuse or neglect (see box)

Obtain history of event, being alert for discrepancies in descriptions by caregiver and observations

  Note sequence of events, including times, especially time lapse between occurrence of injury and initiation of treatment

  Interview child when appropriate, including verbal quotations and information from drawing or other play activities

Interview parents, witnesses, or other significant persons, including verbal quotations

Observe parent-child interactions (verbal interactions, eye contact, touching, evidence of parental concern)

Observe or obtain information regarding names, ages, and condition of other children in the home (if possible)

Perform developmental test

Assist with diagnostic procedures and tests—Radiology, collection of specimens for examination

MANIFESTATIONS OF MALTREATMENT

Physical Neglect

Physical indicators:

  Failure to thrive

  Signs of malnutrition, such as thin extremities, abdominal distention, lack of subcutaneous fat

  Poor personal hygiene, especially of teeth

  Unclean and/or inappropriate dress

  Evidence of poor health care, such as nonimmunized status, untreated infections, frequent colds

  Frequent injuries from lack of supervision

Behavioral indicators:

  Dull and inactive; excessively passive or sleepy

  Self-stimulatory behaviors, such as finger sucking or rocking

  Begging or stealing food

  Absenteeism from school

  Drug or alcohol addiction } in older child

  Vandalism or shoplifting

Emotional Abuse and Neglect

Physical indicators:

  Failure to thrive

  Feeding disorders, such as rumination

  Enuresis

  Sleep disorders

Behavioral indicators:

  Self-stimulatory behaviors, such as biting, rocking, sucking

  During infancy, lack of social smile and stranger anxiety

  Withdrawal

  Unusual fearfulness

  Antisocial behavior, such as destructiveness, stealing, cruelty

  Extremes of behavior, such as overcompliant and passive or aggressive and demanding

  Lags in emotional and intellectual development, especially language

  Suicide attempts

Physical Abuse

Physical indicators:

  Bruises and welts

    On face, lips, mouth, back, buttocks, thighs, or areas of torso

    Regular patterns descriptive of object used, such as belt buckle, hand, wire hanger, chain, wooden spoon, squeeze or pinch marks

    May be present in various stages of healing

MANIFESTATIONS OF MALTREATMENT—cont'd

Burns
  On soles of feet, palms of hands, back, or buttocks
  Patterns descriptive of object used, such as round cigar or cigarette burns, "glovelike" sharply demarcated areas from immersion in scalding water, rope burns on wrists or ankles from being bound, burns in the shape of an iron, radiator, or electric stove burner
  Absence of "splash" marks and presence of symmetric burns
Fractures and dislocations
  Skull, nose, or facial structures
  Injury may denote type of abuse, such as spiral fracture or dislocation from twisting of an extremity or whiplash from shaking the child
  Multiple new or old fractures in various stages of healing
Lacerations and abrasions
  On backs of arms, legs, torso, face, or external genitalia
  Unusual symptoms, such as abdominal swelling, pain, and vomiting from punching
  Descriptive marks such as from human bites or pulling the hair out
Chemical
  Unexplained repeated poisoning, especially drug overdose
  Unexplained sudden illness, such as hypoglycemia from insulin administration
Behavioral indicators:
  Wary of physical contact with adults
  Apparent fear of parents or going home
  Lying very still while surveying environment
  Inappropriate reaction to injury, such as failure to cry from pain
  Lack of reaction to frightening events
  Apprehensive when hearing other children cry
  Indiscriminate friendliness and displays of affection
  Superficial relationships
  Acting-out behavior, such as aggression, to seek attention
  Withdrawal behavior

Sexual Abuse
Physical indicators:
  Bruises, bleeding, lacerations or irritation of external genitalia, anus, mouth, or throat
  Torn, stained, or bloody underclothing
  Pain on urination or pain, swelling, and itching of genital area
  Penile discharge
  Sexually transmitted disease, nonspecific vaginitis, or venereal warts
  Difficulty in walking or sitting
  Unusual odor in the genital area
  Recurrent urinary tract infections
  Pregnancy in young adolescent
Behavioral indicators:
  Withdrawn, excessive daydreaming
  Preoccupied with fantasies, especially in play
  Poor relationships with peers
  Sudden changes, such as anxiety, loss or gain of weight, clinging behavior
  In incestuous relationships, excessive anger at mother for not protecting daughter
  Regressive behavior, such as bed-wetting or thumbsucking
  Sudden onset of phobias or fears, particularly fears of the dark, men, strangers, or particular settings or situations (e.g., undue fear of leaving the house or staying at the daycare center or the baby-sitter's house)
  Running away from home
  Sudden emergence of sexually-related problems, including excessive or public masturbation, age-inappropriate sexual play, promiscuity, or overtly seductive behavior
  Substance abuse, particularly of alcohol or mood-elevating drugs
  Profound and rapid personality changes, especially extreme depression, hostility, and aggression (often accompanied by social withdrawal)
  Rapidly declining school performance
  Suicidal attempts or ideation

NURSING DIAGNOSIS: Potential for trauma related to characteristics of child, caregiver(s), environment

GOAL

Protect from further abuse

INTERVENTIONS

Implement measures to prevent abuse
  Report suspicions to appropriate authorities
  Assist in removing child from unsafe environment and establishing in a safe environment
  Establish protective measures for the hospitalized child as indicated

Keep factual, objective records of
  The child's physical condition
  The child's behavioral response to parents, others, and environment
  Interviews with family members
*Report suspected child abuse to local authorities

EXPECTED OUTCOME

Suspected child abuse victim is removed from abusive environment

---

*Telephone numbers are usually listed under "Child abuse" in the business white pages of the local directory, or call the emergency child abuse hotline: 1-800-422-4453 (1-800-4-A-CHILD).

GOAL

Prevent recurrence

INTERVENTIONS

Collaborate efforts of multidisciplinary team to continually evaluate progress of child in foster home or in return to own family

Be alert for signs of continued abuse or neglect

Help parents identify those circumstances that precipitate an abusive act and ways in which to deal with the release of anger in ways other than attacking child

Refer for alternative placement when indicated

EXPECTED OUTCOME

Child is free of injury or neglect

NURSING DIAGNOSIS: Fear/anxiety related to negative interpersonal interaction, repeated maltreatment, powerlessness

GOAL

Relieve or reduce anxiety and stress

INTERVENTIONS

Provide consistent caregiver and therapeutic environment during hospitalization

Demonstrate acceptance of child while not expecting same in return

Show attention while not reinforcing inappropriate behavior

Plan appropriate activities for attention with nurse, other adults, and other children; use play to work through relationships

Avoid displacing anger on child, such as shouting or yelling, as method of dealing with own frustration toward child's negative behavior

Praise child's abilities in order to promote self-esteem

Treat child as one who has a specific physical problem for hospitalization, not as "abused" victim

Avoid asking too many questions

Use play, especially family or doll house activity, to investigate kind of relationships perceived by child

Provide one consistent person to whom child relates regarding events of abuse

EXPECTED OUTCOMES

Child exhibits minimal or no evidence of distress

Child engages in positive relationships with caregivers

NURSING DIAGNOSIS: Altered parenting related to child, caregiver, or situational characteristics that precipitate abusive behavior

GOAL

Prevent abuse

INTERVENTIONS

Identify families at risk for potential abuse

Promote parental attachment to child

Emphasize child-rearing practices, especially effective methods of discipline

Increase parents' feeling of adequacy and self-esteem

Encourage support systems that lessen stress and total responsibility of child care on one or both parents

EXPECTED OUTCOME

Families exhibit evidence of positive interaction with children

GOAL

Support parents

INTERVENTIONS

Provide "mothering" by directing attention to parent, taking over child-care responsibilities until parent feels ready to participate, and focusing on parent's needs

*Refer parents to special support groups and/or counseling

Help identify a support group for parents, such as extended family or nearby neighbors; help these significant others understand their important role in also preventing further abuse

EXPECTED OUTCOMES

Parents demonstrate appropriate parenting activities

Parents seek group and individual support

GOAL

Educate parents regarding normal child growth and development

INTERVENTIONS

Teach realistic expectations of child's behavior and capabilities

Emphasize alternate methods of discipline, such as reward and verbal disapproval

Suggest methods of handling developmental problems or goals, such as toddler negativism, toilet training, independence

Teach through demonstration and role modeling, rather than lecture; avoid authoritarian approach

EXPECTED OUTCOME

Parents demonstrate an understanding of normal expectations for their child

GOAL

Reduce environmental crises

INTERVENTIONS

Refer to social agencies that can provide assistance in areas such as financial support, adequate housing, and employment

EXPECTED OUTCOME

Parents receive assistance with problems

---

*Physical abuse: **Parents Anonymous,** 6733 Sepulvida, Suite 270, Los Angeles, CA 90045; call 1-800-352-0386.

Sexual abuse: **Parents United** and the adjunct **Daughters and Sons United,** P.O. Box 952, San Jose, CA 95108; call 1-408-280-5055.

GOAL

Promote a sense of parental adequacy during child's hospitalization

INTERVENTIONS

Orient parents to hospital unit and help them feel welcomed and an important part of child's care and recovery

Reinforce competent child care activities

Focus on the abuse as a problem that requires therapeutic intervention, not as a behavior characteristic or deficiency of the parent

Empathize with difficulties of rearing children, especially with additional life crises, while not condoning the act of abuse or neglect

Foster healthy aspects of parent-child relationship

EXPECTED OUTCOME

Parents demonstrate an attitude of concern for and ability to care for the child

GOAL

Plan for discharge

INTERVENTIONS

Prepare for discharge as soon as disposition is finalized

Home placement:

Encourage parents to visit as much as possible during hospitalization

Plan for close supervision and counseling of family

Foster home placement:

Encourage foster family members to visit child before discharge

Stress to them child's need to regress in order to complete missed stages of development

Help child grieve this loss, if parents' rights are being terminated permanently, especially if it entails separation from siblings (long-term counseling is optimum goal)

EXPECTED OUTCOMES

Parents demonstrate ability and desire to care for child

Child is placed in appropriate environment

NURSING CARE PLAN
THE ADOLESCENT WITH ANOREXIA NERVOSA

A disorder characterized by severe weight loss in the absence of obvious physical cause

ASSESSMENT

Perform physical assessment

Obtain history of eating behaviors; explore body image perception

Assess family interpersonal relationships

Observe for manifestations of anorexia nervosa (AN):

Severe and profound weight loss

Signs of altered metabolic activity:

Secondary amenorrhea (if menarche attained)

Primary amenorrhea (if menarche not attained)

Bradycardia

Lowered body temperature

Decreased blood pressure

Cold intolerance

Dry skin and brittle nails

Appearance of lanugo hair

---

*From Diagnostic and statistical manual of mental disorders, ed. 3-revised (DSM-III-R), Washington, DC, 1987, American Psychiatric Association.

Assist with diagnostic procedures and tests including assessment based on the following diagnostic criteria:*

A. Refusal to maintain body weight over a minimal normal weight for age and height, e.g., weight loss leading to maintenance of body weight 15% below that expected; or failure to make expected weight gain during period of growth, leading to body weight 15% below that expected

B. Intense fear of gaining weight or becoming fat, even though underweight

C. Disturbance in the way in which one's body weight, size, or shape is experienced, e.g., the person claims to "feel fat" even when emaciated, believes that one area of the body is "too fat" even when obviously underweight

D. In females, absence of at least three consecutive menstrual cycles when otherwise expected to occur (primary or secondary amenorrhea). (A woman is considered to have amenorrhea if her periods occur only following hormone, e.g., estrogen, administration.)

NURSING DIAGNOSIS: Altered nutrition: less than body requirements related to self-starvation

GOAL

Restore nutritional status

INTERVENTIONS

Implement high-calorie diet as prescribed
Explain nutritional plan to child and family
With dietitian and patient select balanced diet with the prescribed incremental increase in calories
Help patient prepare a dietary diary

EXPECTED OUTCOME

Child evidences weight gain

GOAL

Enforce behavior modification plan (if implemented)

INTERVENTIONS

Make certain all members of the health team determine an approach, understand the plan, and adhere to it consistently
Involve all team members, including the patient
Ensure continuity of caregivers (team members)
Provide for clear communication among team members and with the patient so that patient understands precisely what is expected
Consult with patient regarding progress
Avoid coercive techniques
Avoid extensive discussion of food
Support the patient in efforts (e.g., positive feedback for accomplishments).

EXPECTED OUTCOME

Expectations are met consistently (specify)

GOAL

Reduce energy expenditure

INTERVENTIONS

Monitor physical activity
Supervise selection and performance of activity
Be alert to evidence of secretive exercising

EXPECTED OUTCOME

Child engages in quiet and specified activities

NURSING DIAGNOSIS: Body image disturbance related to altered perception

GOAL

Provide patient with appropriate feeling of control

INTERVENTIONS

Channel need for control and feeling of effectiveness in appropriate directions (rather than control of weight)
Obtain psychiatric referral as indicated
Encourage patient to monitor own care as appropriate

EXPECTED OUTCOME

Child expresses self in acceptable ways

GOAL

Support child

INTERVENTIONS

Maintain open communications with child
Convey an attitude of caring and protection to child
Avoid conveying an attitude of intrusion
Encourage participation in own care

EXPECTED OUTCOMES

Child expresses feelings and concerns
Child becomes actively involved in own care and management

GOAL

Alter distorted self-image

INTERVENTIONS

Support psychiatric plan of care

EXPECTED OUTCOME

Child displays evidence of developing a positive self-image

NURSING DIAGNOSIS: Ineffective individual coping related to unrealistic perceptions

GOAL

Prevent relapse

INTERVENTIONS

Maintain consistency in therapeutic approach selected
Maintain vigilance to detect signs of sabotaging the therapeutic plan, such as self-induced vomiting, hoarding food, disposing of food, placing weighted material in clothing for weigh-in
Provide positive reinforcement for progress
Be alert for signs of depression
Support psychotherapeutic measures
Help arrange for follow-up care

EXPECTED OUTCOME

Child and family conform to therapeutic program (specify behaviors)

NURSING DIAGNOSIS: Family coping: potential for growth related to ambivalent family relationships

GOAL

Resolve disturbed pattern of family interaction

INTERVENTIONS

Observe family interaction
Explore feelings and attitudes of family members
Support psychotherapeutic measures for redirecting malfunctioning family processes
Help arrange for referral to individuals and groups that further therapeutic goals

EXPECTED OUTCOME

Family patterns of interaction are outlined and evaluated

GOAL

Prepare for home care

INTERVENTIONS

Make certain both patient and family understand therapeutic plan
Arrange for follow-up care
*Refer to special agencies for additional information and support

EXPECTED OUTCOME

Family demonstrates an understanding of the etiology of the disorder and conforms to therapeutic program

---

*National Association of Anorexia Nervosa and Associated Disorders, Inc., Box 7, Highland Park, IL 60035; (312) 831-3438. American Anorexia/Bulimia Association, Inc., 133 Cedar Lane, Teaneck, NJ 07666, 201-836-1800.

NURSING CARE PLAN
THE CHILD WHO IS OBESE

An increase in body weight resulting from an excessive accumulation of fat or simply the state of being too fat

Unit 4

ASSESSMENT

Perform physical assessment
Observe for manifestations of obesity:
 Child appears overweight
 Weight over established standards
 Skinfold thickness greater than established standard, p. 111
 Body fat increased above established standards as determined by densitometric, hydrometric, and radiopotassium measurements
Obtain family history of obesity and diet habits and food preferences
Obtain health history including analysis of weight charts, eating habits, behaviors, especially relative to physical activity
Interview child and family to elicit psychologic factors that might contribute to obesity—Cultural standards, use of food for pacification, peer and family interpersonal relationships, use of food as a reward
Assist with diagnostic procedures and tests—Anthropomorphic measurements, biochemical studies for evidence of disease

NURSING DIAGNOSIS: Altered nutrition: more than body requirements related to dysfunctional eating patterns, hereditary factors

GOAL

Identify eating patterns and behaviors

INTERVENTIONS

Instruct child and family to:
 Keep a record of everything eaten, including
 Time eaten
 Amount eaten
 Where food was consumed
 Activity engaged in while eating
 With whom the food was eaten or if it was eaten alone
 Feelings at the time food was eaten, for example, angry, depressed, lonely, elated
Identify food stimuli
 Feelings of hunger
 Television commercials
 Smell or sight of food
Assess eating environments
 Where food is eaten
 With whom food is eaten, or eaten alone
 Feelings at time of food consumption

Activity in which engaged while eating

Analyze preceding data for patterns of eating and relationships of other factors as a basis for making adjustments

EXPECTED OUTCOME

Child's eating patterns become apparent

GOAL

Control food stimuli

INTERVENTIONS

Encourage child to:

Separate eating from other activities

Minimize food cues

Get rid of "junk" food

Prepare and serve only amounts to be eaten

Put snacks out of sight

Avoid purchase of problem foods such as "fast foods" (see box, p. 520)

Serve food from stove or other place out of reach of the established eating place

EXPECTED OUTCOME

Child demonstrates an understanding of eating patterns and endeavors to alter destructive patterns

GOAL

Change eating patterns

INTERVENTIONS

Encourage child to:

Eat at a specific place reserved just for eating

Eat orderly meals at regular hours

Use smaller plates to make amounts of food appear larger

Eat at slow pace

Leave a small amount of food on plate

Eliminate eating during television viewing

Substitute raw vegetables for "junk" food snacks

EXPECTED OUTCOME

Child alters eating behaviors

GOAL

Alter activity patterns

INTERVENTIONS

Encourage child to:

Use activities other than eating to deal with emotional stress, boredom, and fatigue

Engage in hobby activity, take a walk, straighten up room

Become involved in activities away from food

EXPECTED OUTCOME

Child engages in suitable activities according to age and interest

GOAL

Eat the prescribed diet

INTERVENTIONS

Assist the child with meal planning

Employ strategies outlined above

EXPECTED OUTCOMES

Child conforms to prescribed diet plan

Child evidences a steady weight loss (or weight maintenance in a growing child)

NURSING DIAGNOSIS: Activity intolerance related to sedentary life-style, physical bulk

GOAL

Increase physical activity

INTERVENTIONS

Arrange programmed activity such as running, swimming, cycling

Encourage routine activity such as walking, climbing stairs

EXPECTED OUTCOME

Child engages in preferred exercise and activities regularly (specify)

NURSING DIAGNOSIS: Ineffective individual coping related to little or no exercise, poor nutrition, personal vulnerability

GOAL

Promote goal attainment

INTERVENTIONS

Implement a school weight-loss program

Employ a buddy system

Use peers as sponsors and positive reinforcers

Employ frequent weigh-ins conducted by involved adult, nurse, teacher, physical education instructor

Provide reinforcement for weight change

Social—Praise

Tangible—Contract that earns simple rewards

Graph positive weight changes and display where others in the program can see it

Provide nutrition education

Have a family member serve as a monitor at home to help in progress toward goals and to encourage child with positive statements daily

EXPECTED OUTCOME

Child engages in school-based program (specify)

NURSING DIAGNOSIS: Self-esteem disturbance related to perception of physical appearance, internalization of negative feedback

GOAL

Promote goal attainment

INTERVENTIONS

Encourage child to discuss his or her feelings and concerns
Reinforce accomplishments

EXPECTED OUTCOMES

Child expresses feelings and concerns regarding problems
Child maintains a positive attitude toward the weight-loss program

GOAL

Maximize positive aspects of appearance

INTERVENTIONS

Encourage good grooming, hygiene, and posture
Assist with exploring positive aspects of appearance and ways to enhance these aspects

EXPECTED OUTCOME

Child makes measurable efforts to improve appearance (specify)

GOAL

Improve self-esteem

INTERVENTIONS

Relate to child as an important, worthwhile individual
Encourage to set small, attainable goals for self
Encourage and support positive thinking (overweight persons are negative thinkers)
Encourage in activities to relieve boredom
Encourage interaction with peers

EXPECTED OUTCOMES

Child sets realistic short-term goals for self-improvement (specify)
Child voices positive attitudes toward self
Child engages in appropriate activities and interaction with peers (specify)

NURSING DIAGNOSIS: Altered family processes related to management of an obese child

GOAL

Involve family in child's weight-loss program

INTERVENTIONS

Educate family regarding weight-loss program, including nutrition, relationship of food intake and exercise, psychologic support
Encourage family to:
    Use appropriate reinforcement
    Alter food and eating environment
    Maintain proper attitudes regarding program
    Assist in monitoring eating behavior, food intake, physical activity, weight change
    Eliminate food as a reward
    Encourage youngster with positive statements only

EXPECTED OUTCOME

Family becomes actively involved in child's weight-loss program

Unit 4

CALORIC VALUES FOR SELECTED FAST FOOD

Food	Caloric value	Food	Caloric value
Burger King		Cookies and cakes—cont'd	
Cheeseburger	317	Brownie	200
Hamburger	275	Fig Newton, 1	60
Whopper, regular	640	Doughnut, regular, 1 oz	113
w/cheese	723	old fashioned, 1 oz	151
Double beef, plain	850	powdered, 1 oz	117
w/cheese	950	**Crackers**	
French fries, regular	227	Cheese balls & curls, 1 oz	160
Onion rings, regular	274	Corn chips, 1 oz	150-160
Chocolate shake	320	Graham crackers, 1 piece	30
McDonald's		Pretzels, 1 oz	110-116
Big Mac	570	Rye Krisp, 1 triple	25
Hamburger	263	Saltine, 1 piece	12-18
Cheeseburger	328	Tortilla chips, 1 oz	130-140
Chicken McNuggets (6 pieces)	323	Trisket, 1 piece	20
Quarter Pounder	427	Wheat Thins, 1 piece	9
w/cheese	525	**Candy**	
Egg McMuffin	340	Heath, 2½ oz	334
French fries, regular	220	Hershey's, 1.2 oz bar	187
Filet-O-Fish	435	Nestle's, 1.1 oz bar	159
Milk shake, vanilla	352	Hershey's Kisses, 1 piece	27
chocolate	383	Krackle bar, .35 oz	52
Wendy's		Life Savers, 1 piece	10
Hamburger, single	350	Milk Duds, ¾ oz box	89
Hamburger, double	570	1¼ oz box	148
Chicken sandwich	320	M & Ms, peanut, 1½ oz	219
French fries	280	plain, 1½ oz	202
Frosty	400	Mr. Goodbar, 1½ oz	233
Long John Silver's		Snickers, 1.8 oz	247
Fish, 2 pieces & fries	651	Crackerjack, ¾ oz	90
3 pieces & fries	853	**Chewing gum**	
Fish sandwich	337	Any brand, 1 stick	10
Cole slaw	180	Dentyne, 1 stick	4
Hushpuppies (3)	145	Chiclets, Beechies, 1 piece	6
Taco Bell		**Miscellaneous snacks**	
Beef Burrito	466	Potato chips, 1 oz	150-160
Burrito Supreme	457	Pringles, 1 oz	172
Beefy Tostado	291	Yogurt, plain, 8 oz	150-160
Dairy Queen		fruit, 8 oz	230-262
Super Hot Dog/chili	570	Popcorn, plain, 1 cup	54
Super Hot Dog w/cheese	580	**Nuts**	
Fries, small	200	Almonds, 1 oz	170-178
Pizza Hut		Peanuts, dry roasted, 1 oz	160-173
Thin 'n Crispy (¼ medium)		oil roasted, 1 oz	179
Standard cheese	340	Pecans, 1 oz	190-220
Superstyle cheese	410	Pistachios, 1 oz	174
Standard pepperoni	370	Pumpkin seeds, unshelled, 1 oz	116
Superstyle pepperoni	430	Sunflower seeds, shelled, 1 oz	164
Thick 'n Chewy (¼ medium)		unshelled, 1 oz	86
Standard cheese	390	**Dessert snacks**	
Superstyle cheese	450	Popsicle, 1 twin pop	70
Standard pepperoni	450	Turnover	310-340
Superstyle pepperoni	490	Pop Tart	200-220
Supreme	480	**Baskin-Robbins**	
Super Supreme	590	Ice cream, 1 scoop	
Fruit		vanilla	147
Apple w/skin, 2½ in. diameter	66	French vanilla	181
Banana, medium	100	chocolate	165
Peach w/skin, 2 in. diameter	38	chocolate fudge	178
Cookies and cakes		Sherbet, 1 scoop	99-139
Hostess, 1 cup cake		**Beverages**	
orange	151	Chocolate milk, 8 oz	213
chocolate	166	Skim milk, 8 oz	88
Hostess Twinkie, 1	147	Whole milk, 8 oz	159
Oreo, each	50	Coca Cola, 8 oz	96
Chocolate chip	50-80	Sprite, 8 oz	95

NURSING CARE PLAN
THE CHILD WHO IS SUICIDAL

The deliberate act of self-injury with the intent that the injury should kill

Suicidal gesture—Suicidal act without any real attempt to cause either serious injury or death but rather to send out a signal that something is wrong

Suicidal attempt—Suicidal act intended to cause injury or death

ASSESSMENT

Be alert to manifestations of suicidal youth:

Mood/Affect
Marked persistent depression
Feelings of hopelessness, helplessness, isolation
Deteriorating schoolwork
Remains distant, sad, remote
Flat affect—has "frozen" facial expression
Persistently looks or sounds sad and unhappy
Describes self as worthless
Feelings of self-hatred or excessive guilt
Feelings of humiliation, often brought on by inadequate performance at school
Sudden cheerfulness following deep depression
Wish to be punished

Behavior
Changes in physical appearance—A child previously neat and well-groomed will stop bathing and begin to look slovenly
Loss of function due to illness or trauma
Loss of energy—Loss of interest, listlessness, exhaustion without obvious cause
Sleep disturbances—Going to sleep or sleeping excessively, takes voluntary naps during afternoon or evening
Increased irritability, argumentativeness, or stubbornness
Physical complaints—Recurrent stomachaches, headaches
Repeated visits to doctor's office or emergency room for treatment of injuries
Antisocial behavior—Engages in drinking, uses drugs, fights, commits acts of vandalism, runs away from home, becomes sexually promiscuous
*Preoccupation with death—Focuses on morbid thoughts; speaks repeatedly about people getting killed
May begin referring to own death

School and Interpersonal Relationships
Resists or refuses to go to school
May become truant, cuts classes, does not complete assignments
Social withdrawal from friends, activities, interests that were previously enjoyed
*Wants to give away cherished possessions
Lacks an effective social support system

Coping Skills
Loses reality boundaries
Withdraws and isolates self
No use of support systems
Sees self as totally helpless, a victim of fate

*Absolute danger signals.

NURSING DIAGNOSIS: Potential for injury related to acute depression

GOAL

Prevent injury

INTERVENTIONS

Take suicide threat seriously
Convey to the youth an attitude of caring
Listen to the youngster
Encourage the youngster to discuss feelings and concerns
Refer suicidal youngster to the nearest crisis center
  *Maintain current telephone number of 24-hour crisis intervention center
Refer to local center (e.g., school suicide prevention center, community health services) for specialized counseling

EXPECTED OUTCOME

Child receives prompt attention

*Youth Suicide National Center, 1825 I St. N.W., Washington, DC 20006, (202) 429-0190.

NURSING CARE OF THE CHILD WITH POISONING

NURSING CARE PLAN
THE CHILD WITH POISONING

The condition or physical state produced when a substance, in relatively small amounts, is applied to body surfaces, ingested, injected, inhaled, or absorbed and subsequently causes structural damage or disturbance of function

ASSESSMENT

Perform physical assessment with particular attention to vital signs, breath odor, state of consciousness, skin changes, neurologic signs

Obtain careful and detailed history regarding what, when, and how much of toxic substance has entered the body

Look for evidence of poison (container, plant, vomitus)

Observe for evidence of ingestion, inhalation, or absorption of toxic substances:

Skin manifestations
   Pallor
   Redness
   Evidence of burning
   Pain

Mucous membrane manifestations
   Evidence of irritation
   Red discoloration
   White discoloration
   Swelling

Gastrointestinal manifestations
   Salivation
   Inability to clear secretions
   Dry mouth
   Nausea and vomiting
   Diarrhea
   Constipation
   Abdominal pain

Cardiovascular manifestations
   Arrhythmias
   Increased blood pressure
   Decreased blood pressure
   Tachycardia
   Bradycardia
   Evidence of shock

Respiratory manifestations
   Gagging, choking, coughing
   Tachypnea
   Bradypnea
   Cyanosis
   Grunting

Renal manifestations
   Oliguria
   Hematuria

Metabolic/autonomic manifestations
   Sweating
   Hyperthermia
   Hypothermia
   Metabolic acidosis

Neuromuscular manifestations
   Weakness
   Involuntary movements
   Teeth gnashing
   Ataxia
   Dilated pupils
   Constricted pupils
   Seizures

Altered sensorium
   Anxiety, agitation
   Hallucinations
   Confusion
   Coma

Assist with diagnostic tests—Blood levels of toxins, radiograph to determine presence of masses of undissolved tablets remaining in GI tract

Observe for latent symptoms of poisoning

NURSING DIAGNOSIS: Potential for poisoning related to presence of toxic substance, immature judgment of child

GOAL

Prevent occurrence and/or recurrence

INTERVENTIONS

Assess possible contributing factors in occurrence of injury, such as discipline, parent-child relationship, developmental ability, environmental factors, behavior problems, and so on

Refer to visiting nurse agency to evaluate home environment and need for safe-proofing measures

Provide assistance with environmental manipulation when necessary

Institute anticipatory guidance for possible future injuries based on child's age and maturational level

    Assess possible contributing factors in occurrence of injury, such as discipline, parent-child relationship, developmental ability, environmental factors, and behavior problems

    Institute anticipatory guidance for possible future injuries based on child's age and maturational level

    Refer to visiting nurse agency to evaluate home environment and need for safe-proofing measures

    Provide assistance with environmental manipulation when necessary, such as lead removal

    Educate parents regarding safe storage of toxic substances (see Child Safety Home Checklist in the box on p. 184)

    Advise parents to take drugs out of sight of children

    Advise parents to replace *immediately* all toxic substances to safe storage

    Teach children the hazards of ingesting nonfood items without supervision

    Advise parents against using plants for teas or medicine

    Discuss problems of discipline and children's noncompliance and offer strategies for effective discipline

    Instruct parents regarding correct administration of drugs for therapeutic purposes and to discontinue drug if there is evidence of mild toxicity

    Have syrup of ipecac available—Two doses for each child in the family

    Encourage grandparents or other frequent caregivers to keep syrup of ipecac in the home

    *Post number of local Poison Control Center with emergency phone list at the telephone

EXPECTED OUTCOME

Child does not swallow potentially poisonous substance

NURSING DIAGNOSIS: Potential for injury related to presence of toxic substance

Ingested poisons

GOAL

Determine that a poisoning has occurred

INTERVENTIONS

Save any evidence of ingested substance (e.g., empty container, tablets in child's mouth, parts of plants)

Call local Poison Control Center, emergency facility, or physician for immediate advice regarding treatment

EXPECTED OUTCOMES

†Poison is identified
†Appropriate therapy is determined

GOAL

Dilute poisonous substance

INTERVENTION

Give water unless contraindicated

EXPECTED OUTCOME

Child swallows preferred water

GOAL

Remove drug from stomach

INTERVENTIONS

Induce vomiting in alert child unless contraindicated
    *Administer ipecac syrup (15 ml) followed by water
Repeat *once* in 20 minutes if vomiting has not occurred
Perform or assist with gastric lavage when inducing emesis unless contraindicated

EXPECTED OUTCOMES

Child swallows ipecac and water
Child vomits
Stomach contents are removed

GOAL

Prevent aspiration of vomitus

INTERVENTION

Keep child's head lower than chest, place head between the legs, or position child on side

EXPECTED OUTCOME

Stomach is emptied without aspiration

GOAL

Adsorb drug remaining in stomach

INTERVENTION

*Administer activated charcoal only *after* inducing vomiting

EXPECTED OUTCOME

Child swallows charcoal mix

GOAL

Eliminate toxin from body

INTERVENTIONS

*Administer cathartics as ordered
Assist with exchange transfusion
Assist with hemodialysis
Assist with hemoperfusion
*Administer chelating agents as ordered

EXPECTED OUTCOME

Toxin is eliminated

---

*Call 1-800-555-1212 to obtain number of Poison Control Center for any state.
†Nursing outcome

*Dependent nursing action.

Cutaneously absorbed poisons

GOAL

Reduce absorption

INTERVENTIONS

Remove child's clothing
Cleanse skin thoroughly but carefully with tepid water and mild soap
Wear protective gloves during handling of child

EXPECTED OUTCOME

Harmful substance is removed from skin

Inhaled poisons

GOAL

Reduce absorption

INTERVENTIONS

Remove child from source of inhalant
Assist ventilation as needed (humidified air, oxygen)
Assist with intubation and/or respiratory support as indicated

EXPECTED OUTCOME

Respirations are within normal limits (see inside front cover for normal variations)

NURSING DIAGNOSIS: Fear/anxiety related to sudden hospitalization and treatment

GOAL

Support child

INTERVENTIONS

Explain procedures and tests according to developmental level of the child
Allow for expression of feelings
Provide comfort measures
Encourage parents to visit

EXPECTED OUTCOMES

Child expresses feelings and concerns
Child cooperates with procedures
Family remains with child as much as possible

NURSING DIAGNOSIS: Altered family processes related to sudden hospitalization and emergency aspects of illness

GOAL

Support family

INTERVENTIONS

Keep child and parents calm
Do not admonish or accuse child or parent of wrongdoing
Allow expression of feelings regarding circumstances related to the poisoning
Provide reassurance as appropriate
Explain therapies and tests
Keep family informed of child's progress
Avoid placing blame

EXPECTED OUTCOMES

Child and parents exhibit an attitude of confidence in care
Family verbalizes feelings and concerns
Family demonstrates an understanding of therapies

See also:
Nursing care plan: The child in the hospital, p. 246
Nursing care plan: The family of the ill or hospitalized child, p. 254

NURSING CARE PLAN
THE CHILD WITH LEAD POISONING

Chronic ingestion of lead-containing substances resulting in
physical and mental dysfunction

ASSESSMENT

Perform physical assessment
Obtain history of possible sources of lead in the child's environment:

Ingested

*Lead-based paint
   Interior: walls, windowsills, floors, furniture
   Exterior: door frames, fences, porches, siding
Plaster, caulking
Unglazed pottery
Colored newsprint
Painted food wrappers
Cigarette butts and ashes
Water from leaded pipes
Foods or liquids from cans soldered with lead
Household dust
Soil, especially along heavily trafficked roadways
Food grown in contaminated soil
Urban playgrounds
Folk remedies
Pewter vessels or dishes
Hobby materials, e.g., leaded paint or solder for stained glass
windows

Inhaled

*Sanding and scraping of lead-based painted surfaces
Burning of leaded objects
   Automobile batteries
   Newspaper logs of colored paper
Automobile exhaust
Cigarette smoke
Sniffing leaded gasoline
Dust
   Poorly cleaned urban housing
Contaminated clothing and skin of household members work-
ing in smelting factories or working as urban policemen

Obtain history of pica or evidence of this behavior during assessment
Observe for manifestations of lead poisoning:

General Signs

  Anemia
  Acute crampy abdominal pain

---

*Most common sources.

Vomiting
Constipation
Anorexia
Headache
Fever
Short stature (long term)
Decreased weight (long term)

Central Nervous System Signs (early)

  Hyperactivity
  Aggression
  Impulsiveness
  Decreased interest in play
  Lethargy
  Irritability
  Delay or reversal in verbal maturation
  Loss of newly acquired motor skills
  Clumsiness
  Deficits in sensory perception
  Learning difficulties
  Short attention span
  Distractibility

Central Nervous System Signs (late)

  Mental retardation
  Paralysis
  Blindness
  Convulsions
  Coma
  Death

Signs of Gasoline Sniffing

  Irritability
  Tremor
  Hallucinations
  Confusion
  Lack of impulse control
  Depression
  Delirium
  Chorea
  Ataxia
  Sleep disturbances

Assist with diagnostic procedures and tests—Blood-lead concentration, erythrocyte-protoporphyrin level, bone radiography, urinalysis, hemoglobin and complete blood count,
lead mobilization test

Unit 4

NURSING DIAGNOSIS: Potential for poisoning related to sources of lead in the environment

GOAL

Prevent further exposure to lead

INTERVENTIONS

Help family identify and remove sources of lead from the environment at home or other care environments (e.g., day care, relatives, neighbors)

Remove child during deleading procedures, especially sanding of painted surfaces

Supervise children at play and guide toward activity other than pica

EXPECTED OUTCOME

Child no longer ingests or inhales lead from environment

NURSING DIAGNOSIS: Potential for injury related to ingested or inhaled lead

GOAL

Help remove lead from body

INTERVENTIONS

*Administer chelating agents as prescribed

Plan and carry out a systematic rotation plan for administration of chelating agent

EXPECTED OUTCOME

Child receives medication without local complications

---

*Dependent nursing action

NURSING DIAGNOSIS: Fear related to multiple injections

GOAL

Reduce fear of injections

INTERVENTIONS

Prepare child for injections (see p. 211)

Reassure child that injections are a treatment, not a punishment for lead ingestion

Administer medication in place not perceived as "safe" (e.g., treatment room or similar area other than room or play area)

*Administer local anesthetic in conjunction with medication, if possible

See p. 224 for other measures to reduce discomfort from injections

EXPECTED OUTCOME

Child receives medication with minimal distress

NURSING DIAGNOSIS: Altered family processes related to child's access to lead in the environment

GOAL

Support family

INTERVENTIONS

Avoid blame or criticism regarding the child's exposure to lead sources

Assist family to obtain sources of help for removing lead from the environment

Offer praise for positive behaviors in directing child's activity away from pica

Be available to answer questions and offer suggestions

EXPECTED OUTCOME

Family demonstrates a positive attitude toward the child and reducing the risk of lead poisoning

---

*Dependent nursing action

SELECTED POISONINGS IN CHILDREN

Poison	Clinical manifestations	Comments/treatment
Corrosives (strong acids or alkali) Drain, toilet, or oven cleaners Electric dishwasher detergent Mildew remover Batteries Clinitest tablets Denture cleaners	Severe burning pain in mouth, throat, and stomach White, swollen mucous membranes, edema of lips, tongue, and pharynx (respiratory obstruction) Violent vomiting (hemoptysis) Drooling and inability to clear secretions Signs of shock Anxiety and agitation	Household bleach is a frequently ingested corrosive but rarely causes serious damage Liquid preparations cause more damage than granular preparations (e.g., dishwasher detergent, drain or toilet cleaner) **Treatment:** Inducing emesis is contraindicated (vomiting redamages the mucosa) Dilute corrosive with water, not milk (coats membranes, making assessment difficult) Provide patent airway, if needed Administer analgesics Keep NPO or place on clear liquid diet Esophageal stricture may require repeated dilations and/or surgery
Hydrocarbons Gasoline Kerosene Lamp oil Mineral seal oil (found in furniture polish) Lighter fluid Turpentine Paint thinner and remover (some types)	Gagging, choking, and coughing Nausea Vomiting Alterations in sensorium, such as lethargy Weakness Respiratory symptoms of pulmonary involvement Tachypnea Cyanosis Retractions Grunting	Immediate danger is aspiration (even small amounts can cause bronchitis and chemical pneumonia) Gasoline, kerosene, lighter fluid, mineral seal oil, and turpentine cause severe pneumonia **Treatment** (controversial): Inducing emesis is generally contraindicated Gastric lavage may be used Symptomatic treatment of chemical pneumonia includes high humidity, oxygen, hydration, and antibiotics for secondary infection

Acetaminophen	Occurs in 4 stages:
	1. Initial period (2 to 4 hours after ingestion)
	  Nausea
	  Vomiting
	  Sweating
	  Pallor
	2. Latent period (24 to 36 hours)
	  Patient improves
	3. Hepatic involvement (may last up to 7 days)
	  Pain in right upper quadrant
	  Jaundice
	  Confusion
	  Stupor
	  Coagulation abnormalities
	4. Patients who do not die in hepatic stage gradually recover
		Most common drug poisoning in children
		Occurs from acute ingestion, not chronic overdose
		Toxic dose is 140 mg/kg (see also p. 285)
		Treatment:
		Emesis, lavage
		Antidote N-acetylcystcine is given, usually by nasogastric tube because of the antidote's offensive odor (smells like rotten eggs)

Unit 4

Continued.

SELECTED POISONINGS IN CHILDREN—cont'd

Poison	Clinical manifestations	Comments/treatment
Aspirin	Acute poisoning 　Nausea 　Disorientation 　Vomiting 　Dehydration 　Diaphoresis 　Hyperpnea 　Hyperpyrexia 　Oliguria 　Tinnitus 　Coma 　Convulsions Chronic poisoning 　Same as above but subtle onset (often confused with illness being treated) Dehydration, coma, and seizures may be more severe Bleeding tendencies	May be caused by acute ingestion (severe toxicity occurs with 300 to 500 mg/kg [4 to 7 gr/kg]) May be caused by chronic ingestion (i.e., more than 100 mg/kg/day for 2 or more days); can be more serious than acute ingestion **Treatment:** Home use of ipecac for moderate toxicity Hospitalization for severe toxicity Emesis, lavage, activated charcoal, and/or cathartic Sodium bicarbonate transfusions to correct metabolic acidosis External cooling for hyperpyrexia Diazepam for seizures Oxygen and ventilation for respiratory depression Vitamin K for bleeding Dialysis for severest toxicity
Plants (see box, p. 529)	Depends on type of plants ingested May cause local irritation of oropharynx and entire gastrointestinal tract May cause respiratory, renal, and central nervous system symptoms Topical contact with plants can cause dermatitis	Some of most frequently ingested substances Rarely cause serious problems, although some plant ingestions can be fatal **Treatment:** Remove plant parts (emesis) Supportive care as needed
Iron (mineral supplement or vitamin containing iron)	Occurs in 5 stages 1. Initial period (½ to 6 hours after ingestion) 　Vomiting 　Hematemesis 　Diarrhea 　Hematochezia (bloody stools) 　Gastric pain 2. Latency (2 to 12 hours) 　Patient improves 3. Systemic toxicity (4 to 24 hours after ingestion) 　Metabolic acidosis 　Fever 　Hyperglycemia 　Bleeding 　Shock 　Death (may occur) 4. Hepatic injury (48 to 96 hours) 　Seizures 　Coma 5. Rarely pyloric stenosis develops at 2 to 5 weeks	Factors related to frequency of iron poisoning include: 　Widespread availability 　Packaging of large quantities in individual containers 　Lack of parental awareness of iron toxicity 　Resemblance of iron tablets to candy (i.e., M & Ms) **Treatment:** Emesis or lavage Chelation therapy with deferoxamine in severe intoxication

Unit 4

POISONOUS AND NONPOISONOUS PLANTS

Poisonous plants	Toxic parts	Nonpoisonous plants
Apple	Leaves, seeds	African violet
Apricot	Leaves, stem, seed pits	Aluminum plant
Azalea	Foliage and flowers	Asparagus fern
		Begonia
Buttercup	All parts	Boston fern
Cherry (wild or cultivated)	Twigs, seeds, foliage	Christmas cactus
Chrysanthemum	All parts	Coleus
Daffodil	Bulbs	Gardenia
Dumb cane, dieffenbachia	All parts	Grape ivy
		Jade plant
Elephant ear	All parts	Piggyback begonia
English ivy	All parts	
Foxglove	Leaves, seeds, flowers	Piggyback plant
Holly, mistletoe	Berries	Poinsettia*
Honeysuckle	All parts	Prayer plant
Hyacinth	Bulbs	Rubber tree
Ivy	Leaves	Snake plant
Mistletoe	Berries	Spider plant
Oak tree	Acorn, foliage	Swedish ivy
Philodendron	All parts	Wax plant
Plum	Pit	Weeping fig
Poison ivy, poison oak	Leaves, fruit, stems, smoke from burning plants	Zebra plant
Pothos	All parts	
Rhubarb	Leaves	
Tulip	Bulbs	
Water hemlock	All parts	
Wisteria	Seeds, pods	
Yew	All parts	

*Mildly toxic if ingested in massive quantities.

REFERENCES

Beyer JE: The Oucher: a user's manual and technical report, Denver, Colo, 1988, University of Colorado.

Bibace R and Walsh ME: Development of children's concepts of illness, Pediatrics 66(6):912-917, 1980.

Bluebond-Langner M: The private worlds of dying children, Princeton, NJ, 1978, Princeton University Press.

Craig KD, and others: Developmental changes in infant pain expression during immunization injections, Soc Sci Med 19(12):1331-1337, 1984.

Eland JM: The child who is hurting, Semin in Oncol Nurs 1(2):116-122, 1985.

Golden GS: The developmentally disabled child: detection, assessment, referral and treatment, Child Care Newsletter 3(1):8-11, 1984.

Gordon M: Nursing diagnosis and the nursing process, Am J Nurs 76:1298-1300, 1976.

Hester N: The preoperational child's reaction to immunization, Nurs Res 28(4):250-255, 1979.

Hester N: Personal communication, 1989.

Wong D and Baker C: Pain in children: comparison of assessment scales, Pediatr Nurs 14(1):9-17, 1988.

Hobbs N and Perrin JM, editors: Issues in the care of children with chronic illness, San Francisco, 1985, Jossey-Bass Inc.

Hurley A and Whelan FG: Cognitive development and children's perception of pain, Pediatr Nurs 14(1):21-24, 1988.

International Association for the Study of Pain: Pain terms: a current list with definitions and notes on usage, Pain 3:S216-S221, 1986.

Katz FR, Kellerman J, and Siegel SE: Behavioral distress in children with cancer undergoing medical procedures: developmental considerations, J Consult Clin Psychol 48(3):356-365, 1980.

Kim MJ, McFarland GK, and McLane AM: Pocket guide to nursing diagnosis, ed 2, 1987, The CV Mosby Co.

Lindemann E: Symptomatology and management of acute grief, Am J Psychiatry 101:141-143, 1944.

Marion RW and others: Human T-cell lymphotropic virus type III (HTLV-III) embryopathy, Am J Dis Child 140:638-640, 1986.

Mauksch H: A social science basis for conceptualizing family health, Soc Sci Med 8:521-527, 1974.

McCaffery M and Beebe A: Pain: clinical manual for nursing practice, St. Louis, 1989, The CV Mosby Co.

Reynolds MC: The educational needs of disabled children and youths. In Blum, R, editor: Chronic illness and disabilities in childhood and adolescence, New York, 1984, Grune & Stratton, Inc.

Shoemaker J: Essential features of nursing diagnosis. In Kim MJ, McFarland GK, and McLane AM: Pocket guide to nursing diagnosis, ed 2, 1987, The CV Mosby Co.

Unit 4

5

Home Care Instructions

Unit 5

PREPARING THE FAMILY FOR HOME CARE

The Home Care Instructions (HCI) in this unit are provided as a supplement to assist the nurse in preparing the family to manage the child's care at home. These instructions provide a written reference that the family can use when performing the procedure in the absence of a health professional. The HCI can be used as a teaching aid in preparing the patient for discharge from an acute care setting, or in the home when increasing the family's participation in the child's care.

The process of patient education involves giving the family information about the child's condition, the regimen that must be followed, and other health teaching as indicated. The goal of this education is to enable the family to modify behaviors and adhere to the regimen that has been mutually established.

One common problem with patient education is that the health professional delivers the information and the family listens. This one-way flow of material may not achieve the goal of the education. It is estimated that there is only a 50% compliance rate following patient education. Research has also shown that if the family is provided written information that they can understand, they are more likely to comply with the regimen. The HCIs are written in clear, simple language and accomodates those with a low reading level.

To maximize the benefits of patient teaching, these guidelines should be followed:
1. Establish a rapport with the family.
2. Avoid using *any* jargon. Clarify all terms with the family.
3. When possible, allow the family to decide how they want to be taught, for example, all at once or over a day or two. This gives the family a chance to incorporate the information at a rate that is comfortable.
4. Teach the family about the illness.
5. Assist the family in identifying obstacles in their ability to comply with the regimen and the means to overcome those obstacles. Then help the family find ways to incorporate the regimen into their daily lives.

HOW TO USE THE HCI

The home care instructions are based on currently available research. For example, CPR, choking infant and child, and suctioning reflect the latest research-based findings. However, some HCIs, such as obtaining urine for culture, describe conventional approaches that are commonly used, despite research that suggests the practice is unnecessary (see p. 536). The practitioner should be aware that new information may become available after the publication of these instructions. This may be particularly true of the instructions for CPR and choking. These instructions are meant to supplement, not replace, the teaching that reflects current guidelines.

Thoroughly review the HCI that will be given to the family. Make two photocopies, one for the family and one to attach to the nursing care plan. Fill in any blanks (for example, medication name or frequency of dressing change) and individualize the instructions as necessary. If equipment will be needed at home (for example, suction machines or syringes), begin making the necessary arrangements so that discharge can proceed smoothly. Whenever possible, make arrangements for the family to use the same equipment in the home that they are using in the hospital. This allows them to become familiar with the items; in addition the staff can help "troubleshoot" the equipment in a controlled environment. When the family is being taught at home, individualize the instructions and include any adaptations that will be necessary for the family. Plan the teaching sessions well in advance of the time the family will be responsible for performing the care. The more complex the procedure, the more time is needed.

Review the instructions with the family. Allow ample practice time under supervision. At least one family member, but preferably two members, should demonstrate or discuss the care before they are expected to care for the child at home. Provide the family with the telephone numbers of resource individuals who are available to assist them in the event of a problem.

MEASURING YOUR CHILD'S TEMPERATURE

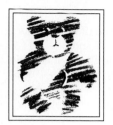

Your temperature changes during the day. Usually body temperature is higher in the afternoon than in the early morning. If you are very active, your temperature may be higher than normal. Fever is a protection for the body. A rise in body temperature above normal (usually 98.6° F) lets you know that there may be an infection somewhere in the body. Fever also helps the body fight the infection. Someone has a fever if the body temperature is higher than 100° F (oral or axillary temperature) or 100.4° F (rectal temperature).

You should measure a child's temperature:

1 When he feels warm to your touch.
2 When the child is not acting like himself.
3 Before calling your health professional to say that the child is sick.

HOW TO READ A THERMOMETER

There are two types of glass thermometers, oral and rectal (Fig. 1). The only difference between the two kinds is the shape of the silver tip. A rectal thermometer has a short rounded tip. It is shaped this way to prevent any damage to the rectum. The oral thermometer has a longer slender tip. Either can be used for an axillary temperature.

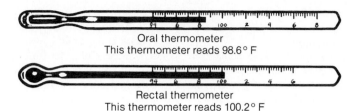

Oral thermometer
This thermometer reads 98.6° F

Rectal thermometer
This thermometer reads 100.2° F

Fig. 1

While holding the clear (or white) end of the thermometer at eye level, slowly turn the thermometer until you can see the silver line (mercury) (Fig. 2). The lower numbers on the thermometer will be on the left. The amount the mercury moves from left to right will depend on your child's temperature. The highest number that the silver line reaches is the right temperature. Before using the thermometer, make sure it reads 96° F or less. If not, while holding the clear end, shake the thermometer sharply above a soft surface, such as a bed or sofa, in case it should fall. Look at the reading again. If it is below 96° F, measure the temperature. If not, repeat the shaking until the reading is below 96° F.

Equipment

Glass thermometer
Clock/watch

HOW TO MEASURE AXILLARY TEMPERATURE

Measuring temperature in the axilla (armpit) is the safest way to check if your child has a fever.

1 Tell the child that you are going to measure his temperature.
2 Wash your hands.
3 Have the thermometer and watch ready.
4 Look at the thermometer to make sure it is reading below 96° F.
5 Place the thermometer under the child's arm. The thermometer's silver tip should rest in the center of your child's armpit (Fig. 3).

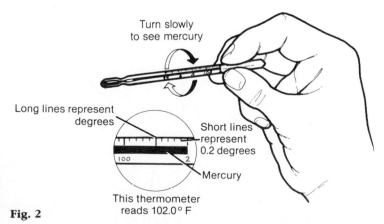

Turn slowly
to see mercury

Long lines represent degrees

Short lines represent 0.2 degrees

Mercury

This thermometer reads 102.0° F

Fig. 2

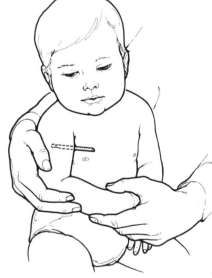

Fig. 3

From Wong D and Whaley L: Clinical manual of pediatric nursing, ed 3. Copyright © 1990 The CV Mosby Co, St Louis.

6 Hold the child's arm firmly against his body.

7 Look at the time.

8 The thermometer must remain in place for 3 to 4 minutes. This may seem like a long time. To help make the time seem to go faster, read a story or watch television with the child. Make sure you hold the thermometer securely.

9 Remove the thermometer and read.

10 PRAISE THE CHILD FOR HIS HELP.

11 Write down the thermometer reading and the time of day.

HOW TO MEASURE ORAL TEMPERATURES

By 5 or 6 years of age, a child can understand how to safely hold the thermometer in his mouth. If the child has had something to eat or drink, wait 15 minutes before you measure an oral temperature.

1 Tell the child why you want to measure his temperature.

2 Wash your hands.

3 Have the thermometer and watch ready.

4 Look at the thermometer to make sure it is reading less than 96° F.

5 Place the thermometer in the child's mouth, far back under the tongue (Fig. 4). Tell him to breathe through the nose and not to talk.

6 Make sure the child does not bite the thermometer.

7 Look at the time.

8 Tell the child that the thermometer must stay in place for 2 to 3 minutes. Read a story or watch TV with him.

9 Remove the thermometer and read.

10 PRAISE THE CHILD FOR HIS HELP.

11 Write down the thermometer reading and the time of day.

HOW TO MEASURE RECTAL TEMPERATURES

Note that rectal temperatures should not be taken if the child has diarrhea or is less than 1 year old. In taking a child's temperature, use the following procedure:

1 Tell the child that you are going to measure his temperature.

2 Wash your hands.

3 Have the thermometer and watch ready (and a clean diaper if needed).

4 Look at the thermometer to make sure it is reading less than 96° F.

5 Measure 1 inch on the thermometer or ⅙ of the thermometer's length.

6 Place the child on his stomach (Fig. 5), on one side with the upper leg bent, or on back with both legs up.

7 Dip the thermometer's silver tip in a lubricant such as petroleum jelly (Vaseline).

8 Place the silver end of the thermometer into the child's anus.

9 Do not insert the thermometer any further than 1 inch.

10 Look at the time.

11 Hold the thermometer in place for 2 to 3 minutes. Always hold the child so that he cannot twist around.

12 Remove the thermometer and read.

13 PRAISE THE CHILD FOR HIS HELP.

14 Wash your hands with soap and water. Count to 10 while washing, then rinse with clear water and dry.

15 Write down the thermometer reading and the time of day.

WHEN A FEVER IS PRESENT

Call your health professional *as soon as possible* if (1) the child has a temperature higher than 105° F or (2) a fever (oral or axillary temperature above 100° F or 100.4° F rectally) is present and the child:

■ Is less than 2 months of age.

■ Has a stiff neck, severe headache, stomach pain, persistent vomiting, purple spots on his skin, or earache with the temperature.

■ Has a serious illness in addition to the fever.

■ Is confused or delirious.

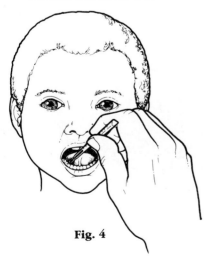

Fig. 4

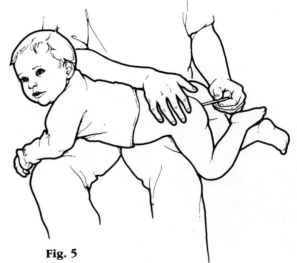

Fig. 5

- Has had a convulsion.
- Has trouble breathing after you have cleaned his nose.
- Is hard to awaken.
- Seems sicker than you would expect.
- Cannot be comforted.
- Has a temperature that continues to rise after medicine has been given.

Call your health professional *during office hours* if:

- The temperature is between 104° F and 105° F, especially if the child is less than 2 years old.
- Burning or pain with urination.
- The fever has been present for more than 72 hours.
- The fever has been present for more than 24 hours without a known cause.
- The fever went away for more than 24 hours, then returned.
- The child has a history of febrile seizures.
- You have some questions.

The most important thing to remember is not to bundle up the child with extra clothes and blankets. Dress him in light clothing. This will help cool him by letting air circulate and heat leave the body.

When a fever is present, it increases the amount of liquid that is needed by the body. It is important to encourage the sick child to drink fluids. Some things that may help encourage him to drink are straws, small cups instead of a big glass, popsicles, jello, and soft drinks with the fizz removed (stale). The carbonation can be removed by leaving the soft drink uncovered, by warming the soda in a microwave or on a stove, or by stirring in ¼ teaspoon sugar.

Medicines should not be used routinely to lower the temperature. If the child is uncomfortable and the fever needs to be treated with more than light clothes and increasing fluids, then drugs can be used.

Recommended dosages of acetaminophen for each age/weight child*

Age	3 mo	4-11 mo	12-23 mo	2-3 yr	4-5 yr	6-8 yr	9-10 yr	11-12 yr
Weight (lb)		12-17	18-23	24-35	36-45	44-64	66-76	77
Dose (mg)		80	120	160	240	320	400	480
TYPE OF MEDICINE								
Liquids								
Drops (1 dropper = 80 mg/0.8 ml)		1	1½	2	3	4	5	
Elixir/syrup 160 mg/ 5 ml (1 tsp)		½ tsp	¾ tsp	1 tsp	1½ tsp	2 tsp	2½ tsp	3 tsp
Tablets								
Chewable tablets (80 mg/tablet)			1-½	2	3	4	5	6
Swallowable tablets (160 mg/tablet)						2	2½	3

Acetaminophen brand names:	**Drops**	**Tablets**
	Panadol	Chewable Anacin 3
	Tylenol	Chewable Tylenol
	Tempra	St. Joseph Aspirin Free Chewable
		Junior Strength Tylenol

*Give the dose that is recommended for the child's weight if his weight is higher or lower than the weight listed for his age.

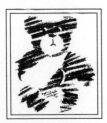

OBTAINING A URINE SAMPLE

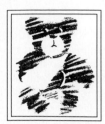

Children who are 8 years of age and older may be able to obtain the sample by themselves. Tell the child how to clean himself and how to obtain the sample. Help the child if needed. Children under 8 years of age will need your help. Young children may not be able to urinate on request. Use the child's words and usual place for obtaining the urine sample if possible. To help the child urinate, have him blow through a straw or listen to running water while you hold the specimen cup. Do not give the child more than one glass of liquid to drink. Large amounts of liquid can affect the result of the urine test. If you think the child does not understand, have him practice one time, then collect the specimen the next time.

INSTRUCTIONS FOR THE TOILET-TRAINED CHILD

Equipment

Urine cup
Potty chair or toilet
Soap and water
Washcloth or paper wipes

Routine urine sample (boys)

1 Tell the child that you need to obtain a urine sample. Use the word the child uses for urine.
2 If the child is able to obtain the sample of urine, have him wash his hands.
3 Wash your hands.
4 Gather the equipment needed.
5 Open the urine container, being careful not to touch the inside of the cup or lid.
6 Have the child urinate directly into the cup.
7 Replace the lid on the cup.
8 Label the cup with the child's first and last name.
9 PRAISE THE CHILD FOR HIS HELP.

10 Wash your hands with soap and water. Count to 10 while washing, then rinse with clear water and dry.

Urine sample for culture (boys)

If you are told that a "clean catch" specimen is needed, follow previous steps 1 through 5, then:

1 If paper wipes have been provided, use these instead of the washcloth; rinsing is not necessary with the wipes.
2 Wash the tip of the penis with a wipe or soap and water. Rinse well if soap is used. If the child is uncircumcised, pull back the foreskin only as far as it will go and then wash and rinse the tip of the penis with a clean part of the washcloth.
3 Have the child begin to urinate in the potty chair or toilet.
4 Tell him to stop.
5 Then have the child begin to urinate into the cup. If he cannot stop the flow of urine, place the urine cup so that you can "catch" some of the urine.
6 Replace the lid on the cup.
7 Label the cup with the child's first and last name.
8 PRAISE THE CHILD FOR HIS HELP.
9 Wash your hands with soap and water. Count to 10 while washing, then rinse with clear water and dry.

Routine urine sample (girls)

1 Tell the child that you need to obtain a urine sample. Use the word the child uses for urine.
2 If the child is able to obtain the sample of urine, have her wash her hands.
3 Wash your hands.
4 Open the urine cup, being careful not to touch the inside of the jar or lid.
5 Place the child on the potty chair or toilet.
6 Hold the cup in place while the child urinates.
7 Replace the lid on the cup.
8 Label the cup with the child's first and last name.
9 PRAISE THE CHILD FOR HER HELP.

Urine sample for culture (girls)

If you are told that a "clean catch" specimen is needed, follow steps 1 through 5, then:

1 If paper wipes are provided, use them instead of a washcloth; rinsing is not necessary with the wipes.
2 Spread the child's labia (lips) (Fig. 1) with your fingers. Wash the area with a paper wipe or soap and water; rinse if soap is used. Wash from front to back, rinsing well with a clean part of the washcloth.
3 Have the child begin to urinate into the potty chair or toilet.
4 Tell her to stop.
5 Then hold the cup in place and tell her to start to urinate into the cup. If she cannot stop the flow of urine, place the cup so that you can "catch" some of the urine.
6 Replace the lid on the cup.
7 Label the cup with the child's first and last name.
8 PRAISE THE CHILD FOR HER HELP.
9 Wash your hands with soap and water. Count to 10 while washing, then rinse with clear water and dry.

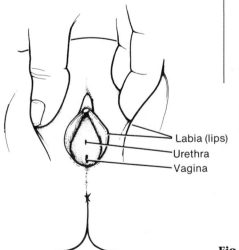

Labia (lips)
Urethra
Vagina

Fig. 1

INSTRUCTIONS FOR THE CHILD WHO IS NOT TOILET TRAINED

Equipment

Urine cup
Urine collector or "bag" or "U-bag"
Soap and water
Washcloths or paper wipes
Clean diaper

Instructions

If the child is very active, you will need help to put on the urine bag.

1 Wash your hands with soap and water. Count to 10 while washing, then rinse with clear water and dry. Your helper should also wash his hands.
2 Tell the child what you are going to do.
3 Gather the needed equipment.
4 Place the child on his back.
5 Remove the child's diaper.
6 If the urine sample is for culture, clean the child's genital area with soap and water as described on the previous page.
7 Rinse thoroughly and pat dry.
8 Have your helper hold the child's legs apart while you apply the bag.
9 Hold the urine collector with the bag portion downward.
10 Remove the bottom half of the adhesive protector.

For girls

1 Spread the labia and buttocks, keeping the skin tight.
2 Begin with the bottom of the adhesive. Place the sticky portion of the bag as flat as possible against the skin (Fig. 2).
3 Smooth the plastic to avoid any wrinkles.
4 Remove the top half of the adhesive protector and smooth it also on the labia.

For boys

1 Place the boy's penis and scrotum into the bag (Fig. 3).
2 Smooth the sticky portion of the bag on the skin, taking care to avoid making any wrinkles.
3 Remove the top half of the adhesive protector and smooth the top part on the skin, to remove any wrinkles.

Check the bag often and remove it as soon as the child urinates.

To remove the bag, hold it against the child's skin at the bottom and carefully peel it off from top to bottom. Pour the urine into the urine cup provided.

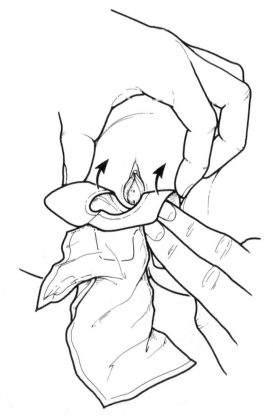

Fig. 2

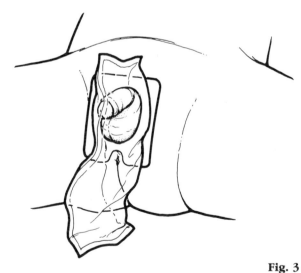

Fig. 3

CARING FOR THE CHILD IN A CAST

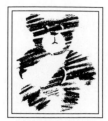

Casts are made from many different types of material and used on different parts of the body. A cast was put on your child so that the injured area could heal well. The care of the cast will change a little based on the type of cast that was put on.

Before the cast is applied, a smooth material is used to protect the skin. The cast is then put on over this material. At first, the cast will feel warm; this will last for about 10 to 15 minutes. A plaster cast will remain damp for many hours, while a synthetic cast will dry within 30 minutes. Do not put anything in the cast while it is drying or afterwards. During the drying time, touch the cast as little as possible. If you have to touch the cast, use the palms of your hands, not the fingers (Fig. 1). Turning the child in a plaster body cast at least every 2 hours will help the cast dry. Do not use a heated fan or dryer. A regular fan can be used to circulate the air in humid weather.

Check the skin around the cast frequently. Notify your health professional, if any of these occur:

- Numbness
- Tingling
- Unrelieved pain
- Odor
- Strange feelings
- Temperature change
- Cast becomes soft, broken, or cracked.
- Toes cannot be seen at edge of cast after correction of club foot.

If it is a leg or arm cast, check the color of the toes or fingers. They should be warm to the touch. When the skin in these areas is lightly pressed and released, the color should return quickly. To help prevent swelling, raise the arm/leg in the cast above the level of the child's heart (Fig. 2) by resting the cast on several pillows or blankets. If an arm is casted, a sling may be of help to support the arm during the day and pillows can be used at night. For leg casts, at nighttime, the covers on the bed can be loosened or a pillow

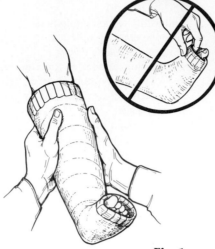

Fig. 1

folded to keep the blanket from putting pressure on the toes.

Some leg casts (weight bearing) are made so that the child can walk with the cast. If this type of cast cannot be used, the older child can be taught how to walk with crutches. When crutches are needed, follow your health professional guidelines for the correct size and padding of the crutches. If the child can move around independently, the presence of the cast is less of a problem.

The cast will be on for about _____ weeks. During this time, the child should exercise the joints and muscles that are not casted. Games like "Simon Says" can make the movement more enjoyable. Your health professional can give suggestions on appropriate exercises for your child.

SKIN CARE

During the time the cast is on, special care must be taken to keep the skin around the cast healthy. Rubbing alcohol can be used if the skin around the cast becomes reddish in color. Apply a small amount to the skin and let it dry. The back of the leg may be irritated when the child is in a short leg cast, and the skin between the thumb and the index finger often is a problem. If the cast rubs against the skin, tape can be used to cover the rough edges on a plaster cast. This is called petalling and includes these steps (Fig. 3):

1. Band-aids or cut several 3-inch strips of 1 to 2 inch wide adhesive tape.
2. Tape one end of the strip to the inside of the cast.
3. Tape the other end to the outside of the cast covering the cast edge.
4. Repeat with the other strips of tape. Overlap the edges to make a smooth surface.

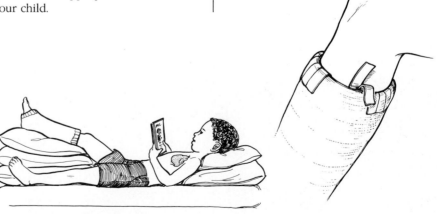

Fig. 2   **Fig. 3**

Itching

Sometimes the skin under the cast will feel itchy. Do not put anything inside the cast to scratch the skin. Children are often tempted to put forks, knives, crumbs, combs, and other objects in the cast. Notify your health professional if any object is stuck in the cast. If the skin itches, some things that may make the child more comfortable include:

1 Blow COOL air from a hair dryer into the cast.
2 Rub the opposite arm or leg.
3 Rub the skin around the cast edges.

BATHS

Children in body casts and full leg casts should receive sponge baths. A child with a lower leg or arm cast may be bathed or may take a shower if the cast is well covered or kept out of the water. The cast must remain dry. It can be wrapped with a plastic covering or a waterproof cast cover. The plastic cover should be removed and stored safely after the bath or shower. If a plaster cast becomes wet, it will soften and may need to be replaced. When a synthetic cast becomes wet, it should be thoroughly dried with a fan or hair dryer on the cool setting.

CAST CARE

If the cast will be on for a long time, some things can be done to keep it clean. The surface of synthetic casts can easily be wiped clean with a damp cloth. However, plaster casts cannot be cleaned. Cloth coverings such as a large, stretchy sock or stockinette can be used to protect the cast. These coverings can then be washed and replaced. If a cover is used, it must be fabric and not plastic so that air can circulate through the cast.

SPICA CASTS (BODY CAST)

Body casts are designed to immobilize the child's hips and thighs. Special care must be taken since the cast covers the child's abdomen and the child is usually unable to move about. A "window" may be cut in the cast to allow the stomach to expand after meals. The genital area will be left open to allow the child to urinate and have a bowel movement without soiling the cast. To protect the cast, plastic sheeting or disposable diapers (plastic side out) may be taped to the cast around this opening. This allows urine and stool to be easily wiped off. The other edges of the cast can be "petalled" to keep rough edges from harming the child's skin. Also, cotton padding, available from beauty supply stores, can be used as disposable cushioning inside the edges of the cast.

The child should be lifted with support under the shoulders and hips. Two people may be needed to safely lift the older infant and child (Fig. 4). When lifting, avoid any twisting of the child's body. Never use the bar that keeps the legs separated to lift the child. Placing pressure on this bar can damage the cast. A new cast must be put on if the cast is badly damaged.

Since the child cannot move much, diet changes may be needed. Two problems that may occur with body casts are constipation and too much weight gain. The older infant and child should be given extra liquids and a diet high in fiber, such as fresh fruits, vegetables, beans, and whole grains such as oatmeal and whole wheat bread. To prevent too much weight gain, avoid sugared drinks and candy since they add "empty" calories and may keep the child from eating foods needed for healing and growth.

While in a body cast, the young child cannot move around. You must be responsible for positioning the child and meeting all other needs. If the child was able to crawl or walk, a car mechanics' dolly (flatbed wagon on wheels) can be used to help the child move around. Make sure there are no stairs or loose rugs that can cause injury.

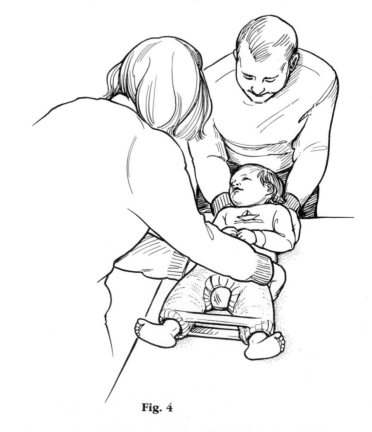

Fig. 4

INFANTS

Feeding the infant in a body cast requires some planning. You can support the child with your arm under the neck and head. The infant's hips and legs can be placed on a pillow at your side. This position can be used for bottle- or breast-feeding. You can also hold the child's head and shoulders in front of you with the legs behind your back. If the child is able to sit, a chair or table can be padded to help the child eat and play in a semi-sitting position.

For infants who are heavy wetters or for nighttime, a sanitary napkin can be placed inside a smaller diaper for extra absorbency. Both napkin and diaper are then changed after each wetting. Diaper liners and ultra absorbent diapers may also be helpful.

Children in body casts must be safely restrained while riding in cars. Some approved car seats can be modified, and a specially designed car restraint is available for purchase. [Jerome Koziatek and Associates, Inc., 190 W. Boston Rd., Hinckley, Ohio 44233-9631; (216) 659-4961.]

OLDER CHILDREN

Allow the child to help set the daily schedule. Within reason, the child can decide when meals, activities, schoolwork, and visits from friends take place. Since most clothing will not fit over the cast, some changes must be made. Loose-fitting shorts can be slit on the side seams and Velcro or other simple fasteners attached so that these can be easily placed on the child.

It is too difficult for the child to use the bathroom. A bedpan or urinal should be available for the child to use.

When it is necessary to travel with the child in a car, seat belts should be used if at all possible. If the child can lie on the back seat, a special vest can be used to restrain the child with the car seat belts. [The E-Z On vest is available from E-Z On Products, 500 Commerce Way West, Jupiter, FL 33458; (305) 747-6920 or (800) 323-6598 (outside Florida).]

CAST REMOVAL

When the injury is healed, the cast will be removed. A cast is removed by rapid vibrations of the cast cutter. Although the machine makes a loud noise that can be scary, there is little chance that the child can be hurt by it. However, the child should be prepared for the cast removal. If possible, show the child how the cutter vibrates and give him a chance to get used to the noise.

The skin will appear dry, pale, and scaly when the cast is removed. To soften and remove the dead skin, soak the skin in warm water and use skin moisturizers. Never scrub the skin in an effort to remove the scales. As the old skin comes off, new skin will grow.

PREVENTING AIDS AND HEPATITIS INFECTION

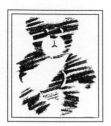

The child has an infection that can be harmful to other people in the home. To protect all people who come near the child, certain guidelines must be followed. The germ that caused the child's illness can be spread to others by contact with some of the child's body fluids. These may include blood and bloody body fluids.

Your best protection against infection is good handwashing after you have taken care of the child. Always wash your hands with soap and water. Count to 10 while you are washing, then rinse with clear water and dry. If there are any cuts or other open areas on your hands, you need to wear gloves when handling any of the child's body fluids. Always follow any contact with the child's body fluids with good handwashing, even if gloves are worn.

Each time you care for the child, you must decide what type of safeguard to use. If the child wears diapers, the disposable kind should be used. During a diaper change, if the child does not have loose, watery stools, and your hands will not come in contact with the urine or stool, then good handwashing after changing the diaper is sufficient. However, if the child has large, loose stools, gloves should be worn to provide added protection. You must wash your hands when you are finished, even if gloves were worn. Place all diapers, gloves, tissues, and used dressings in a leakproof bag for disposal.

When feeding an infant, protect your clothes with a waterproof apron or cloth in case the infant has a "wet burp" or vomits.

CLEANING BODY FLUID SPILLS

If the child vomits, has a nose bleed, or has a loose stool that needs to be cleaned, you should wear gloves. First, using paper towels, blot the spill to decrease the amount of liquid to be cleaned. Dispose of these towels in a plastic garbage bag. Pour a bleach solution (1 part household bleach mixed in 9 parts water) onto the spill area. Carefully blot with paper towels. Place these towels into a plastic leakproof bag. Soiled linens and clothes should be washed separately in hot water with detergent. If the child requires special care such as suctioning, refer to the appropriate home care instruction.

GIVING MEDICATIONS TO CHILDREN

It is necessary for you to give the child medicine called _____. This medicine will have the following benefits: _____

You will need to give the drug as follows:

    Amount _____

    How often _____

    Special instructions _____

Your health professional has written on the chart below when the medicine should be given. Give the drug at the same time each day so that it becomes part of the daily routine for you and the child.

For the child to have the most value from this medicine, it must be given until your health professional tells you to stop. Even though the child does not seem ill any longer, the medicine must be given for the prescribed time period.

Some common side effects of the drug are: _____.

If you have any problems that concern you or notice any unexpected reactions from the medicine, notify your health professional at _____

Drug schedule

	Sunday	Monday	Tuesday	Wednesday	Thursday	Friday	Saturday
When child wakes up							
Breakfast 1 hr before							
with							
2 hr after							
Lunch 1 hr before							
with							
2 hr after							
Dinner 1 hr before							
with							
2 hr after							
Bedtime							
During night							

    Check the box for the correct day and time. If the drug is given at times that differ from the suggested ones, write in the hour where appropriate.

GIVING ORAL MEDICATIONS

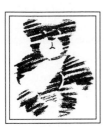

Your health professional has prescribed special medicine for the child, which must be given by mouth. This is a good time to teach the child about medicines as special things we take to get better. Do not tell him that the drug is candy. If the child thinks that the medicine is candy, and if the bottle is ever left in a place where he can reach it, he may take an overdose. Tell the child to take drugs ONLY from you or other special people, such as grandparents or baby-sitter. Store ALL drugs in a safe place, such as a locked cabinet. The storage area should be cool and dry. Bathrooms are usually too warm and moist for storing tablets or capsules. Always keep drugs in the original container, tightly closed. Place drugs that need to be refrigerated on a high shelf toward the back of the refrigerator, not on the door.

Unpleasant-tasting drugs can be mixed with a small amount of a pleasant-tasting food such as applesauce, juice, jelly, ice cream, or other more flavorful foods. Tell the child what you have done so that he does not think the food always tastes like the drug-food combination. Do not add drugs to essential foods and liquids (milk, formula, orange juice, cereal) to encourage him to take the medicine. When mixing a drug with food or liquids, add it to a *small* amount so the child will only have to eat or drink a little to take all of the medicine.

TO ENCOURAGE THE CHILD

If the drug tastes unpleasant, you can cut a straw in half and have the child sip the medicine through a straw. Some drugs taste better if served cold rather than at room temperature.

If medicine is mixed with a teaspoon of a pleasant-tasting food, allow the child to choose the food to which the drug will be added. This will help him to eat or drink all of the medicine.

Give the child a gold star or sticker for taking the drug. These can be placed

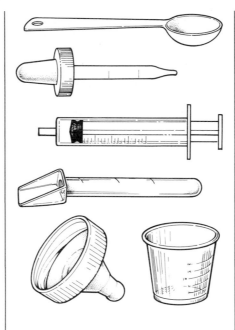

Fig. 1

on the drug schedule sheet that you were given. The child can keep track of the number of times he has taken the medicine and how many doses are left. The stars or stickers also provide a record of his help.

Offer the child a drink of water or other liquid to rinse the taste of the drug from his mouth.

Liquid medications-equipment

Measuring spoon, dropper, syringe, calibrated spoon, nipple, or medicine cup (Fig. 1)
Medicine

Instructions

1 Read the label to make certain you have the right drug and to check the right amount of drug to give the child.
2 Do NOT use household teaspoons or tablespoons. These are not standard sizes and will not measure the correct amount of medicine. Use a measuring spoon or the special measuring device sometimes supplied with the drug.

Measuring spoon	Metric equivalent
¼ teaspoon	1¼ cc
½ teaspoon	2½ cc
¾ teaspoon	3¾ cc
1 teaspoon	5 cc
1 tablespoon	15 cc
1 ounce	30 cc

3 Give the medicine to the child in a quiet place so that you will not be disturbed.
4 Tell the child what you are going to do.
5 Pour out the exact amount of the drug into the measuring spoon.
6 Allow the child to sip the drug from the spoon.
7 If it is a large amount of medicine and the child can drink from a cup, you can measure the drug into a small cup. Make sure that the child takes all of the drug. You may have to add a small amount of water to rinse the drug from the sides of the cup.
8 Return the drug to a safe place out of the child's reach.
9 Write down the time you gave the child the drug and check for the time you need to give the next dose.

LIQUID MEDICINES FOR INFANTS AND YOUNG TODDLERS

Very young children are not able to take drugs from a spoon. Methods exist to give drugs to this age-group. These include a dropper or syringe, or placing the drug in a baby bottle nipple and allowing the child to suck the drug from the nipple.

1 Read the label to make certain you have the right drug and to check the right amount of medicine to give the child.
2 Fill the syringe or dropper with the drug to the right amount. Read the amount of liquid at the bottom of the semicircle at the top of the liquid (Fig. 2).
3 Give the medicine to the child in a quiet place so that you will not be disturbed.
4 Tell the child what you are going to do.

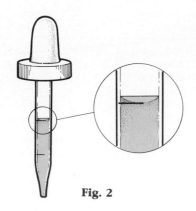

Fig. 2

5 Hold the child in your lap. Place his arm closest to you behind your back. Firmly hug his other arm and hand with your arm and hand; snuggle his head between your body and your arm (Fig. 3). Sometimes you may also want to grasp his legs between yours. Your other hand remains free to give the child the drug.

6 Gently place the dropper or syringe in the child's mouth along the inside of the cheek (Fig. 4). Allow the child to suck the liquid from the dropper or syringe. If the child does not suck, squeeze a small amount of the drug at a time. This takes longer, but the child will swallow the medicine and he is less likely to spit it out or choke on it.

OR

Place an empty bottle nipple in the child's mouth, add the drug to the nipple, and allow the child to suck the nipple (Fig. 5).

7 Rinse the child's mouth with plain water to remove any of the drug from his gums and teeth. This can be done by wrapping a paper towel around your finger, soaking it in plain water, and then swabbing the gums, cheeks, palate, and tongue.

8 Return the drug to a safe place out of the child's reach.

9 Write down the time you gave the child the medicine and check for the time you need to give the next dose.

10 PRAISE THE CHILD FOR HIS HELP.

TABLETS AND CAPSULES

Many tablets are pleasantly flavored, and the child can either swallow the tablet whole or chew the tablet. If a half-tablet is prescribed, only scored tablets (those with a visible groove on the tablet) can be broken in half. An unscored tablet may break into unequal portions. This does not matter if the child is taking the whole tablet. If the tablet has an unpleasant taste or the child cannot swallow the tablet, you can crush the tablet between two spoons or a spoon and a piece of wax paper. However, before crushing any tablet, check with your health professional or pharmacist to make sure the tablet can be crushed. After the tablet is crushed, you can mix it with a nonessential food such as applesauce, jam, or fruit juice. Make sure all of the crushed tablet is added. If you have added medicine to the food, tell the child.

If the medicine is a capsule, do not open the capsule unless you have been told to do so by the pharmacist or your health professional. If it can be opened, add it to food as described above. Praise the child after he has taken the medicine.

Fig. 3

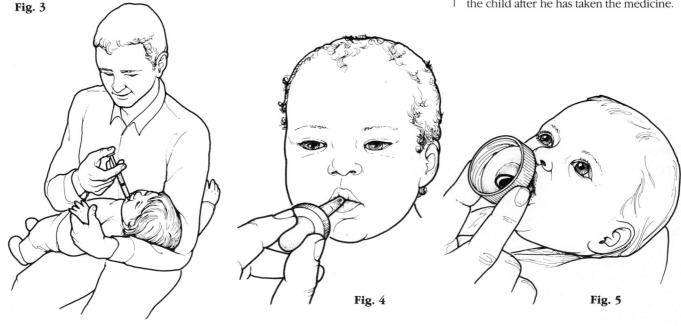

Fig. 4   **Fig. 5**

GIVING INTRAMUSCULAR (IM) INJECTIONS

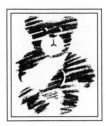

Your health professional has prescribed special medicine for the child, which must be given by injection. This is a good time to teach the child about medicines as special things that we need to get better. Several things can be done to make the injection less painful:

1 Give the child something to do, such as squeezing someone's hand, humming, or counting.
2 Keep the child involved in talking or singing.
3 Place a wrapped ice cube on the injection site for about 1 minute to numb the area before you give the injection.

Equipment

Alcohol swabs
Syringe and needles
Drug stored at room temperature

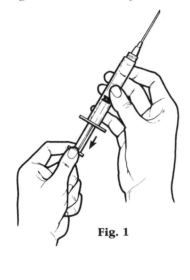

Fig. 1

Instructions

1 Gather all equipment
2 Wash your hands with soap and water. Count to 10 while washing, then rinse with clear water and dry.
3 Open the packet of a new syringe.
4 Clean the top of the drug bottle with alcohol.
5 Remove the cap from the syringe. Do not touch the needle.
6 Pull back the plunger and fill with the same amount of air as the drug dose (Fig. 1).
7 Put the needle into the drug bottle. Turn the bottle upside down. Push the plunger to inject the air into the drug bottle (Fig. 2).
8 With the tip of the needle in the drug, pull back the plunger to fill the syringe with the amount needed (Fig. 3).
9 Remove the syringe from the bottle.
10 Remove any air bubbles in the syringe. Hold the syringe with the needle pointing upward and firmly tap the syringe with the finger of the free hand. When all of the bubbles are at the top of the syringe, push the plunger gently to remove the bubbles.

11 Make sure the drug is the right amount (Fig. 4).
12 Put the cap back on the needle loosely.
13 Use the injection spot circled in the accompanying diagram (Fig. 5).
14 Have the child lie or sit down and remove all clothing from the injection area.
15 Have someone hold the child if you think the child will not be able to lie still.
16 Using a circular motion, clean the injection spot with the alcohol.
17 Let the skin dry.
18 Place your hand on the landmarks shown in the picture to locate the correct injection spot.
19 Grasp the muscle firmly between your thumb and fingers. This steadies the muscle and allows for the drug to be injected into the deepest part of the muscle.
20 Remove the cap from the needle. Slip the cap between the two fingers that arc grasping the skin and pull out the syringe.

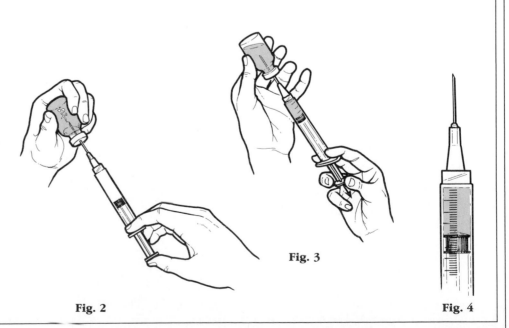

Fig. 2

Fig. 3

Fig. 4

545

21 With a quick darting motion, insert the needle into the injection spot at a 90-degree angle (Fig. 6).

22 Pull back the plunger and check to see if there is any blood in the syringe.

   a. If there is blood, remove the needle, change needles, and begin again after making sure the medication dose is still right.

   b. If there is no blood, push the plunger slowly until the syringe is empty.

23 Remove the syringe quickly from the site, and gently rub the area with a clean tissue.

24 Place a small Band-aid on the injection spot.

25 Comfort the child and make sure that he knows the drug is necessary to get better. It is important that he does not think that the injections are punishment.

26 PRAISE THE CHILD FOR HIS HELP.

27 Return the drug to a safe place out of the child's reach.

28 Throw the used needle and syringe into a puncture-resistant container, such as an empty plastic milk carton.

29 Write down the date and time of the dose and which injection site was used. Check the time that the next dose needs to be given.

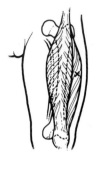

Vastus lateralis (outer thigh)

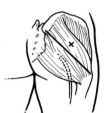

Dorsogluteal (outer hip)

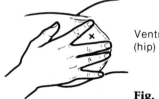

Ventrogluteal (hip)

Fig. 5

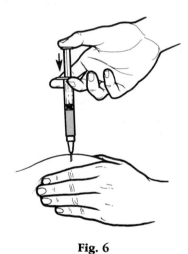

Fig. 6

NOTES

GIVING SUBCUTANEOUS (SUB Q) INJECTIONS

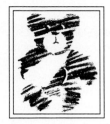

Your health professional has prescribed special medicine for the child, which must be given by injection. This is a good time to teach the child about medicines as special things we take to get better. Several things can be done to make the injection of medicine less painful:

1 Give the child something to do, such as squeezing someone's hand, humming, or counting.
2 Keep the child involved in talking or singing.
3 Place a wrapped ice cube on the injection site for about 1 minute to numb the area before you give the injection.

Equipment

Alcohol swabs
Syringe and needles
Medicine stored at room temperature

Instructions

1 Gather all equipment.
2 Wash your hands with soap and water. Count to 10 while washing, then rinse with clear water and dry.
3 Open the packet of a new syringe.
4 Clean the top of the drug bottle with alcohol.

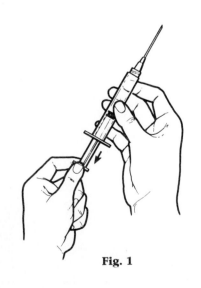

Fig. 1

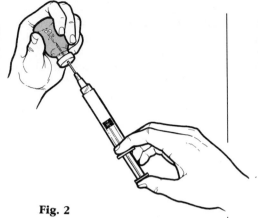

Fig. 2

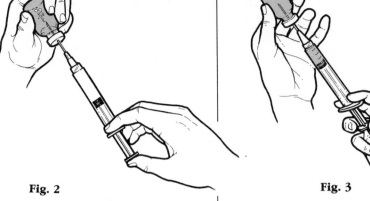

Fig. 3

5 Remove the cap from the syringe. Do not touch the needle.
6 Pull back the plunger and fill with the same amount of air as the drug dose (Fig. 1).
7 Put the needle into the drug bottle. Turn the bottle upside down. Push the plunger to inject the air into the medication bottle (Fig. 2).
8 With the tip of the needle in the drug, pull back the plunger to fill the syringe with the amount needed (Fig. 3).
9 Remove the syringe from the bottle.
10 Remove any air bubbles in the syringe. Hold the syringe with the needle pointing up and firmly tap the syringe with the finger of the free hand. When all of the bubbles are at the top of the syringe, push the plunger gently to remove the bubbles.
11 Make sure the drug is the right amount (Fig. 4).
12 Put the cap back on the needle loosely.
13 Have the child lie or sit down and remove all clothing from the injection area.
14 Have someone hold the child if you think the child will not be able to lie still.
15 Using a circular motion, clean the injection spot with the alcohol.
16 Let the skin dry.
17 Grasp the skin around the injection spot firmly, raising only the skin ½ to 1 inch (Fig. 5).

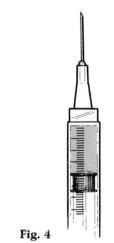

Fig. 4

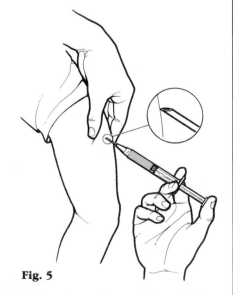

Fig. 5

From Wong D and Whaley L: Clinical manual of pediatric nursing, ed 3. Copyright © 1990 The CV Mosby Co, St Louis.

18 Remove the cap from the needle. Slip the cap between the two fingers that are grasping the skin and pull out the syringe.

19 With a quick darting motion, insert the needle (bevel up—see insert) into the injection site at a 45-degree angle.

20 Release your grasp on the child's skin.

21 Pull back the plunger and check to see if there is any blood in the syringe.

 a. If there is blood, remove the needle, change needles, and begin again after making sure the medication dose is still right.

 b. If there is no blood, push the plunger slowly until the syringe is empty.

22 Remove the syringe quickly from the site, and gently rub the area with a clean tissue.

23 Place a small Band-aid on the injection spot.

24 Comfort the child and make sure that he knows the drug is necessary to get better. It is important that he does not think that the injections are punishment.

25 PRAISE THE CHILD FOR HIS HELP.

26 Return the drug to a safe place out of the child's reach.

27 Throw the used needle and syringe into a puncture-resistant container, such as an empty plastic milk carton.

28 Write down the date and time of the dose and which injection spot was used. Check the time that the next dose needs to be given.

NOTES

CARING FOR A HEPARIN LOCK

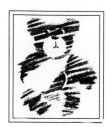

A small tube (catheter) was placed in the child for the administration of intravenous (IV) drugs at home. This tube is known as a heparin lock. Look at the spot where the tube enters the skin several times each day. Notify your health professional if you observe any of the following signs around the heparin lock:

- Redness
- Swelling/puffiness
- Leaking/drainage
- Red streak along the skin near the heparin lock
- Pain around the entry spot
- A clean gauze dressing or bandage can be kept taped over the heparin lock as protection. The child may wash around the entry spot, but he should be careful not to get the tube itself wet. During a bath or shower, cover the tube with plastic that is taped to the skin to prevent the tube from becoming wet. The heparin lock will need to be changed by your health professional every _____ days or if any problems develop.

FLUSHING

The inside of the catheter must be rinsed (flushed) with a heparin solution (a special drug called an anticoagulant) to prevent any blood clots from forming, which can clog the tube. The small amount of heparin that you are using will rinse the entire length of the tube. The tube must be flushed _____ time(s) each day and after any drug or fluid is given through the tube.

Equipment

Needle and syringe
Alcohol swabs
Bottle of heparin solution at room temperature.

Instructions

1. Gather equipment that you will need on a clean dry surface.
2. Wash your hands with soap and water.

Fig. 1

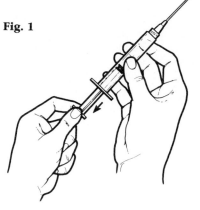

Count to 10 while washing, then rinse with clear water and dry.

3. Open the package of alcohol swabs.
4. With one of the swabs, wipe the top of the heparin bottle. (This is not necessary the first time the heparin bottle is used, when the metal tab is removed.)
5. With the second swab, wipe the cap on the catheter.
6. Remember not to touch the bottle top or the injection cap after you have cleaned them.
7. Open the packet of a new syringe.
8. Remove the cap from the syringe. Do not touch the needle.
9. Pull back the plunger and fill with the same amount of air as the heparin dose (Fig. 1).

Fig. 2

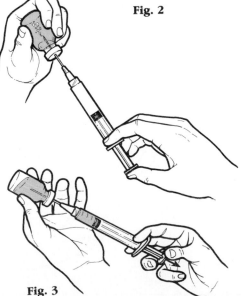

Fig. 3

10. Put the needle into the heparin bottle. Turn the bottle upside down. Push the plunger to inject the air into the heparin bottle (Fig. 2).
11. With the tip of the needle in the heparin, pull back the plunger to fill the syringe with the amount needed (Fig. 3).
12. Remove the syringe from the bottle.
13. Remove any air bubbles in the syringe. Hold the syringe with the needle pointing up and firmly tap the syringe with the finger of the free hand. When all of the bubbles are at the top of the syringe, push the plunger gently to remove the bubbles.
14. Make sure the heparin is the right amount (Fig. 4).
15. Inject the heparin into the center of the cap (Fig. 5).

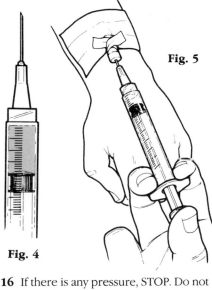

Fig. 5

Fig. 4

16. If there is any pressure, STOP. Do not force the plunger forward. Call your health professional.
17. Remove the syringe from the heparin lock.
18. PRAISE THE CHILD FOR HIS HELP.
19. Return the heparin to a safe place out of the child's reach.
20. Throw the used needle and syringes into a puncture-resistant container, such as an empty plastic milk carton.
21. Write down the date and time of the dose and check the time that the next heparin dose needs to be given.

CARING FOR A CENTRAL VENOUS CATHETER

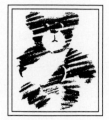

A catheter (tube) was placed in your child so that an intravenous line is available for long-term treatment. This tube can be used to give medications, fluids, nutrients, and possibly for obtaining blood specimens. Several different types of catheters can be used, such as the Broviac or the Groshong. Both types of catheters are inserted under the skin and into a major blood vessel near the heart.

SPECIAL CONSIDERATIONS

A young child, either the child with the tube or a playmate, may want to handle the tube and accidentally pull it out. To prevent the child from playing with the tube, keep a T-shirt on the child, use one-piece outfits such as overalls, or outfits that open in the back. Never leave the child alone when he is undressed. Keep all sharp objects, especially scissors, out of the reach of young children in the home.

When the child is bathed, keep the skin dry where the tube enters the body. Plastic wrap can be taped over a gauze dressing or a transparent dressing can be used to protect the site.

All people who care for the child should be taught about the catheter. At school tell both the child's teacher and the school nurse so that an adult can help the child if needed.

Your health professional should be notified if the tube becomes damaged. The tube should be repaired as soon as possible because of the risk of infection. If the child has a Broviac catheter, clamp the tube at once. The Groshong catheter does not need to be clamped.

FLUSHING THE TUBE

The care of each catheter is slightly different. These written instructions will help you to care for the tube at home. Catheter care should always be done in a quiet place where you will not be disturbed. If the child is active, you will need a helper. The helper can keep the child still while you do the catheter care.

The inside of the Broviac must be flushed (rinsed) with a heparin (a special drug called an anticoagulant) solution. This will help prevent any blood clots from forming. If blood clots form, the tube may become plugged. The small amount of heparin that you are using will rinse the entire length of the tube. If the child has a Groshong catheter, no heparin flushes are needed, only weekly saline rinses. The Broviac must be flushed _____ time(s) each day and either tube is rinsed after giving any drug or fluid through the tube.

Equipment

Needle and syringe
2 antiseptic swabs
Bottle of heparin at room temperature (Broviac)
Bottle of sterile saline at room temperature (Groshong)

Instructions

1 Gather equipment that you will need and place on a clean, dry surface.
2 Wash your hands with soap and water. Count to 10 while washing, then rinse with clear water and dry.
3 Open the package of antiseptic swabs.
4 With one of the swabs, scrub the top of the solution bottle. (This is not necessary the first time the heparin or saline bottle is used.)

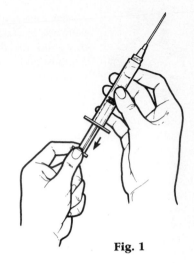

Fig. 1

5 Open the package of a new syringe.
6 Remove the cap from the syringe. Do not touch the needle.
7 Pull back the plunger and fill the syringe with the same amount of air as needed (Fig. 1).
8 Insert the needle into the rubber stopper of the bottle. Turn the bottle upside down. Push the plunger to inject the air into the bottle (Fig. 2).
9 With the tip of the needle in the solution, pull back the plunger to fill the syringe with the amount needed (Fig. 3).
10 Remove the syringe from the bottle.
11 Remove any air bubbles in the syringe. Hold the syringe with the needle pointing up and firmly tap the syringe with the finger of the free

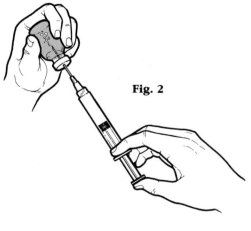

Fig. 2

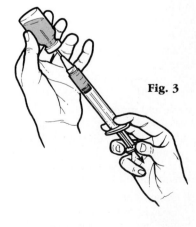

Fig. 3

From Wong D and Whaley L: Clinical manual of pediatric nursing, ed 3. Copyright © 1990 The CV Mosby Co, St Louis.

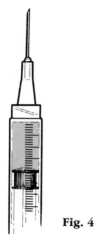

Fig. 4

hand. When all the bubbles are at the top of the syringe, push the plunger gently to remove the bubbles.

12 Make sure the heparin or saline is the right amount (Fig. 4).

13 Place the needle cover over the needle and set aside.

14 With the second swab, scrub the injection cap on the catheter.

15 Remove the needle cap.

16 Insert the needle into the center of the injection cap. Inject the solution by pushing the plunger (Fig. 5).

17 If there is any pressure, STOP. Do not force the plunger forward. Call your health professional at once.

18 Remove the needle and syringe. With the Broviac catheter remove the needle as the last 0.2 ml of fluid is injected.

CHANGING THE INJECTION CAP

This should be done _____ time(s) per week. If the cap is changed at the time of rinsing, the heparin or saline is given through the new injection cap.

Equipment

Antiseptic swab
Injection cap
Padded clamp

Procedure

1 Gather the equipment you will need.

2 Wash your hands with soap and water. Count to 10 while washing, then rinse with clear water and dry.

3 Clamp the tube midway between the skin and the end of the tube or on the reinforced clamping sleeve that is on some catheters (Fig. 6); do not clamp a Groshong catheter.

4 With the antiseptic swab, clean around the tip of the tube below the injection cap.

5 Open the new injection cap package.

6 Remove the used injection cap from the tube and attach the new injection cap (Fig. 7 and 8).

7 Remove the clamp from the catheter (not needed with Groshong).

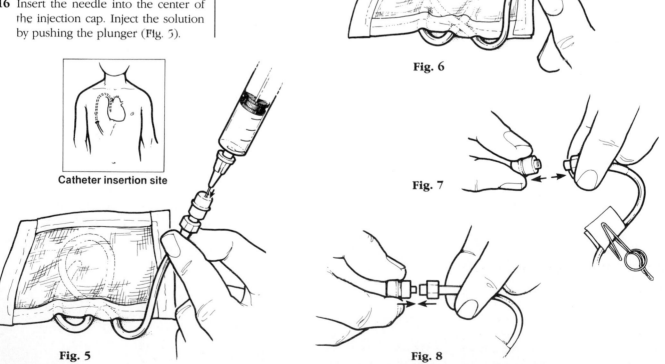

Fig. 6

Catheter insertion site

Fig. 5

Fig. 7

Fig. 8

DRESSING CHANGE

Both gauze and transparent dressings are used to protect the catheter. Your health professional will instruct you on the preferred dressing type for your child. Directions for the care of each dressing are included. The dressing is placed over the site where the tube leaves the child's body. The dressing must be changed every _____ days/week, or if it becomes loose or dirty. Germs may be able to grow where the tube enters the skin and cause an infection if the dressing is not clean and secure.

Transparent dressing

The clear dressing lets you see the child's skin around the tube. Look at the skin around the tube each day. Call your health professional at once if you see any redness, drainage, or swelling, if the area around the tube is painful, or if the child has a temperature above 100° F orally or axillary (100.4° F rectally).

Equipment

Adhesive remover pad
Transparent dressing
1 package antiseptic ointment
Antiseptic swabs
Bag for disposing of used supplies and
    dressing
Cotton swabs and hydrogen peroxide in
    a clear paper cup

OR

Alcohol-acetone swabs
Suggested skin preparation solution
Tape

Instructions

1. Gather the equipment on a clean, dry surface.
2. Wash your hands with soap and water. Count to 10 while washing, then rinse with clear water and dry.
3. Gently peel off the old dressing using adhesive remover, if necessary.
4. Carefully look at the skin around the tube.
5. Using either the alcohol-acetone swabs or cotton swabs dipped in hy-

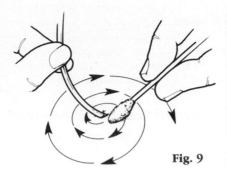

Fig. 9

drogen peroxide, clean the skin where the tube enters the body. Use a circular motion starting at the tube and moving out about 3 inches from the tube. Use each swab only *once* and do not dip the swab a second time in the hydrogen peroxide after it has touched the skin (Fig. 9). Start at the center with each new swab.

6. Using the antiseptic swabs, repeat the cleaning process. Move outward from the tube in a circular motion.
7. Allow the antiseptic to dry on the skin.
8. Using the skin preparation solution paint a "window frame" or square around the tube where the clear dressing will meet the skin. Be careful not to touch the skin close to the catheter (Fig. 10).

9. Loop the tube around the entry site, leaving the injection cap below the bottom of the "window frame."
10. Carefully place the dressing on the child's skin. Hold the dressing in both hands. Start at the top of the "window frame" being careful not to let any air bubbles occur. When the top of the dressing is on the skin, slowly bring the dressing toward the bottom of the window frame making sure that it attaches to the skin. Pinch the dressing around the tube to make a tight seal (Fig. 11).
11. Secure the end of the tube with tape to keep it from dangling.
12. Place all used items in a paper bag. Close the bag and throw it away.
13. PRAISE THE CHILD FOR HIS HELP.

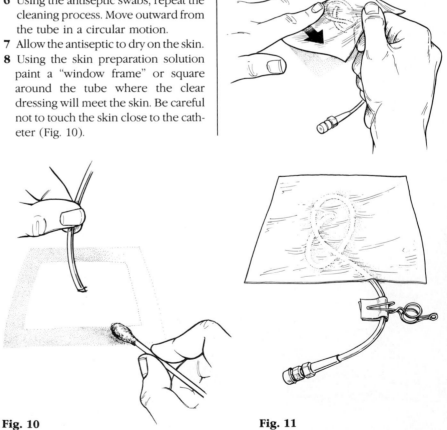

Fig. 10

Fig. 11

Gauze dressing

Dressing changes are a good time to look at the child's skin for any signs of redness, irritation, or infection. Call your health professional at once if you notice any redness, drainage, or swelling, if the area around the tube is painful, or if the child has an oral or axillary temperature above 100° F (100.4° F rectally).

Equipment

4 × 4 gauze pads; 1 with a slit
1 package antiseptic ointment
Antiseptic swabs
Adhesive remover
Padded clamp
Tape
Bag for disposing of used supplies and dressing
Cotton swabs and hydrogen peroxide in a clean paper cup

OR

Alcohol-acetone swabs

Instructions

1 Gather the equipment on a clean, dry surface.
2 Wash your hands with soap and water. Count to 10 while washing, then rinse with clear water and dry.
3 Gently peel off the old dressing, using adhesive remover if necessary.
4 Carefully look at the skin around the catheter entry site.
5 Using either the alcohol-acetone swabs or the cotton swabs dipped in hydrogen peroxide, clean the catheter site. Use a circular motion, starting at the catheter and moving approximately 3 inches from the catheter. Use each swab only *once,* and do not dip the swab a second time in the hydrogen peroxide after it has touched the skin (see Fig. 9).
6 Using the antiseptic swabs, repeat the cleaning process. Move outward from the catheter in a circular motion.
7 Allow the antiseptic to dry on the skin.
8 Open the ointment.
9 Squeeze ointment onto the catheter site without touching the catheter or the skin with the ointment container (Fig. 12).

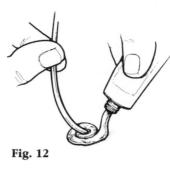

Fig. 12

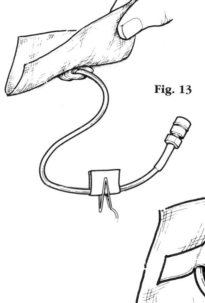

Fig. 13

10 Place a gauze sponge over the catheter insertion site (Fig. 13).
11 Loop the catheter *over* this gauze sponge (Fig. 14).
12 Cover the catheter with another gauze sponge.
13 Tape the edges of the gauze dressing securely to the skin, leaving the cap exposed (Fig. 15).
14 PRAISE THE CHILD FOR HIS HELP.
15 Place all used items in a paper bag. Close the bag and throw it away.

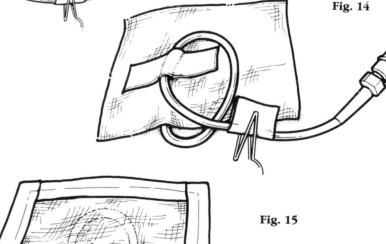

Fig. 14

Fig. 15

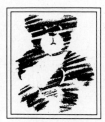

Medicines can be given rectally if the child cannot eat or drink. If you have been told to give only half of a suppository, cut the suppository in half *lengthwise*.

Equipment

Suppository
Warm water

Instructions

1 Gather equipment.
2 Wash your hands with soap and water. Count to 10 while washing, then rinse with clear water and dry.
3 Remove the wrapper from the suppository.
4 The index finger or pinky (fifth finger) should be used to put in the suppository. The pinky is preferred if the child is small. Make sure the fingernail is short and smooth. As a covering, you can use plastic wrap or a plastic sandwich bag on the finger. Finger cots can also be bought and used.
5 Remove the child's underpants or diaper.
6 With water, wet the finger or covering you will use to insert the suppository.
7 Wet the suppository with warm (not hot) water. Do not use Vaseline or any other kind of grease or lubricant. These may affect how the medicine works.
8 Insert the suppository, pointed end first, into the child's rectum 1 inch (Fig. 1).
9 If the child is too young to help, hold the buttocks together for at least 5 minutes. This prevents him from pushing the suppository out.
10 Wash your hands as above.
11 PRAISE THE CHILD FOR HIS HELP.

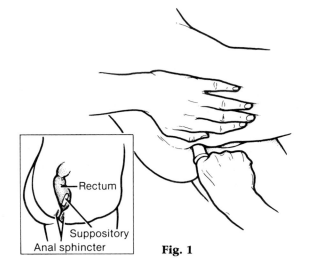

Fig. 1

NOTES

GIVING EYE MEDICATIONS

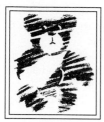

A special drug has been prescribed by your health professional for the child's eye(s). For this drug to have the most benefit, it is important that you closely follow these procedures.

Equipment

Dropper
Medicine at room temperature
Clean tissue, clean washcloth, warm water

Instructions for eye drops

1 Gather equipment.
2 Wash your hands with soap and water. Count to 10 while washing, then rinse with clear water and dry.
3 Remove any discharge from the eye with a clean tissue.
4 If the eye has crusted material around it, wet a washcloth with warm water and place this over the eye. Wait about 1 minute. Gently wipe the eye with the washcloth, place it on the eye, and wait again. If you cannot remove the crusting, rewet the washcloth. Then try to gently remove the crusted drainage. Continue using the warm, moist washcloth and gently wiping until all of the crusting is removed. Launder the washcloth before using it again.
5 Have the child lie on his back on a flat surface. If the child will not lie still, you can hold the child by sitting on a flat surface such as the floor or bed. Place the child on his back with his head between your legs and his arms under your legs. If needed, you can cross your lower legs over the child's legs to keep him from moving. Place a pillow under the child's shoulders, or a rolled up towel under his neck, so that his head is tilted back and to the same side as the eye to be treated (right eye, turn head to right; left eye, turn head to left). The eye drops should flow *away* from the child's nose.

6 Carefully remove the eye dropper from the drug bottle. The dropper portion should not touch anything but the inside of the bottle.
7 Make sure the right amount of drug is in the dropper.
8 Tell the child to look up and to the other side (away from the eye into which you are putting the drops). If the child is young, you can make a game of giving the eye drops. Tell the child to open his eyes on the count of 3. Then count to 3. When you say 3, drop the eye drops into the child's eye.
9 Note that the wrist of the hand you will be using to give the drops should be placed on the child's forehead. This will help steady your hand.
10 Gently pull down the child's lower eyelid with the other hand by placing gentle downward pressure below the eyelashes (Fig. 1).
11 Position the dropper so that the drug will fall into the lower eyelid, *never* directly onto the eyeball.
12 Squeeze the dropper for the required number of drops.
13 Tell the child to close the eye, then to blink. This helps spread the drug around the eye.

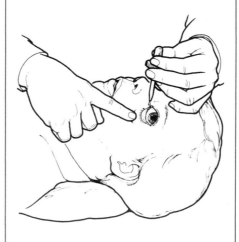

Fig. 1

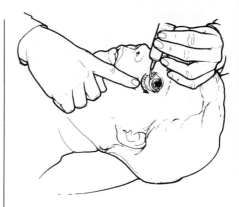

Fig. 2

14 Remove any extra drug with a clean tissue, wiping from the nose outward. Putting gentle pressure on the inner corner of the eye for 1 minute prevents any medicine from dripping into the back of the throat and causing an unpleasant taste.
15 If both eyes are to be given the drug, repeat with the other eye.
16 PRAISE THE CHILD FOR HIS HELP.
17 Write down the time you gave the child the drug and check for the time you need to give the next dose.

Instructions for ointments

When both drops and ointment are to be given, the drops are always applied before the ointment. If the ointment is to be used only once each day, it is better to apply the ointment at bedtime, since it will blur the child's vision.

1 Follow steps 1-10 for eye drops.
2 Position the tube at the inner part of the eye near the nose.
3 Squeeze a ribbon of the ointment onto the inside of lower eyelid. Begin at the side of the eye near the nose and go toward the outer edge of the eye.
4 Give the tube a half-turn. This helps "cut" the ribbon of medicine.
5 Finish with steps 13-17 for eye drops.

GIVING EAR MEDICATIONS

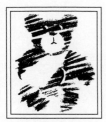

A special drug has been prescribed by your health professional for the child's ear(s). For this drug to have the most benefit, it is important that you follow these instructions.

Equipment

Medicine
Container of warm water
Clean tissue or cotton-tipped applicator and cotton ball if desired

Instructions

1 Gather equipment.
2 Wash your hands with soap and water. Count to 10 while washing, then rinse with clear water and dry.
3 Place the drug bottle in warm water.
4 Feel the drops to make sure the drug is warm, not too cold or hot.
5 Have the child lie on the side opposite the ear into which you will be putting the drug (right ear, on left side; left ear, on right side). If the child will not lie still, you can hold the child by sitting on a flat surface, such as the floor or bed. Place the child on his back with his head between your legs and his arms under your legs. If needed, you can cross your lower legs over the child's legs to keep him from moving.
6 Check the ear to see if any drainage is present. If there is drainage, remove it with a clean tissue or cotton-tipped applicator. Do NOT clean any more than the outer ear.
7 Carefully remove the dropper from the bottle. The dropper portion should not touch anything but the inside of the bottle.
8 Make sure there is enough drug in the dropper.
9 Note that the wrist of the hand you will be using should be placed on the cheek or head. This will help steady your hand.
10 You will need to straighten the child's ear canal. For children who are 3 years old and under, pull the outer ear *down* and toward the *back* of the head (Fig. 1). For older children, pull the outer ear *up* and toward the *back* (Fig. 2).
11 Position the dropper so that the drops will fall against the side of the ear canal (Fig. 3).
12 Squeeze the dropper for the right number of drops.
13 Keep the child lying on that side with the medicated ear up for 1 minute. Gently rub the skin in front of the ear (Fig. 4). This helps the drug flow to the inside of the ear.
14 If any drug has spilled onto the skin, wipe the outer ear. A cotton ball can be loosely placed in the ear, but it must be changed each time drops are given.
15 If both ears are to receive the drug, repeat with the other ear after the 1-minute wait.
16 PRAISE THE CHILD FOR HIS HELP.
17 Write down the time you gave the child the drug and check for the time you need to give the next dose.

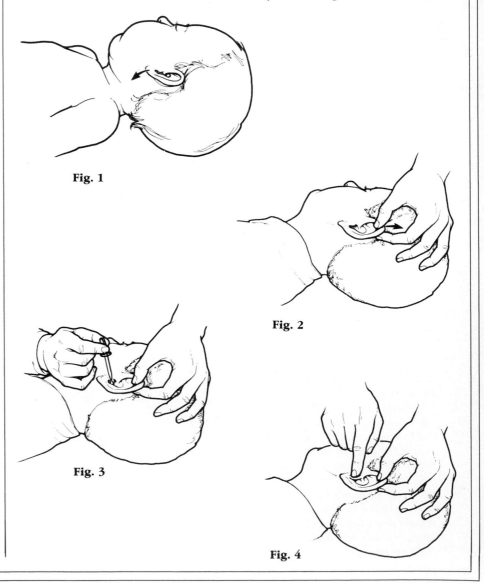

Fig. 1

Fig. 2

Fig. 3

Fig. 4

GIVING NOSE DROPS

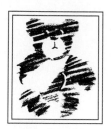

A special drug has been prescribed by your health professional. This drug is placed in the child's nose. If the child is having trouble breathing and eating because of a "stuffy nose," these drops may help the child. For this drug to have the most benefit, you should follow these instructions.

Equipment

Dropper

Drug at room temperature

Clean tissues, clean washcloth, warm water

Instructions

1 Gather equipment.

2 Wash your hands with soap and water. Count to 10 while washing, then rinse with clear water and dry.

3 Remove any mucus from the nose with a clean tissue.

4 If the nose has crusted material around it, wet a washcloth with warm water and place this around the nose. Wait about 1 minute. Gently wipe the nose with the washcloth. If you cannot remove the crusting, rewet the washcloth and again place it around the nose. Continue using the warm moist washcloth and gently wiping until all of the crusting is removed. Launder the washcloth before using it again.

5 Place the child on his back.

6 If the child will not lie still, have a helper hold the child. If you are alone, you can hold the child by sitting on a flat surface such as the floor or a bed. Place the child on his back with his head between your legs and his arms under your legs. If needed, you can cross your lower legs over the child's legs to keep him from moving (Fig. 1).

7 Tilt the child's head backward by placing a pillow or rolled up towel under the child's shoulders or letting his head hang over the side of a bed or your lap (Fig. 2).

8 Open the bottle of nose drops.

9 Make sure the right amount of drug is in the dropper.

10 Place the right number of drops in each side of the nose.

11 Keep the child's head tilted back for at least 1 minute (slowly count to 60) to prevent gagging or tasting the drug.

12 Hold and comfort the child.

13 PRAISE THE CHILD FOR HIS HELP.

14 Return the drug to a safe place out of the child's reach.

15 Write down the time you gave the child the nose drops and check for the time you need to give the next dose.

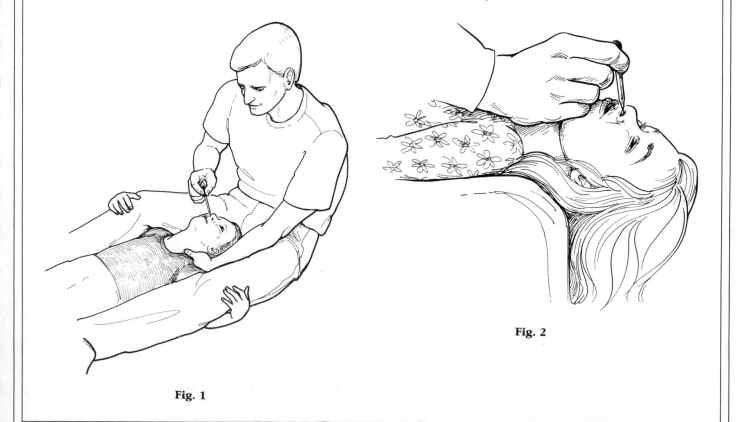

Fig. 1

Fig. 2

557

From Wong D and Whaley L: Clinical manual of pediatric nursing, ed 3. Copyright © 1990 The CV Mosby Co, St Louis.

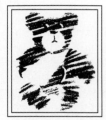

For the child to obtain enough food to grow, you must feed him by tube. If the child is active, you will need someone to hold the child while you insert the tube. After the tube is securely in place, you should hold and cuddle the child during the feeding.

You should give the child _____ ounces of _____ every _____ hours.

Call your health professional at _____ if any of the following occur:

- Vomiting
- Change in color of stomach contents
- Increased amount of stomach contents before feeding
- Increased bowel movements
- You are unable to put in the tube
- The child becomes very irritable

Equipment

Liquid food at room temperature and water in pour container
Feeding tube
½-inch tape
Water
Syringe
Stethoscope

Instructions

1 Gather equipment.
2 Wash your hands with soap and water. Count to 10 while washing, then rinse with clear water and dry.
3 Cut a piece of tape. You will need this to mark the right distance and to hold the tube in place during the feeding.
4 Tell the child (even if infant) what you will be doing.
5 Place the child on your lap, on his right side, or reclining in an infant seat.
6 Measure the tube for the exact distance you will have to insert it.
   a. Hold the tip of the tube on the child's stomach (midway between the belly button and the highest point of the lower rib cage).

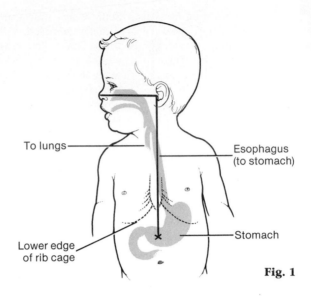

To lungs

Esophagus (to stomach)

Lower edge of rib cage

Stomach

Fig. 1

b. Extend the tube up to the child's ear lobe then out to his nose (Fig. 1).
   c. Mark the spot at the nose with the piece of tape.
7 Dip the tip of the tube in clear water to moisten.
8 Insert the tip of the tube into one nostril guiding it toward the back of the child's throat.
9 If the child is able to help, have him swallow the tube to help it pass.
10 Quickly insert the tube to the tape mark on the tube.
   If the child begins coughing or has any other problems, remove the tube at once.
11 Tape the tube to the child's upper lip and cheek (Fig. 2).
12 Check the placement of the tube:
   a. Place 5 cc of air in the syringe. Connect the syringe to the tube.
   b. Place the stethoscope over the child's stomach area.
   c. Inject the air into the tube while listening for the sound of gurgling through the stethoscope.
   d. Remove the air.
   e. With the syringe connected to the tube, gently pull back the plunger. If stomach contents appear in the tube, it is in the correct place.

f. If you are unable to see any stomach contents in the tube, place the child on the left side or advance the tube a short distance. Pull back on plunger again to check for stomach contents.
   g. Return the stomach contents.
13 Check the temperature of the food; it should be room temperature.
14 Disconnect the syringe from the tube and remove the plunger from the syringe.

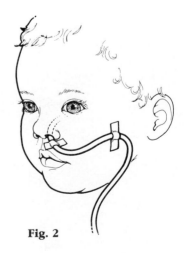

Fig. 2

This section may be photocopied and distributed to families.
From Wong D and Whaley L: Clinical manual of pediatric nursing, ed 3. Copyright © 1990 The CV Mosby Co, St Louis.

15 Reconnect the syringe to the tube.
16 Fill the syringe with the right amount of food.
17 If necessary, push gently with the plunger to start the flow of food. Then remove the plunger and allow the food to flow by gravity.
18 The bottom of the syringe should never be held higher than the child's chin, or 6 inches above the level of the child's stomach (Fig. 3).
19 Continue adding food until the right amount has been fed. Do not allow the syringe to become empty.
20 When the food is at the bottom of the syringe, add 1 teaspoon (5 ml) of water to rinse the tube.
21 Place the clamp on the tube if it will be left in place between feedings.
22 Hold, cuddle, and burp the child.
23 Write down the time and amount of the child's feeding.

TO REMOVE THE TUBE

1 Loosen the tape that is holding the tube.
2 Fold the tube and pinch it tightly together.
3 Pull the tube out quickly.
4 Hold, cuddle, and burp the child.

CARE OF THE NASOGASTRIC TUBE AND SYRINGE

Wash with soap and water, and rinse the inside well with clear water. Dry and store in a clean, dry container (e.g., plastic bag, margarine container).

If the tube remains in place between feedings, *always* check to make sure the tube is in the right place before adding formula (step 12).

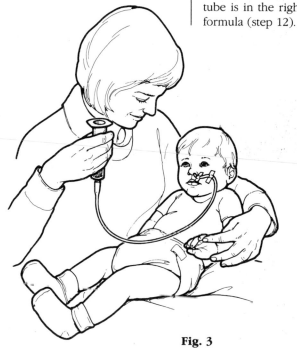

Fig. 3

NOTES

GIVING GASTROSTOMY TUBE FEEDINGS

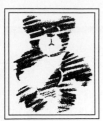

To help the child get enough food to grow, an opening was made into the child's stomach. The gastrostomy tube has been put into this opening. You can now feed the child through this gastrostomy tube. You should hold and cuddle the child during the feeding.

You should give the child _____ ounces of _____ every _____ hours.

Call your health professional at _____ if any of the following occur.

- Vomiting
- Change in color of stomach contents
- Increased amount of stomach contents before feeding
- Increased bowel movements
- The child becomes very irritable

Equipment

Liquid food at room temperature in pour container
Water to rinse tube
Syringe

Instructions

1 Gather equipment.
2 Wash your hands with soap and water. Count to 10 while washing, then rinse with clear water and dry.
3 Tell the child (even if infant) what you will be doing.
4 Place the child on your lap or reclining in an infant seat.
5 Attach the syringe with the plunger removed to the gastrostomy tube.
6 Unclamp the tube.
7 Fill syringe with the right amount of food.
8 A gentle push with the plunger of the syringe may be necesssary to start the flow of food. Then remove the plunger and allow the food to flow by gravity.
9 Never hold the bottom of the syringe higher than the child's chin (Fig. 1).
10 Continue adding food to the syringe until you have finished the right amount. Do not allow the syringe to become empty.
11 When the food is at the bottom of the syringe add 1 teaspoon (5 ml) of water to rinse the tube and keep it from clogging.
12 Clamp the tube and remove the syringe.
13 Gently pull the tube to allow the balloon to rest against the inside of the stomach at the opening.
14 Secure the tube to prevent it from advancing or allowing stomach contents to leak on the skin.
15 Hold and cuddle child after the feeding.

Wash the syringe in warm soap and water. Rinse the inside well with clear water. Dry the syringe and store in a clean dry container between feedings (e.g., plastic bag, margarine container).

CARE OF A GASTROSTOMY TUBE

The gastrostomy tube should be changed _____. If the tube accidentally comes out, it should be replaced. A gauze bandage can be placed over the opening until you can get to a quiet place where you can reinsert the tube. When you are away from home and the child will need to be fed, you should carry an extra gastrostomy tube with you in case something happens to the tube that is in place.

Equipment

Gastrostomy tube
Water for lubricant
Small syringe
Water or air if needed for balloon
Tape

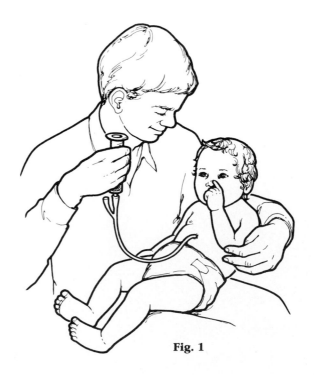

Fig. 1

Removing the tube

Remove the tube just before feeding so that there will be only a small amount of liquid in the child's stomach:

1 Gather equipment.
2 Wash your hands with soap and water. Count to 10 while washing, then rinse with clear water and dry.
3 Tell the child what you will be doing.
4 Place the child on the right side or semisitting in an infant seat.
5 Attach small syringe to the tube at point A (Fig. 2).
6 Withdraw the air/water from the balloon.
7 With the tube still clamped, quickly remove it holding the tip up to prevent stomach contents from dripping.
8 Place it out of the child's reach while you push in the new tube.

Insertion of tube

The rubber portion of a baby bottle nipple may be used to support the gastrostomy tube. Cut several holes (air vents) in the base of the nipple. Put the tube into the base of the nipple and pull it through the hold at the top. It may be necessary to make the hole in the top of the nipple slightly larger or use tweezers to pull the tube snugly through the hole. Slide the nipple up about 4 to 5 inches so you can comfortably handle the tube.

1 Wet the tip of the clean tube with water.
2 Put the tip of the tube through the opening into the child's stomach.
3 Insert the tube beyond the balloon on the tip (Fig. 3).
4 Connect the syringe, containing _____ cc of air or water, to point A.
5 Inject the air or water into the tube.
6 Gently pull on the tube to make sure the balloon is inflated and the tube is in position.
7 Tape the tube securely to the child's abdomen.
8 Clamp the new tube until you are ready for the next feeding

The gastrostomy tube that you have removed should be cleaned in soap and water. Rinse the inside of the tube well with clear water. Dry the tube and store in a clean dry container (e.g., plastic bag, margarine container).

SKIN CARE

Keep the skin around the gastrostomy tube clean and dry. A bandage does not have to be put over the area, but this may be needed to keep the child from pulling on the tube. A cloth diaper can also be wrapped around the child's abdomen and secured with tape. This will keep the child from playing with the tube.

Petrolatum (Vaseline) can be used on the skin around the tube. This will provide protection for the skin in case there is a small leakage of gastric fluid. If the area becomes reddened or sore, call your health professionals at _____ for further directions.

CLOTHING

Dress the child in loose fitting clothing that does not press the gastrostomy tube against the skin. Bib-type overalls are preferable to pants. The overalls cover the tube, make it less likely that the child or other children will play with the tube. Also the overalls avoid tight elastic around the child's waist.

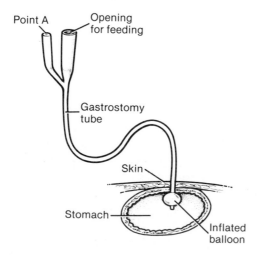

Fig. 2

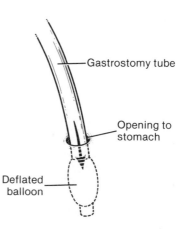

Fig. 3

HOME CARE INSTRUCTIONS

PERFORMING CLEAN INTERMITTENT SELF-CATHETERIZATION

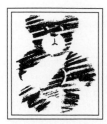

This will help the child to remain dry and will help prevent bladder infections. Catheterization should be done when the child wakes up in the morning, before bedtime, and every ____ hours during the day. If the child is unable to do the catheterization alone, someone at school should be taught to help the child. Stopping fluids 2 hours before bedtime will help the child stay dry through the night.

A record should be kept of all that the child drinks and the amount of urine that was obtained by catheterization (see sample below). A description of the urine is helpful so you can notice changes that may be caused by an infection. Look at the urine to see if it is cloudy or clear, or pale yellow or dark amber, smell it to tell if a strange odor is present.

Call your health professional at ____ if any of these occur:
- Temperature above 100° F orally or axillary or 100.4° F rectally
- Trouble inserting the tube
- Change in the amount of urine
- Change in the way the urine looks or smells

Equipment

Catheter and storage container
Soap and water/towelettes
Urine container
Lubricant for boys

Instructions for boys

1 Have equipment ready; keep the tube in its container until you are ready to use it.
2 Wash your hands with soap and water. Count to 10 while washing, then rinse with clear water and dry.
3 Tell the child what you will be doing.
4 Remove or arrange the child's clothing so it will not get wet and the urine can flow.
5 Wet the first 2 inches of the tube either by placing lubricant on your finger and spreading it on the tube or by dipping the catheter into the lubricant on a clean tissue.
6 Hold penis straight; if the child is uncircumcised, pull the foreskin back as far as it will go without forcing it.
7 Put the tube into the urinary opening; insert it until urine begins to flow (Fig. 1).
8 If you have trouble passing the tube stop; do not force the tube. Call your health professional ____.
9 Let all of the urine flow out.
10 Tell the child to squeeze his belly as if he were having a bowel movement. This helps empty all of the urine out of the bladder.

SAMPLE RECORD

Time	Fluid in	Wet/dry	Amount out	Appearance

562

From Wong D and Whaley L: Clinical manual of pediatric nursing, ed 3. Copyright © 1990 The CV Mosby Co, St Louis.

11 Slowly remove the tube; if urine begins to flow again, stop removing the tube and allow it to empty.

12 Remove the tube holding the tip up so that any urine in the tube will not spill.

13 Wash your hands and the catheter with soap and water. Rinse the inside of the tube well with clear water.

14 Dry the catheter and store in a clean dry container (e.g., plastic bag, margarine container).

15 PRAISE THE CHILD FOR HIS HELP.

16 Write down the time and the amount and the way the urine looks.

Instructions for girls

1 Gather equipment; keep the tube in its container until you are ready to use it.

2 Wash your hands with soap and water. Count to 10 while washing, then rinse with clear water and dry.

3 Tell the child what you will be doing.

4 Remove or arrange the child's clothing so it will not get wet and urine can flow.

5 Locate the urinary opening: for self-catheterization, a mirror can be used, but it should not be required. If you wipe the area between the labia with a downward stroke, a small slit or V indicates the opening.

6 Put the tube into the urinary opening; insert it until urine begins to flow (Fig. 2)

7 Allow all of the urine to flow out.

8 Tell the child to squeeze her belly as if she were having a bowel movement. This helps empty all of the urine out of the bladder.

9 Slowly remove the tube; if urine begins to flow again, stop removing the tube and allow it to empty.

10 Remove the tube holding the tip up so that any urine in the tube will not spill.

11 Wash your hands and the catheter with soap and water. Rinse the inside of the tube well with clear water.

12 Dry the tube and store in a clean dry container (e.g., plastic bag, margarine container).

13 Write down the time, amount, and the way the urine looks.

14 PRAISE THE CHILD FOR HER HELP.

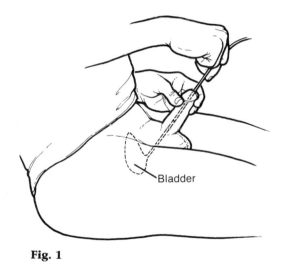

Fig. 1

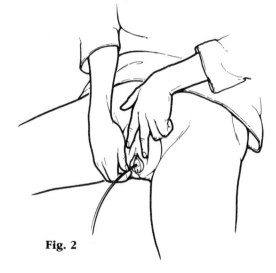

Fig. 2

NOTES

CARING FOR THE CHILD WITH A COLOSTOMY

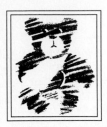

The child has had surgery that has changed the way in which he has a bowel movement. An opening was made in the abdomen and the bowel was attached to the skin. This allows the bowel to empty through the opening (stoma) instead of the rectum. Therefore the area must be kept clean to prevent the skin from becoming irritated. This can be done by using a barrier on the skin and keeping the stool from spreading over the child and clothing. School age children should wear a pouch.

You will need to do the ostomy care for the infant and young child. The child can assist according to his level. For example, he can gather the equipment and hand you supplies. As the child grows, allow him to increase his responsibility in the care of his ostomy. By the age of 8 or 10, most children can do the care by themselves.

Ostomy care should be taught to other people who will be caring for the child. At school, tell both the child's teacher and the school nurse so that adult help is available if needed. An extra set of clothing can be kept at the school in case the ostomy appliance leaks. This will help spare the child any embarrassment.

If the skin around the ostomy becomes irritated (moist or red in color), it is important to help the area heal as fast as possible. Leaving the child's abdomen and stoma uncovered as often as possible and keeping the skin clean and dry helps the healing. When the child has a bowel movement, remove the stool by gently patting the area with a cloth or paper towel or by rinsing it with warm water from a squeeze bottle. Gently pat the area dry and leave open to the air. A hair dryer on the cool setting can be used to dry the skin around the stoma.

Dress the child in loose-fitting clothing that does not press on the colostomy. Bib-type overalls or dresses are preferable to pants. The overalls or dress will cover the ostomy and avoid the elastic waistband on pants, which may irritate the ostomy.

Call your health professional if any of these occur:

- Bleeding from the stoma more than usual when cleaning stoma
- Bleeding from skin around stoma
- Change in bowel pattern
- Change in the size of the stoma
- Temperature above 100.4° F

OSTOMY CARE (WITHOUT A POUCH/APPLIANCE)

Ostomy care should be done whenever the child has a bowel movement. Every 1-2 days the area should be well cleaned and a new barrier applied. During the day, the stool can be removed/rinsed from the barrier and if the barrier is still intact a clean diaper applied.

Equipment

Washcloth or paper towels
Skin barrier
Cloth diaper; Diaper pins/tape

Instructions

1 Gather equipment
2 Wash your hands with soap and water. Count to 10 while washing, then rinse with clear water and dry.
3 Clean the stool off of the child's skin with a warm, wet washcloth, or paper towels.
4 Pat the skin around the stoma dry.
5 Apply the skin barrier recommended by your health professional:
   a. Stomadhesive* wafer cut to fit around the stoma.
   b. Thick layer of zinc oxide ointment with gauze, soft tissue, or karaya powder around the stoma.
   c. Thick layer of petroleum based ointment with karaya powder sprinkled around the stoma.
6 Wrap cloth diaper around child's stomach. Secure with diaper pins or tape.
7 Wash your hands as above.

OSTOMY CARE (WITH A POUCH/APPLIANCE)

The pouch will remain intact for different periods of time. The pouch should

*Manufactured by E.R. Squibb & Sons, Princeton, New Jersey.

be changed on a routine schedule or sooner, if it leaks. Each time the pouch is changed the area needs to be clean and dry and a new barrier must be applied. During the day, the stool can be removed/rinsed from the pouch, and then it can be clamped. Two-piece pouches are also available.

Equipment

Washcloth	Pouch/appliance
Skin barrier/wafer	Rinse bottle
Stoma paste	

Instructions

1 Gather equipment.
2 Wash your hands with soap and water. Count to 10 while washing, then rinse with clear water and dry.
3 Tell child what you are going to do. (Have him do it if old enough.)
4 Remove old pouch and skin barrier.
5 Wash the skin and gently pat dry.
6 Look for any redness or irritation.
7 Cut the skin barrier to size.
8 Apply the skin barrier. If using the type with an adhesive backing, remove the paper seal first.
9 Remove the covering from adhesive backing on the pouch.
10 Center the pouch over the stoma and press gently beginning from the stoma edge out.
11 Close the end of the pouch with a clamp or rubber band.
12 Wash your hands as above.

Emptying the pouch

1 When the pouch is one-third filled with stool, open the lower end of the pouch over the toilet or another container and let the stool drain out.
2 Rinse the inside of the pouch each day with a squeeze bottle of cool water to remove all the stool. Fill the pouch with a small amount of clear water and swish it around to thoroughly clean pouch. Then empty pouch over the toilet or a diaper.
3 Make a wick from toilet tissue to dry the inside lower 1 inch of the pouch. Wipe off the outside and reattach the clamp or rubber band.
4 Wash your hands as above.

GIVING AN ENEMA

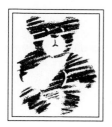

An enema is needed when stool must be removed from the bowel or intestine. However, simple constipation in children should not be treated with enemas but with changes in the child's diet. Increasing the amount of liquids to at least 1 quart each day and the amount of fiber in foods (especially whole grains, bran cereals, fresh vegetables, and fruit with the skin on) should increase the size and number of the child's bowel movements. If the child has persistent constipation, a complete medical evaluation is necessary to determine the cause. If you have been told to give an enema to the child by a health professional, use these instructions.

Equipment

Lukewarm water (water that feels comfortably warm)
Salt
Measuring spoon
Enema kit/prepackaged enema
Lubricant such as Vaseline
Potty chair or toilet

Age	Amount of lukewarm water	Approximate amount of salt	Distance to insert tube
Infant	4 ounces-1 cup (120 ml-240 ml)	¼ tsp-½ tsp (1.25 ml-2.5 ml)	1 in (2.5 cm)
2-4 yr	1 cup-1½ cups (240 ml-360 ml)	½ tsp-¾ tsp (2.5 ml-3.75 ml)	2 in (5.0 cm)
4-10 yr	1½ cup-2 cups (360 ml-480 ml)	¾ tsp-1 tsp (3.75 ml-5.0 ml)	3 in (7.5 cm)
11 yr	2 cups-3 cups (480 ml-720 ml)	1 tsp-1½ tsp (5.0 ml-7.5 ml)	4 in (10 cm)

Instructions (for non-prepackaged enemas)

1 Gather equipment.
2 Wash your hands with soap and water. Count to 10 while washing, then rinse with clear water and dry.
3 Refer to the above chart for the right amount of water and salt for the child's age; never use plain tap water.
4 Mix the lukewarm water and salt.
5 Measure the rectal tube for the correct distance.
6 Check to make sure the tube is clamped shut. Then fill the enema container with the solution.
7 Place the child in one of the following positions:
   a. Lying face down on belly with the knees and hips bent toward the chest (Fig. 1).
   b. Lying on the left side with the left leg straight and the right leg bent at the hip and knee and placed comfortably on top of the left leg (Fig. 2).
   c. Sitting on the potty chair or toilet (Fig. 3).
8 Allow the liquid to flow through the tube to remove air that is present. Clamp the tube.
9 Place a small amount of lubricant on your finger or on a tissue and spread the lubricant around the tip of the tube, being careful not to plug the holes with lubricant (Fig. 4).
10 Gently put the tube into the child's rectum to the marked distance (Fig. 5).
11 Holding the bottom of the container no more than 4 inches above the child, open the clamp and allow the liquid to flow. You may have to hold the tube in place.
12 When the container is empty, remove the tube.
13 Have the child keep the liquid inside for 3 to 5 minutes. If the child is too young to follow instructions, then hold the buttocks together to keep the liquid inside.
14 Help the child to the toilet or potty chair, or allow the child to release the liquid into a diaper.
15 PRAISE THE CHILD FOR HIS HELP.
16 Write down the appearance of the results of the enema.
17 Wash your hands as above.

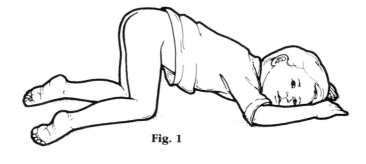

Fig. 1

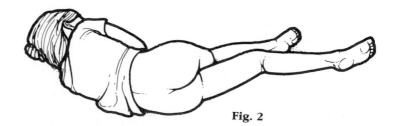

Fig. 2

565

PREPACKAGED ENEMAS

Ready-to-use enemas are available in varying amounts and solutions for infants, children, and adults. Use the amount and type of solution recommended by your health professional.

Instructions

1 Warm the liquid in a basin of warm water.
2 Wash your hands with soap and water. Count to 10 while washing, then rinse with clear water and dry.

3 Place the child in one of the following positions:
   a. Lying face down on belly with the knees and hips bent toward the chest (Fig. 1).
   b. Lying on the left side with the left leg straight and the right leg bent at the hip and knee and placed comfortably on top of the left leg (Fig. 2).
   c. Sitting on the potty chair or toilet (Fig. 3).
4 Remove the cap (Fig. 6). Put the tip that is already lubricated into the child's rectum the right distance (Fig. 7).

5 Gently squeeze the enema container to empty. A small amount will remain in the container after squeezing.
6 Remove the tip.
7 Have the child keep the liquid inside for 3 to 5 minutes. If the child is too young to follow instructions, then hold the buttocks together to keep the liquid inside.
8 Help the child to the toilet or potty chair or allow the child to release the solution into a diaper.
9 PRAISE THE CHILD FOR HIS HELP.
10 Write down the appearance of the results of the enema.
11 Wash your hands as above.

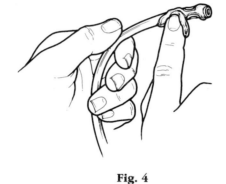

Fig. 4

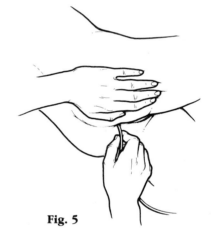

Fig. 5

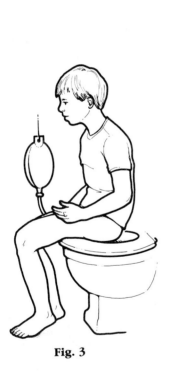

Fig. 3

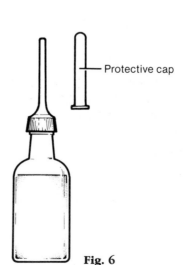

Protective cap

Fig. 6

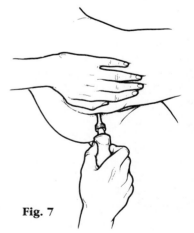

Fig. 7

PERFORMING POSTURAL DRAINAGE

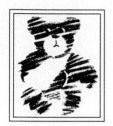

Mucus is a protective covering of the inside of the lungs and airways. Mucus traps dust and dirt in the air that we breathe and helps prevent these from irritating the lung. When an infection or other irritation is present, the body produces more thick mucus to help the lungs get rid of the infection. When this thick mucus blocks the airways, breathing becomes more difficult. To help the body get rid of the extra mucus, postural drainage is done. This series of activities helps move thick mucus from the lungs into the trachea (windpipe) where it can be coughed out. The airways can be compared to a freshly opened catsup bottle. Even when the bottle is held upside down, it takes several sharp blows to the bottom of the bottle to make the catsup start flowing.

The postural drainage needs to be carried out ____ times per day. This should be done when the child wakes up, before bedtime, and about 1½ hours before lunch and the evening meal. It should not be done after meals since the exercises and coughing may cause the child to vomit. The exercises should be finished 30 to 45 minutes before the meal, so that the child has a chance to rest and feel like eating.

The child must be placed in several different positions for the postural drainage. You must adapt the procedure for the child's age and strength. Each session should usually last 20 to 30 minutes and involve only four to six positions. The remaining positions are then used at the other postural drainage times throughout the day.

TECHNIQUES YOU WILL NEED
Cupping (percussion)

Place your hand as if you were holding a liquid or powder (but reversed) (Fig. 1). When the child is in the drainage position, rapidly strike the child's chest with your hand. The entire oval of your hand should make contact with the child's chest. The bottom of a baby bottle nipple can be padded with tissue and then secured with adhesive tape (Fig. 2). This can be used for cupping an infant. The drawings that follow have a shaded area to show where to place your hand for each position. Cupping is carried out for about 1 minute in each position. Have the child wear a shirt so your hand does not touch the child's bare skin during cupping. Remember, cupping is not the same as hitting. When done right, cupping does not hurt the child or cause the skin to become red, which occurs when the skin is slapped.

Vibration

Learning to vibrate may take a little practice. First, place one of your hands on top of the other, then rapidly tighten and loosen the muscles of your lower arm (Fig. 3). This creates a vibration that, when applied to the skin, is passed through to the lungs to loosen mucus. Now, have the child take a deep breath and while he is breathing out, place your hands over the lung segment to be drained and vibrated. An electric vibrator, a padded electric toothbrush (for infants), as well as your hands can be used for vibration.

POSITIONING AIDS

Infants and small children can be positioned in your lap. For older children a padded slant board can be used. If a slant board is not available, a bed or couch at a comfortable height can be used. Pillows are helpful to position the child comfortably.

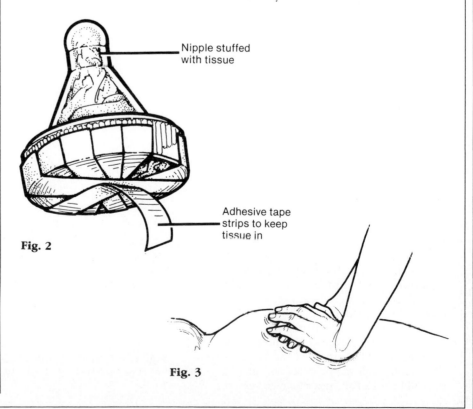

Nipple stuffed with tissue

Adhesive tape strips to keep tissue in

Fig. 2

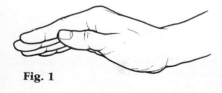

Fig. 1

Fig. 3

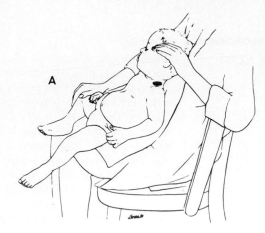

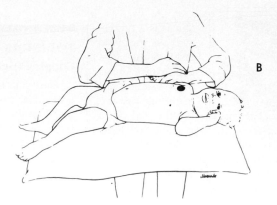

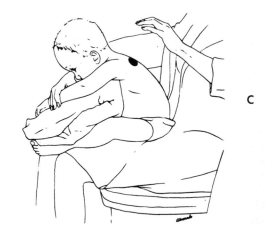

Instructions

1 Place the child in the position in Fig. 4, *A*.

2 Tell the child to take several deep breaths. The child can also use special blow bottles or try to blow up a balloon. These help the child to take deep breaths and may cause the child to cough.

3 Cup the area shaded in the picture for about 1 minute.

4 After cupping have the child take a deep breath and vibrate the area as he breathes out. Repeat this for 3 breaths. If the child is too young to understand how to breathe deeply and slowly, just vibrate during a few breaths.

5 Tell the child to cough. Since he may not be able to cough when lying down, help him to a sitting position to produce a good deep cough.

6 Repeat steps 1 through 5 for each of the other positions.

7 Only one side is shown above, but remember that the procedure must be repeated for both left and right sides.

REMEMBER: Spend about 20 to 30 minutes at each session. Watch the child carefully for signs of tiredness. The postural drainage should be stopped before he becomes tired. It can be continued after the child has had an opportunity to rest.

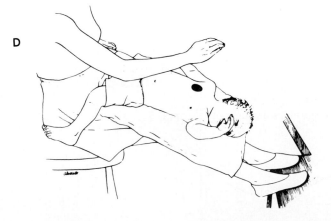

Fig. 4, A-I, modified from Infant Segmental Bronchial Drainage. Reprinted with the permission of Cystic Fibrosis Foundation, Rockville, Maryland.

Fig. 4, cont'd

SUCTIONING THE NOSE AND MOUTH

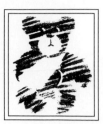

The child needs help to keep the mouth and nose clear of mucus. Suctioning equipment, a humidifier, and other supplies will be needed. While the child is in the hospital, you should use the same suction machine that you will be using at home. This allows you a chance to become familiar with the equipment. You will also need a mucus trap or nasal aspirator that can be used to remove mucus when you and the child are away from home. Practice with these items while the child is in the hospital.

Certain guidelines are helpful for the child who has problems clearing mucus from the nose and mouth. To keep the mucus liquid so that it is easy to remove by both suctioning and coughing, added moisture is needed. Encourage the child to drink at least 1 quart (4 8-ounce cups) of liquid each day and place a cool mist humidifier in the room where the child sleeps. Change the water in the humidifier each day and clean the humidifier with white vinegar at least once a week.

All of the people who provide care for the child must know how to suction the child so that they can assist you. Tape the emergency phone numbers, such as 911 (if available in your area), the local hospital, your health professional, and any numbers that are necessary, to each telephone in the house. Notify your health professional if any of the following occur:

- Temperature above 100.4° F
- Presence of yellow or green mucus
- Change in the smell of the mucus
- Increased amount of mucus
- The child is very irritable
- The child is having difficulty breathing

SUCTIONING

Suctioning keeps the airway (nose and mouth) (Fig. 1) clear of mucus to help the child breathe more easily. Suctioning should not be done routinely, but only when needed. Suction when:

- The child is having trouble breathing
- The child appears very restless
- The child has difficulty eating or sucking
- The child's color becomes paler
- The child's nostrils flare (spread out)
- You hear the sound of air bubbling through the mucus

When the child has a cold, more mucus is produced, so you will probably need to suction more often. The child may cough or gag when you insert or remove the suction catheter. Gently tell the child when you are almost finished. If the child is old enough, teach him how to help you by holding the supplies.

Preparing the supplies

Clean jars and containers:

Wash plastic whipped cream or margarine containers and glass jars with lids in a dishwasher or hot, soapy water and rinse well. Use a clean towel to dry or allow to air dry. Keep a supply washed and dried.

Salt solution (saline):

Boil water for 5 minutes. Add ¾ teaspoon of salt to each 2 cups of water when you are heating the water. Let cool, then pour into a clean glass jar and cover. Store the sterile saline in the refrigerator.

Equipment

Suction machine with tubing
Suction catheters
Saline (cool)
Clean container for rinsing catheter

Instructions

1 Gather all the equipment you will need.
2 Wash your hands with soap and water. Count to 10 while washing, then rinse with clear water and dry.
3 Open the suction catheter package and connect the catheter to the suction machine.
4 Make sure the suction machine is plugged in and working.
5 Measure the tube for the distance you will have to insert it. Place the tip of the catheter at the child's ear lobe and mark the distance to the tip of the child's nose. Hold the catheter at this mark (Fig. 2).
6 Place the tip of the catheter in the sterile saline and place your thumb over the opening to obtain suction. The saline wets the catheter (Fig. 3).
7 Tell the child to take a deep breath.
8 With your thumb off the opening (no suction), insert the suction catheter in one nostril up to the measured distance (Fig. 4, A).

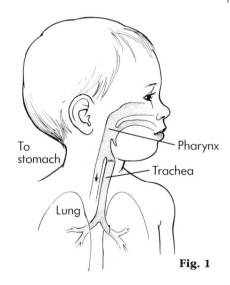

To stomach
Pharynx
Trachea
Lung

Fig. 1

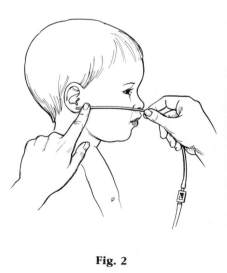

Fig. 2

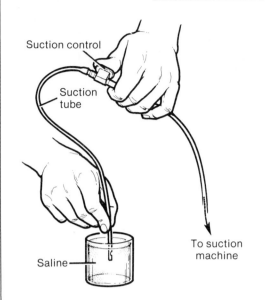

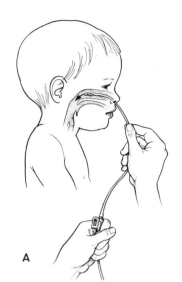

Fig. 3

Fig. 4

9 Place your thumb on the suction port to obtain suction.

10 Rotate or twist the catheter as you remove it with a slow steady motion (Fig. 4, *B*). Both inserting the catheter and suctioning should take no longer than 5 seconds. Remember, the child may not breathe while you are suctioning. Try holding your breath whenever your thumb is on the suction port. This will be a reminder to you for timing.

11 Look at the mucus. Check the color, smell, and consistency for any change.

12 Rinse the suction catheter in the sterile saline with your thumb on the suction port.

13 Allow the child to take a few deep breaths.

14 Repeat steps 7 through 14 up to 2 times, then repeat for the other nostril.

15 After suctioning the nose, you can use the same catheter to clear the child's mouth.

16 Place the tip of the catheter in the saline and place your thumb over the opening to obtain suction.

17 Tell the child to take a deep breath.

18 With your thumb off the opening (no suction), insert the suction catheter in the child's mouth along one side of the mouth until it reaches the back of the throat. A tongue blade may be needed to keep the tongue out of the way and to keep the child from biting the catheter (Fig. 5).

19 Place your thumb on the suction port to obtain suction.

20 Rotate or twist the catheter as you remove it with a slow steady motion. Both inserting the catheter and suctioning should take no longer than 5 seconds. Remember, the child may not breathe while you are suctioning. Try holding your breath whenever your thumb is on the suction port. This will be a reminder to you for timing

21 Look at the mucus. Check the color, smell, and consistency for any change.

22 Rinse the suction catheter in the saline with your thumb on the suction port.

23 Allow the child a chance to take a few deep breaths.

24 Repeat steps 17 through 23 up to three times.

25 Hold and comfort the child.

26 PRAISE THE CHILD FOR HIS HELP.

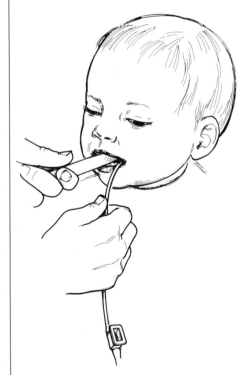

Fig. 5

27 After each use, throw away the saline and clean the container. The suction machine should be clean and ready for the next time that you will have to use it.

28 Your health professional will instruct you on the care of the suction catheters or use the method described below.

29 Wash your hands with soap and water. Count to 10 while washing your hands, then rinse with clear water and dry.

INSTRUCTIONS FOR CLEANING THE SUCTION CATHETERS

1 Rinse the suction catheters in cool tap water. Do not use hot water because it "cooks" the mucus, which makes it more difficult to remove.

2 Place the catheters in a clean jar filled with hot, soapy water.

3 Rinse both the inside and outside of the tube under hot, running water. Hold the tube with kitchen tongs so that you don't burn yourself.

4 Shake off the excess water.

5 Place on a clean paper towel to dry. When the tube is completely dry, place it in a clean plastic bag.

6 Close the bag and store until the next time you suction the child.

7 If you notice any moisture in the bag, repeat the entire cleaning procedure.

INSTRUCTIONS FOR USING A NASAL ASPIRATOR

When the child's nose is plugged with loose, runny mucus, the nasal aspirator is very helpful in removing it. The aspirator can also be used when the nose is plugged with dry, crusted mucus. Nose drops must first be used to moisten the mucus before it can be removed. Saline nose drops are the safest product to use. These can be purchased or made at home. To make the nose drops at home, mix ¾ teaspoon salt with 1 pint (2 cups) tap water or the mixture prescribed by

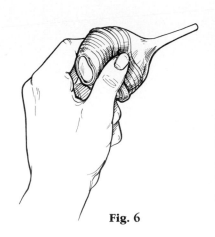

Fig. 6

your health professional. The solution can be stored in any clean covered container, but should be mixed fresh each day. Use a clean eye dropper to put the solution in the child's nose, or wet a cotton ball and let the saline drip into the nose. Once the dried mucus is removed, then the nasal aspirator can be used.

Instructions

1 Squeeze the rounded end of the bulb (Fig. 6).

2 Place the tip of the bulb snugly into one side of the nose (nostril).

3 Let go of the bulb slowly; the bulb will suck the mucus out of the nose (Fig. 7).

4 When the bulb is reinflated, remove it from the nose (Fig. 8).

5 Squeeze the bulb into a tissue to get rid of the mucus.

6 Repeat steps 1-5 for the other side of the nose.

7 Repeat this process as often as needed to keep the nose clear.

Cleaning the nasal aspirator

Clean the nasal aspirator by filling it with tap water. Then squeeze the bulb to remove the water and the mucus. Refill the bulb with water and boil for 10 minutes. Let the bulb cool and squeeze out the water before using it again.

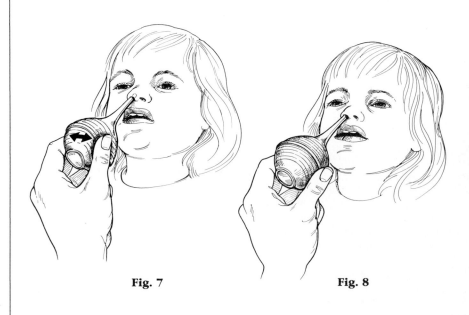

Fig. 7   **Fig. 8**

CARING FOR THE CHILD WITH A TRACHEOSTOMY

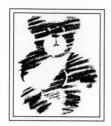

A small opening (stoma) was made in the child's windpipe (or trachea) (Fig. 1) to help him breathe easier. The tracheostomy ("trach") will require special care while you are at home. Suctioning equipment, a humidifier, and other supplies will be needed. While the child is in the hospital, you should use the same suction machine (and monitor) that you will be using at home. This helps you to become familiar with the equipment. You will also need a mucous trap that can be used to remove mucus from the child's trach when you are on short trips. Other supplies needed when outside the home are a trach tube with ties and scissors. Practice with these items while the child is in the hospital.

SPECIAL CONSIDERATIONS

Certain precautions are needed for the child with a trach. Since the air that the child breathes no longer passes through the nose and mouth, it is no longer warmed, moistened, and filtered before it enters the lungs. To keep the mucus liquid, so that it is easy to remove by both suctioning and coughing, added moisture is needed. Have the child drink at least 1 quart (4-8 oz cups) of liquid each day and place a cool mist humidifier in the room where the child sleeps. Change the water in the humidifier each day and clean well with white vinegar at least once a week.

When the child is out in hot, dry, or cold weather or on very windy days, wrap a handkerchief or scarf around the child's neck. This will help warm and filter the air the child breathes. Humidifying/filtering devices can also be bought.* To keep food and liquids from falling into the trach, use a cloth bib with short ties when the child is eating.

NOTE: For some children, additional instructions on stoma care and/or use of monitor may be needed. Home Care Instructions are available for CPR and postural drainage.

*Manufactured by Portex, Inc., 42 Industrial Way, Wilmington, MA 01887.

Any smoke, aerosol sprays, powder, or dust can irritate the lining of the child's trachea. Therefore the child should not be in the same room with anyone who is smoking or where aerosol sprays such as hairspray and antiperspirants are being used. Strong cleaning liquids such as ammonia are also irritating. Hair from animals that are fuzzy and that shed can clog the child's trachea. Avoid stuffed animals and toys with small parts that can be removed and put into the trach by a curious child.

The moist secretions from the trach can irritate the skin. It is important to keep the area around the tracheostomy clean and dry to prevent skin irritation and infection. Change the trach ties each day or if they become wet or dirty. Tie the knot in a new place each time, to keep from irritating the skin. Do not apply any ointments or other medications on the skin unless you are told by your health professional.

Careful adult supervision is needed when the child is near water. Tub baths can be given, but be careful not to allow water into the trach. Swimming and boating must be avoided. However, the child can use a wading pool with supervision.

All of the people who provide care for the child must be aware of how to suction the trach so that they can help you. Anyone caring for the child alone must also know cardiopulmonary resuscitation (CPR). Tape the emergency phone numbers to each telephone in the house. Include 911 (if available in your area), the local hospital, your health professional, and any others that are needed. Call your health professional if any of the following occur for 12 to 24 hours:

- Temperature above 100.4° F
- Yellow or green mucus from trach or stoma
- Bright red blood from the trach
- Change in the smell of the mucus
- Increased amount of mucus
- The child is very irritable
- The child is having trouble breathing

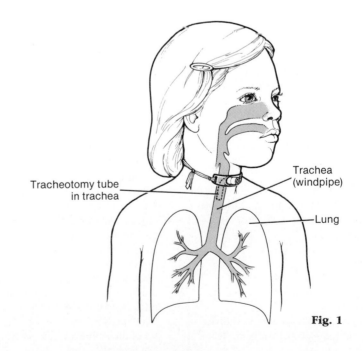

Fig. 1

SUCTIONING

You will need to suction the child's trach to keep the airway clear of mucus. Suctioning helps the child to breathe more easily. Suctioning should be done when the child wakes up and before sleep. Suction the child when any of the following occur:

- He is having trouble breathing
- He appears very restless
- He has trouble eating or sucking
- His color becomes paler
- His nostrils flare (spread out)
- You hear the sound of air bubbling through the mucus or stridor (whistling)

When the child has a cold, more mucus is produced so you will need to suction more often.

Preparing the supplies

Clean jars and containers:

Wash plastic whipped cream or margarine containers and glass jars with lids in a dishwasher or hot soapy water and rinse well. Use a clean towel to dry or allow to air dry. Keep a supply washed and dried.

Sterile saline:

Boil water for 5 minutes. Add ¾ teaspoon of noniodized salt (check the ingredients on the box) to each 16 oz (2 cups) of water when you are heating the water. Let cool, then pour into a clean glass jar and cover. Store the sterile saline in the refrigerator.

Tracheostomy ties:

Use ½-inch seam binding, which is available in the sewing department of many stores.

Equipment

Suction machine with tubing
Cardiorespiratory monitor (if ordered)
Suction catheters
Sterile saline (cool) (available in individual containers or clean syringe or dropper)
Clean plastic container for rinsing catheter

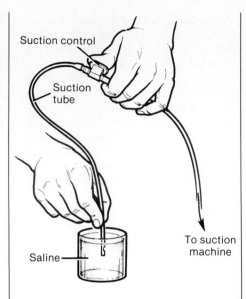

Suction control

Suction tube

Saline

To suction machine

Fig. 2

Instructions

1 Gather all the equipment you will need.
2 Wash your hands with soap and water. Count to 10 while washing, then rinse with clear water and dry.
3 Open the suction catheter package and connect the catheter to the suction machine.
4 Make sure the suction machine is plugged in and working. Check that the suction pressure is not above 100 mm Hg for infants or 120 mm Hg for older children.
5 If the mucus is thick, place normal saline in the trach. Use up to 0.5 cc for infants, 1-2 cc for toddlers, and 2-3 cc for older children.
6 Before suctioning, you must measure the right distance to insert the tube. Holding the extra trach in one hand, place the suction catheter next to the trach tube. Slowly push the catheter until it is ¼ inch longer than the trach tube. Hold this spot with your fingers. Now measure the distance from the tip of the catheter to the spot you are holding. Write it down ___. This is how far you should place the catheter each time you suction.

7 Place the tip of the catheter in the sterile saline and place your thumb over the opening to get suction. The sterile saline lubricates the catheter (Fig. 2).
8 With your thumb off the opening (no suction), insert the suction catheter to a distance ¼ inch longer than the tube (about 2 to 3 inches in an infant and small child) (Fig. 3).
9 Place your thumb on the suction port to obtain suction. Rotate or twist the catheter as you remove it with a slow steady motion (Fig. 4). Both inserting the catheter and suctioning should take no longer than 3 or 4 seconds. Remember, the child cannot breathe during suctioning. As a reminder, count 1-one thousand, 2-one thousand, and so on.
10 Look at the secretions. Check the color, smell, and thickness for any change.

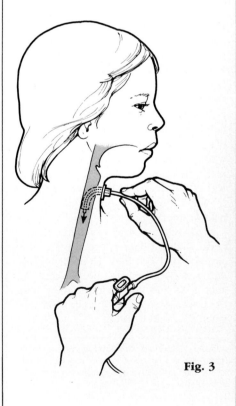

Fig. 3

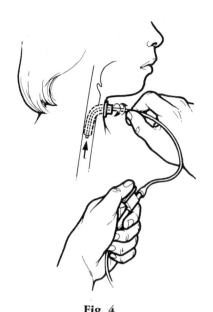

Fig. 4

11 Rinse the suction catheter in the sterile saline with your thumb on the suction port.
12 Allow about 30 seconds before suctioning again.
13 Repeat steps 5 through 12 up to 3 times.
14 Hold and comfort the child.
15 PRAISE THE CHILD FOR HIS HELP.
16 After each use, discard the saline and clean the container. Clean the suction machine to have it ready for the next time.
17 Use the following instructions, or your health professional will discuss the care of the suction catheters.
18 Wash your hands with soap and water. Count to 10 while washing, then rinse with clear water and dry.

CHANGING THE TRACHEOSTOMY TUBE

The tracheostomy tube is changed routinely to allow for a thorough cleaning of the tube. The change should be done 2 to 3 hours after meals to avoid any chance of the child vomiting. When you change the tube, check the skin around the trach for any redness, swelling, cuts, or bruises.

Change the trach tube in a quiet place where you will not be disturbed. If the child is active, you will need someone to hold the child.

Equipment

Clean trach tube with trach ties attached (Fig. 5) and obturator, if needed
Suction machine with catheters
Sterile saline in clean container
Pipe cleaners
Hot soapy water

Instructions for changing the tube

1 Gather all the equipment you will need.
2 Wash your hands with soap and water. Count to 10 while washing, then rinse with clear water and dry.
3 Place the child in an infant seat or sitting upright.
4 If the child is unable to help, have your helper hold the child's arms while the tube is being changed.
5 Suction the trach until it is clear (see instructions for suctioning).
6 Untie or carefully cut the old trach ties. Use scissors with a rounded tip.
7 Remove the trach tube (Fig. 6).

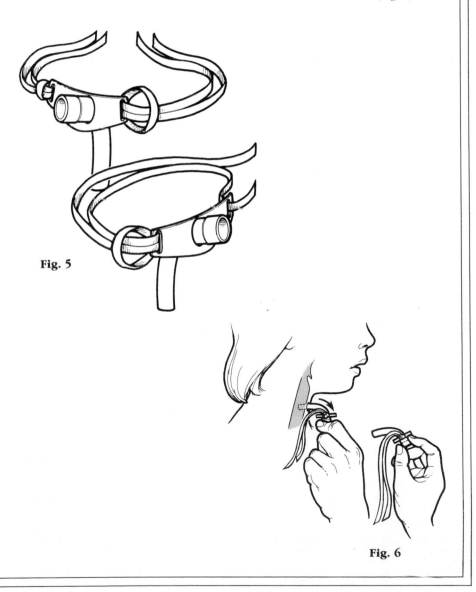

Fig. 5

Fig. 6

8 Quickly check the skin.

9 Quickly dip the clean trach tube in the sterile saline and shake to remove excess water.

10 Insert the clean tracheostomy tube (with or without an obturator) into the opening (stoma).

11 Secure the tracheostomy ties, either at the side or back of the neck. Change the position of the knot each time the tube or ties are changed.

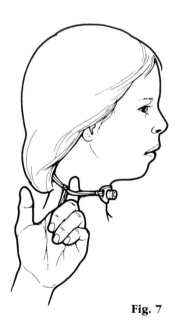

Fig. 7

Make sure that the ties are snug enough to allow you to put only one finger under them (Fig. 7).

12 Hold and comfort the child.

13 PRAISE THE CHILD FOR HIS HELP.

14 Wash your hands with soap and water. Count to 10 while washing, then rinse with clear water and dry.

The child may cough or gag during the insertion or removal of the tracheostomy tube. Gently tell the child when you are almost finished. If the child is old enough, teach him how to help you by handing you the supplies.

INSTRUCTIONS FOR CLEANING THE SUCTION CATHETERS

1 Rinse the suction catheters in cool tap water. Do not use hot water because it "cooks" the mucus and makes it more difficult to remove.

2 Place the catheters in a clean jar filled with hot, soapy water.

3 Rinse both the inside and outside of the tube under hot, running water. Hold the tube with kitchen tongs so that you don't burn yourself.

4 Shake off the excess water.

5 Place on a clean paper towel to dry. When the tube is completely dry, place it in a clean plastic bag.

6 Close the bag and store until the next time you suction the child.

7 If you notice any moisture in the bag, repeat the entire cleaning procedure.

INSTRUCTIONS FOR CLEANING THE TRACHEOSTOMY TUBE

1 Rinse the trach tube in cool tap water. Hot water "cooks" the mucus, which makes it harder to remove.

2 Place the trach tube in a clean jar filled with hot soapy water.

3 Scrub the tube with pipe cleaners while it is in the jar.

4 While holding it by the area where the ties are attached, rinse both the inside and outside of the tube under hot running water. You can hold it with kitchen tongs so that you do not burn yourself.

5 Rinse the inside and outside of the tube with sterile saline.

6 Shake off the excess water.

7 Place inside a clean paper towel to dry. Keep the trach tube in a safe place so that it can dry undisturbed.

8 When the tube is completely dry, place it in a clean plastic bag.

9 Close the bag and store until the next tube change.

10 If you notice any moisture in the bag, repeat the entire cleaning procedure.

NOTES

HOME APNEA MONITORING

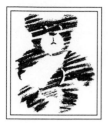

Prolonged apnea is defined as a lack of breathing for 20 seconds or more or a shorter time period if the child develops a bluish or pale color or the heart rate drops or both. Many infants will not breathe for approximately 15 seconds. This is considered normal when the child does not have any color change or a significant drop in heart rate and begins breathing without stimulation.

When the child has apnea, it is necessary for his breathing and heart rate to be monitored at home by using special equipment called an apnea monitor. You also need to keep a record sheet and write down a description of each apneic episode. This description includes the date, time, and the child's condition. This record will help your health professional to evaluate the need for continued home monitoring.

Equipment

Apnea monitor (respiratory and heart rate)

Electrodes/belt

Clock or watch with second hand in the room where the baby sleeps

Apnea recording sheet and pencil or pen near monitor

Emergency numbers attached to all telephones in the house

The monitor that will be used at home should be the same one that is used in the hospital. This allows you to become familiar with that monitor before you take the child home. Follow the manufacturer's instructions for application of the electrodes or belt to the child and the "set-up" of the monitor. The monitor requires electricity to operate. Most monitors are equipped with battery packs that allow you to take short trips with the child. Carefully read the manufacturer's instructions for the care of the batteries. All adults in the home should be familiar with the monitor and the following information.

The monitor can be used anywhere in the home and is easily moved. Place the monitor on a sturdy flat surface in the room, out of the reach of any other children. The monitor will sound an alarm if breathing stops for more than 20 seconds. When an alarm sounds, you must determine if infant has stopped breathing, if child is able to self-correct and begin breathing without stimulation, and if machine is working properly.

Care of skin electrodes

If skin electrodes are used, they should be changed every 2 to 3 days or when they become loose. To change the electrodes, carefully peel them off the child's chest. Wash the skin with soap and water to remove all of the adhesive and dry it thoroughly. Attach the monitor leads to the new electrodes before you apply them to the skin. Peel the backing of one of the electrodes and apply it to the skin. Attach the other electrode in the same manner. Notify your health professional if there are signs of redness at the site of the electrodes.

Procedure for alarms sounding

1 Calmly check the time.
2 Do not touch the child. Observe the child for 10 seconds. If the child is not awake:
   a. Look at the child's color to see if it is the usual color.
   b. Place your ear by the child's nose and mouth and listen for air moving.
   c. Look to see if the child's chest is moving.
3 If the child's color is good and the child is breathing without difficulty, wait 10 seconds, check the monitor to make sure the connections are intact, and reset the alarms. Write down the event on the record sheet.
4 If there is a change in the skin color or the child has not resumed breathing, rub the child's back or chest. Wait 10 seconds and look to see if the infant begins breathing. If he does, observe him for another 10 seconds. If the color and breathing have returned to normal, check the monitor to make

sure the connections are intact and reset the alarms. Write down the event on the record sheet.
5 If the child has not resumed breathing, slap the bottom of his feet. Wait 10 seconds and look to see if he begins breathing. If he does, observe for another 10 seconds. If the color and breathing have returned to normal, check the monitor to make sure the connections are tight and reset the alarms. Write down the event on the record sheet.
6 If the child has not responded to measures such as slapping the feet, begin CPR.

HOME CARE INSTRUCTIONS

INFANT CARDIOPULMONARY RESUSCITATION (CPR)

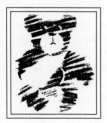

Cardiopulmonary resuscitation (CPR) is a way to do the work of the heart and lungs. The heart pumps the blood around the body to provide oxygen and nutrients to the different body systems. The lungs are a transfer spot. As the blood flows through the lungs, oxygen is picked up by the blood and carbon dioxide is released. When the infant breathes, oxygen is brought into the body and carbon dioxide is breathed out.

Before beginning CPR you must assess the infant to determine if both breathing and the heart have stopped. CPR is done when the infant's heart and breathing have stopped. You can breathe for the infant by blowing air into the lungs. Between breaths, the chest falls and air flows out of the lungs. The heart can be squeezed between the breastbone and the backbone to force blood out of the heart and into the arteries that carry it to the rest of the body. When you remove the pressure, the heart fills with blood so that the next squeeze (compression) will force additional blood to the body.

All of the infant's caregivers must be able to perform CPR so that you can have relief and help if needed. Prepare for an emergency before it happens. In case someone else has to call for help, tape emergency telephone numbers to each phone in the house. Include 911 (if available in your area), the phone number that you are calling from, the address, directions to the house, what happened, who is involved, and the condition of the infant. When calling in an emergency be sure to give all of this information and be the last to hang up.

Equipment

Emergency telephone numbers
Bulb syringe

Figures (except 1 and 4) reproduced with permission. © Healthcare Providers Manual for Basic Life Support, 1988, American Heart Association, Dallas TX.

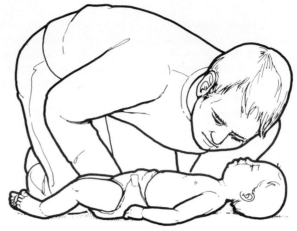

Fig. 1

ASSESSMENT

1 Look at the infant's color to see if it is normal (Fig. 1).
2 Look at the infant again to determine if he or she is breathing.
3 Look to see if the infant's chest is moving.
4 Place your ear by the infant's nose and mouth and listen for air moving.
5 Slap the bottom of the infant's feet if there is a change in skin color or if the infant is not breathing.
6 Begin CPR at once if the infant has not started breathing after his or her feet were slapped.
7 If there is someone else with you, have that person call the emergency telephone numbers for help. If you are alone, do not stop to call, but begin CPR immediately. Do CPR for 1 minute, then call the emergency numbers as quickly as possible.

AIRWAY

1 Place the infant on his back on a firm surface.
2 Properly position the head and open the airway by placing your hand on the forehead and place the fingers (not thumb) of your other hand under the bony part of the lower jaw near the middle of the chin. Then lift and slightly tilt the head backward to a sniffing or nose pointing to the ceil-

ing position. Proper positioning is essential to allow air to enter the windpipe to the lungs (Fig. 2).
3 If vomit is present, you must clear the infant's mouth before you breathe for the infant.

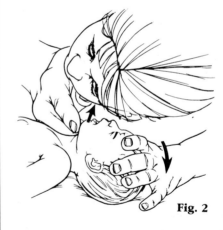

Fig. 2

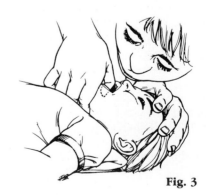

Fig. 3

4 Quickly remove any mucus or vomit with your fingers or a bulb syringe after turning the infant's head to the side. If using a bulb syringe, squeeze it before placing it in the mouth, then release the pressure in the bulb to remove the material.

   a. Open the infant's mouth by grasping the tongue and lower jaw between your thumb and fingers (Fig. 3).

   b. If you see an object, vomit, or mucus, insert the index or little finger of your other hand inside the mouth on the side farthest from you (Fig. 4).

   c. Move your finger across the back of the throat toward you. This sweeping action will help remove foreign objects.

5 Once the mouth is clear, reposition the head and observe the chest to determine if the infant has begun breathing. Place your ear close to the infant's mouth and look, listen, and feel for breathing for 3 to 5 seconds.

BREATHING

6 If breathing has not begun, you must breathe for the infant.

   a. Open your mouth wide. Cover both the nose and mouth with your mouth (Fig. 5). If the infant is large, cover his mouth with yours and press your cheek against his nose so air cannot escape from there.

   b. Give two slow breaths about 1 to 1½ seconds in length, pausing to inhale between them. Each breath should be just enough to make the chest rise.

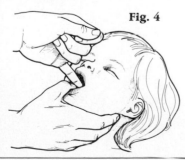

Fig. 4

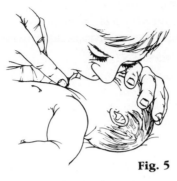

Fig. 5

7 If you do not see the chest rise, reposition the head and try again. After repositioning the head, if you still cannot see the chest rise, then follow the instructions for Caring for the choking infant (p. 583)

8 If the infant vomits, turn his head to the side and clean out the mouth with your finger or the bulb syringe.

CIRCULATION

9 After giving two breaths and seeing the chest rise, if the infant does not start breathing on his own, check his pulse.

10 Lightly place your index and middle fingers on the inside of the infant's elbow on the side closest to his body (Fig. 6). Feel for a pulse for 5 to 10 seconds. Practice this before an emergency arises to become used to finding the pulse.

11 When there is a pulse but no breathing, rescue breathing should be started and continued until the infant

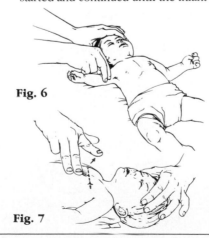

Fig. 6

Fig. 7

resumes breathing. For an infant, the rate should be 1 breath every 3 seconds, or 20 per minute. Rescue breathing may be all that is needed to restart the infant's breathing.

12 Begin cardiac compressions if there is no pulse.

13 Locate the correct position for chest compressions. Draw an imaginary line connecting the infant's nipples. While holding the head in the correct position (see step 2), place two fingers one finger width below the imaginary line on the breastbone (Fig. 7).

14 Using your index and middle finger, press straight down on the breast bone from ½ to 1 inch. Repeat this 5 times. After each 5 compressions, stop and give the infant one breath of air (Fig. 8).

15 Compress the chest at least 100 times per minute. To keep from going too fast, count 1 and 2 and 3 and 4 and 5 in your head.

16 After 10 cycles of 5 compressions for each breath, stop and check the pulse for 5 seconds. (Remember to always stop and start with a breath.) Call the emergency numbers if you are alone. If you need to move the infant to get help or to get out of danger, try not to stop CPR for more than 5 seconds.

17 CPR may be stopped only if:

   a. The infant begins breathing and the heart rate returns to normal.

   b. You are relieved by someone who can do CPR.

   c. You reach medical assistance and other action is begun.

If the infant begins breathing on his own, write down a description of what occurred and immediately notify your health professional.

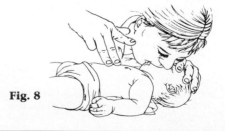

Fig. 8

CHILD CARDIOPULMONARY RESUSCITATION (CPR)*

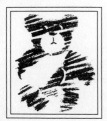

Cardiopulmonary resuscitation (CPR) is a way to do the work of the heart and lungs. The heart pumps the blood around the body to provide oxygen and nutrients to the different body systems. The lungs are a transfer spot. As the blood flows through the lungs, oxygen is picked up by the blood and carbon dioxide is released. When the child breathes, oxygen is brought into the body and carbon dioxide is breathed out.

Before beginning CPR you must assess the child to determine if both breathing and the heart have stopped. CPR is done when the child's heart and breathing have stopped. You can breathe for the child by blowing air into the lungs. Between breaths, the chest falls and air flows out of the lungs. The heart can be squeezed between the breastbone and the backbone to force blood out of the heart and into the arteries that carry it to the rest of the body. When you remove the pressure, the heart fills with blood so that the next squeeze (compression) will force additional blood to the body.

All of the child's caregivers must be able to perform CPR so that you can have relief and help if needed. Prepare for an emergency before it happens. In case someone else has to call for help, tape emergency telephone numbers to each phone in the house. Include 911 (if available in your area), the phone number that you are calling from, the address, directions to the house, what happened, who is involved, and the condition of the child. When calling in an emergency be sure to give all of this information and be the last to hang up.

Figures (except 2) reproduced with permission. © Healthcare Provider's Manual for Basic Life Support, 1988, American Heart Association, Dallas, TX.
Figure 2 reproduced with permission. Heartsaver Manual: A Student Handbook for Cardiopulmonary Resuscitationh and First Aid for Choking, 1987, American Heart Association.

*Instructions are for children between 1 and 8 years old. The sections in italics are for children older than 8 years.

Equipment

Emergency telephone numbers

ASSESSMENT

1 Look at the child's color to see if it is normal.
2 Look at the child again to determine if the child is breathing.
3 Look to see if the child's chest is moving.
4 Place your ear by the child's nose and mouth and listen for air moving.
5 Gently shake the child and call his name if there is a change in skin color or the child is not breathing.
6 Begin CPR at once if the child has not started breathing after gentle shaking.
7 If there is someone else with you, have him call the emergency telephone numbers for help. If you are alone, do not stop to call, but begin CPR immediately. Do CPR for 1 minute, then call the emergency numbers as quickly as possible.

AIRWAY

1 Place the child on his back on a firm surface.
2 Properly position the head and open the airway by placing your hand on the forehead and place the fingers (not thumb) of your other hand under bony part of the lower jaw near the middle of the chin. Then lift and slightly tilt the head backward to a sniffing or nose pointing to the ceiling position. Proper positioning is essential to allow air to enter the windpipe to the lungs (Fig. 1).

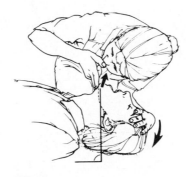

Fig. 1

3 If vomit is present, you must clear the child's mouth before you breathe for the child.
4 Quickly remove any mucus or vomit with your fingers after turning the child's head to the side.
   a. Open the child's mouth by grasping the tongue and lower jaw between your thumb and fingers (Fig. 2).
   b. If you see an object, vomit, or mucus, insert the index or little finger of your other hand inside the mouth on the side farthest from you (Fig. 3).
   c. Move your finger across the back of the throat toward you. This sweeping action will help remove foreign objects.

BREATHING

5 Once the mouth is clear, reposition the child's head and observe the chest to determine if breathing has begun. Place your ear close to the child's mouth and look, listen, and feel for breathing for 3 to 5 seconds.

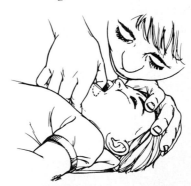

Fig. 2

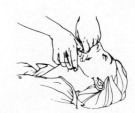

Fig. 3

CHILD CARDIOPULMONARY RESUSCITATION
(CPR)—cont'd

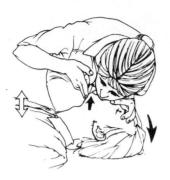

Fig. 4

6 If breathing has not begun, you must breathe for the child.

   a. Open your mouth and cover the child's mouth with your mouth (Fig. 4). If the child is small, cover his mouth with yours and press your cheek against his nose so air cannot escape from there. For a larger child, pinch the child's nose closed with the thumb and forefinger of the hand you have on the forehead.

   b. Give two slow breaths about 1 to 1½ seconds in length, pausing to inhale between them. Each breath should be just enough to make the chest rise.

7 If you do not see the chest rise, reposition the head and try again. After repositioning the head, if you still cannot see the chest rise, then follow the instructions for Caring for the choking child (p. 585).

8 If the child vomits, turn his head to the side and clean out the mouth with your finger.

CIRCULATION

9 After giving two breaths and seeing the chest rise, if the child does not start breathing on his own, check his pulse.

10 Lightly place your index and middle fingers on the child's windpipe. Slide your fingers into the groove between the windpipe and the neck muscles (Fig. 5). Feel for a pulse for 5 to 10 seconds. Practice this before an emergency arises to become used to finding the pulse.

11 When there is a pulse but no breathing, rescue breathing should be started and continued until the child resumes breathing. For a child 1 to 8 years old, the rate should be 1 breath every 4 seconds, or 15 per minute. *For children 8 years and older, the rate should be 1 breath every 5 seconds or 12 per minute.* Rescue breathing may be all that is needed to restart the child's breathing.

12 Begin cardiac compressions if there is no pulse.

13 Locate the correct position for chest compressions. Using the hand that is closer to the child's feet find the place on the child's lower chest where the ribs meet the breastbone. Locate this spot with your middle finger. Place your index finger on the breastbone next to your middle finger. Look at the spot where your index finger is placed. Now take away that hand and put the bottom of that hand on the breastbone next to the place where

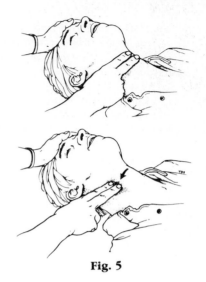

Fig. 5

you had your index finger. The fingers of the hand that is on the chest should be pointed away from you, across the child's chest (Fig. 6.) *For children 8 years and older place the hand closest to the child's head on the breastbone next to the index finger on the chest. Then place the hand that you used to mark the place on*

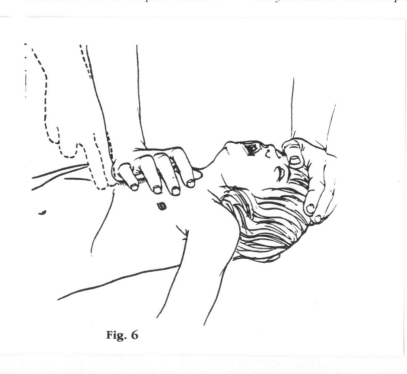

Fig. 6

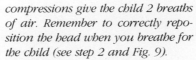

the child's chest on top of your other hand. Your fingers can be interlaced or straight; your arms must be straight and your shoulders above your hands (Figs. 7 & 8).

14 Using one hand, press straight down on the breastbone from 1 to 1½ inches. Repeat this 5 times. After each 5 compressions, stop and give the child one breath of air. Keep your other hand on the head to maintain the head in the right position.

For children 8 years and older, using both hands, press straight down on the breastbone from 1½ to 2 inches. Repeat this 15 times. After each 15

compressions give the child 2 breaths of air. Remember to correctly reposition the head when you breathe for the child (see step 2 and Fig. 9).

15 Compress the chest at least 80 to 100 times per minute. To keep from going too fast, count 1 and 2 and 3 and 4 and 5 in your head.

16 After 10 cycles of 5 compressions for each breath, stop and check the pulse for 5 seconds. (Remember always stop and start with a breath.)

For children 8 years and older, after 4 cycles of 15 compressions and 2 breaths, stop and check the pulse.

Call the emergency numbers as

quickly as possible if you are alone. If you need to move the child to get help or to get out of danger, try not to stop CPR for more than 5 seconds.

17 CPR may be stopped only if:
   a. The child begins breathing and the heart rate returns to normal.
   b. You are relieved by someone who can do CPR.
   c. You reach medical assistance and other action is begun.

If the child begins breathing on his own, write down a description of what occurred and immediately notify your health professional.

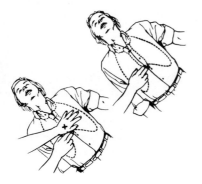

Fig. 7

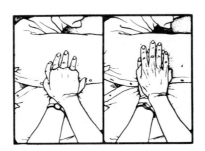

Fig. 8

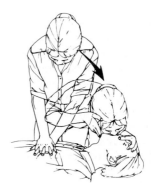

Fig. 9

NOTES

CARING FOR THE CHOKING INFANT

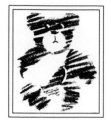

Choking is a very serious, life-threatening event. If the infant begins to choke or is having difficulty breathing, immediate action is needed. When the airway is blocked, the infant cannot cry or make sounds. If the infant is coughing, his color is pink, and he can make sounds, no action may be needed.

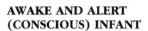

AWAKE AND ALERT (CONSCIOUS) INFANT

1 Look at the infant to see if he is having difficulty breathing.
2 If the infant is not breathing, take action immediately:
   a. Position the infant face down on your forearm. Hold the head and neck firmly with one hand. If the infant is large, it may be necessary to support his weight on your thigh.
   b. Give 4 quick blows between the shoulder blades with the heel of your hand (Fig. 1).
3 If this does not remove the object, give 4 chest thrusts.
   a. Draw an imaginary line connecting the child's nipples.
   b. Place your fingers on the breastbone, one finger width below the imaginary line (Fig. 2).
   c. Using your index and middle finger, thrust straight down on the breastbone from ½ to 1 inch (Fig. 3).
4 Repeat steps 2 and 3 until the airway is clear and the infant begins breathing or the infant becomes unconscious. If the infant becomes unconscious, call the emergency numbers at once.

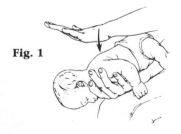

Fig. 1

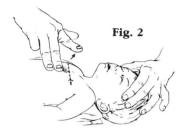

Fig. 2

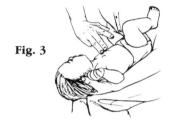

Fig. 3

Figures (except 5) reproduced with permission. © Heartsaver Manual: A Student Handbook for Cardiopulmonary Resuscitation and First Aid for Choking, 1987, American Heart Association, Dallas, TX.

INFANT BECOMES UNCONSCIOUS

1 If the infant becomes unconscious, place him on a firm flat surface.
2 Check the inside of the infant's mouth to see if there is a foreign object.
3 Open the infant's mouth using your thumb and fingers to grasp both the tongue and lower jaw and lift up gently (Fig. 4).
4 If you see an object, insert the index or little finger of your other hand inside the child's mouth on the side farthest from you and move your finger across the back of the infant's throat toward you. This sweeping action will help remove the foreign object. Be careful not to push it farther into the throat (Fig. 5.)
5 If the infant does not begin breathing, properly position the head and open the airway by placing your hand on the forehead and place the fingers (not thumb) of your other hand under the bony part of the lower jaw near the middle of the chin. Then lift and slightly tilt the head backward to a sniffing or nose pointing to ceiling position. Proper positioning is essential to allow the air to enter the windpipe to the lungs (Fig. 6).

6 If vomit is present, you must clear the infant's mouth before you give the breath.
7 Cover the infant's mouth and nose with your mouth. Give one breath and watch to see if the chest rises (Fig. 7). If the chest does not rise with the breath, place the infant on your fore-

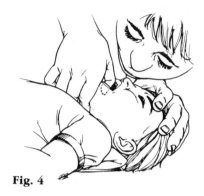

Fig. 4

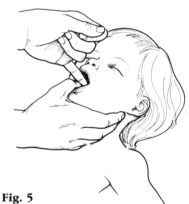

Fig. 5

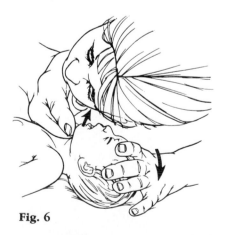

Fig. 6

From Wong D and Whaley L: Clinical manual of pediatric nursing, ed 3. Copyright © 1990 The CV Mosby Co, St Louis.

arm with his face down. Give him 4 quick blows between the shoulder blades with the heel of your hand (Fig. 1).

8 Quickly turn the infant onto his back and give four chest compressions.
   a. Draw an imaginary line connecting the child's nipples.
   b. Place your finger on the breastbone, one finger width below the imaginary line (Fig. 2).
   c. Using your index and middle finger, thrust straight down on the breastbone from ½ to 1 inch (Fig. 3).

9 Quickly place the infant on a firm flat surface and check the infant's mouth again. If an object is seen, attempt to remove it with a finger sweep. (See steps 3 and 4.)

10 Properly position the head (see step 5) and give a breath. Watch to see if the chest rises (Fig. 7).

11 Keep repeating steps 2 through 10 until the infant's airway is cleared and you can see his chest rise with your breath. Give a second breath.

12 When the obstruction is removed, check the brachial pulse for 5 to 10 seconds by placing your fingers on the inside of the upper arm (Fig. 8).

13 If the pulse is present but breathing is absent, breathe for the infant once every 3 seconds or 20 times each minute (Fig. 7).

14 If the pulse is absent, start cycles of compressions and breaths (Fig. 9). Continue your actions until the infant begins breathing and the pulse returns, or emergency help arrives.

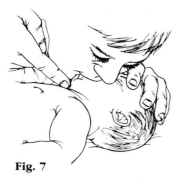

Fig. 7

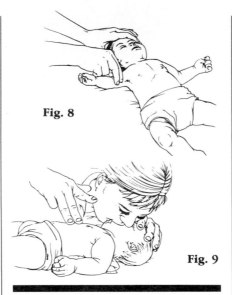

Fig. 8

Fig. 9

INFANT FOUND UNCONSCIOUS

1 Look at the infant to see if he is breathing.

2 Look to see if the chest is moving.

3 Place your ear by the infant's nose and mouth and listen for air moving.

4 Slap the bottom of the infant's feet if there is a change in skin color or if the infant is not breathing.

5 If there is someone else with you, have him or her call the emergency telephone numbers for help. If you are alone, do not stop to call, but begin treatment immediately.

6 Place the infant on his back on a firm surface.

7 Properly position the head and open the airway by placing your hand on the forehead and place the fingers (not thumb) of your other hand under bony part of the lower jaw near the middle of the chin. Then lift and slightly tilt the head backward to a sniffing or nose pointing to ceiling position. Proper positioning is essential to allow air to enter the windpipe to the lungs (Fig. 6).

8 Look, listen, and feel for breathing for 5 seconds.

9 If the infant does not begin breathing, give him a breath. Watch to see if the chest rises (Fig. 7).

10 If vomit is present, you must clear the infant's mouth before you open the airway.

11 If the chest does not rise, reposition the infant's head and try to breathe again.

12 If the chest still does not rise, place the infant on your forearm with his face down. Give him four quick blows between the shoulder blades with the heel of your hand (Fig. 1).

13 Quickly turn the infant onto his back and give four chest compressions.
   a. Draw an imaginary line connecting the child's nipples.
   b. Place your finger on the breastbone, one finger width below the imaginary line (Fig. 2).
   c. Using your index and middle finger, thrust straight down on the breastbone from ½ to 1 inch (Fig. 3).

14 Check the infant's mouth again. If an object is seen, attempt to remove it with a finger sweep.
   a. Open the infant's mouth by grasping the tongue and lower jaw between your thumb and fingers (Fig. 4).
   b. If you see an object, insert the index or little finger of your other hand inside the mouth on the side farthest from you and move your finger across the back of the infant's throat toward you. This sweeping motion will help remove the foreign object. Be careful not to push it farther into the throat (Fig. 5).

15 Properly position the head and give a breath. Watch to see if the chest rises (Fig. 7).

16 Keep repeating steps 8 through 15 until the infant's airway is cleared and you can see that his chest rises with your breath. Give a second breath.

17 Check the brachial pulse for 5 to 10 seconds by placing your fingers on the inside of the upper arm (Fig. 8).

18 If the pulse is present but breathing is absent, breathe for the infant once every 3 seconds or 20 times each minute (Fig. 7).

19 If the pulse is absent, start compressions (Fig. 9). Continue your actions until the infant begins breathing and the pulse returns, or emergency help arrives.

CARING FOR THE CHOKING CHILD

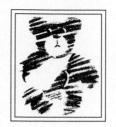

Choking is a very serious life-threatening event. If a child begins to choke or is having difficulty breathing, immediate action is needed. When the airway is blocked, the child cannot talk or make noises. If the child is coughing forcefully and can make sounds, no action is needed. If the child is not awake and alert, begin immediately with the directions for the unconscious child.

AWAKE AND ALERT (CONSCIOUS) CHILD— SITTING OR STANDING

1 Ask the child if he is choking. Check if he can talk or make noise. If the child cannot make any sounds, then begin emergency treatment.
2 Stand behind the child (Fig. 1).
3 Wrap your arms around the child's waist. Make one hand into a fist.
4 Put your fist, with the thumb side against the child's skin, on the abdomen just above the belly button. Make sure you are well below the breast bone.

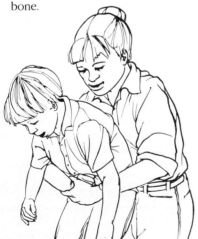

Fig. 1

Figures (except 1) reproduced with permission. Heartsaver Manual: A Student Handbook for Cardiopulmanary Resuscitation and First Aid for Choking, 1987, American Heart Association. Figure 1 reproduced with permission. Healthcare Provider's Manual for Basic Life Support, 1988, American Heart Association, Dallas, TX.

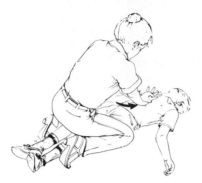

Fig. 2

5 Grab the fist with your other hand. Press into the child's abdomen with 6 to 10 upward thrusts.
6 Each thrust should be a separate movement. This allows enough force to help the child expel the object.
7 If the child still cannot breathe, continue the thrusting while calling for help.
8 Continue your actions until the object is removed, help arrives, or the child becomes unconscious. If the child becomes unconscious, call the emergency telephone numbers at once.

AWAKE AND ALERT (CONSCIOUS) CHILD— LYING DOWN

1 If the child is on the floor, ask if the child is okay. If he cannot breathe or talk, place the child flat on his back.
2 Kneel on the floor at the child's feet. On a larger child you can straddle his or her legs.
3 Put the heel of one hand on the child's abdomen just above the belly button. Make sure you are well below the breastbone.
4 Put your other hand on top of the first hand and press into the child's abdomen with a quick upward thrust (Fig. 2).
5 Repeat the thrusts 6 to 10 times if needed. Each thrust should be a separate movement. This allows enough force to help the child expel the object.
6 Repeat steps 3, 4, and 5 until the object is removed, help arrives, or the child becomes unconscious. If the child becomes unconscious, call the emergency numbers at once.

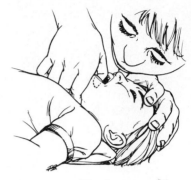

Fig. 3

CHILD BECOMES UNCONSCIOUS

1 If the child is not already on the floor, place the child on a firm, flat surface such as the floor.
2 Kneel on the floor next to the child.
3 Open the child's mouth. Use your thumb and fingers to grasp both the tongue and lower jaw and lift (Fig. 3).
4 If you can see an object, insert the index or little finger of your other hand inside the mouth on the side farthest from you. Move your finger across the back of the throat toward you and remove the object (Fig. 4).
5 If the child does not begin breathing, open the airway and try to breathe for the child.
  a. To open the airway, gently lift the chin with the fingers of one hand on the lower jaw near the middle of the chin, while pushing down on the forehead with your other hand. Tilt the child's head into a sniffing or nose pointing to ceiling position.
  b. Lift the chin so the teeth are almost together while listening for breathing (Fig. 5).

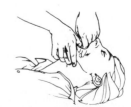

Fig. 4

HOME CARE INSTRUCTIONS

CARING FOR THE CHOKING CHILD—cont'd

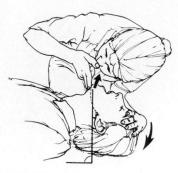

Fig. 5

c. If the child does not begin breathing at once, pinch the child's nostrils with your thumb and forefinger, while keeping the child's head in the right position.

d. Open your mouth wide, take a deep breath and make a tight seal over the child's mouth, and try to breathe for child (Fig. 6).

e. Watch to see if the child's chest rises with your breath.

f. If the child's chest still does not rise, get ready to do abdominal thrusts.

6 Kneel on the floor at the child's feet. On a larger child you can straddle the child's legs (Fig. 2).

7 Put the heel of one hand on the child's abdomen just above the belly button. Make sure you are well below the breastbone.

8 Put your other hand on top of the first hand and press into the child's abdomen with a quick upward thrust.

9 Repeat the thrusts 6 to 10 times if needed. Each thrust should be a separate movement. This allows enough

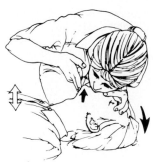

Fig. 6

force to help the child expel the object.

10 Repeat steps 3-9 until the object is removed and the child is breathing, or emergency help arrives. As soon as the obstruction is removed, give the child one breath. If the chest rises, give another breath, then check for a pulse.

If a pulse is present and the child is not breathing, give one rescue breath every 4 seconds until the child resumes breathing. If the pulse is absent, begin chest compressions as described in Child cardiopulmonary resuscitation (p. 580). Continue CPR until emergency help arrives or the child begins breathing and the pulse returns.

CHILD FOUND UNCONSCIOUS

1 Tap the child's shoulder and call by name. Ask the child if he is okay.

2 If the child is not already on the floor, place the child on a firm, flat surface such as the floor.

3 Call for help. If someone comes to help, tell them to call the emergency telephone number in your area.

4 Kneel on the floor next to the child.

5 If the child is not breathing, open the airway and try to breathe for the child.

a. To open the airway, gently lift the chin with one hand, while pushing down on the forehead with your other hand. Tilt the child's head into a sniffing or neutral position.

b. Lift the chin so the teeth are almost together while listening for breathing (Fig. 5).

c. If the child does not breathe after 5 seconds, pinch the child's nostrils with your thumb and forefinger, while keeping the child's head in the right position.

d. Open your mouth wide, take a deep breath and make a tight seal over the child's mouth, and attempt to breathe for the child (Fig. 6).

e. Watch to see if the child's chest rises with your breath.

f. If the child's chest does not rise, reposition the head and try to give a second breath. If the chest still does not rise, get ready to do abdominal thrusts.

g. If you are alone, call the emergency telephone numbers now.

6 Kneel on the floor at the child's feet. On a larger child you can straddle the child's legs (Fig. 2).

7 Put the heel of one hand on the child's abdomen just above the belly button. Make sure you are well below the breastbone.

8 Put your other hand on top of the first hand and press into the child's abdomen with a quick upward thrust (Fig. 2).

9 Repeat the thrusts 6 to 10 times if needed. Each thrust should be a separate movement. This allows enough force to help the child expel the object.

10 Open the child's mouth and check for a foreign object. Use your thumb and fingers to grasp both the tongue and lower jaw and lift (Fig. 3).

11 If you can see an object, put the index or little finger of your other hand inside the mouth on the side farthest from you. Move your finger across the back of the throat toward you and remove the object (Fig. 4).

12 Repeat steps 5-11 until the object is removed and the child is breathing, or emergency help arrives. As soon as the obstruction is removed, give the child one breath. If the chest rises give another breath, then check for a pulse.

If a pulse is present and the child is not breathing, give one rescue breath every 4 seconds until the child resumes breathing. If the pulse is absent, begin chest compressions as described in Child cardiopulmonary resuscitation (p. 580). Continue CPR until emergency help or the child begins breathing and the pulse returns.

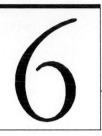

Reference Data

Unit 6

PREFIXES DENOTING DECIMAL FACTORS	
Prefix	**Symbol**
mega	M
kilo	k
hecto	h
deka	da
deci	d
centi	c
milli	m
micro	μ
nano	n
pico	p
femto	f

ABBREVIATIONS USED IN LABORATORY TESTS	
Prefix	**Symbol**
AU	arbitrary unit
CNS	central nervous system
conc.	concentration
d	day; diem
EDTA	ethylenediaminetetraacetate
F	female
g	gram
M	male
m	meter
hr	hour
Hb	hemoglobin
IU	International units of hormone activity
L	liter
mEq	milliequivalent
min	minute(s)
mm	millimeter
mm^3	cubic millimeter
mo	month
mol	mole
RBC	red blood cell(s)
RIA	radioimmunoassay
RID	radial immunodiffusion
RT	room temperature
s	second(s)
Therap.	therapeutic
U	International units of enzyme activity
V	volume
wk	week
yr	year
>	greater than
$\geq$	greater than or equal to
<	less than
$\leq$	less than or equal to
$\pm$	plus/minus
$\simeq$	approximately equal to

Common laboratory tests

Test/specimen	Age/sex/reference	Conventional units	International units
		Normal ranges	
Acetaminophen			
Serum, plasma	Therap. conc.	10-30 μg/ml	66-200 μmol/L
	Toxic conc.	>200 μg/ml	>1300 μmol/L
Ammonia nitrogen			
Plasma or serum	Newborn	90-150 μg/dL	64-107 μmol/L
	0-2 weeks	79-129 μg/dL	56-92 μmol/L
	>1 month	29-70 μg/dL	21-50 μmol/L
	Thereafter	15-45 μ/dL	11-32 μmol/L
Urine, 24 hr		500-1200 mg/d	36-86 mmol/d
Amylase	Newborn	5-65 U/L	5-65 U/L
Serum	>1 yr	25-125 U/L	25-125 U/L
Urine, timed specimen		1-17 U/hr	1-17 U/hr
Antistreptolysin O titer (ASO)		<166 Todd units	
Serum	School-age children	170-330 Todd units	
Base excess			
Whole blood	Newborn	(−10)-(−2) mmol/L	(−10)-(−2) mmol/L
	Infant	(−7)-(−1) mmol/L	(−7)-(−1) mmol/L
	Child	(−4)-(+2) mmol/L	(−4)-(+2) mmol/L
	Thereafter	(−3)-(+3) mmol/L	(−3)-(+3) mmol/L
Bicarbonate (HCO$_3$)			
Serum	Arterial	21-28 mmol/L	21-28 mmol/L
	Venous	22-29 mmol/L	22-29 mmol/L

Test/specimen	Age/sex/reference	Premature (mg/dL0)	Full-term (mg/dL)	Premature (μmolL)	Full-term (μmolL)
Bilirubin, total					
Serum	Cord	<2.0	<2.0	<34	<34
	0-1 day	8.0	<6.0	<137	<103
	1-2 days	12.0	<8.0	<205	<137
	2-5 days	16.0	<12.0	<274	<205
	Thereafter	2.0	0.2-1.0	<34	3.4-17.1

Test/specimen	Age/sex/reference	Conventional units	International units
Bilirubin, direct (conjugated)			
Serum		0.0-0.2 mg/dL	0-3.4 μmol/L
Bleeding time			
Blood from skin puncture			
Ivy	Normal:	2-7 min	2-7 min
	Borderline:	7-11 min	7-11 min
Simplate (G-D)		2.75-8 min	2.75-8 min
Blood volume			
Whole blood	Male	52-83 mL/kg	0.052-0.083 L/kg
	Female	50-75 mL/kg	0.050-0.075 L/kg
C-reactive protein (CRP)			
Serum	Cord	10-350 ng/mL	10-350 μg/L
	Adult	68-8200 ng/mL	68-8200 μg/L
Calcium, ionized			
Serum, plasma, or whole blood	Cord	5.0-6.0 mg/dL	1.25-1.50 mmol/L
	Newborn	4.3-5.1 mg/dL	1.07-1.27 mmol/L
	24-48 hr	4.0-4.7 mg/dL	1.00-1.17 mmol/L
	Thereafter	4.48-4.92 mg/dL or 2.24-2.46 mEq/L	1.12-1.23 mmol/L

Modified from Behrman RE and Vaughan VC, III, editors: Nelson Textbook of Pediatrics, ed 13, Philadelphia, 1987, WB Saunders Co.

Unit 6

Common laboratory tests—cont'd

Test/specimen	Age/sex/reference	Conventional units	International units
		Normal ranges	
Calcium, total			
Serum	Cord	9.0-11.5 mg/dL	2.25-2.88 mmol/L
	Newborn, 3-24 hr	9.0-10.6 mg/dL	2.3-2.68 mmol/L
	24-48 hr	7.0-12.0 mg/dL	1.75-3.0 mmol/L
	4-7 d	9.0-10.9 mg/dL	2.25-2.73 mmol/L
	Child	8.8-10.8 mg/dL	2.2-2.70 mmol/L
	Thereafter	8.4-10.2 mg/dL	2.1-2.55 mmol/L
Urine (24 hr)	Ca free diet:	5-40 mg/d	0.13-1.0 mmol/d
	Low to average Ca in diet:	50-150 mg/d	1.25-3.8 mmol/d
	Average Ca in diet:	100-300 mg/d	2.5-7.5 mmol/d
CSF		4.2-5.4 mg/dL or 2.1-2.7 mEq/L	1.05-1.35 mmol/L
Feces	Average	0.64 g/d	16 mmol/d
Carbon dioxide, partial pressure (Pco_2)			
Whole blood, arterial	Newborn	27-40 mm Hg	3.6-5.3 kPa
	Infant	27-41 mm Hg	3.6-5.3 kPa
	Thereafter: Male	35-48 mm Hg	4.7-6.4 kPa
	Female	32-45 mm Hg	4.3-6.0 kPa
Carbon dioxide, total (tCO_2)			
Serum or plasma	Cord	14-22 mmol/L	14-22 mmol/L
	Premature (1 week)	14-27 mmol/L	14-27 mmol/L
	Newborn	13-22 mmol/L	13-22 mmol/L
	Infant	20-28 mmol/L	20-28 mmol/L
	Child	20-28 mmol/L	20-28 mmol/L
	Thereafter	23-30 mmol/L	23-30 mmol/L
Cerebrospinal fluid pressure			
CSF		70-180 mm water	70-180 mm water
Cerebrospinal fluid volume			
CSF	Child	60-100 mL	0.006-0.10 L
	Adult	100-160 mL	0.1-0.16 L
Chloride			
Serum or plasma	Cord	96-104 mmol/L	96-104 mmol/L
	Newborn	97-110 mmol/L	97-110 mmol/L
	Thereafter	98-106 mmol/L	98-106 mmol/L
CSF		118-132 mmol/L	118-132 mmol/L
Urine, 24 hr	Infant	2-10 mmol/d (diet-dependent)	2-10 mmol/d
	Child	15-40 mmol/d	15-40 mmol/d
	Thereafter	110-250 mmol/d (varies with Cl intake)	110-250 mmol/d
Sweat	Normal (homozygote)	0-35 mmol/L	0-35 mmol/L
	Marginal (e.g., asthma, Addison disease, malnutrition)	30-60 mmol/L	30-60 mmol/L
	Cystic fibrosis	60-200 mmol/L	60-200 mmol/L
*Cholesterol, total			
Serum or plasma	Cord	45-100 mg/dL	1.17-2.59 mmol/L
	Newborn	53-135 mg/dL	1.37-3.50 mmol/L
	Infant	70-175 mg/dL	1.81-4.53 mmol/L
	Child	120-200 mg/dL	3.11-5.18 mmol/L
	Adolescent	120-210 mg/dL	3.11-5.44 mmol/L

*Normal cholesterol values for children are not universally defined. The mean cholesterol levels for children ages 1 to 19 are reported as 160.9 mg/dl to 166.4 mg/dl (as cited in Resnicow, Morley-Kotchen, and Wynder, 1989). Cutoff values for determining risk for future coronary heart disease in children are inconsistent. The American Academy of Pediatrics (1989) recommends a cutoff value of 176 mg/dl (75th percentile) for children 0 to 19 years of age.

Common laboratory tests— cont'd

Test/specimen	Age/sex/reference	Conventional units	International units
		Normal ranges	
Clotting time (Lee-White)			
Whole blood		5-8 minutes (glass tubes)	5-8 min
		5-15 minutes (room temp)	5-15 min
		30 minutes (silicone tube)	30 min
Copper			
Serum	Birth-6 mo	20-70 μg/dL	3.14-10.99 μmol/L
	6 yr	90-190 μg/dL	14.13-29.83 μmol/L
	12 yr	80-160 μg/dL	12.56-25.12 μmol/L
	Adult: Male	70-140 μg/dL	10.99-21.98 μmol/L
	Female	80-155 μg/dL	12.56-24.34 μmol/L
Creatine kinase (CK, CPK)			
Serum	Newborn	68-580 U/L	68-580 U/L
	Adult: Male	12-70 U/L	12-70 U/L
	Female	10-55 U/L	10-55 U/L
	Ambulatory: Male	25-90 U/L	25-90 U/L
	Female	10-70 U/L	10-70 U/L
		Higher after exercise	Higher after exercise
Creatinine			
Serum	Cord	0.6-1.2 mg/dL	53-106 μmol/L
	Newborn	0.3-1.0 mg/dL	27-88 μmol/L
	Infant	0.2-0.4 mg/dL	18-35 μmol/L
	Child	0.3-0.7 mg/dL	27-62 μmol/L
	Adolescent	0.5-1.0 mg/dL	44-88 μmol/L
	Adult: Male	0.6-1.2 mg/dL	53-106 μmol/L
	Female	0.5-1.1 mg/dL	44-97 μmol/L
Urine, 24 hr	Infant	8-20 mg/kg/d	71-180 μmol/kg/d
	Child	8-22 mg/kg/d	71-195 μmol/kg/d
	Adolescent	8-30 mg/kg/d	71-265 μmol/kg/d
	Adult	14-26 mg/kg/d	124-230 μmol/kg/d
Creatinine clearance (endogenous)			
Serum or plasma and urine	Newborn	40-65 ml/min/1.73 m²	
	<40 yr: Male	97-137 ml/min/1.73 m²	
	Female	88-128 ml/min/1.73 m²	
Digoxin			
Serum, plasma; collect at least 12 hr after dose	Therap. conc.		
	CHF	0.8-1.5 ng/ml	1.0-1.9 nmol/L
	Arrhythmias:	1.5-2.0 ng/ml	1.9-2.6 nmol/L
	Toxic conc.		
	Child	>2.5 ng/mL	>3.2 nmol/L
	Adult	>3.0 ng/mL	>3.8 nmol/L
Eosinophil count			
Whole blood, capillary blood		50-350 cells/mm³ (μL)	50-350 × 10⁶ cells/L
Erythrocyte (RBC) count			
Whole blood	cord	3.9-5.5 million/mm³	3.9-5.5 × 10¹² cells/L
	1-3 d	4.0-6.6 million/mm³	4.0-6.6 × 10¹² cells/L
	1 wk	3.9-6.3 million/mm³	3.9-6.3 × 10¹² cells/L
	2 wk	3.6-6.2 million/mm³	3.6-6.2 × 10¹² cells/L
	1 mo	3.0-5.4 million/mm³	3.0-5.4 × 10¹² cells/L
	2 mo	2.7-4.9 million/mm³	2.7-4.5 × 10¹² cells/L
	3-6 mo	3.1-4.5 million/mm³	3.1-4.5 × 10¹² cells/L
	0.5-2 yr	3.7-5.3 million/mm³	3.7-5.3 × 10¹² cells/L
	2-6 yr	3.9-5.3 million/mm³	3.9-5.3 × 10¹² cells/L
	6-12 yr	4.0-5.2 million/mm³	4.0-5.2 × 10¹² cells/L
	12-18 yr: Male	4.5-5.3 million/mm³	4.5-5.3 × 10¹² cells/L
	Female	4.1-5.1 million/mm³	4.1-5.1 × 10¹² cells/L

Unit 6

Common laboratory tests—cont'd

Test/specimen	Age/sex/reference	Conventional units	International units
		Normal ranges	
Erythrocyte sedimentation rate (ESR) Whole blood			
Westergren (modified)	Child	0-10 mm/hr	0-10 mm/hr
	<50 yr: Male	0-15 mm/hr	0-15 mm/hr
	Female	0-20 mm/hr	0-20 mm/hr
Wintrobe	Child	0-13 mm/hr	0-13 mm/hr
	Adult: Male	0-9 mm/hr	0-9 mm/hr
	Female	0-20 mm/hr	0-20 mm/hr
ZETA		41-54%	41-54 AU
Fat, fecal			
Feces (72 hr)	Infant, breast-fed	<1 g/d	<1 g/d
	0-6 yr	<2 g/d	<2 g/d
	Adult	<7 g/d	<7 g/d
Fatty acids, free			
Serum or plasma	Adults	8-25 mg/dL	0.30-0.90 mmol/L
	Children and obese adults	<31 mg/dL	<1.10 mmol/L
Fibrinogen			
Plasma	Newborn	125-300 mg/dL	1.25-3.00 g/L
	Thereafter	200-400 mg/dL	2.00-4.00 g/L
Galactose			
Serum	Newborn	0-20 mg/dL	0-1.11 mmol/L
	Thereafter	<5 mg/dL	<0.28 mmol/L
Urine	Newborn	≤60 mg/dL	≤3.33 mmol/L
	Thereafter	<14 mg/dL	<0.08 mmol/L
Glucose			
Serum	Cord	45-96 mg/dL	2.5-5.3 mmol/L
	Premature	20-60 mg/dL	1.1-3.3 mmol/L
	Neonate	30-60 mg/dL	1.7-3.3 mmol/L
	Newborn, 1 d	40-60 mg/dL	2.2-3.3 mmol/L
	Newborn, >1 d	50-90 mg/dL	2.8-5.0 mmol/L
	Child	60-100 mg/dL	3.3-5.5 mmol/L
	Thereafter	70-105 mg/dL	3.9-5.8 mmol/L
Whole blood	Adult	65-95 mg/dL	3.6-5.3 mmol/L
CSF	Adult	40-70 mg/dL	2.2-3.9 mmol/L
Urine (quantitative)		<0.5 g/d	<2.8 mmol/d
(Qualitative)		Negative	Negative
Glucose tolerance test (GTT), oral Serum			

Dosages		Normal	Diabetic	Normal	Diabetic
Adult: 75 g	Fasting	70-105 mg/dL	>115 mg/dL	3.9-5.8 mmol/L	>6.4 mmol/L
Child: 1.75 g/kg of ideal	60 min	120-170 mg/dL	≥200 mg/dL	6.7-9.4 mmol/L	≥11 mmol/L
weight up to maximum of	90 min	100-140 mg/dL	≥200 mg/dL	5.6-7.8 mmol/L	≥11 mmol/L
75 g	120 min	70-120 mg/dL	≥140 mg/dL	3.9-6.7 mmol/L	≥7.8 mmol/L

Growth hormone (hGH, Somatotropin)					
Plasma	Cord	10-50 ng/mL		10-50 µg/L	
Fasting, at rest	Newborn	10-40 ng/mL		10-40 µg/L	
	Child	<5 ng/mL		<5 µg/L	
	Adult: Male	<5 ng/mL		<5 µg/L	
	Female	<8 ng/mL		<8 µg/L	

Common laboratory tests—cont'd

Test/specimen	Age/sex/reference	Conventional units	International units
		Normal ranges	
Hematocrit (HCT, Hct)			
Whole blood	1 d (cap)	48-69%	0.48-0.69 vol. fraction
	2 d	48-75%	0.48-0.75 vol. fraction
	3 d	44-72%	0.44-0.72 vol. fraction
	2 mo	28-42%	0.28-0.42 vol. fraction
	6-12 yr	35-45%	0.35-0.45 vol. fraction
	12-18 yr: Male	37-49%	0.37-0.49 vol. fraction
	Female	36-46%	0.36-0.46 vol. fraction
Hemoglobin (Hb)			
Whole blood	1-3 d (cap)	14.5-22.5 g/dL	2.25-3.49 mmol/L
	2 mo	9.0-14.0 g/dL	1.40-2.17 mmol/L
	6-12 yr	11.5-15.5 g/dL	1.78-2.40 mmol/L
	12-18 yr: Male	13.0-16.0 g/dL	2.02-2.48 mmol/L
	Female	12.0-16.0 g/dL	1.86-2.48 mmol/L
Hemoglobin A			
Whole blood		>95% of total	0.95 fraction of Hb
Hemoglobin F			
Whole blood	1 d	63-92% HbF	0.62-0.92 mass fraction HbF
	5 d	65-88% HbF	0.65-0.88 mass fraction HbF
	3 wk	55-85% HbF	0.55-0.85 mass fraction HbF
	6-9 wk	31-75% HbF	0.31-0.75 mass fraction HbF
	3-4 mo	<2-59% HbF	<0.02-0.59 mass fraction HbF
	6 mo	<2-9% HbF	<0.02-0.09 mass fraction HbF
	Adult	<2.0% HbF	<0.02 mass fraction HbF
Immunoglobulin A (IgA)			
Serum	Cord	0-5 mg/dL	0-50 mg/L
	Newborn	0-2.2 mg/dL	0-22 mg/L
	½-6 mo	3-82 mg/dL	30-820 mg/L
	6 mo-2 yr	14-108 mg/dL	140-1080 mg/L
	2-6 yr	23-190 mg/dL	230-1900 mg/L
	6-12 yr	29-270 mg/dL	290-2700 mg/L
	12-16 yr	81-232 mg/dL	810-2320 mg/L
	Thereafter	60-380 mg/dL	600-3800 mg/L
Immunoglobulin D (IgD)			
Serum	Newborn	None detected	None detected
	Thereafter	0-8 mg/dL	0-0.44 μmol/L
Immunoglobulin E (IgE)			
Serum	Male	0-230 IU/mL	0-230 k/U/L
	Female	0-170 IU/mL	0-170 k/U/L
Immunoglobulin G (IgG)			
Serum	Cord	760-1700 mg/dL	7.6-17 g/L
	Newborn	700-1480 mg/dL	7-14.8 g/L
	½-6 mo	300-1000 mg/dL	3-10 g/L
	6 mo-2 yr	500-1200 mg/dL	5-12 g/L
	2-6 yr	500-1300 mg/dL	5-13 g/L
	6-12 yr	700-1650 mg/dL	7-16.5 g/L
	12-16 yr	700-1550 mg/dL	7-15.5 g/L
	Adults	600-1600 mg/dL (higher in blacks)	6-16 g/L
Immunoglobulin M (IgM)			
Serum	Cord	4-24 mg/dL	40-240 mg/L
	Newborn	5-30 mg/dL	50-300 mg/L
	½-6 mo	15-109 mg/dL	150-1090 mg/L
	6 mo-2 yr	43-239 mg/dL	430-2390 mg/L
	2-6 yr	50-199 mg/dL	500-1990 mg/L
	6-12 yr	50-260 mg/dL	500-2600 mg/L
	12-16 yr	45-240 mg/dL	450-2400 mg/L
	Thereafter	40-345 mg/dL	400-3450 mg/L

Common laboratory tests—cont'd

Test/specimen	Age/sex/reference	Conventional units		International units	
		Normal ranges			
Iron					
Serum	Newborn	100-250 μg/dL		17.90-44.75 μmol/L	
	Infant	40-100 μg/dL		7.16-17.90 μmol/L	
	Child	50-120 μg/dL		8.95-21.48 μmol/L	
	Thereafter, Male	50-160 μg/dL		8.95-28.64 μmol/L	
	Female	40-150 μg/dL		7.16-26.85 μmol/L	
	Intoxicated child	280-2550 μg/dL		50.12-456.5 μmol/L	
	Fatally poisoned child	>1800 μg/dL		>322.2 μmol/L	
Iron-binding capacity, total (TIBC)					
Serum	Infant	100-400 μg/dL		17.90-71.60 μmol/L	
	Thereafter	250-400 μg/dL		44.75-71.60 μmol/L	
Lead					
Whole blood	Child	<25 μg/dL		<1.21 μmol/L	
	Adult	<40 μg/dL		<1.93 μmol/L	
	Acceptable for industrial exposure	<60 μg/dL		<2.90 μmol/L	
	Toxic	≥100 μg/dL		≤4.83 μmol/L	
Urine, 24 hr		<80 μg/L		<0.39 μmol/L	
Leukocyte count (WBC count)		×1000 cells/mm³ (μL)		×10⁹ cells/L	
Whole blood	Birth	9.0-30.0		9.0-30.0	
	24 hr	9.4-34.0		9.4-34.0	
	1 mo	5.0-19.5		5.0-19.5	
	1-3 yr	6.0-17.5		6.0-17.5	
	4-7 yr	5.5-15.5		5.5-15.5	
	8-13 yr	4.5-13.5		4.5-13.5	
	Adult	4.5-11.0		4.5-11.0	
		×1000 cells/mm³ (μL)		×10⁶ cells/L	
CSF	Premature	0-25 mononuclear		0-25	
		0-100 polymorphonuclear		0-100	
		0-1000 RBC		0-1000	
	Newborn	0-20 mononuclear		0-20	
		0-70 polymorphonuclear		0-70	
		0-800 RBC		0-800	
	Neonate	0-5 mononuclear		0-5	
		0-25 polymorphonuclear		0-25	
		0-50 RBC		0-50	
	Thereafter	0-5 mononuclear		0-5	
Leukocyte differential count					
Whole blood	Myelocytes	0%	0 Cells/mm³ (μL)	number fraction 0	
	Neutrophils—"bands"	3-5%	150-400 Cells/ mm³ (μL)	number fraction 0.03-0.05	
	Neutrophils—"segs"	54-62%	3000-5800 Cells/ mm³ (μL)	number fraction 0.54-0.62	
	Lymphocytes	25-33%	1500-3000 Cells/ mm³ (μL)	number fraction 0.25-0.33	
	Monocytes	3-7%	285-500 Cells/ mm³ (μL)	number fraction 0.03-0.07	
	Eosinophils	1-3%	50-250 Cells/ mm³ (μL)	number fraction 0.01-0.03	
	Basophils	0-0.75%	15-50 Cells/mm³ (μL)	number fraction 0-0.0075	

Common laboratory tests—cont'd

Test/specimen	Age/sex/reference	Conventional units	International units
		Normal ranges	
Mean corpuscular hemoglobin (MCH)			
Whole blood	Birth	31-37 pg/cell	0.48-0.57 fmol/L
	1-3 d (cap)	31-37 pg/cell	0.48-0.57 fmol/L
	1 wk-1 mo	28-40 pg/cell	0.43-0.62 fmol/L
	2 mo	26-34 pg/cell	0.40-0.53 fmol/L
	3-6 mo	25-35 pg/cell	0.39-0.54 fmol/L
	0.5-2 yr	23-31 pg/cell	0.36-0.48 fmol/L
	2-6 yr	24-30 pg/cell	0.37-0.47 fmol/L
	6-12 yr	25-33 pg/cell	0.39-0.51 fmol/L
	12-18 yr	25-35 pg/cell	0.39-0.54 fmol/L
	18-49 yr	26-34 pg/cell	0.40-0.53 fmol/L
Mean corpuscular hemoglobin concentration (MCHC)			
Whole blood	Birth	30-36% Hb/cell or g Hb/dL RBC	4.65-5.58 mmol or Hb/L RBC
	1-3 d (cap)	29-37% Hb/cell or g Hb/dL RBC	4.50-5.74 mmol or Hb/L RBC
	1-2 wk	28-38% Hb/cell or g Hb/dL RBC	4.34-5.89 mmol or Hb/L RBC
	1-2 mo	29-37% Hb/cell or g Hb/dL RBC	4.50-5.74 mmol or Hb/L RBC
	3 mo-2 yr	30-36% Hb/cell or g Hb/dL RBC	4.65-5.58 mmol or Hb/L RBC
	2-18 yr	31-37% Hb/cell or g Hb/dL RBC	4.81-5.74 mmol or Hb/L RBC
	>18 yr	31-37% Hb/cell or g Hb/dL RBC	4.81-5.74 mmol or Hb/L RBC
Mean corpuscular volume (MCV)			
Whole blood	1-3 d (cap)	95-121 μm^3	95-121 fL
	0.5-2 yr	70-86 μm^3	70-86 fL
	6-12 yr	77-95 μm^3	77-95 fL
	12-18 yr: Male	78-98 μm^3	78-98 fL
	Female	78-102 μm^3	78-102 fL
Osmolality			
Serum	Child, adult:	275-295 mOsmol/kg H_2O	
Urine, random		50-1400 mOsmol/kg H_2O, depending on fluid intake. After 12 hr fluid restriction: ≥850 mOsmol/kg H_2O	
Urine, 24 hr		≃300-900 mOsmol/kg H_2O	
Oxygen, partial pressure (pO_2)			
Whole blood, arterial	Birth	8-24 mm Hg	1.1-3.2 kPa
	5-10 min	33-75 mm Hg	4.4-10.0 kPa
	30 min	31-85 mm Hg	4.1-11.3 kPa
	>1 hr	55-80 mm Hg	7.3-10.6 kPa
	1 d	54-95 mm Hg	7.2-12.6 kPa
	Thereafter (decreased with age)	83-108 mm Hg	11-14.4 kPa
Oxygen saturation			
Whole blood, arterial	Newborn	40-90%	Fraction saturated 0.40-0.90
	Thereafter	95-99%	Fraction saturated 0.95-0.99
Partial thromboplastin time (PTT)			
Whole blood (Na citrate)			
Nonactivated		60-85 s (Platelin)	60-85 s
Activated		25-35 s (differs with method)	25-35 s

Unit 6

Common laboratory tests—cont'd

Test/specimen	Age/sex/reference	Conventional units	International units
		Normal ranges	
pH			H$^+$ concentration:
Whole blood, arterial	Premature (48 hr)	7.35-7.50	31-40 nmol/L
	Birth, full term	7.11-7.36	43-77 nmol/L
	5-10 min	7.09-7.30	50-81 nmol/L
	30 min	7.21-7.38	41-61 nmol/L
	>1 hr	7.26-7.49	32-54 nmol/L
	1 d	7.29-7.45	35-51 nmol/L
	Thereafter	7.35-7.45	35-44 nmol/L
	Must be corrected for body temperature		
Urine, random	Newborn/neonate	5-7	0.1-10 μmol/L
	Thereafter (average ≃6)	4.5-8	0.01-32 μmol/L (average ≃1.0 μmol/L)
Stool		7.0-7.5	31-100 nmol/L
Phenylalanine			
Serum	Premature	2.0-7.5 mg/dL	0.12-0.45 mmol/L
	Newborn	1.2-3.4 mg/dL	0.07-0.21 mmol/L
	Thereafter	0.8-1.8 mg/dL	0.05-0.11 mmol/L
Urine, 24 hr	10 d-2 wk	1-2 mg/d	6-12 μmol/d
	3-12 yr	4-18 mg/d	24-110 μmol/d
	Thereafter	trace-17 mg/d	trace-103 μmol/d
Plasma volume			
Plasma	Male	25-43 mL/kg	0.025-0.043 L/kg
	Female	28-45 mL/kg	0.028-0.045 L/kg
Platelet count (thrombocyte count)			
Whole blood (EDTA)	Newborn (After 1 wk, same as adult)	84-478 × 10^3/mm^3 (μL)	84-478 × 10^9/L
	Adult	150-400 × 10^3/mm^3 (μL)	150-400 × 10^9/L
Potassium			
Serum	Newborn	3.9-5.9 mmol/L	3.9-5.9 mmol/L
	Infant	4.1-5.3 mmol/L	4.1-5.3 mmol/L
	Child	3.4-4.7 mmol/L	3.4-4.7 mmol/L
	Thereafter	3.5-5.1 mmol/L	3.5-5.1 mmol/L
Plasma (heparin)		3.4-4.5 mmol/L	
Urine, 24 hr		2.5-125 mmol/d varies with diet	
Protein			
Serum Total			
	Premature	4.3-7.6 g/dL	43.0-76.0 g/L
	Newborn	4.6-7.4 g/dL	46.0-74.0 g/L
	Child	6.2-8.0 g/dL	62.0-80.0 g/L
Electrophoresis			
Albumin	Premature	3.0-4.2 g/dL	30-42 g/L
	Newborn	3.6-5.4 g/dL	36-54 g/L
	Infant	4.0-5.0 g/dL	40-50 g/L
	Thereafter	3.5-5.0 g/dL	35-50 g/L
α$_1$-Globulin	Premature	0.1-0.5 g/dL	1-5 g/L
	Newborn	0.1-0.3 g/dL	1-3 g/L
	Infant	0.2-0.4 g/dL	2-4 g/L
	Thereafter	0.2-0.3 g/dL	2-3 g/L
α$_2$-Globulin	Premature	0.3-0.7 g/dL	3-7 g/L
	Newborn	0.3-0.5 g/dL	3-5 g/L
	Infant	0.5-0.8 g/dL	5-8 g/L
	Thereafter	0.4-1.0 g/dL	4-10 g/L

Common laboratory tests—cont'd

Test/specimen	Age/sex/reference	Conventional units	International units
		Normal ranges	
β-Globulin	Premature	0.3-1.2 g/dL	3-12 g/L
	Newborn	0.2-0.6 g/dL	2-6 g/L
	Infant	0.5-0.8 g/dL	5-8 g/L
	Thereafter	0.5-1.1 g/dL	5-11 g/L
γ-Globulin	Premature	0.3-1.4 g/dL	3-14 g/L
	Newborn	0.2-1.0 g/dL	2-10 g/L
	Infant	0.3-1.2 g/dL	3-12 g/L
	Thereafter	0.7-1.2 g/dL	7-12 g/L
		Higher in blacks	Higher in blacks
Total			
Urine, 24 hr		1-14 mg/dL	10-140 mg/L
		50-80 mg/d (at rest)	50-80 mg/L
		<250 mg/d after intense exercise	<250 mg/L after exercise
Total			
CSF		Lumbar: 8-32 mg/dL	80-320 mg/L
Prothrombin time (PT)			
One-stage (Quick)			
Whole blood (Na citrate)	In general	11-15 s (varies with type of thromboplastin)	11-15 s
	Newborn	Prolonged by 2-3 sec	Prolonged by 2-3 sec
Two-stage modified (Ware and Seegers)			
Whole blood (Na citrate)		18-22 sec	18-22 sec
RBC count, see erythrocyte count			
Red cell volume			
Whole blood	Male	20-36 mL/kg	0.020-0.036 L/kg
	Female	19-31 mL/kg	0.019-0.031 L/kg
Reticulocyte count			
Whole blood	Adults	0.5-1.5% of erythrocytes or 25,000-75,000/mm³ (μL)	0.005-0.015 (number fraction) 25,000-75,000 × 10⁶/L
Capillary	1 d	0.4-6.0%	0.004-0.060 (number fraction)
	7 d	<0.1-1.3%	<0.001-0.013 (number fraction)
	1-4 wk	<0.1-1.2%	<0.001-0.012 (number fraction)
	5-6 wk	<0.1-2.4	<0.001-0.024 (number fraction)
	7-8 wk	0.1-2.9%	0.001-0.029 (number fraction)
	9-10 wk	<0.1-2.6%	<0.001-0.026 (number fraction)
	11-12 wk	0.1-1.3%	0.001-0.013 (number fraction)
Salicylates			
Serum, plasma	Therap. conc.:	15-30 mg/dL	1.1-2.2 mmol/L
	Toxic conc.:	>30 mg/dL	>2.2 mmol/L
Sedimentation rate, see erythrocyte sedimentation rate			
Sodium			
Serum or plasma	Newborn	136-146 mmol/L	134-146 mmol/L
	Infant	139-146 mmol/L	139-146 mmol/L
	Child	138-145 mmol/L	138-145 mmol/L
	Thereafter	136-146 mmol/L	136-146 mmol/L
Urine, 24 hr		40-220 mmol/L (diet dependent)	40-220 mmol/L
Sweat	Cystic fibrosis	10-40 mmol/L >70 mmol/L	10-40 mmol/L >70 mmol/L

Unit 6

Common laboratory tests—cont'd

Test/specimen	Age/sex/reference	Conventional units	International units
		Normal ranges	
Specific gravity			
Urine, random	Adult	1.002-1.030	1.002-1.030
		>1.025	>1.025
Urine, 24 h	After 12 hr fluid restriction	1.015-1.025	
Theophylline			
Serum, plasma	Therap. conc.		
	Bronchodilator	8-20 µg/mL	44-110 µmol/L
	Prem. apnea	6-13 µg/mL	33-72 µmol/L
	Toxic conc.	>20	>110 µmol/L
Thrombin time			
Whole blood (Na citrate)		Control time ± 2 sec when control is 9-13 sec	Control time ± 2 sec when control is 9-13 sec
Thyroxine, total (T_4)			
Serum	Cord	8-13 µg/dL	103-168 nmol/L
	Newborn	11.5-24 (lower in low birth weight infants)	148-310 nmol/L
	Neonate	9-18 µg/dL	116-232 nmol/L
	Infant	7-15 µg/dL	90-194 nmol/L
	1-5 yr	7.3-15 µg/dL	94-194 nmol/L
	5-10 yr	6.4-13.3 µg/dL	83-172 nmol/L
	Thereafter	5-12 µg/dL	65-155 nmol/L
	Newborn screen (filter paper)	6.2-22 µg/dL	80-284 nmol/L
Tourniquet test (capillary fragility)		<5-10 petechiae in 2.5 cm circle on forearm (halfway between systolic and diastolic pressure for 5 min); 0-8 petechiae in 6 cm circle (50 torr for 15 min); 10-20 petechiae in 5 cm circle (80 mm Hg)	<5-10 petechiae in 2.5 cm circle on forearm (halfway between systolic and diastolic pressure for 5 min); 0-8 petechiae in 6 cm circle (50 torr for 15 min); 10-20 petechiae in 5 cm circle (80 mm Hg)

Test/specimen	Age/sex/reference	mg/dL		g/L	
		M	F	M	F
Triglycerides (TG)					
Serum, after ≥12 hr fast					
	Cord blood	10-98	10-98	0.10-0.98	0.10-0.98
	0-5 yr	30-86	32-99	0.30-0.86	0.32-0.99
	6-11 yr	31-108	35-114	0.31-1.08	0.35-1.14
	12-15 yr	36-138	41-138	0.36-1.38	0.41-1.38
	16-19 yr	40-163	40-128	0.40-1.63	0.40-1.28

Test/specimen	Age/sex/reference	Conventional units	International units
Triiodothyronine, free			
Serum	Cord	20-240 pg/dL	0.3-3.7 pmol/L
	1-3 d	200-610 pg/dL	3.1-9.4 pmol/L
	6 wk	240-560 pg/dL	3.7-8.6 pmol/L
	Adults (20-50 yr)	230-660 pg/dL	3.5-10.0 pmol/L
Triiodothyronine, total (T_3-RIA)			
Serum	Cord	30-70 ng/dL	0.46-1.08 nmol/L
	Newborn	72-260 ng/dL	1.16-4.00 nmol/L
	1-5 yr	100-260 ng/dL	1.54-4.00 nmol/L
	5-10 yr	90-240 ng/dL	1.39-3.70 nmol/L
	10-15 yr	80-210 ng/dL	1.23-3.23 nmol/L
	Thereafter	115-190 ng/dL	1.77-2.93 nmol/L

Unit 6

Common laboratory tests—cont'd

Test/specimen	Age/sex/reference	Conventional units	International units
		Normal ranges	
Urea nitrogen			
Serum or plasma	Cord	21-40 mg/dL	7.5-14.3 mmol urea/L
	Premature (1 wk)	3-25 mg/dL	1.1-9 mmol urea/L
	Newborn	3-12 mg/dL	1.1-4.3 mmol urea/L
	Infant/Child	5-18 mg/dL	1.8-6.4 mmol urea/L
	Thereafter	7-18 mg/dL	2.5-6.4 mmol urea/L
Uric acid (serum)	Newborn	2.0-6.2 mg/dL	119-369 µmol/L
Phosphotungstate	Adult: Male	4.5-8.2 mg/dL	268-488 µmol/L
	Female	3.0-6.5 mg/dL	178-387 µmol/L
Uricase	Child	2.0-5.5 mg/dL	119-327 µmol/L
	Adult: Male	3.5-7.2 mg/dL	208-428 µmol/L
	Female	2.6-6.0 mg/dL	155-357 µmol/L
Urine volume			
Urine, 24 hr	Newborn	50-300 mL/d	0.050-0.300 L/d
	Infant	350-550 mL/d	0.350-0.500 L/d
	Child	500-1000 mL/d	0.500-1.000 L/d
	Adolescent	700-1400 mL/d	0.700-1.400 L/d
	Thereafter: Male	800-1800 mL/d	0.800-1.800 L/d
	Female	600-1600 mL/d (varies with intake and other factors)	0.600-1.600 L/d

WBC, see Leukocyte

REFERENCES

1. Committe on nutrition: Indications for cholesterol testing in children, Pediatrics 83(1):141-142, 1989.
2. Resnicow K, Morley-Kotchen J, and Wynder E: Plasma cholesterol levels of 6585 children in the United States: Results of the know your body screening in five states, Pediatrics 84(6):969-976, 1989.

Unit 6

Resources for families and health care professionals
*General resources: Child health and special services**

American Academy of Pediatrics
Publications Department
P.O. Box 927
141 Northwest Point Blvd.
Elk Grove Village, IL 60007
(708)228-5005
(800)433-9016
(800)421-0589

American Dietetic Association
216 W. Jackson Blvd., Ste. 800
Chicago, IL 60606
(312) 899-0040

American Hospital Association
840 N. Lake Shore Drive
Chicago, IL 60611
(312) 280-6000

Association of Birth Defects in Children
3526 Emerywood Lane
Orlando, FL 32812
(407) 859-2821

Association for the Care of Children's Health
3615 Wisconsin Ave. N.W.
Washington, DC 20016
(202) 244-1801

Association for Neuro-Metabolic Disorders
5223 Brookfield Lane
Sylvania, OH 43560
(419) 885-1497

Boys Town
Communications and Public Service Division
Father Flanagan's Boys' Home
Boys Town, NE 68010
(402) 498-1111
(800) 448-3000 (hotline)

Canadian Institute of Child Health
17 York St., Ste. 105
Ottawa, Ontario K1N 557
(613) 238-8425

Cancer Information Services
National Cancer Institute
Office of Cancer Communications
Building 31, Room 10A-24
9000 Rockville Pike
Bethesda, MD 20892
(301) 496-5583
(800) 4-CANCER (hotline)

Centering Corporation
P.O. Box 3367
Omaha, NE 68103-0367
(402) 553-1200

Children's Defense Fund
122 'C' St. N.W., Ste. 400
Washington, DC 20001
(202) 628-8787

Child and Youth Services Administration
1120 19th St. N.W., Ste. 700
Washington, DC 20036
(202) 673-7783

Child Welfare League of America
440 First St. N.W., Ste. 310
Washington, DC 20001
(202) 638-2952

Federation for Children with Special Needs, Inc.
95 Berkeley St., Ste. 104
Boston, MA 02116
(617) 482-2915

Government Printing Office
Superintendent of Documents
Washington, DC 20402-9325
(202) 275-3050

Human Resource Center
201 I.U. Willets Rd.
Albertson, NY 11507
(516) 747-5400

March of Dimes Birth Defects Foundation
1275 Mamaroneck Ave.
White Plains, NY 10605
(914) 428-7100

Mead Johnson
Nutritional Division
2400 W. Lloyd Expressway
Evansville, IN 47721
(812) 429-5000

Medic-Alert Foundation International
P.O. Box 1009
Turlock, CA 95381
(209) 668-3333
(800) 344-3226

National Center for Education in Maternal and Child Health
38th and 'R' Streets N.W.
Washington, DC 20057
(202) 625-8400

National Center for Health Statistics
Department of Health and Human Services
Public Health Services
3700 East-West Highway, Room 157
Hyattsville, MD 20782
(301) 436-8500

National Dairy Council
6300 N. River Rd.
Rosement, IL 60018-4233
(708) 696-1020

National Easter Seal Society for Crippled Children
70 E. Lake St.
Chicago, IL 60612
(312) 726-6200
(312) 726-4258 (TDD)
(800) 221-6827

*Organizations serving the needs of children and families with specific disorders are listed as appropriate throughout Unit 4.

National Foundation for Jewish Genetic Diseases, Inc.
250 Park Ave., Ste. 1000
New York, NY 10177
(212) 371-1030

National Heart, Lung and Blood Institute
National Institutes of Health
9000 Rockville Pike
Building 31, Room 4A21
Bethesda, MD 20892
(301) 496-4236

National Information Center for Children and Youth with Hand-
    icaps (NICHCY)
P.O. Box 1492
Washington, DC 20013
(703) 893-6061 (Virginia Telephone Number)
(800) 999-5599

National Information System for Health Related Services
University of South Carolina
Benson Building
Columbia, SC 29208
(800) 922-9234

National Institutes of Child Health and Human Development
Building 31, Room 2A-32
9000 Rockville Pike
Bethesda, MD 20892
(301) 496-5133

National Institute of Marriage and Family Relations
6116 Rolling Rd., Ste. 306
Springfield, VA 22152
(703) 569-2400

National Mental Health Association
1021 Prince St.
Alexandria, VA 22314
(703) 684-7722

National Rehabilitation Association
633 S. Washington St,
Alexandria, VA 22314
(703) 836-0850

National Safety Council
444 N. Michigan Ave.
Chicago, IL 60611
(312) 527-4800
(800) 621-7615

Pediatric Projects
P.O. Box 1880
Santa Monica, CA 90406
(213) 828-8963

"Plain Talk" and "Caring about Kids" Series
U.S. Department of Health and Human Services
Public Health Service
Alcohol, Drug Abuse, and Mental Health Association
5600 Fishers Lane
Rockville, MD 20857
(301) 443-3875

Public Affairs Information Services
521 W. 43rd St., 5th Floor.
New York, NY 10036
(212) 736-6629

Ross Laboratories
Division Abbott Laboratories
Creative Services and Information
625 Cleveland Ave.
Columbus, OH 43215
(614) 227-3333

Sarah K. Davidson Family–Patient Health Education Library
Strong Children's Medical Center
University of Rochester Medical Center
P.O. Box 777
601 Elmwood Ave.
Rochester, NY 14642
(716) 275-7129

SKIP (Sick Kids Need Involved People) of New York
990 2nd Ave.
New York, NY 10022
(212) 421-9161

Sudden Infant Death Syndrome National Headquarters
10500 Little Patuxen Parkway
Columbia, MD 21044
(301) 964-8000
(800) 221-SIDS

U.S. Consumer Product Safety Commission
5401 Westbard Ave.
Washington, DC 20207
(301) 492-5500
(800) 492-8104 (Maryland only)
(800) 638-CPSC (Outside Maryland)
(800) 638-8270 (TDD)

U.S. Department of Agriculture
Office of Public Information
Food and Nutrition Service
3101 Park Center Dr.
Alexandria, VA 22302
(703) 756-3276

Wyeth Laboratories
P.O. Box 8299
145 King of Prussia
Radnor, PA 19087
(215) 383-0600

Unit 6

National clearinghouses

Clearinghouse on Child Abuse and Neglect
P.O. Box 1182
Washington, DC 20013
(703) 821-2086 (Virginia telephone number)

Consumer Information Catalog
P.O. Box 100
Pueblo, CO 81009
(719) 948-3334

Food and Drug Administration
Office of Consumer Affairs
5600 Fishers Lane
Rockville, MD 20857
(301) 443-1544

High Blood Pressure Information Center
120/80 National Institutes of Health
Bethesda, MD 20892
(301) 496-2411

Human Nutrition Information Service
Department of Agiculture
6505 Belcrest Rd., Room 360
Hyattsville, MD 20782
(301) 436-7725

National Digestive Diseases Information Clearinghouse
Box NDDIC
Bethesda, MD 20892
(301) 468-6344

National Health Information Clearinghouse "Healthfinder"
ONHIC
P.O. Box 1133
Washington, DC 20013-1133
(301) 565-4167 (Maryland telephone number)
(800) 336-4797

National Highway Traffic Safety Administration
NES-11 HL
U.S. Department of Transportation
400 7th St., S.W.
Washington, DC 20590
(202) 366-9550

National Information System and Clearinghouse
University of South Carolina
Benson Building
Columbia, SC 29208
(800) 922-9234

National Institute of Mental Health
Public Inquiries Branch
Parklawn Building, Room 15C-05
5600 Fishers Lane
Rockville, MD 20857
(301) 443-4513

National Library Service for the Blind and
Physically Handicapped
Library of Congress
1291 Taylor Street, N.W.
Washington, DC 20542
(202) 707-5100

National Maternal and Child Health Clearinghouse
38th and 'R' Streets, N.W.
Washington, DC 20057
(202) 625-8400

National Rehabilitation Information Center
8455 Colesville Rd., Ste. 935
Silver Spring, MD 20910-3319
(301) 588-9284
(800) 346-2742

National Self-Help Clearinghouse
33 W. 42nd St., Room 620N
New York, NY 10036
(212) 642-2944

National Technical Information Service
Agency of the Department of Commerce
5285 Port Royal Rd.
Springfield, VA 22161
(703) 487-4650

Self-Help Center
1600 Dodge Ave., Ste. S-122
Evanston, IL 60201
(708) 328-0470

Sudden Infant Death Syndrome Clearinghouse
8201 Greensboro Dr., Ste. 600
McLean, VA 22102
(703) 821-8955

Information has been verified as of January 1990.

ABBREVIATIONS AND ACRONYMS

In nursing practice a substantial number of words and phrases have been abbreviated for convenience in communication. Although most of the abbreviations are familiar to health professionals, many are not. In addition, students unfamiliar with the vocabulary used by health professionals are at a particular disadvantage when interpreting communications. This extensive list is compiled to facilitate this process. Because many of the abbreviations can represent several different words or phrases, the user is advised to use caution in their interpretation. For example, *per os* can be interpreted as give *by mouth* or give in *left eye*; *D/C* can mean *discharge* or *discontinue*. Other common abbreviations with multiple meanings include AS, CP, DPT, HS, LOC, MD, MS, NP, OD, OT, PA, PAP, PE, PR, RA, SD, SR, and TLC.

AA	Automobile accident; Alcoholics Anonymous
AAMD	American Association for Mental Deficiency
Ab	Antibody
ABG	Arterial blood gases
ABR	Auditory brainstem response
ac	*Ante cibum* (before meals)
ACCH	Association for the Care of Children's Health
ACLS	Advanced cardiac life support
ACT	Activated clotting time
ACTH	Adrenocorticotropic hormone
AD	Autosomal dominant; atopic dermatitis; auris dextra (right ear)
ADA	Adenosine deaminase (deficiency disease)
ADC	Aid to Dependent Children
ADD	Attention deficit disorder
ADDH	Attention deficit disorder, hyperactivity
ADH	Antidiuretic hormone
ADHD	Attention deficit-hyperactivity disorder
ADI	Acceptable daily intake
ADL	Activities of daily living
ad lib	*Ad libitum* (as desired)
ADP	Adenosine diphosphate
ADR	Adverse drug reaction
ADS	Attention deficit syndrome; antidiuretic substance
AEP	Auditory evoked potential
AF	Atrial fibrillation
AFB	Acid fast bacillus
AFDC	Aid to families of dependent children
AFP	Alpha fetoprotein
Ag	Antigen
AGA	Appropriate for gestational age
AGC	Absolute granulocyte count
AGN	Acute glomerulonephritis
AHC	Acute hemorrhagic conjunctivitis
AHD	Autoimmune hemolytic disease
AHF	Antihemophilic factor; antihemolytic factor
AHG	Antihemophilic globulin; antihuman globulin
AI	Aortic insufficiency
AID	Artificial insemination by donor
AIDS	Acquired immune deficiency syndrome
AIH	Artificial insemination by husband
AJ	Ankle jerk
ALG	Antilymphocytic globulin
ALL	Acute lymphoid leukemia
ALS	Advanced life support
ALT	Alanine aminotransferase
AMA	Against medical advice; American Medical Association
AMI	Acute myocardial infarction
AML	Acute myelogenous leukemia
amp	Ampule
AMP	Adenosine monophosphate
ANA	Antinuclear antibody; American Nurses' Association
ANLL	Acute nonlymphocytic leukemia
ANS	Autonomic nervous system; anterior nasal spine
AODM	Adult onset diabetes mellitus
AOM	Acute otitis media
AP	Anterior-posterior; antepartum; atrioperitoneal
APON	Association of Pediatric Oncology Nurses
aq	Aqua (water)
AR	Autosomal-recessive
ARC	AIDS-related complex
ARD	Acute respiratory distress
ARDS	Adult respiratory distress syndrome
ARF	Acute renal failure; acute respiratory failure
ARV	AIDS-associated retrovirus
AS	Aortic stenosis; aortic sounds; aqueous solution; aqueous suspension; astigmatism; ankylosing spondylitis; *auris sinistra* (left ear)
ASAP	As soon as possible
ASD	Atrial septal defect
ASDH	Acute subdural hematoma
ASH	Asymmetric septal hypertrophy
ASK	Antistreptokinase
ASO	Antistreptolysin O
ATC	Certified athletic trainer; around the clock
ATG	Antithymocyte globulin
ATN	Acute tubular necrosis
ATO	Alimentary tract obstruction
ATP	Autoimmune thrombocytopenia (purpura); adenosine triphosphate
ATPS	Ambient temperature and pressure saturated (with water)
ATV	All terrain vehicles
AU	*Auris uterque* (each ear)
Av	Average; avoirdupois
AV (A-V)	Atrioventricular
AVM	Arteriovenous malformation
AWD	Abdominal wall defect
BA	Bronchial asthma; bone age
BAEP	Brainstem auditory evoked potential
BAER	Brainstem auditory evoked response
BAT	Brown adipose tissue
BBB	Blood-brain barrier
BBT	Basal body temperature
BCG	Bacille Calmette Guerin (tuberculin vaccine)
BCS	Battered child syndrome
BD	Bronchial drainage; birthday
BE	Barium enema
BEAM	Brain electrical activity map
BEI	Butanol-extractable iodine
BFP	Biologic false positive
BG	Blood glucose
BHI	Biosynthetic human insulin
bid	*Bis in die* (twice a day)
BJ	Biceps jerk
BM	Bowel movement; bone marrow
BMD	Bone marrow depression
BMR	Basal metabolic rate
BNBAS	Brazelton Neonatal Behavioral Assessment Scale
BOA	Behavioral observation audiometry; born out of asepsis
BPD	Bronchopulmonary dysplasia
BRP	Bathroom privileges
BS	Blood sugar; bowel sounds; breath sounds
BSA	Body surface area; bovine serum albumin
BSE	Breast self-examination
BSER	Brainstem-evoked response
BSI	Biologic substance(s) isolation; body substance isolation
BSID	Bayley Scales of Infant Development
BT	Bleeding time
BTPS	Body temperature and pressure saturated (with water)
BUN	Blood urea nitrogen

Unit 6

BWF	Basic waking frequency
BWS	Battered woman syndrome
Bx	Biopsy
c	*Con* (with)
CA (Ca)	Cancer; chronologic age
cAMP	Cyclic adenosine monophosphate
CAL	Chronic airflow limitation
CAH	Congenital adrenal hyperplasia; chronic active hepatitis
cap	Capsule
CAPD	Continuous ambulatory peritoneal dialysis
CAT	Computerized axial tomography
CAVH	Continuous arteriovenous hemofiltration
CBA	Congenital biliary atresia
CBC	Complete blood count
CBD	Closed bladder drainage
CBF	Cerebral blood flow
CBV	Cerebral blood volume; cerebral blood (flow) velocity
CBPU	Care by parent unit
CC	Chief complaint; caucasian child; common cold; critical condition; color and circulation; creatinine clearance; gas chromatography
CCMS	Clean-catch midstream specimen
Ccr	Creatinine clearance
CCS	Crippled Children's Services
CD	Communicable disease; celiac disease
CDC	Centers for Disease Control
CDGA	Constitutional delay of growth and adolescence
CDH	Congenital dislocated hip; congenital diaphragmatic hernia
CDP	Continuous distending pressure
C-E	Croup-epiglottitis syndrome
CF	Cystic fibrosis; cardiac failure; complement fixation
CFU	Colony-forming units
CHAP	Child Health Assessment Program
CHB	Complete heart block
CHC	Child health conference; community health center
CHD	Congenital heart disease; childhood disease; coronary heart disease
CHF	Congestive heart failure
CHL	Crown-heel length
CI	Cardiac index; cardiac insufficiency; cerebral infarction
CID	Cytomegalic inclusion disease; combined immune deficiency
CIE	Countercurrent immunoelectrophoresis
CINAHL	Cumulative Index to Nursing and Allied Health Literature
CK	Creatine kinase
CL	Cleft lip
CLBBB	Complete left bundle branch block
CLD	Chronic lung disease; chronic liver disease
CL (P)	Cleft lip with or without cleft palate
CLP	Cleft lip and palate
CMA	Cow's milk allergy
CMI	Cell-mediated immunity
CML	Chronic myelocytic leukemia
CMPI	Cow's milk protein intolerance
CMR	Cerebral metabolic rate
CMV	Cytomegalovirus
CN	Clinical Nurse
CNA	Canadian Nurses' Association
CNM	Certified Nurse Midwife
CNS	Central nervous system; Clinical Nurse Specialist
CNSD	Chronic nonspecific diarrhea
CO	Cardiac output
COA	Children of alcoholics
Cocci	Coccidioidomycosis
COHb	Carboxyhemoglobin
COLD	Chronic obstructive lung disease
COPD	Chronic obstructive pulmonary disease
COR	Conditioned orientation reflex
CP	Cleft palate; cerebral palsy; capillary pressure; cor pulmonale; Certified Prosthetist; constant pressure;
	child psychiatrist; closing pressure (spinal tap); chronic pyelonephritis
CPAP	Continuous positive airway pressure
CPAV	Continuous positive airway ventilation
CPD	Cephalopelvic disproportion; childhood polycystic disease
CPK	Creatine phosphokinase
CPM	Continuous passive motion
CPN	Certified Pediatric Nurse
CPP	Cerebral perfusion pressure
CPPV	Continuous positive pressure ventilation
CPR	Cardiopulmonary resuscitation
CPS	Cycles per second; child protective services
CPSC	Consumer Product Safety Commission
CPT	Chest physiotherapy
CRBBB	Complete right bundle branch block
CRD	Child restraint devices
CRF	Corticotropin releasing factor
CRP	C-reactive protein
CS	Clinical Specialist
CSA	Colony stimulating activity
CSD	Sickle cell disease; cat scratch disease
CSF	Cerebral spinal fluid; cerebrospinal fluid
CSII	Continuous subcutaneous insulin infusion
CT	Computerized tomography; circulation time; clotting time; coated tablet; compressed tablet; corneal transplant
CTT	Computerized transaxial tomography
CUG	Cystourethrogram
CV	Closing volume
CVA	Cerebrovascular accident; costal vertebral angle
CVI	Common variable immunodeficiency
CVP	Central venous pressure
CVR	Cerebral vascular resistance
CVS	Clean voided specimen; chorionic villi sampling
CW	Crutch walking
C/W	Consistent with
CXR	Chest x-ray
DA	Developmental age
DASE	Denver Articulation Screening Examination
DAW	Dispense as written
db	Decibel
DC D/C	Discontinue; discharge; dichorionic
D & C	Dilatation and curettage
DD	Dry dressing; differential diagnosis; discharge diagnosis; discharge by death
DDST	Denver Developmental Screening Test
DDST-R	Denver Developmental Screening Test, revised
DFA	Diet for age
DH	Diaphragmatic hernia
DHHS	Department of Health and Human Services
DI	Diabetes insipidus
D/I	Direct/indirect ratio (bilirubin)
DIC	Disseminated intravascular coagulation
DIP	Desquamated interstitial pneumonitis
DKA	Diabetic ketoacidosis
DLIS	Digoxin-like immunoreactive substance
DM	Diabetes mellitus; diastolic murmur
DMD	Duchenne muscular dystrophy
DNHW	Department of National Health and Welfare (Canada)
DNR	Do not resuscitate
DOA	Date of admission; dead on arrival
DOB	Date of birth
DOD	Date of discharge; date of death
DOE	Dyspnea on exertion
DP	Dorsalis pedis (artery)
DPNB	Dorsal penile nerve block
DPT	Diphtheria-pertussis-tetanus (vaccine); Demerol-Phenergan-Thorazine
DQ	Developmental quotient
DRG	Diagnosis-related group(s)

DS	Down syndrome		**FBS**	Fasting blood sugar
DSA	Digital subtraction angiography		**FDA**	Food and Drug Administration
DSD	Dry sterile dressing		**FEP**	Free erythrocyte porphyrins
DSDB	Direct self-destructive behavior		**FET**	Forced expiratory technique
DSM	Diagnostic & Statistical Manual of Mental Disorders		**FEV₁**	Forced expiratory volume, 1 second
DT	Diphtheria toxoid; diphtheria and tetanus toxoid; delirium tremens		**FEV₅**	Forced expiratory volume, 5 seconds
DTP	Diphtheria-tetanus-pertussis		**FEVC**	Forced expiratory volume capacity
DTR	Deep tendon reflex		**FFA**	Free fatty acids
DU	Diagnosis undetermined		**FFP**	Fresh-frozen plasma
DV	Dilute volume		**FH, FHx**	Family history
DW	Distilled water		**FHS**	Fetal hydantoin syndrome
D5W	Distilled water with 5% glucose		**Fio₂, FIO₂**	Forced inspiratory oxygen; fraction of inspired oxygen
Dx	Diagnosis		**FLK**	Funny looking kid
DZ	Dizygotic		**FMD**	Fibromuscular dysplasia
EA	Esophageal atresia		**FMH**	Family medical history
EBL	Estimated blood loss		**FMS**	Fat-mobilizing substance
EBV	Epstein-Barr virus		**FNP**	Family Nurse Practitioner
ECC	Emergency cardiac care		**FRC**	Functional residual capacity
ECD	Endocardial cushion defect		**FS**	Full strength
ECF	Extracellular fluid; extended care facility		**FSH**	Follicle-stimulating hormone
ECG	Electrocardiogram		**FSP**	Fibrin split products
ECM	Erythema chronicum migrans		**FSS**	Family short stature
ECMO	Extracorporeal cardiopulmonary bypass with membrane oxygenation		**FTA-ABS**	Fluorescent treponemal antibody absorption (test)
ED	Emergency department		**FTSG**	Full-thickness skin graft
EDC	Estimated date of confinement		**FTT**	Failure to thrive
EDD	Estimated date of delivery		**FUE**	Fever of unknown etiology
EEE	Eastern equine encephalitis		**F/U**	Follow up
EEG	Electroencephalogram		**FUO**	Fever of unknown origin
EF	Extended field (irradiation)		**FVC**	Forced vital capacity
EFA	Essential fatty acid		**FWB**	Full weight bearing
EFE	Endocardial fibroelastosis		**Fx**	Fracture
EFM	Electronic fetal monitoring		**FYI**	For your information
EGS	Electric galvanic stimulator		**GA**	General anesthesia
EHBA	Extrahepatic biliary atresia		**GABHS**	Group A beta hemolytic streptococci
E-IPV	Enhanced (potency) - IPV		**GAS**	Group A streptococci
ELISA	Enzyme-linked immunosorbent assay		**GBM**	Glomerular basement membrane
elix	Elixir		**GC**	Gonococci (gonorrhea); general condition; general circulation
EMG	Electromyogram		**GCS**	Glasgow coma scale
EMI	Electromagnetic interference		**G & D**	Growth and development
EMM	Expressed mother's milk		**GDM**	Gestational diabetes mellitus
EMR	Educable mentally retarded		**GER**	Gastroesophageal reflux
EMS	Emergency medical services		**GFR**	Glomerular filtration rate
EMT	Emergency medical technology		**GGT**	Gamma glutamyltranspeptidase
ENA	Extractable nuclear antigens		**GGTP**	Gamma glutamyltranspeptidase
EOA	Examination, opinion, and advice		**GH**	Growth hormone
EOM	Extraocular movement; extraocular muscle		**GHB, GHb**	Glycosylated hemoglobin
EP	Extraperitoneal; evoked potential; erythrocyte protoporphyrin		**GHD**	Growth hormone deficiency
			GHRF	Growth hormone releasing factor
EPA	Erect posteroanterior		**GH-RH**	Growth hormone releasing hormone
EPI	Echo-planar imaging		**GI**	Gastrointestinal
EPSDT	Early and Periodic Screening, Diagnosis, and Treatment		**GOT**	Glutamic-oxaloacetic transaminase
ER	Emergency room; external rotation; expiratory reserve; equivalent roentgen		**G6PD**	Glucose-6-phosphate dehydrogenase
			GSE	Gluten sensitive enteropathy
ERA	Electric response audiometry		**GSW**	Gunshot wound
ERG	Electroretinography		**GTT**	Glucose tolerance test
ERPF	Effective renal plasma flow		**GU**	Genitourinary
ERV	Expiratory reserve volume		**GVH**	Graft-vs-host
ESI	Early Screening Inventory		**GVHD**	Graft-vs-host disease
ESR	Erythrocyte sedimentation rate		**GVHR**	Graft-vs-host reaction
ESRD	End-stage renal disease		**h**	*Hora* (hour)
ET	Endotracheal		**HA**	Headache
ETA	Estimated time of arrival		**H-A**	Hartmannella-Acanthamoeba
ETOH	Alcohol		**HAV**	Hepatitis A virus
ETT	Endotracheal tube		**Hb**	Hemoglobin
EV	Enterovirus		**HB**	Heart block
FAAN	Fellow in American Academy of Nursing		**HBGM**	Home blood glucose monitoring
FAB	French-American-British		**HBIG**	Hepatitis B immune globulin
FAS	Fetal alcohol syndrome		**HBO**	Hyperbaric oxygen
FB	Foreign body		**HbOC**	Haemophilus b conjugate vaccine (diphtheria CRM₁₉-protein conjugate)
FBA	Foreign body aspiration		**HBsAg**	Hepatitis B surface antigen

HBV	Hepatitis B virus; honey bee venom
HC	Hyperosmolar coma
hCG	Human chorionic gonadotropin
HCI	Home care instructions
HCM	Health care management
Hct	Hematocrit
HD	Heart disease
HDCV	Human diploid cell virus
HDL	High-density lipoprotein
HDN	Hemorrhagic disease of the newborn
HEENT	Head, eye, ear, nose, & throat
HFJV	High-frequency jet ventilation
HFO	High-frequency oscillation
HFOV	High-frequency oscillatory ventilation
HFPPV	High-frequency positive pressure ventilation
HFV	High-frequency ventilation
Hgb	Hemoglobin
HGH (hGH)	Human growth hormone
HHHO	Hypothyroidism, hypoxia, hypogonadism, obesity
HHNC	Hyperosmolar, hyperglycemic, nonketogenic coma
HHNK	Hyperosmolar, hyperglycemic, nonketotic dehydration
H/I	Hypoxia-ischemia
Hib (HIB)	*Haemophilus influenzae type* B
HIE	Hypoxic-ischemic encephalopathy
HISG	Human immune serum globulin
HIV	Human immunodeficiency viruses
HL	Hearing level
HLA	Human leukocytic antigen; histocompatibility locus antigen
HMD	Hyaline membrane disease
HMO	Health maintenance organization; high molecular weight
HO	House officer
HOB	Head of bed
HOME	Home Observation for Measurement of the Environment Inventory
HOPI	History of previous (prior) illness
HPA	Hypothalamic-pituitary-adrenal (axis)
HPB	Health Protection Branch (of DNHW, Canada)
HPC	Healed primary complex
HPLC	High-power liquid chromatography
HPN	Hypertension
HPV	Human parvovirus; human papilloma virus
HR	Heart rate
HRA	Health risk appraisal
HRF	Health-related facility
HRIG	Human rabies immune globulin
hs	*Hora somni* (hour of sleep; bedtime)
HS	Heart sounds; herpes simplex; house surgeon
HSA	Health systems agency; human serum albumin
HSBG	Heal stick blood gases
HSE	Herpes simplex encephalitis
HSP	Henoch-Schönlein purpura
HSV	Herpes simplex virus
HTLV-III	Human T-lymphotropic virus type III
HTN	Hypertensive; hypertension
HTPN	Home total parenteral nutrition
HTSI	Human thyroid stimulator immunoglobulin
HUS	Hemolytic uremic syndrome
Hx	History
IA	Imperforate anus; internal auditory; intraarterial; intraarticular; infantile apnea
IAA	Insulin autoantibodies
IABP	Intraaortic balloon pump
IAFI	Infantile amaurotic familial idiocy
IAR	Interagency referral
IBC	Iron-binding capacity
IBD	Inflammatory bowel disease
IBO	In behalf of
IBS	Irritable bowel syndrome
IBW	Ideal body weight

IC	Intracutaneous
ICA	Islet cell antibodies
ICC	Intermittent clean catheterization
ICD	International Classification of Diseases
ICF	Intracellular fluid
ICN	Intensive care nursery
ICP	Intermittent catheterization program; intracranial pressure
ICS	Intercostal space
ICSH	Interstitial cell-stimulating hormone
ICU	Intensive care unit
ID	Identification; intradermal; initial dose; infective dose; ineffective dose; inside diameter
IDD	Insulin dependent diabetes
IDDM	Insulin dependent diabetes mellitus
IDM	Infant of diabetic mother
IDP	Infant development program
IEP	Individualized education program; immunoelectrophoresis
I/E ratio	Inspiratory-expiratory ratio
IF	Involved field (irradiation); immunofluorescence
IFA	Indirect fluorescent antibody
Ig (IG)	Immune globulin
IGIV	Immune globulin intravenous
IgS	Immunoglobulin system
IGT	Impaired glucose tolerance
IH	Infectious hepatitis
IHA	Indirect hemagglutination
IHSS	Idiopathic hypertrophic subaortic stenosis
IIA	Interrupted infantile apnea
IM	Intramuscular; internal medicine; infectious mononucleosis; intramedullary
IMV	Intermittent mandatory ventilation
IND	Investigational new drug
INV	Influenza vaccine
IOL	Intraocular lens implant
IPH	Intraparenchymal hemorrhage
IPPB	Intermittent positive pressure breathing
IPPD	Intermedial purified protein derivative (tuberculin test)
IPV	Inactivated polio virus (vaccine)
IQ	Intelligence quotient
IRB	Institutional Review Board
IRDS	Idiopathic respiratory distress syndrome; infant respiratory distress syndrome
IRV	Inspiratory reserve volume
ISADH	Inappropriate secretion of ADH
ISC	Intermittent self-catheterization
ISDB	Indirect self-destructive behavior
ISF	Interstitial fluid
ISG	Immune serum globulin
ISP	Infant stimulation program
IT	Intrathecal
ITP	Idiopathic thrombocytopenia; idiopathic thrombocytopenic purpura
ITQ	Infant temperament questionnaire
IU	Immunizing unit; international unit
IUCD	Intrauterine contraceptive device
IUD	Intrauterine device
IUGR	Intrauterine growth retardation
IV	Intravenous
IVC	Inferior vena cava
IVCD	Intraventricular conduction defect
IVDU	Intravenous drug use
IVGG	Intravenous gamma globulin
IVH	Intraventricular hemorrhage
IVP	Intravenous pyelogram
IVT	Intravenous transfusion
IWL	Insensible water loss
JA	Juvenile arthritis
JAS	Juvenile ankylosing spondylitis
JCAH	Joint Commission on the Accreditation of Hospitals
JCP	Juvenile chronic polyarthritis

Unit 6

JND	Just noticeable difference	
JOD	Juvenile-onset diabetes	
JODM	Juvenile-onset diabetes mellitus	
JRA	Juvenile rheumatoid arthritis	
KD	Kawasaki disease	
KIDS	Kansas Infant Development Screen	
17-KGS	Ketogenic steroids	
17-KS	Ketosteroids	
KUB	Kidney, ureters, and bladder	
KVO	Keep vein open	
LA	Left atrium	
LAE	Left atrial enlargement	
LATS	Long-acting thyroid stimulator	
LAV	Lymphadenopathy-associated virus	
LBCD	Left border of cardiac dullness (sternal border)	
LBM	Lean body mass	
LBW	Low birth weight; lean body weight	
LCM	Left costal margin	
LD	Lethal dose; light difference (perception)	
LDH	Lactic dehydrogenase	
LDL	Low-density lipoprotein	
L&D	Labor and delivery	
LE	Lupus erythematosus; left eye; LE prep; lower extremity	
LES	Lower esophageal sphincter; Life Expectancy Survey	
LFD	Light for dates	
LGA	Large for gestational age	
LH	Luteinizing hormone	
LH-RH	Luteinizing hormone releasing hormone	
LIP	Lymphoid interstitial pneumonitis	
LJM	Limited joint movement	
LKS	Liver, kidney, spleen	
LLBCD	Left lower border of cardiac dullness	
LLE	Left lower extremity	
LLL	Left lower lobe	
LLQ	Left lower quadrant	
LMC	Left midclavicular line	
LMD	Local medical doctor	
LMN	Lower motor neuron	
LMP	Last menstrual period	
LNMP	Last normal menstrual period	
LOC	Level of consciousness; loss of consciousness; locus of control	
LOM	Left otitis media; loss of movement; limitation of motion	
LP	Lumbar puncture	
LPN	Licensed practical nurse	
LQ	Lower quadrant	
LRE	Least restrictive environment	
LRI	Lower respiratory tract infection	
LSB	Left sternal border; left scapular border	
LTB	Laryngotracheobronchitis	
LTH	Luteotropic hormone	
LUE	Left upper extremity	
LUL	Left upper lobe	
LUQ	Left upper quadrant	
LV	Left ventricle	
LVH	Left ventricular hypertrophy	
LVN	Licensed vocational nurse	
LVO	Left ventricular output	
M	Molar; mean	
M²	Meters squared (square meters)	
MA	Mental age; menstrual age	
MABP	Mean arterial blood pressure	
MAC	Maximum allowable concentration	
MAMC	Midarm muscle circumference	
MAP	Mean arterial pressure; mean airway pressure; most appropriate placement	
MAS	Meconium aspiration syndrome	
MAWP	Mean arterial wedge pressure	
MBC	Minimum bactericidal concentration	
MBP	Mean blood pressure	
MC	Mucocutaneous lymph node syndrome; maternal child; monochorionic	

MCDI	Minnesota Child Development Inventory
mcg	Microgram
MCH	Mean corpuscular (cell) hemoglobin; maternal and child health
MCHC	Mean corpuscular (cell) hemoglobin concentration
MCL	Mid-clavicular line
MCNS	Minimal change nephrotic syndrome
MCSI	McCarthy Scales of Children's Abilities
MCT	Medium-chain triglyceride; mean circulatory time
MCV	Mean corpuscular (cell) volume; mean clinical value
MD	Muscular dystrophy; medical doctor; manic depression; myocardial disease
MDA	Minimal daily allowance
MDI	Medium dose inhalants; metered dose inhaler
MDR	Minimal daily requirement
MED	Minimal effective dose; minimal erythema dose
mEQ	Milliequivalents
MFD	Minimal fatal dose
MGN	Membranous glomerulonephritis
MH	Melanocytic hormone
MHC	Major histocompatibility complex
MI	Mitral insufficiency; myocardial infarction; myocardial ischemia; mental illness
MIC	Minimum inhibitory concentration
MID	Minimum infective dose
MIF	Migration inhibiting factor
MLC	Mixed lymphocyte culture
MLD	Minimum lethal dose; median lethal dose
MLNS	Minimal lesion nephrotic syndrome
MM	Mucous membrane; malignant melanoma; myocardial infarction; myocardial ischemia; mitral insufficiency
MMEF	Maximal midexpiratory flow
MMPI	Minnesota Multiphasic Personality Inventory
MMR	Mumps, measles, rubella; Morbidity and Mortality Report
MNP	Mononuclear phagocyte
MO	Medical officer
MOD	March of Dimes
MODM	Mature-onset diabetes mellitus
MOF	Multiple organ failure
MOSF	Multiple organ system failure
MPAP	Mean pulmonary artery pressure
MPD	Maximum permissible dose
MPI	Minnesota Preschool Inventory
MPS	Mucopolysaccharidosis
MR	Mental retardation; may repeat; measles, rubella; mitral regurgitation
MRD	Minimum reacting dose
MRI	Magnetic resonance imaging
MS	Mitral stenosis; multiple sclerosis; mitral sounds; morphine sulfate; musculoskeletal
MS-1	Hepatitis A
MS-2	Hepatitis B
MSAFP	Maternal serum alpha-fetoprotein
MSL	Midsternal line
MSP	Münchausen syndrome by proxy
MST	McCarthy Screening Tests
MTT	Mean transit time
MVA	Motor vehicle accident
MVP	Moisture vapor permeable (dressing)
MVV	Maximum voluntary ventilation
MZ	Monozygotic
N	Normal
n	Number
NA	Nutritional assessment
NAD	No abnormalities noted; no appreciable disease
NAI	Nonaccidental injury
NANB	Non-A, non-B
NAPNAP	National Association of Pediatric Nurse Associates & Practitioners
NASN	National Association of School Nurses
NB	Newborn

Unit 6

NBAS	Newborn behavioral assessment scale	**OTC**	Over the counter
NBN	Newborn nursery	**OU**	*Oculi unitas* (both eyes)
NCDB	National Center Drugs and Biologics	**OV**	Oculovestibular (cold water caloric test)
NCDC	National Center for Disease Control	**p**	Probability
NCHS	National Center for Health Statistics	**PA**	Posteroanterior; pernicious anemia; primary amenor-
NCV	Nerve conduction velocity		rhea; pulmonary artery; prolonged action; physi-
ND	Not done		cian's assistant
NEC	Necrotizing enterocolitis	**PAC**	Premature atrial contraction
NFT	Nonorganic failure to thrive	**Paco$_2$**	Carbon dioxide pressure (tension), arterial
NG	Nasogastric	**PACU**	Postanesthesia care unit
NGU	Nongonorrheal urethritis	**PAIDS**	Pediatric AIDS
NH	Neonatal hepatitis	**PANESS**	Physical and neurologic examination for soft signs
NHL	Non-Hodgkin lymphoma	**Pao$_2$**	Oxygen pressure (tension), arterial
NICU	Newborn intensive care unit	**PAP**	Primary atypical pneumonia; Papanicolaou smear; pas-
NIDDM	Noninsulin dependent diabetes mellitus		sive aggressive personality; pulmonary artery pres-
NIH	National Institutes of Health		sure
NIMH	National Institute of Mental Health	**PAPVR**	Partial anomalous pulmonary venous return
NKA	No known allergies	**PAR**	Post anesthesia room
nl	Normal (value)	**PAT**	Paroxysmal atrial tachycardia
NLN	National League for Nursing	**PBB**	Polybrominated biphenyls
NLTR	Non-life-threatening reaction	**PBGT**	Personal blood glucose testing
NM	Neonatal mortality	**PBI**	Protein-bound iodine
NMR	Nuclear magnetic resonance; neonatal mortality rates	**Paw**	Mean airway pressure
NND	New and non-official drugs	**PAWP**	Pulmonary artery wedge pressure
NNS	Non-nutritive sucking	**PB**	Peripheral blood
NOFT	Nonorganic failure to thrive	**PBS**	Phosphate-buffered saline solution
NOP	Not otherwise provided for	**pc**	Postprandial (after meals)
NOS	Not otherwise specified	**PC**	Purulent conjunctivitis; present complaint
NP	Nasopharynx; new patient; not palpable; nerve palsy;	**PCA**	Patient controlled analgesia
	nurse practitioner	**PCB**	Polycholorinated biphenyls
NPN	Nonprotein nitrogen	**PCM**	Protein-calorie malnutrition
NR	Normal range; nonreactive; no report; no respirations;	**Pco$_2$**	Partial pressure (tension), carbon dioxide
	not remarkable; no resuscitation; not refillable; nor-	**PCP**	Patient care plan; *Pneumocystis carinii* pneumonia
	mal reaction	**PCT**	Prothrombin consumption test
NREM	Nonrapid eye movement	**PCV**	Packed cell volume
NS	Normal saline; not significant	**PCWP**	Pulmonary capillary wedge pressure
NSAID	Nonsteroidal antiinflammatory drug	**PD**	Pupillary distance
NSFTD	Normal spontaneous full-term delivery	**PDA**	Patent ductus arteriosus
NSR	Normal sinus rhythm	**PDC**	Private diagnostic clinic
NSU	Nonspecific urethritis	**PDI**	Preschool Development Inventory
NT	Nasotracheal	**PDNB**	Penile dorsal newborn; Penile dorsal nerve block
NTB	Necrotizing tracheobronchitis	**PDQ**	Prescreening Developmental Questionnaire
NTD	Neural tube defects	**PDR**	Physician's Desk Reference
NTM	Nontuberculous mycobacterium	**PE**	Physical examination; pressure equalizing; probable er-
NTP	Normal temperature and pressure		ror; pulmonary embolism; port of entry; point of
NUG	Necrotizing ulcerative gingivitis		entry; physical education; pelvic examination
NVSS	Normal variant short stature	**PEEP**	Positive end-expiratory pressure
NWB	Non-weight-bearing	**PEEX**	Pediatric Early Elementary Examination
NYD	Not yet diagnosed	**PEFR**	Peak expiratory flow rate
OASDL	Ordinary activities and skills of daily living	**PEG**	Percutaneous endoscopic gastrostomy; pneumoen-
OBS	Organic brain syndrome		cephalogram
OC	Oral contraceptive; oculocephalic (doll's eye reflex)	**PEN**	Parenteral/enteral nutrition
OCD	Over-the-counter drug; obsessive-compulsive disorder	**PERL**	Pupils equal and react to light
OCP	Ova, cysts, and parasites	**per os**	By mouth
OD	*Oculus dexter* (right eye); once daily; overdose; outside	**PERRLA**	Pupils equal, round, react to light and accommodation
	diameter; optical density	**PET**	Positron emission tomography
OFC	Occipitofrontal circumference	**PETT**	Positron emission transaxial tomography
OHS	Orally administered hydration solution(s)	**PF**	Pulmonary flow
OI	Opportunistic infection; osteogenesis imperfecta	**PFC**	Persistent fetal circulation
OJ	Orange juice	**PFNB**	Percutaneous fine needle biopsy
OM	Otitis media; opportunistic mycoses	**PFT**	Pulmonary function tests
OME	Otitis media with effusion	**PG**	Prostaglandin
OOB	Out of bed	**PH**	Past history; previous history; public health
O&P	Ova and parasites	**pH**	Power of hydrogen
OPC	Outpatient clinic	**PHA**	Phytohemagglutinin
OPD	Outpatient department	**PHN**	Public health nurse
OR	Operating room	**PHV**	Peak height velocity
ORIF	Open reduction internal fixation	**PI**	Pulmonary insufficiency; present illness
OS	*Oculus sinister* (left eye)	**PICU**	Pediatric intensive care unit
OSA	Obstructive sleep apnea	**PID**	Pelvic inflammatory disease
OSB	Open spina bifida	**PIE**	Pulmonary interstitial emphysema
OT	Ocupational therapy; orotracheal; old tuberculin; old	**PIH**	Pregnancy-induced hypertension
	term	**PIP**	Peak inspiratory pressure

PIPP	Peak inspiratory plateau pressure
PKD	Polycystic kidney disease
PKU	Phenylketonuria
PLH	Pulmonary lymphoid hyperplasia
PLT	Psittacosis-lymphogranuloma venereum-trachoma
PM	Postmortem; post meridian
PMC	Pseudomembranous colitis
PMD	Private medical doctor; past (previous) medical doctor
PMH	Past medical history
PMI	Point of maximum impulse (intensity)
PMN	Polymorphonuclear neutrophil
PMR	Psychomotor retardation; perinatal mortality rate; physical, medical, and rehabilitation
PNA	Pediatric nurse associate
PND	Paroxysmal nocturnal dyspnea; postnasal drip
PNM	Postnatal mortality
PNP	Pediatric nurse practitioner
PNPR	Positive-negative pressure respiration
po	*Per os* (by mouth)
PO	Postoperative; phone order
Po₂	Partial pressure (tension), oxygen
POA	Primary optic atrophy
POMR	Problem oriented medical record
POR	Problem oriented record
PP	Partial pressure; patient profile; peripheral pulses; postpartum; postprandial; presenting problem
PPC	Progressive patient care
PPD	Purified protein derivative
PPHN	Persistent pulmonary hypertension
PPLO	Pleuropneumonia-like organisms
PPPA	Poison Prevention Packaging Act
PPS	Peripheral pulmonic stenosis
PPT	Partial prothrombin time
PR	Perfusion rate; peripheral resistance; progress report; pulse rate; public relations
PRA	Plasma renin activity
PRBC	Packed red blood cells
PRESS	Preschool Readiness Experimental Screening Scale
PRN, prn	*Pro re nata* (as necessary); as circumstance may require
PROM	Passive range of motion; premature rupture of membranes
PRP	Persistent recurrent pneumonia
PRP-D	Polysaccharide of haemophilus influenza type b conjugated to diptheria toxoid
PS	Pulmonic stenosis; pyloric stenosis
P/SH	Personal social history
PSP	Phenolsulfonphthalein test
PSMA	Progressive spinal muscular atrophy
PSR	Psychological Stimulus Response
PSRO	Professional Standards Review Organization
PSSD	Psychosocial dwarfism
PT	Physical therapy (therapist); prothrombin time
PTA	Prior to admission; plasma thromboplastin antecedent
PTC	Plasma thromboplastin component; phenyltheocarbamide
PTH	Parathyroid hormone; pseudohyperparathyroidism
PTT	Partial thromboplastin time
PUD	Peptic ulcer disease
PUO	Pyrexia of undetermined (unknown) origin
PV	Parainfluenza virus
PVC	Premature ventricular contraction; polyvinyl chloride
PVD	Percussion, vibration, and drainage
PVH	Periventricular hemorrhage
PVP	Pulmonary venous pressure
PVR	Peripheral vascular resistance; pulmonary vascular resistance
PVS	Percussion, vibration, and suction
PWB	Partial weight-bearing
PWM	Pokeweed mitogen
PWP	Pulmonary wedge pressure
PWS	Port wine stain; Prader-Willi syndrome
Px	Prognosis; pneumothorax
q	*Quaque* (every)
qd	*Quaque die* (every day)

qh	*Quaque hora* (every hour)
qid	*Quater in die* (four times a day)
qn	Every night
qns	Quantity not sufficient
qod	Every other day
q2h	Every 2 hours
QPIT	Quantitative pilocarpine iontophoresis test
qs	Quantity sufficient
RA	Rheumatoid arthritis; return appointment; renal artery; right arm; right atrium; rectal atresia; repeat action; room air
RAE	Right atrial enlargement
RAST	Radioallergosorbent test
RATG	Rabbit anti-thymocytic globulin
RBC	Red blood cell
RBD	Right border dullness
RBE	Relative biologic effectiveness
RBF	Renal blood flow
RBS	Random blood sugar
RC	Rice cereal
RCC	Red cell concentrate
RCM	Right costal margin
RD	Retinal detachment; respiratory disease; right deltoid
RDA	Recommended daily allowance
RDS	Respiratory distress syndrome
RDSI	Revised Developmental Screening Inventory
RE	Regional enteritis; rear end (accident); right eye; rectal examination
REE	Resting energy expenditure
REM	Rapid eye movement
RF	Rheumatic fever
RHD	Rheumatic heart disease; relative hepatic dullness
RIA	Radioimmunoassay; radioactive immunoassay
RICE	Rest, ice, compression, elevation
RICM	Right intercostal margin
RIG	Rabies immune globulin
RLE	Right lower extremity
RLF	Retrolental fibroplasia
RLQ	Right lower quadrant
RMA	Rhythmic motor activities
RML	Right mediolateral; right middle lobe
RMR	Resting metabolic rate
RMSF	Rocky Mountain spotted fever
RN	Registered Nurse
RN,C	Registered Nurse, Certified
RN,CS	Registered Nurse, Certified Specialist
RO	Rule out; routine order
ROM	Range of motion; right otitis media
ROP	Retinopathy of prematurity
ROS	Review of systems
R-PDQ	Revised Prescreening Developmental Questionnaire
RPF	Renal plasma flow
RPR	Rapid plasma reagin
RR	Respiratory rate; recovery room; radiation response
RS	Review of symptoms; Reye syndrome; Reiter syndrome
RSB	Right sternal border
RSV	Respiratory syncytial virus
RT	Respiratory therapy (therapist); room temperature
RTA	Renal tubular acidosis
RTI	Respiratory tract infection
RTUS	Real-time ultrasound
RUE	Right upper extremity
RUL	Right upper lobe
RUQ	Right upper quadrant
RV	Residual volume; right ventricle
RVH	Right ventricular hypertrophy
Rx	Prescription
s	*Sans* (without)
SAC	Short arm cast
SAD	Sugar and acetone determination
SAH	Subarachnoid hemorrhage
SAM	Surface active material; Society for Adolescent Medicine
Sao₂	Saturated arterial oxygen

Unit 6

SBE	Subacute bacterial endocarditis
SC	Subcutaneous
SCB	Strictly confined to bed
SCD	Sudden cardiac death
SCFE	Slipped capital femoral epiphysis
SCID	Severe combined immune deficiency disease
SCM	Sternocleidomastoid muscle
SCU	Special care unit
SCV	Smooth, capsulated, virulent
SD	Standard deviation; septal defect; spontaneous delivery; sudden death; shoulder disarticulation
SEA	Seronegative enthesopathy and arthropathy (syndrome)
SES	Socioeconomic status
SFD	Small for dates
SG	Specific gravity
SGA	Small for gestational age
SGOT	Sergum glutamic-oxaloacetic transaminase
SGPT	Serum glutamic-pyruvic transaminase
SH	Social history; self help; serum hepatitis; shoulder
SI	*Système International*
SIADH	Syndrome of inappropriate ADH
SIDS	Sudden infant death syndrome
SIG	Serum immune globulin
SIMV	Synchronized intermittent mandatory ventilation
SISADH	Syndrome of inappropriate secretion of ADH
SKL	Serum killing levels
SKSD	Streptokinase/streptodornase (control test)
SLC	Short leg cast
SLD	Specific learning disability
SLE	Systemic lupus erythematosus; St. Louis encephalitis
SLUD	Salivation, lacrimation, urination, defecation
SLWC	Short leg walking cast
SMA	Smooth muscle antibodies
SMBG	Self-monitoring blood glucose
SM-C	Somatomedin-C
SNF	Skilled nursing facility
SNP	School nurse practitioner
SNS	Sympathetic nervous system
SOB	Short of breath; see order book
SOM	Serous otitis media
S/P	Status post
SPA	Suprapubic aspiration
SPF	Sun protection factor
SPL	Sound pressure levels
SPT	Sweat patch test
SQ	Subcutaneous
SR	System review; sinus rhythm; sedimentation rate; stretch reflex; schizophrenic reaction; stimulus response
S-R	Stimulus-response
SRI	Systemic reaction index
SRSA	Slow reacting substance of anaphylaxis
ss	*Semis* (one half)
S/S	Signs and symptoms
SSE	Soapsuds enema; soap solution enema
SSEP	Somatosensory evoked potential
SSI	Segmental spinal instrumentation
SSSS	Staphylococcal scalded skin syndrome
stat	*Statim* (immediately)
STC	Serum theophylline concentration
STD	Sexually transmitted disease; skin test dose; standard test dose
STS	Serologic test for syphilis
STSG	Split-thickness skin graft
STU	Skin test unit
SubQ	Subcutaneous
supp	Suppository
susp	Suspension
SV	Stroke volume
SVC	Superior vena cava
SVD	Spontaneous vaginal delivery
SVR	Systemic vascular resistance
SVT	Sinus ventricular tachycardia; supraventricular tachycardia
Sx	Symptoms
SxH	Sexual history
T_3	Tri-iodothyronine
T_4	Thyroxine
TAPVR	Total anomalous pulmonary venous return
TA	Toxin-antitoxin; tricuspid atresia; truncus arteriosus
T & A	Tonsillectomy & adenoidectomy
tab	Tablet
TAT	Tetanus antitoxin
TB (Tbc)	Tuberculosis
TBG	Thyroxine-binding globulin
TBI	Traumatic brain injury; Total body irradiation
TBLC	Term birth, living child
TBM	Total body mass
Tbn	Tuberculin
TBSA	Total body surface area
TBT	Tracheobronchial tree
TBW	Total body water
TcB	Transcutaneous bilirubinometer
TCDB	Turn, cough, deep breathe
$tcPCO_2$	Transcutaneous carbon dioxide pressure (tension)
$tcPO_2$	Transcutaneous oxygen pressure (tension)
TCU	Transitional care unit
Td	Adult tetanus
TD	Typhoid dysentery
TDM	Therapeutic drug monitoring
T_E	Expiratory time
TEF	Tracheoesophageal fistula
TEN	Toxic epidermal necrolysis
TENS	Transcutaneous electrical nerve stimulation
TEV	Talipes equinovarus
Tg	Thyroglobulin
TG	Triglyceride(s)
TGA	Transposition of great arteries
TGE	Theoretical growth evaluation
TGV	Transposition of great vessels
TI	Tricuspid insufficiency
TIA	Transient ischemic attack
tid	*Ter in die* (three times a day)
TIPP	The Injury Prevention Program
TKO	To keep open
TLC	Tender loving care; total lung capacity; total lymphocyte count; thin layer chromatography
TM	Tympanic membrane; temperature by mouth; tender midline; transmetatarsal; temporomandibular
TO	Target organ; telephone order
TOF	Tetralogy of Fallot
TOPV	Trivalent oral poliomyelitis vaccine
TORCH	Toxoplasmosis, (other), rubella, cytomegalovirus, herpes
TORCHES	Toxoplasmosis, rubella, cytomegalovirus, herpes, syphilis
Torr	Millimeters of mercury
TMR	Trainable mentally retarded
TNI	Total nodal irradiation
TNR	Tonic neck reflex
TPN	Total parenteral nutrition
TPR	Temperature, pulse, respiration; total perfusion resistance
TRH	Thyrotropin-releasing hormone
TS	Terminal sensation; test solution; tricuspid stenosis; Tourette syndrome
TSF	Triceps skinfold
TSB	Total serum bilirubin
TSE	Testicular self-examination
TSH	Thyroid stimulating hormone
TSS	Toxic shock syndrome
TT	Transit time; tuberculin tested; tetanus toxoid
TU	Tuberculin units; toxic unit; transmission unit

TV	Total volume; tidal volume
Tx	Treatment; therapy
UA	Urinalysis
UAC	Umbilical artery catheters
UCHD	Usual childhood diseases
UD	Urethral discharge
UDT	Undescended testicle
UGI	Upper gastrointestinal
U/L	Upper/lower body ratio
ULC	Unique looking child
UMN	Upper motor neuron
UNO	United Network for Organ Sharing
UP	Universal precautions
UPC	Unplanned pregnancy counseling
UQ	Upper quadrant
UrA	Uric acid
URI	Upper respiratory infection
US	Ultrasound
USA	Ultrasonic aerosol (nebulization)
USPHS	United States Public Health Service
UTI	Urinary tract infection
UV	Ultraviolet
UVA	Ultraviolet A
UVB	Ultraviolet B
VA	Visual acuity
VAD	Venous access devices
VAR	Visual-aural range
VC	Vital capacity
VCA	Viral capsid antigen
VCG	Vectorcardiography
VCT	Venous clotting time
VCUG	Voiding cystourethrogram
VD	Venereal disease
VDG	Venereal disease, gonorrhea
VDRL	Venereal Disease Research Laboratory
VDRR	Vitamin D-resistant rickets
VDS	Venereal disease, syphilis
VDT	Video display terminal

VE	Vesicular exanthem
VEP	Visual evoked potential
VF	Visual fields
VG	Ventricular gallop
VIG	Vaccinia immune globulin
VLBW	Very low birth weight
VLDL	Very low-density lipoprotein
VM	Vasomotor; vestibular membrane
VNA	Visiting Nurses' Association
VO	Verbal order
VP	Venous pressure
VPC	Ventricular premature complex
VRA	Visual reinforced audiometry
VS	Vital signs
VSD	Ventricular septal defect
VSGA	Very small for gestational age
VSS	Vital signs stable
V_T	Tidal volume
VUR	Vesicoureteral reflux
VZIG	Varicella zoster immune globulin
VZV	Varicella zoster virus
WAIS	Wechsler Adult Intelligence Scale
WB	Whole blood
WBC	White blood count
WEE	Western equine encephalitis
WHM	Women's health movement
WHO	World Health Organization
WIPI	Word intelligibility by picture identification
WISC-R	Wechsler Intelligence Scale for Children—Revised
WNL	Within normal limits
WPPSI	Wechsler Preschool and Primary Scale of Intelligence
WPW	Wolff-Parkinson-White syndrome
WRAT	Wide Range Achievement Test
XLMR	X-linked mental retardation
XLR	X-linked recessive
XTB	X-ray treated blood
ZIG	Zoster immune globulin
ZIP	Zoster immune plasma

Drugs

The use of acronyms or abbreviations to designate drugs is unsafe practice since many abbreviations are similar to others and not universally known to users. Any drug order, written or transcribed, should be written out clearly and legibly. Some notable exceptions are: BAL, EDTA, NPH.

ACh	Acetylcholine
ARA-A	Vidarabine
ARA-C	Cytarabine
ASA	Acetylsalicylic acid (aspirin)
BAL	British Antilewisite (dimercaprol)
CaEDTA	Calcium disodium edetate
CBZ	Carbamazepine
CPZ	Chlorpromazine
DDAVP	Desmopressin acetate
DES	Diethylstilbestrol
DF, DFO	Deferoxamine
DIG	Digoxin
DPT	Demerol-phenergan-thorazine
EDTA	Edetate disodium; ethylenediaminetetraacetic acid
EES	Erythromycin ethylsuccinate
Epi	Epinephrine
HCT	Hydrocortisone; hydrochlorothiazide
HCTZ	Hydrochlorothiazide
INH	Isoniazid

KCl	Potassium chloride
LSD	Lysergic acid diethylamide
MOM	Milk of magnesia
MS	Morphine sulfate
MTX	Methotrexate
MTZ	Tapazole
MVI	Multivitamins (without fat-soluble vitamins)
NPH	Neutral-protamine-Hagedorn; isoprophane
NTG	Nitroglycerine
PABA	Para-aminobenzoic acid
PAS	Aminosalicylic acid
Pb	Phenobarbital
PCN	Penicillin
PCP	Phencyclidine
PTU	Propylthiouracil
PVP	Povidone-iodine solution
PZ	Protamine zinc
SRT	Sustained release theophylline
SSKI	Saturated solution of potassium iodide
TAO	Troleandomycin
THAM	Tromethamine
TRIS	Tris (hydroxymethyl) aminomethane
VMA	Vanillylmandelic acid

Unit 6

INDEX

CONVERSION OF POUNDS TO KILOGRAMS FOR PEDIATRIC WEIGHTS

Pounds→	0	1	2	3	4	5	6	7	8	9
0	0.00	0.45	0.90	1.36	1.81	2.26	2.72	3.17	3.62	4.08
10	4.53	4.98	5.44	5.89	6.35	6.80	7.35	7.71	8.16	8.61
20	9.07	9.52	9.97	10.43	10.88	11.34	11.79	12.24	12.70	13.15
30	13.60	14.06	14.51	14.96	15.42	15.87	16.32	16.78	17.23	17.69
40	18.14	18.59	19.05	19.50	19.95	20.41	20.86	21.31	21.77	22.22
50	22.68	23.13	23.58	24.04	24.49	24.94	25.40	25.85	26.30	26.76
60	27.21	27.66	28.22	28.57	29.03	29.48	29.93	30.39	30.84	31.29
70	31.75	32.20	32.65	33.11	33.56	34.02	34.47	34.92	35.38	35.83
80	36.28	36.74	37.19	37.64	38.10	38.55	39.00	39.46	39.93	40.37
90	40.82	41.27	41.73	42.18	42.63	43.09	43.54	43.99	44.45	44.90
100	45.36	45.81	46.26	46.72	47.17	47.62	48.08	48.53	48.98	49.44
110	49.89	50.34	50.80	51.25	51.71	52.16	52.61	53.07	53.52	53.97
120	54.43	54.88	55.33	55.79	56.24	56.70	57.15	57.60	58.06	58.51
130	58.96	59.42	59.87	60.32	60.78	61.23	61.68	62.14	62.59	63.05
140	63.50	63.95	64.41	64.86	65.31	65.77	66.22	66.67	67.13	67.58
150	68.04	68.49	68.94	69.40	69.85	70.30	70.76	71.21	71.66	72.12
160	72.57	73.02	73.48	73.93	74.39	74.84	75.29	75.75	76.20	76.65
170	77.11	77.56	78.01	78.47	78.92	79.38	79.83	80.28	80.74	81.19
180	81.64	82.10	82.55	83.00	83.46	83.91	84.36	84.82	85.27	85.73
190	86.18	86.68	87.09	87.54	87.99	88.45	88.90	89.35	89.81	90.26
200	90.72	91.17	91.62	92.08	92.53	92.98	93.44	93.89	94.34	94.80

CONVERSION OF POUNDS AND OUNCES TO KILOGRAMS FOR PEDIATRIC WEIGHTS

Pounds	Kilograms	Pounds	Kilograms	Ounces	Kilograms	Ounces	Kilograms
1	0.454	9	4.082	1	0.028	9	0.255
2	0.907	10	4.536	2	0.057	10	0.283
3	1.361	11	4.990	3	0.085	11	0.312
4	1.814	12	5.443	4	0.113	12	0.340
5	2.268	13	5.897	5	0.142	13	0.369
6	2.722			6	0.170	14	0.397
7	3.175			7	0.198	15	0.425
8	3.629			8	0.227		

CONVERSION FACTORS FOR TEMPERATURE*

Celsius	Fahrenheit	Celsius	Fahrenheit	Celsius	Fahrenheit	Celsius	Fahrenheit
34.0	93.2	36.4	97.5	38.6	101.5	41.0	105.9
34.2	93.6	36.6	97.9	38.8	101.8	41.2	106.1
34.4	93.9	36.8	98.2	39.0	102.2	41.4	106.5
34.6	94.3	37.0	98.6	39.2	102.6	41.6	106.8
34.8	94.6	37.2	99.0	39.4	102.9	41.8	107.2
35.0	95.0	37.4	99.3	39.6	103.3	42.0	107.6
35.2	95.4	37.6	99.7	39.8	103.6	42.2	108.0
35.4	95.7	37.8	100.0	40.0	104.0	42.4	108.3
35.6	96.1	38.0	100.4	40.2	104.4	42.6	108.7
35.8	96.4	38.2	100.8	40.4	104.7	42.8	109.0
36.0	96.8	38.4	101.1	40.6	105.2	43.0	109.4
36.2	97.2			40.8	105.4		

*$(°C) \times (9/5) + 32 = °F$

$(°F - 32) \times (5/9) = °C$

°C = temperature in Celsius (centigrade) degrees
°F = temperature in Fahrenheit degrees